Cereal Grains
Laboratory Reference and Procedures Manual

FOOD PRESERVATION TECHNOLOGY SERIES

Series Editor
Gustavo V. Barbosa-Cánovas

Cereal Grains
Laboratory Reference and Procedures Manual

Sergio O. Serna-Saldivar
Tecnológico de Monterrey, Mexico

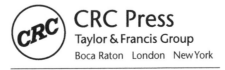

CRC Press
Taylor & Francis Group
Boca Raton   London   New York

CRC Press is an imprint of the
Taylor & Francis Group, an **informa** business

CRC Press
Taylor & Francis Group
6000 Broken Sound Parkway NW, Suite 300
Boca Raton, FL 33487-2742

© 2012 by Taylor & Francis Group, LLC
CRC Press is an imprint of Taylor & Francis Group, an Informa business

No claim to original U.S. Government works

Printed in the United States of America on acid-free paper
Version Date: 20120124

International Standard Book Number: 978-1-4398-5565-2 (Paperback)

Visit the Taylor & Francis Web site at
http://www.taylorandfrancis.com

and the CRC Press Web site at
http://www.crcpress.com

This practical handbook is dedicated to my lovely father Dr. Pablo Serna Treviño, who recently passed away. His love, guidance, motivation, and support throughout my whole life will be always in my heart.

Contents

Preface

This practical laboratory manual complements the book entitled *Cereal Grains: Properties, Processing, and Nutritional Attributes*. Its main goal is to assist students and researchers interested in the fundamentals of analysis, quality control, experimental studies, and product development of the wide array of cereal-based foods. This book is designed to emphasize the essential principles underlying preparation of cereal-based products and to demonstrate the roles of ingredients. The manual is organized in such a way that the student progressively learns and applies the theoretical knowledge described in the parent book. For instructors, this manual will serve as a practical guide to implement and apply quality control measurements of grains, milled products, starches, and an ample array of finished products. The book is designed to facilitate the acquisition of practical knowledge and provides new innovative ideas for new developments. Each chapter contains a set of key references so the reader can broaden the knowledge and study questions planned to motivate students to go beyond the boundaries of the covered material. In addition, each set of related procedures contains at the end research suggestions. A section of weight, volume, density, and other equivalences to convert kitchen and English units to metric measurements and vice versa is included.

The practical manual is divided into fourteen chapters. The first three chapters includes the main quality control measurements used to determine physical, morphological, chemical–nutritional properties, and sensory properties (color, texture, and organoleptic tests) of cereal grains and their products. In these chapters, the student will learn and practice grade and class determination, the most frequently used methods to assess chemical and physical properties and the viewing of the different anatomical parts of cereal grains. In addition, Chapter 3 deals with color, texture, and sensory evaluations of cereal products. The objective of the fourth chapter is to provide the practical knowledge of the most critical factors that affect grain stability throughout prolonged storage, identify the most common insects and pests responsible for grain storage losses, and practice the most common analytical techniques to determine insect fragments, filth, mycotoxins, and other sanitary indicators. The fifth chapter is designed to practice at the laboratory level the various types of dry-milling processes for production of dry-milled fractions of maize, polished rice, refined wheat flour, groats, and decorticated sorghum that are used as raw materials for the production of prepared cereal based end-products. This section includes the most common physical and chemical tests to determine quality of refined products including the determination of dough rheological properties with the mixograph, farinograph, extensigraph,

alveograph, and the new assay with the mixolab. Chapter 6 includes laboratory wet-milling procedures aimed toward the production of maize, rice, and wheat starches and microscopic methods to determine birefringence, starch granule morphology, and types of starches. This section also includes the two most common methods (amylograph and differential scanning calorimetry) to assess starch functionality and the quantification of resistant starch. Chapter 7 is designed to practice production of nixtamalized fresh *masa* and dry *masa* flours used for the manufacturing of maize tortillas and related products. In this part, the reader will be exposed to the production of table tortillas and the most common laboratory methods to assess *nixtamal*, *masa*, and tortilla quality and shelf-life. Chapter 8 focuses in assessing activity of yeast and chemical leavening agents critically important for the elaboration of bakery and other fermented products. The first part of this section thoroughly covers procedures to determine yeast activity using the pressurometer, gasograph, and maturograph, whereas the second part, laboratory procedures, is for the determination of the neutralization values of various types of chemical leavening agents. Chapter 9 describes laboratory and pilot plant procedures for the production of different types of yeast-leavened breads including official methods to test flour for baking purposes. The production of baguettes, Chinese steamed bread, white and whole wheat table bread, yeast-leavened donuts, Arabic breads, bagels, pretzels, sour breads, sweet breads, and pastries such as danish, croissants, cinnamon rolls, and an assort of pastries is covered. The laboratory procedures include different formulations so the student can learn ingredient functionality. Chapter 10 describes laboratory procedures for the production of crackers and different sorts of chemically leavened bakery products including the most common method (spread factor) employed to assess soft wheat flour functionality. The student will have laboratory procedures for the elaboration of different sorts of cookies (rotary molded, wire-cut, laminated) and cakes and other related products such as pancakes, crepes, muffins, biscuits, and coffee donuts. This chapter also thoroughly covered the manufacturing of refined and whole wheat flour tortillas. Chapter 11 depicts laboratory procedures for the production of different types of short and long pasta products from semolina and regular and alkaline oriental noodles produced from refined wheat flour. The next section contains a set of activities so the reader can practice the production of important breakfast cereals and snacks via traditional and extrusion processes. The reader will be exposed to different protocols for the production of flakes, oven-puffed rice, granolas, and extruded products. Likewise, different laboratory and pilot plant procedures are included for the production of popcorn, corn chips, tortilla chips, and second- and third-generation extruded snacks. The last two chapters of the manual contains protocols to bioenzymatically transform starch into modified starches and different types of syrups and sweeteners, laboratory processes for the production of regular and light beers, distilled spirits, and fuel ethanol.

By working carefully through the contents of this book, the reader will acquire the practical side and hands-on experience of many quality control procedures and experimental product development protocols of cereal-based products. Furthermore, from these foundations the developing professional will be able to enhance research skills for product development, process design, and ingredient functionality.

Acknowledgments

The author wishes to thank all former and current undergraduate and graduate students who have shared with him, throughout the past 25 years, their interest in the fascinating fields of cereal science, technology, and processing. Their interest and dynamism is his upmost motivation. The author wishes to especially recognize Dr. Esther Perez-Carrillo, Ana Chew-Guevara, Erick Heredia-Olea, Cristina Chuck-Hernandez, and Alexandra Robles for their skillful assistance in the elaboration of figures and photographs.

Author

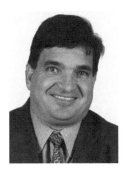

Dr. Sergio O. Serna-Saldivar is head and professor of the Biotechnology and Food Engineering Department, Tecnologico de Monterrey. Before this, he was research scientist at the Soil and Crop Science Department at Texas A&M University, consultant for EMBRAPA at Río de Janeiro, Brazil, and associate professor for the University of Sonora. He is currently the research chair leader of "Nutraceutical Value of Indigenous Mexican Foods and Plants." He has been a member of the American Association of Cereal Chemists for over 25 years and the Institute of Food Technologists and has acted as associate editor for the journals of *Cereal Chemistry* and *Cereal Science*. He was a member of the AACC International Board of Directors. He received his B.S. in Animal Science/ Agricultural Engineering from ITESM and his M.Sc. and Ph.D. degrees in Scientific Nutrition and Food Science and Technology from Texas A&M University. He has published six books, 21 chapters, 80 referred journal articles, six patents, and is the codeveloper of the wheat variety TAM-202. He has directed 52 M.Sc. and five Ph.D. students. His research interests focus on chemistry, nutraceutical/nutritional properties, and biotechnology of maize, sorghum, and other grains. He belongs to the maximum level of the Mexican National Research System and the Mexican Academy of Sciences. In addition, he was awarded the "Luis Elizondo" award in Agricultural and Food Industries, the 2004 AACC Excellence in Teaching award, and is a six-time awardee of the Teaching and Research Award at Tecnologico de Monterrey.

List of Equivalences

Kitchen Unit Conversions

Cup	0.24 L or 240 mL or 0.5 pints or 16 tablespoons
Cup of water	230 mL
Cup of flour	100 g
Cup of powdered chocolate	100 g
Cup of fresh egg	227 g or 0.5 lb
Cup of egg whites	227 g or 0.5 lb
Cup of egg yolks	227 g or 0.5 lb
Cup of fluid milk	230 mL or 0.5 lb
Cup of dry milk	114 g or 0.25 lb
Cup of brown sugar	150 g or 0.33 lb
Cup of powdered sugar	130 g or 0.285 lb
Cup of honey	340 g or 12 oz
Cup of oil	225–230 mL
Cup of shortening	180 g
Teaspoon	0.33 large spoon
Tablespoon	3 teaspoons or 16 = 1 cup
1 butter stick	90–100 g
1 egg (without shell)	45–50 g or approximately 0.1 lb
1 egg white	29–33 g or 0.062 lb
1 egg yolk	17–18 g or 0.04 lb
1 tablespoon of salt	14 g
1 tablespoon of baking powder	11.3 g
1 tablespoon vanilla	14 mL
1 tablespoon of dry yeast	10 g
1 tablespoon of ground cinnamon	6.3 g
1 tablespoon of cream of tartar	9.5 g
1 tablespoon of lemon juice	14 mL

Length Conversion Factors

Meter (m)	100 cm or 39.37 in or 3.28 feet or 1.094 yards
Centimeter (cm)	10 mm
Inch	2.54 cm or 25.4 mm
Foot	12 in or 30.48 cm
Yard	3 ft or 36 in or 0.914 m

Weigh Conversion Factors

Kilogram (kg)	1,000 g or 2.2 lb or 35.3 oz
Gram (g)	0.001 kg or 1,000 mg
Ounce	28.35 g
Pound	454 g or 16 oz

Volume Conversion Factors

Cubic meter (m^3)	1,000 L
Cubic meter (m^3)	33.3 ft^3
Hectoliter	100 L or 0.1 mt^3
Liter (L)	1,000 mL or cm^3 or 4.22 cups or 1.057 pint
Milliliter (mL)	0.001 L
Bushel (bu) USA	8 gal or 35.24 L
Bushel (bu) UK	8 gal or 36.37 L
Pint	0.473 L or 0.125 gal
Quart	0.946 L or 2 pints

Gallon	3.785 L or 8 pints or 4 quarts
Fluid ounce	29.6 mL

Density Conversion Factors

Pounds (lb)/bushel (bu)	1.247 kg/hL

Pressure Conversion Factors

1 kg/cm^2	14.21 psi
1 psi	0.07 kg/cm^2
1 psi	6,894 Pa
1 kPa	0.145 psi

Temperature Conversion Factors

Degrees centigrade	5/9 ($^\circ$F − 32)
Degrees fahrenheit	(9 × $^\circ$C)/5 + 32

1 Physical and Morphological Properties of Cereal Grains

1.1 INTRODUCTION

Cereals are one-seeded fruits of the Gramineae family designed to store nutrients critically important for the perpetuation of the species. Kernels are protected by physical barriers and chemical compounds against external biotic agents. Nevertheless, the different genus, species, and types differ in their grains' physical, chemical, and morphological characteristics. These features are also affected by the environment, especially during maturation in the field, and by storage conditions. The main criteria used to select grains for specific uses are related to their physical properties because they affect chemical composition, functionality, and end use.

Therefore, the determination of the physical properties, grade, and class plays an important and critical role in the market value of any given lot of grain. Grain classification and grading assures that a particular lot of grain meets preestablished quality parameters. Federal governments usually have impartial regulatory agencies in charge of assigning grain quality. Furthermore, the standardization of grain quality allows better and fairer marketing between sellers and buyers and also allows processors to blend lots of grains with similar grade or quality (Kiser 1991). The value of any given lot of grain depends on both grade and class. Grade is an indication of quality and grain health condition whereas class is related to the potential use or functionality of the grain (color, gluten type, hardness, etc.). The classification systems are aimed toward the facilitation of impartial commercialization of grains, providing information related to grain quality for storage and further processing, and providing information that can be further related to yields of products and by-products (milling yields, end-product quality, etc.).

All cereal plants produce protected or covered fruits. The kernel, which is botanically termed a caryopsis, is a monocotyledon. The caryopsis consists of a pericarp (fruit coat) and a true seed. The seed consists of a germ and endosperm covered by a seed coat or *testa* and a single or multilayered aleurone. Some cereal grains, such as oats, rice, and barley, tightly retain the glumes after harvesting and consequently are considered as husked grains. The rest of the cereals are commonly known as naked caryopses because they generally lose the ventral and dorsal glumes known as *lemma* and *palea*, respectively, during harvesting.

To understand the important changes that cereals undergo during processing, it is essential to comprehend the macrostructure and microstructure, physiology, and the composition of each anatomical part of the caryopsis. Among each type of cereal, important variations exist in endosperm hardness due to the different proportions of vitreous and floury endosperm types, pericarp color and thickness, type of starch, and kernel size.

1.2 DETERMINATION OF PHYSICAL PROPERTIES OF CEREAL GRAINS

1.2.1 TEST WEIGHT

The bushel, test or volumetric weight is the most critical criteria to determine grade and class. The test simply consists of first sampling the grain which is then placed in a container with a proven volume. The grain is weighed and the test weight or apparent density is calculated. Test weights are generally expressed in pounds per bushel (2150.42 in.^{3}) or in kilograms per hectoliter (100 L). The conversion factors of pounds per Winchester bushel (2150.42 in.^{3}) and pounds per imperial bushel (2219.36 in.^{3}) to kilograms per hectoliter are 1.297 and 1.247, respectively. The bushel weight is closely related to the true grain density and therefore is affected by grain condition, grain texture, and even grain protein content. This test is very useful because insects, molds, and sprouted or heat-damaged kernels have a lower test weight when compared with healthy or sound counterparts. On the other hand, vitreous or corneous grains with a slightly higher protein content are usually denser. Lots of grains with higher moisture contents usually have a lower test weight because water has a density of 1 g/cm^3, whereas starch has a density of 1.6 g/cm^3. Insect-perforated kernels have a lower apparent density because the air in the perforations has a density of only 0.1 g/cm^3. Both grade and class are affected by test weight. The most common way to measure test weight is by the Winchester bushel meter provided with different cups with a known volume.

1.2.1.1 Test Weight Procedure

Grain test weights are usually measured according to Method 55-10 (American Association of Cereal Chemists; AACC 2000).

A. *Samples, Ingredients, and Reagents*
   - Different lots of grains
B. *Materials and Equipment*
   - Digital scale
   - Boerner divider
   - Ruler
   - Seed clipper or Carter dockage test meter
   - Winchester bushel meter apparatus
   - Strike-off stick

C. *Procedure*

1. Obtain a representative grain sample, preferably by using the Boerner divider.
2. Fill the hopper or the Cox funnel of the Winchester bushel meter with enough grain to fill the cup. Make sure the hopper gate is closed and to place a pan to collect excess grain.
3. Move the hopper so its gate is aligned right in the center of the cup.
4. Open the gate and allow the grain to flow and overfill the cup (Figure 1.1).
5. Carefully remove excess grain from the cup with the aid of a strike-off stick moved vertically over the cup's rim. Excess grain should be removed with a zigzag motion.
6. Weigh the grains in the cup with an accuracy of 0.1 g.
7. Calculate test weight or apparent density by dividing the weight/volume. Express test weight in pounds per bushel (lb/bu) and kilograms per hectoliter (kg/hL). To convert test weight from kilograms per hectoliter to pounds per bushel, multiply the number by 0.6674. One bushel is equal to 0.303 hL.

1.2.2 TRUE DENSITY

True grain density, generally expressed in grams per cubic centimeter, is commonly determined by measuring the weight of a given volume that is displaced by a known weight of test material. True density can be determined by ethanol displacement or by air, nitrogen, or helium displacement using a pycnometer. Nitrogen is the most commonly used gas. Another popular way to determine density is by alcohol displacement. True density values are important because they are closely related to grain condition, endosperm texture, and milling yields. Dense grains are less prone to insect damage and have better handling properties (less susceptible to breakage) during storage, commercialization, and processing. For wheat, density values are strongly associated to class and functional use. The density of other grains, such as maize and sorghum, is also important for dry and wet millers. For dry-milling, the industry selects grains with higher density because they usually yield more and better quality products. The wet-milling industry typically uses less dense or softer kernels because these kernels require shorter steeping requirements and commonly yield more starch.

1.2.2.1 Determination of True Density with the Pycnometer

A. *Samples, Ingredients, and Reagents*

*   Different lots of grains

B. *Materials and Equipment*

*   Scale
*   Multipycnometer (model MUP-1)
*   Boerner divider
*   Nitrogen gas

C. *Procedure*

1. Turn the multipycnometer power on 10 to 15 minutes before testing.
2. Obtain a representative grain sample, preferably by using the Boerner divider. Make sure the sample is free of foreign material, broken kernels, and other types of kernels. If necessary, clean the grain with a clipper, air aspiration system, or a Carter dockage tester.

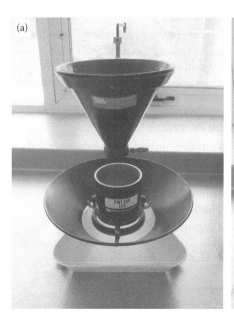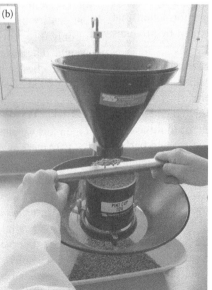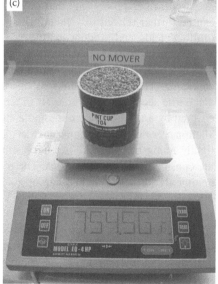

FIGURE 1.1 Determination of test weight. (a) Winchester bushel meter; (b) removal of excess grain; (c) determination of sample weight.

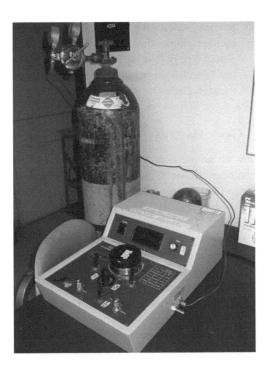

FIGURE 1.2 Pycnometer used to determine grain density.

3. Weigh an 80-g sample to an accuracy of 0.01 g and place it in the pycnometer cup (Figure 1.2). Place cup with grain in the sample cell.

4. With the selector valve at the cell position, open the "gas out" toggle valve and wait for a stable reading near zero.

5. Close the gas out valve and set the meter to zero.

6. Open the "gas in" toggle valve to pressurize the cell to 15 psi to 17 psi. Stop the gas flow by closing the gas in valve.

7. Record the pressure reading as P1 after stabilization and then turn the selector valve to cell position and record the pressure as P2.

8. Release pressure by opening the gas out toggle valve.

9. Calculate the volume of gas using the following equation: volume (cm^3) = Vc − Vr × [(P1/P2) − 1], where Vc = large sample cell volume = 149.67, Vr = large reference volume = 71.60. Calculate the true density by dividing grain weight/volume. Express true density in grams per cubic centimeter (Figure 1.2).

1.2.2.2 Determination of Density with Alcohol Displacement

Density was calculated using the method of Rooney (2007).

A. Samples, Ingredients, and Reagents
- Different lots of grains
- Anhydrous ethanol
- Distilled water

B. Materials and Equipment
- Digital scale
- Air-aspiration system
- Graduated cylinders (100 mL)
- Boerner divider
- Carter dockage tester

C. Procedure
1. Prepare an 80% ethanol solution by mixing 20 mL of water and 80 mL of anhydrous ethanol.

2. Obtain a representative grain sample, preferably by using the Boerner divider. Make sure the sample is free of foreign material, broken kernels, and other types of kernels. If necessary, clean the grain with a clipper, air aspiration system, or a Carter dockage tester. The idea is to test only whole kernels.

3. Determine the weight of the empty graduated cylinder.

4. Fill the graduated cylinder to the 100 mL mark with the whole kernels. Tap the cylinder several times to settle the kernels and then add more kernels to bring the level back to the 100 mL mark.

5. Weigh the filled cylinder and subtract the empty weight to obtain the exact kernel weight.

6. Measure 100 mL of the 80% ethanol solution in the second graduated cylinder.

7. Pour the ethanol slowly into the cylinder containing the whole kernels. Fill this cylinder to the 80 mL mark (the alcohol solution should cover all kernels). Tap the cylinder several times to remove trapped air bubbles and then refill to the 100 mL mark with the 80% ethanol solution.

8. Record the volume (in milliliters) of the ethanol solution left in the second cylinder. This volume is the volume of grain displaced.

9. Calculate the density by dividing the kernel weight by the volume of ethanol left in the second graduated cylinder. Express results within two decimal places in grams per cubic centimeter.

1.2.3 FLOTATION INDEX

The flotation test was originally developed by the Quaker Oats Company as a quick index of grain density and dry-milling quality. The test simply consists of preparing one (i.e., 1.275 g/cm^3) or various sodium nitrate solutions with different specific gravities for the determination of the percentage of floating kernels. The number of floaters increases as moisture content increases, therefore, the percentage of floaters is usually adjusted using a correction chart (Rooney and Suhendro 2001). Soft kernels contain larger quantities of air in the endosperm and float more than hard ones.

1.2.3.1 Determination of Floating Kernels

A. *Samples, Ingredients, and Reagents*
- Different types of maize kernels
- Sodium nitrate
- Water

B. *Materials and Equipment*
- 1 L beaker
- Thermometer
- Hydrometer (1.2–1.42 g/cm³ range)
- 250 mL graduated cylinder
- Hot plate
- Stirring rod
- Wire screen basket
- Chronometer

C. *Procedure*
1. Clean the grain sample and discard broken kernels. Determine moisture content and test and thousand kernel weights (refer to procedures in Sections 2.2.1.1, 1.2.1.1, and 1.2.7.1).
2. Randomly select three sets of 100 sound kernels.
3. Prepare a solution of sodium nitrate (178.9 g in 250 mL of water) with a density of 1.275 g/cm³. Control the temperature of the solution to 21°C, preferably in a water bath (Figure 1.3). Read the density of the resulting solution with the hydrometer. If necessary, adjust density by adding water to reduce it or sodium nitrate to increase it.
4. Deposit 500 mL to 600 mL of the solution tempered to 21°C previously prepared in a 1-L beaker.
5. Add 100 kernels and agitate every 30 seconds for 5 minutes (Figure 1.3).
6. Suspend agitation and after 1 minute, count the number of floating kernels. Express result as percentage of floating kernels = number of floating kernels/number of total kernels. Determine the standard error of the mean.

1.2.4 GRAIN HARDNESS

There are an ample number of subjective tests to estimate grain hardness. Hardness is mainly affected by the ratio of corneous to floury endosperm and apparent and true density values. The most practiced assays consist of subjecting, for a given time, a lot of grain to the abrasive action of a mechanical decorticator such as the tangential abrasive dehulling device or TADD mill. Softer kernels will lose more material or will break into smaller particles during decortication or impaction. There are other tests, mainly used by the wheat industry, in which kernels are milled using a standardized procedure. The particle size distribution of the resulting flour is related to hardness. Softer grains produce finer flours. The principle of determining particle size distribution has gained popularity because it can be adapted to near-infrared reflectance analysis (NIRA). The U.S. Department of Agriculture (USDA) is using this assay for grading wheat. There are many new methods to estimate hardness, especially developed for wheat varying from the estimation of hardness in single kernels and others based on the estimation of time, force, and even noise produced in a standard mill during grinding. Recently, the NIRA has been used to predict hardness when a given ground sample is scanned at 1080 nm to 1180 nm. The NIRA hardness test proved to have a good correlation with kernel vitreousness and different parameters of the Stenvert test (Hoffman et al. 2010).

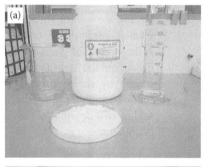
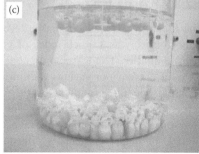
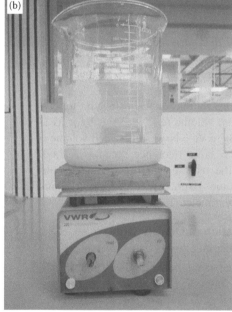

FIGURE 1.3 Procedure to determine percentage of floating kernels. (a) Reagent necessary for sodium nitrate solution; (b) heating solution; (c) determination of floating maize kernels.

1.2.4.1 Subjective Determination of the Ratio of Soft to Hard Endosperm or Endosperm Texture

The subjective evaluation of the relative amount of corneous to floury endosperm is critically important because it is the main factor affecting grain hardness and density. This factor is greatly affected by genetics and environment. The determination of the ratio of soft to hard endosperm is critically important in the wheat industry because different classes of wheat have different ratios of the two types of endosperms. Soft wheats are mostly floury whereas durum wheats contain vitreous endosperms. Most hard wheats contain intermediate endosperm textures. The same applies for maize kernels. The flint or corneous types, in which popcorn is included, contain hard endosperm whereas dent corns may contain genotypes with different proportions of hard to floury endosperms. The ratio of soft to hard endosperm greatly affects dry- and wet-milling operations and optimum cooking times. The subjective method simply consists of bisecting the kernel in preparation for the observation of the hard or vitreous (translucent) to soft or floury (opaque) endosperm. It is recommended that at least 10 kernels should be rated because of natural variations.

A. *Samples, Ingredients, and Reagents*
- Different types of grains
- Distilled water

B. *Materials and Equipment*
- Light box
- Tweezers
- Scalper

C. *Procedure*
1. Obtain a representative grain sample from the lot of grain preferably from the Boerner divider. Randomly select 10 kernels and place them on a light box for viewing.
2. Determine the ratio of soft-floury-chalky to vitreous-hard-glassy endosperm of each kernel using a 1 to 5 scale (1, totally vitreous; 2.5, 50% vitreous and 50% soft; and 5, totally soft or floury). The soft endosperm will have an opaque appearance whereas the vitreous endosperm will have glassy translucent appearance (Figure 1.4).
3. After rating whole kernels, cut each kernel longitudinally with a scalper. Make sure to hold the kernels with a tweezer before cutting. Rate the ratio of soft to hard endosperm using a 1 to 5 scale (1, totally vitreous; 2.5, 50% vitreous and 50% soft; and 5, totally soft or floury).
4. Calculate the average and standard deviation of the 10 observations and the correlation between ratings of whole and longitudinally dissected kernels.

1.2.4.2 Procedure to Determine Grain Hardness Using the TADD Mill

There are several laboratory equipments devised for determining grain hardness. The TADD mill (Oomah et al. 1981)

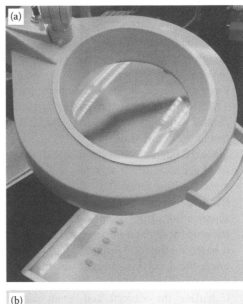

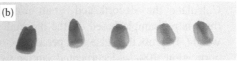

FIGURE 1.4 Subjective determination of ratio of soft to hard endosperm on a light box. (a) Kernels viewed on a light box; (b) kernels with different endosperm textures.

is commonly used to indirectly determine grain hardness especially of coarse grains (maize and sorghum). The procedure simply consists of subjecting samples to the abrasive mechanical action of the mill for a certain time. Hard- and soft-textured grains lose less and more dry matter, respectively, during the fixed and standardized milling procedures. The TADD measures the resistance of the kernels to the abrasive action of a horizontal aluminum oxide wheel surface rotating at a constant speed. The amount of material removed is inversely related to hardness (Rooney 2007).

A. *Samples, Ingredients, and Reagents*
- Different lots of samples (maize, sorghum, or wheat)

B. *Materials and Equipment*
- Digital scale
- Boerner divider
- Aluminum oxide disk
- Chronometer
- Clipper or dockage test meter
- TADD mill (Venables Machine Works, Saskatoon, Canada)
- Eight-hole base

C. *Procedure*
1. Set up the TADD mill with the eight-hole base and verify the condition of the abrasive disk.
2. Clean the lot of grain manually or using a clipper or dockage test meter.
3. Obtain a representative cleaned grain sample and determine its physical properties (test

weight, 1000 kernel weight, and true density) and moisture content. Subsample the lot of grain using the Boerner divider.

4. Weigh exactly 40 g of sample with an accuracy of 0.1 g.

5. Place sample in the round compartment of the TADD mill. Make sure to include a standard or control with a known hardness value and fill the rest of the compartments.

6. Place the lid of the mill and then start the equipment for exactly 10 minutes or the predetermined milling time.

7. Remove samples from each compartment and separate fines from decorticated kernels. Weigh the amount of decorticated kernels and express it based on the total original grain weight. The lower the decorticated grain weight, the softer the grain (Figure 1.5).

8. Calculate the decorticated grain weight of the control sample based on the original grain weight. Express the value as a percentage of decortication: 100—[(decorticated sample weight/original sample weight) × 100]. Calculate the correction factor using the following equation: % decorticated grain weight of control sample/% decorticated grain weight. Correct all experimental values according to the standard sample with a known TADD hardness value (correction factor = original TADD hardness value/new TADD hardness value). This is especially important when the abrasive disk is changed.

1.2.4.3 Procedure to Determine Grain Hardness Using the Stenvert Test

The Stenvert hardness test (SHT) is based on the principle that the time required to grind a sample is directly related to its hardness (Stenvert 1974; Pomeranz et al. 1985, 1986a,b).

It is especially used to evaluate wheat and maize kernels. In this technique, 20 g of kernels at a specific moisture content is milled in a microhammer mill. The parameters used to define hardness index include the resistance time to mill 17 mL of meal, the height of the ground meal in the collection tube, and the weight ratio of coarse to fine particles in the resulting meal (Li et al. 1996). Hard-textured kernels are more resistant to milling, produce less height in the collection tube, and yield coarser particles and higher volume ratios of coarse to fine particles compared with softer counterparts. Li et al. (1996) constructed a computer-based data logging and analysis system to calculate the milling time and transient power consumption during the milling process of 38 maize hybrids and found a strong correlation between the ratio of soft to hard endosperm and bulk density to SHT.

A. Samples, Ingredients, and Reagents
- Different lots of samples (maize, sorghum, or wheat)

B. Materials and Equipment
- Scale
- Boerner divider
- Tester receptacles (125 mm long by 25 mm in diameter)
- Chronometer
- Clipper or dockage test meter
- Glen Creston or Stenvert microhammer mill

C. Procedure

1. Clean the lot of grain manually or using a clipper or dockage test meter.

2. Obtain a representative cleaned grain sample and determine its physical properties (test weight, 1000 kernel weight, and true density) and moisture content.

3. Subsample the lot of grain using the Boerner divider.

4. Weigh exactly 20 g of sample with an accuracy of 0.1 g.

5. Grind sample in the Glen Creston microhammer mill fitted with a 2-mm aperture particle screen. The mill speed is set to 3600 rpm. Make sure to mill a standard or control with a known hardness value.

6. Register the time taken to mill 17 mL of meal and the meal height in the collection tube or tester receptacle at the completion of milling the 20-g grain sample, move samples from each compartment and separate fines from decorticated kernels. In addition, determine the volume of coarse (top layer) and fine particles (bottom layer) and the ratio of coarse to fine particles in the tester receptacles (125 mm long by 25 mm in diameter). Coarse particles are defined as those larger than 0.7 mm in diameter, whereas fines particles are smaller than 0.5 mm in diameter.

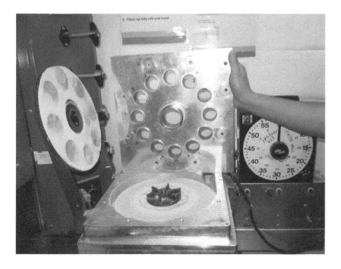

FIGURE 1.5 TADD mill used to determine grain hardness.

1.2.5 BREAKAGE TESTS

Breakage susceptibility is defined as the potential for kernel fragmentation when subjected to impact or mechanical impact forces during handling and transport. Broken kernels play a critical role for grain grading. The breakage susceptibility of kernels generally increases as the rate of artificial drying increases and is directly related to the number of stress cracks or fissures. It can also provide an indication of the relative number of fines that will be generated during handling and the susceptibility of broken kernels to insect and mold attack. Breakage susceptibility is especially important in the rice milling industry because broken rice has a lower price compared with intact white polished kernels (Champagne 2004; Kohlwey 1994). The mechanical properties of maize kernels change with heated air-drying because of the reduction in moisture content and physical changes (e.g., stress cracks) caused by heating. Kernels that are artificially dried generally become more susceptible to breakage when subjected to mechanical stress, and this is undesirable in terms of wet and dry-milling performance because there are physical losses and changes in processing characteristics when the integrity of kernels is destroyed. Kernel breakage is one measure of physical quality necessary in the evaluation of the control system performance. In a grain breakage test, it is desirable to simulate the mechanical stresses encountered by kernels in auger conveyors, bucket elevators, and drop spouts. Different assumptions about the nature of handling stresses have led to the development of several types of breakage testing equipment. It is generally accepted that the impact of kernels on hard surfaces is a primary cause of breakage in maize (Watson and Herum 1986), and most breakage testers have used some method of direct impact testing. However, kernel-to-kernel impact, such as that experienced when grain freefalls into a storage bin from a spout, also causes breakage. Breakage testers can be grouped into three broad categories depending on the way stresses are generated: an impeller rotating in a cup containing many kernels, single kernels impinging against a hard stationary surface, or single kernels impinging on a grain surface. In the first tester category, stresses on each kernel are generated by repeated impact with the impeller as well as by collisions with other kernels. The current standard test method for maize breakage is the AACC approved Method 55-20 (AACC 2000), which requires a Stein model CK-2M breakage tester of the first type (Fred Stein Laboratories, Atchison, KS). The Stein breakage tester (SBT) is a modified laboratory grain mill developed by the U.S. Department of Agriculture (Miller et al. 1979; Thompson and Foster 1963; Stephens and Foster 1976). It has also been the most widely studied commercial breakage tester. A hardened steel impeller, rotating at 1700 rpm to 1800 rpm inside a stainless steel sample cup, propels grain kernels against each other, and against the top and sides of the cup. Maize kernels treated using the SBT typically show a combination of abrasion and impact damage. The design of the impeller for the Stein breakage tester was modified in 1981 to permit more rapid testing and improved repeatability of results (Miller et al. 1981). The other popular method is the Wisconsin breakage tester (WBT) in which individual kernels are impinged against a stationary metal surface at a high velocity and therefore tends to crack or chip small pieces of the kernels.

1.2.5.1 Determination of Breakage Susceptibility with the Stein Breakage Tester (Method 55-20)

The Stein breakage tester (SBT) is the only commercially available breakage susceptibility tester (AACC 2000). It was especially devised for maize testing. Presieved corn samples of 100 g size are impacted by a rotating blade or impeller on a confined grain sample in a special cylindrical cup for a specific time (usually 2 minutes). The action of the impeller causes abrasions on the corn material, which is then removed from the cup and resieved on a 4.76-mm (12/64-in.) round-holed sieve. The percentage of the sample passing though the sieve is the numerical value of the breakage susceptibility. Good sound corn will have breakage values ranging from 2% to 10%, whereas heat-damaged corn may have values of more than 50%. Breakage susceptibility values are also dependent on the moisture content of the sample. As the corn becomes drier, the difference in breakage values between sound kernels and stress content of the maize increases significantly. Conversely, as the moisture content of the kernel increases to approximately 16%, it is not possible to delineate between high-breakage and low-breakage susceptibility corn. Breakage values are not absolute values from the sample but will change as the sample is either rewetted or dehydrated.

A. *Samples, Ingredients, and Reagents*
   - Different lots of samples of maize
B. *Materials and Equipment*
   - Digital scale
   - Boerner divider
   - Sieve with 4.76 mm round holes
   - Chronometer
   - Clipper or dockage test meter
   - Stein breakage tester
   - Gamet shaker
C. *Procedure*
   1. Clean the lot of grain manually or using a clipper or dockage test meter.
   2. Obtain a representative cleaned grain sample and determine its physical properties (test weight, 1000 kernel weight, and true density), stress cracks, and moisture content. The history of dehydration is critically important because drying time and temperature greatly affect breakage susceptibility.
   3. Subsample the lot of grain using the Boerner divider.
   4. Weigh exactly 100 g of the sample with an accuracy of 0.1 g. The grain should be preferably tested at 13% moisture.

5. Break the 100-g sample through the Stein breakage tester for exactly 2 minutes. The action of the SBT impeller causes abrasions on the kernels.

6. Remove sample from the breaker and place contents on a 4.76-mm (12/64-in.) round-hole sieve in a Gamet shaker programmed for 30 cycles.

7. Register the weight of the sample which passed though the sieve and express it as a percentage according to the original sample weight. This is the percentage of the breakage susceptibility.

1.2.5.2 Determination of Breakage Susceptibility with the Wisconsin Breakage Tester

The Wisconsin breakage tester (WBT) is a single-impact device that contains a 254-mm diameter impeller that operates at 1800 rpm (Gunasekaran 1988). As a result, kernels are centrifugally propelled to impact the inside surface of a 305-mm diameter vertical cylinder. The kernels and fragments are collected at the bottom of the housing and are received on a 6.55-(12/64-in.) or 4.76-mm (16/64-in.) round-hole sieve for 30 cycles in a Gamet shaker. The impact force in the WBT is greater than in the SBT, although the SBT has many more total impacts per kernel. The type of damage or broken material created by the two testers is different. The WBT has such a high impact that it often will split a kernel into two pieces but will not create much dust or small particles and correlates strongly with stress cracks. Thus, the WBT can be used as an indirect measure of stress cracks. The WBT is not a commercially available instrument. The instruments used were located at research institutions or commercial grain quality testing laboratories in the United States.

A. *Samples, Ingredients, and Reagents*
   - Different lots of samples of maize
B. *Materials and Equipment*
   - Digital scale
   - Boerner divider
   - Vibratory feeder (400–800 g/min)
   - Gamet shaker
   - Clipper or dockage test meter
   - Wisconsin breakage tester
   - Sieve with a 4.7- or 6.35-mm round holes
   - Chronometer
C. *Procedure*
   1. Clean the lot of maize kernels manually or using a clipper or dockage test meter.
   2. Obtain a representative cleaned grain sample and determine its physical properties (test weight, 1000 kernel weight, and true density), stress cracks, and moisture content. The history of dehydration is critically important because drying time and temperature greatly affect breakage susceptibility.
   3. Subsample the lot of grain using the Boerner divider.

4. Weigh exactly 100 g of sample with an accuracy of 0.1 g. The grain should be preferably tested at 13% moisture.

5. Adjust vibratory feeder to dispense 400 g of maize per minute and impact the sample through the Wisconsin breakage tester.

6. Place contents on a 4.76- (12/64-in.) or 6.35-mm round-hole sieve in a Gamet shaker programmed for 30 cycles.

7. Register the weight of the sample that passed though the sieve and express it as a percentage according to the original sample weight: % WBT = [(original sample weight—amount of sample retained by the sieve)/original sample weight] × 100. Express results based on the chosen sieve. The larger sieve will give higher WBT values.

1.2.6 Stress Cracks and Fissures

Stress cracks are internal fissures in the vitreous or hard endosperm of cereal grains. Grain lots with a high incidence of stress cracks are more susceptible to breakage. This is especially important in rice because a high incidence of stress cracks lowers milling yields (Chapter 5). Stress cracks are mainly generated because of moisture gradients inside the kernels during artificial drying, especially when the air temperature exceeds 60°C. Stress cracks are determined by a careful examination of a representative sample of the grain lot. The naked caryopses are placed onto a light box and the number of fissures counted. Each kernel is individually inspected for single, double, or multiple cracks.

1.2.6.1 Determination of Stress Cracks or Fissures
A. *Samples, Ingredients, and Reagents*
   - Different types of grains (rice)
B. *Materials and Equipment*
   - Light box
   - Rice dehuller
   - Magnifying lens
C. *Procedure*
   1. Obtain a representative grain sample from the lot of grain preferably obtained from the Boerner divider. If rice was selected, run a representative sample through the rice dehuller (refer to Chapter 5) to obtain brown rice. Randomly select 10 kernels and place them on a light box for viewing.
   2. Determine the number and size of stress cracks or fissures of each kernel.
   3. After rating, calculate the average number and size of fissures and standard deviations of the 10 observations.

1.2.7 Thousand Kernel Weight

This parameter is frequently used because within type of cereal is an excellent indicator of grain size and is correlated to the amount of shriveled kernels. In addition, 1000 kernel weight is related to dry- and wet-milling yields. The industry prefers uniform and large kernels because they contain a higher proportion of endosperm and starch. The test is simple, practical, and fast, and is usually performed using an automatic seed counter.

1.2.7.1 Determination of Kernel Weight

A. Samples, Ingredients, and Reagents
- Different types of grains

B. Materials and Equipment
- Scale
- Clipper or Carter dockage tester
- Automatic seed counter

C. Procedure
1. Before counting caryopses, clean the grain sample, making sure to remove foreign material and broken kernels.
2. With an automatic seed counter, program the equipment to count exactly 100 kernels. Alternatively, manually count 100 randomly selected kernels.
3. Weigh the sample with an accuracy of 0.01 g.
4. Multiply the resulting weight by 10 to obtain the 1000 kernel weight in grams. Calculate the average kernel weight in milligrams.

1.2.8 Foreign or Extraneous Material

The dockage is defined as the foreign material (other grains, stones, sticks, metals, pieces of glass, etc.) contaminating a particular lot of grain. For obvious reasons, dockage greatly affects the grading and market value of the grain. The amount of foreign material is inversely related to product yield. Grains with higher dockage contents imply a higher management cost because kernels will require cleaning before storage. Furthermore, if the amount of foreign material is too high, the price is penalized because the grain will be more prone to deterioration during storage. It is recognized that grains with higher dockage are less stable during storage because the foreign material fosters insects. Some foreign seeds negatively affect the quality of milled products, and consequently, the quality of the end-products. In some cereals, such as maize and sorghum, the foreign material also comprises broken kernels (Keiser 1991; USDA 1993; USDA-Grain Inspection, Packers and Stockyards Administration [GIPSA] 1999).

1.2.8.1 Determination of Dockage or Foreign Material

Foreign material is any material other than the grain that remains in a sample. In maize and sorghum, the foreign material is evaluated with the broken kernels. In wheat, the foreign material (other grains and weed seeds) is evaluated after removing dockage and shrunken kernels.

A. Samples, Ingredients, and Reagents
- Different types and classes of kernels

B. Materials and Equipment
- Digital scale
- Tweezers
- Boerner divider
- Clipper or Carter dockage tester

C. Procedure
1. Divide the lot of grain using the Boerner divider.
2. Select and weigh, with a precision of 0.1 g, the amount of grain to be cleaned (1000 g).
3. Make all the adjustments suggested by the equipment manufacturer according to the grain to be cleaned. Make sure that the equipment is furnished with the set of sieves for the specific type of grain and the recommended air speed of the aspiration system.
4. Turn on the machine and pour the sample into the hopper. Turn off the machine after the sample has passed through the last sieve.
5. Weigh the foreign material and express the amount based on the original simple weight. If needed, sort the foreign material into other seeds, vegetative dockage chaff, stones, pieces of glass, or even metal impurities. Express as a percentage of foreign material = [(weight of foreign material/sample weight) × 100].

1.2.8.2 Test for Maize Breakage and Damaged Kernels

The test is aimed toward the determination of cracked, broken, and nicked maize kernels (Rooney 2007).

A. Samples, Ingredients, and Reagents
- Different lots of grain
- Fast green FCF dye solution (0.1% w/w)

B. Materials and Equipment
- Digital scale
- Beaker (100 mL)
- Chronometer
- Boerner divider
- Wire sieves (0.6 cm and 0.3 cm openings)

C. Procedure
1. Screen the corn sample over a 0.6-cm round-holed sieve. Randomly select and count 100 kernels.
2. Weigh the 100 kernels and multiply by 10 to estimate the 1000 kernel weight.
3. Immerse the maize sample in fast green dye solution for 4 minutes. After staining, pour into a sieve and wash the resulting kernels in running water for 30 seconds. The fast green dye will stain any break.
4. Spread out kernels and examine individually. Sort kernels into three categories: intact or unstained, major damage (open cracks, chipped, severe pericarp damage) that is noticeable without the green dye, and minor damage that is noticeable with the dye (fissures or cracks).
5. Express each category of kernels as a percentage of the original weight.

1.2.9 DAMAGED KERNELS

Damaged kernels are considered those that have an evident visual damage and negatively affect their value for cereal processors. The determination of damaged kernels is made after the removal of foreign material and fines. The main types of damage are due to insects, heat, molds, and weathering, sprouted, frost, and lack of grain filling known as shrunken. Insect-damaged kernels are easily identified because they have perforations or web-like material that aggregate kernels. These grains could lose more than half of their weight and have lower test and thousand kernel weights. The insects puncture grains for feeding and reproduction purposes. Heat damage is considered as one of the most important categories because it is generally produced by faulty storage. Most heat-damaged kernels are generated when grains are stored at high moisture and therefore have high respiration rates. High grain temperature and the generation of soluble sugars due to the activation of intrinsic enzymes produce Maillard reactions and off-colors and, in some instances, the loss of seed viability. These kernels usually have high diastatic activity and contain degraded starch and other enzyme-degraded nutrients that negatively affect functionality. The germ damage is usually associated with heat damage because the heat generated during storage causes important changes in the color or appearance of the germ. The so-called black tip or blue eye grains are not viable and have higher quantities of damaged starch and reducing sugars that enhances Maillard reactions. In addition, these grains have higher fat acidity and oxidative rancidity, indicating hydrolysis of fats due to lipases. Sprouted kernels usually germinate in the spike or panicle in the field or during storage providing that they found the appropriate moisture and temperature conditions. Sprouted kernels are straightforwardly identified because they contain rootlets and, in some instances, even acrospires. Sprouted grains have high diastatic, lypolitic, and proteolytic activities because of the generation of amylases, lipases, and proteases, respectively. Therefore the starch, lipids, and proteins are hydrolyzed or damaged, generating higher amounts of reducing sugars, free fatty acids, and alpha amino nitrogens, respectively. The use of sprouted kernels yields sticky doughs and off-colored products. Mold-infested or weathered kernels are easily detected because of the color change on the pericarp and germ tissues. These kernels usually acquire a dirty off-coloration. Molds have potent enzymes that degrade reserve tissues of the *scutellum* and endosperm. Grain inspectors are trained to detect mold-infested or weathered kernels through visual inspection and the moldy stench of infested grains. Kernels infested with *Fusarium* and *Aspergillus* molds will probably contain significant amounts of mycotoxins that can harm human or animal health. For the specific case of sorghum, field-weathered kernels have a typical grayish or darker coloration. Sorghum is susceptible to weathering because it generally grows in hot and humid environments. A high environmental humidity postanthesis and during grain filling tends to increase the susceptibility to weathering. Frost damage occurs when maturing grains in the spike or panicle halt their normal growth due to low or freezing temperatures. These grains have a lighter coloration and usually lower thousand kernel weights because they did not fill properly in the field or are badly shrunken. Shrunken kernels have a wrinkled pericarp and a relatively low amount of endosperm and, therefore, a relatively low thousand kernel weight. These grains are produced when environmental conditions do not favor the development of the grain during inflorescence such as the lack of water or nutrients, heat stress, early frosts, and plant diseases. A high incidence of wrinkled kernels produces low milling yields.

1.2.9.1 Determination of Damaged Kernels

There are several reasons why a kernel may be damaged in the field or during storage. For instance, weather or bad environmental conditions during grain maturation in the field can cause discolored, weathered, frost, or sprouted kernels. Heat, insect, mold, and germ damage usually occurs during faulty storage.

A. *Samples, Ingredients, and Reagents*
- Different types and classes of sound and damaged kernels

B. *Materials and Equipment*
- Digital scale
- Tweezers
- Boerner divider
- Carter dockage tester

C. *Procedure*
1. Divide the lot of grain using the Boerner divider.
2. Select and weigh 200 g to 250 g of the cereal.
3. Manually separate damaged kernels into the following categories:
   a. Heat-damaged. Recognized by the darker coloration compared with sound or healthy counterparts.
   b. Insect-damaged. Recognized by visual perforations and the presence of live insects or web-like material.
   c. Germ-damaged or black tip. Kernels that have a dark or black germ that is not viable.
   d. Sprouted kernels. Recognized by the presence of rootlets and, in some instances, acrospires.
   e. Mold-damaged and weathered. Easily detected because of the moldy stench and color changes on the pericarp and germ tissues. These kernels usually acquire dirty off-colorations.
   f. Frost-damaged. Kernels have lighter colorations and usually lower thousand kernel weights because they did not fill properly in the field or are badly shrunken. Frost-damaged wheat and barley have a waxy appearance and a light green, brown, or even black coloration. In these cereals, the

pericarp is generally wrinkled and blistered in the dorsal and creased parts of the caryopsis.

  g. Shrunken kernels. These have wrinkled pericarp and a relatively low amount of endosperm and therefore a relatively low thousand kernel weight.

4. Weigh each category of damaged kernels and express results as a percentage of the original sample weight [(weight of damaged kernels/ original sample weight) × 100].

1.2.9.2 Tetrazolium Test for Germ Viability (Dead Germ)

The tetrazolium test is a quick test widely recognized as an accurate means of estimating germ viability. This method was developed in Germany in the 1940s by Professor G. Lakon, who had been trying to distinguish between live and dead seeds. Today, the test is used throughout the world as a highly regarded method of estimating seed viability. Kernels that have been overheated during uncontrolled sprouting or drying test negatively because they have dead germs which are unable to germinate. The tetrazolium reagent stains live germ and is used for the determination of viable or dead germs, especially in barley, for the brewing industry. It is based on the fact that viable kernels have aerobic respiration that includes electron and oxygen transport. During these oxidation metabolic events, energy is produced as adenosine 5 triphosphate. The elimination of electrons is catalyzed by dehydrogenases, enzymes that transfer electrons to other organic compounds that are not present in live cells such as 2,3,5-triphenyl tetrazolium chloride. This reagent is reduced in viable cells by dehydrogenases into a red complex called triphenil formazan. On the other hand, the nonrespiring dead cells are not capable of forming this colored compound because they do not have dehydrogenase activity (Association of Official Seed Analysts (AOSA) 2000; Moore 1985).

A. Samples, Ingredients, and Reagents
- Different types and classes of sound and damaged kernels
- 2,3,5-Triphenyl tetrazolium
- Distilled water

B. Materials and Equipment
- Boerner divider
- Scale
- Razor blade or dissecting knife
- 100 mL graduated cylinder
- Thermometer
- Different types and classes of kernels
- Tweezers
- 250 mL beaker
- Oven
- Chronometer

C. Procedure
1. Dissolve 1 g of 2,3,5-triphenyl tetrazolium in 100 mL of distilled water.

2. Divide the lot of grain using the Boerner divider.
3. Take 50 randomly selected kernels and carefully cut longitudinally in half to expose the germ. Discard the other half of the kernel.
4. Place kernel halves in the 1% tetrazolium solution and leave in an oven set at 70°C for 2 to 4 hours until color develops.
5. Remove samples from the oven and decant the tetrazolium solution.
6. Spread kernel halves onto paper towels and examine each sample. Viable or live germs will stain pink or reddish. Express the number of viable or dead kernels as a percentage: viable kernels = (number of live germs/total number of kernels) × 100, or dead germ or kernels = (number of unstained halves/total number of kernels) × 100.
   a. 85–100%, normal viability
   b. 75–84%, regular viability
   c. 50–74%, medium viability
   d. 0–49%, bad viability

1.2.10 RESEARCH SUGGESTIONS

1.2.10.1 Test Weight

1. Compare test weights of samples before and after cleaning with the clipper or Carter dockage tester.
2. Temper a given lot of grain to 16%, 18%, and 20% moisture and determine test weights after 8 hours of equilibration.
3. Compare test weight of a given lot of sound grain that has been purposely insect- or mold-damaged (refer to Chapter 4).
4. Compare test weighs of paddy, brown, and white polished rice or whole oats and groats (refer to Chapter 5).
5. Determine and compare test weights of soft, hard, and durum wheats.
6. Determine and compare test weights of unpopped and popped popcorn.

1.2.10.2 True Density

1. Compare true density values of a given grain sample conditioned to 16%, 18%, and 20% moisture after 8 hours of equilibration.
2. Compare true density of a given lot of sound grain that has been purposely insect- or mold-damaged (refer to Chapter 4).
3. Compare true densities of paddy, brown, and white polished rice or whole oats and groats (refer to Chapter 5).
4. Determine and compare true density values of soft, hard, and durum wheats.
5. Determine and compare true densities of unpopped and popped popcorn.

1.2.10.3 Flotation Index

1. Compare flotation index values of a soft dent, intermediate-textured, and hard maize kernels.
2. Determine the ideal density of the solution for determining flotation indexes of oats.
3. Temper a given lot of grain to 16%, 18%, and 20% moisture and determine their flotation indexes after 8 hours of equilibration.
4. Compare flotation indexes of a given lot of sound grain that has been purposely insect- or mold-damaged (refer to Chapter 4).
5. Determine and compare flotation indexes of soft, hard, and durum wheats.

1.2.10.4 Endosperm Texture

1. Compare endosperm texture and hardness of a soft dent, intermediate-textured, and hard samples of maize or soft, hard, and durum wheats. How do hardness and texture values relate?
2. Determine endosperm texture and hardness of soft and hard wheats and then mill the wheats into flours. Compare milling yields and particle size distribution of the resulting flours.
3. Determine endosperm texture and hardness of soft and hard sorghums and then decorticate kernels to remove 15% of the kernel weight. Compare decorticated kernel milling yields, amount of brokens, and the milling time required to achieve 15% weight removal.
4. Select two paddy rices with contrasting endosperm textures and mill them separately into white polished rice. Which sort of rice yielded higher amounts of polished rice? Why?
5. Compare hardness values determined with the TADD and Stenvert testers of a given lot of maize first artificially dried at three different temperatures (35°C, 50°C, and 65°C) and then conditioned to contain 14% moisture.

1.2.10.5 Breakage Susceptibility

1. Compare breakage susceptibility of a soft, intermediate-textured, and hard samples of dent maize before and after drying at 60°C. How do endosperm texture and drying affect breakage susceptibility?
2. Select two rough rices with contrasting breakage susceptibility values and mill them separately into white polished rice. Which sort of rice yielded higher amounts of polished rice? Which one yielded higher amounts of second head and brokens? Why?
3. Select an intermediate-textured sorghum and then subject part of the sample to artificial drying (60°C for 2 hours). Allow the dehydrated sample to equilibrate for at least 12 hours before milling. Determine the breakage susceptibility of the two samples and then decorticate the regular and artificially dehydrated sorghum samples separately for a fixed

milling time (i.e., time necessary to remove 15% of the regular sorghum weight). After milling, determine the amount of decorticated kernels and broken kernels. Determine which sort of sorghum yielded higher amounts of broken kernels.
4. Compare the breakage susceptibility with the Stein or Wisconsin breakage tester of a given lot of maize first artificially dried at three different temperatures (35°C, 50°C, and 65°C) and then conditioned to contain 14% moisture content.

1.2.10.6 Stress Cracks

1. Dry a lot of paddy rice or hard maize or durum wheat at 35°C, 45°C, and 55°C for 2 hours and then allow samples to equilibrate at room temperature for an additional 2 hours. Then, determine the average number and size of the stress cracks or fissures of the control, 35°C, 45°C, and 55°C dehydrated samples. Remember to dehull the rice sample before determining stress cracks (refer to procedure in Section 1.2.6.1).
2. Experimentally mill paddy rice samples with a contrasting number of stress cracks and determine the yield of white polished rice, second heads, and brokens.
3. Place a lot of durum wheat or dent maize in a sealed container to subject samples to mechanical damage. Determine the number of stress cracks as affected by time of mechanical damage.

1.2.10.7 Kernel Weight

1. Determine the average kernel weight of two- and six-rowed barley samples.
2. Compare thousand kernel weights of a given lot of sound grain that has been purposely germinated or sprouted, insect-, mold-, or frost-damaged (refer to Chapter 4).
3. Compare the average size (length/width) and 1000 kernel weights of long and short paddy, brown, and white polished rices. Determine the difference between the two rice classes and the effect of dehulling and decortication-polishing on kernel weights.
4. Compare the 1000 kernel weight of a given lot of barley before and after malting (make sure to compare samples at equivalent moisture contents).
5. Compare the 1000 kernel weight of a given lot of dent maize before and after nixtamalization (make sure to compare samples at equivalent moisture contents).
6. Compare thousand kernel weight values of soft, hard, and durum wheats.
7. Compare thousand kernel weight values from sound and shriveled wheat samples.
8. Determine milling yields or flour extraction rates of two wheats that greatly differ in thousand kernel weight (for instance, compare 22 g/1000 vs. 34 g/1000 kernels).

1.2.10.8 Foreign Material and Dockage

1. Prepare two lots of the same type of maize or wheat tempered to 17.5% moisture that greatly differ in amount of foreign material (i.e., 1% vs. 7% foreign material) and then subject the two lots to storage at room temperature for at least 1 month (refer to procedure in Section 4.2.1.2). At the end of the programmed storage, compare the grain's physical properties and insect and mold damage.
2. Clean and mill (refer to procedure in Section 5.2.2.1) two lots of the same type of wheat containing contrasting amounts of foreign material and then determine milling yields based on uncleaned and cleaned sample weights.
3. Place a lot of dent maize in a sealed container to subject samples to mechanical damage. Determine the amount of dockage as affected by mechanical damage.

1.2.10.9 Grain Damage

1. Mill a given lot of wheat that was purposely insect-, mold-damaged or sprouted. Determine milling yield or extraction rate, color of resulting flours, number of insect fragments, mycotoxins, diastatic activity, or falling number and other flour quality parameters such as farinograph or alveograph.
2. Process a given lot of white maize that was purposely insect-damaged into tortillas. Determine dry matter losses during the nixtamalization process, *masa* texture, tortilla yield, and quality especially in terms of starch content, color, texture, and amount of insect fragments (refer to Chapters 4 and 7).
3. Determine germ viability (tetrazolium test), percentage of germination, diastatic activity, and malting losses of two lots of barleys with different amounts of damaged kernels (refer to Chapter 14).
4. Process a given lot of malting barley that was purposely insect- and mold-damaged into lager beer. Determine percentage of germination, diastatic activity of the two barleys after malting, dry matter losses after malting, and lager beer quality especially in terms of extraction, color, alcohol content, and organoleptic properties (refer to Chapters 3 and 14).

1.2.11 Research Questions

1.2.11.1 Test Weight

1. What are the main intrinsic factors in the grain that affect test weight?
2. Why is the test weight widely used to grade and classify grains?
3. What is the conversion factor of pounds per bushel to kilograms per hectoliter?
4. How much wheat or oats with test weights of 56 lb/bu and 30 lb/bu can you place in a storage bin with the following dimensions: 15 m wide, 10 m high,

and 60 m long? Express results in pounds and tons (1000 kg).
5. Explain why the test weights of hulled oats and groats greatly differ.
6. Explain why the test weights of popcorn and yellow dent maize greatly differ.
7. What is the effect of moisture content on test weight of a given lot of grain? Why do they differ?

1.2.11.2 True Density

1. What are the main grain intrinsic factors that affect true density?
2. What are the differences and similarities between test weight and true density? How do these tests relate?
3. Explain why the true densities of popcorn and yellow dent maize differ.
4. What is the effect of moisture content on true density of a given lot of grain? Why do they differ?
5. How do insect and mold damage affect true density values?

1.2.11.3 Flotation Index

1. What are the main grain intrinsic factors that affect flotation index?
2. How will you modify the flotation index procedure to screen different lots of popcorns?
3. How does temperature affect flotation index?
4. What are the differences and similarities between flotation index and true density? How do these tests relate?
5. Do you think that flotation index can be used to determine wheat class? Why?
6. What is the effect of insect damage on the flotation index of a given lot of grain? Why do they differ?

1.2.11.4 Endosperm Texture

1. Explain how endosperm texture and grain hardness relate.
2. What would happen to the hardness of a given lot of barley after malting?
3. What would happen to the hardness of a given lot of sorghum after weathering?
4. What kind of maize, especially in terms of endosperm texture and hardness, would you select for wet-milling (starch) and production of refined flaking grits?
5. How does grain hardness relate to test weight, true density, and flotation index?
6. Investigate how grain hardness can be effectively measured with the NIRA.

1.2.11.5 Breakage Susceptibility

1. Explain how endosperm texture and grain hardness affect breakage susceptibility.
2. Compare the storability of a given lot of maize with contrasting breakage susceptibilities.

3. Explain how artificial drying affects breakage susceptibility and milling yields of rough rice.

4. What would happen to the breakage susceptibility of a given lot of popcorn if it is not properly harvested (threshed) and dehydrated on the field? How would it affect popcorn expansion rate?

1.2.11.6   Stress Cracks

1. Explain how grain hardness affects susceptibility to stress cracks.

2. How would you prevent the generation of stress cracks in a lot of rough rice during drying and handling?

3. Explain how parboiling affects stress cracks and milling yields of white polished rice.

4. What would happen to the susceptibility to stress cracks of a given lot of popcorn if it is not properly harvested (threshed) and dehydrated on the field? How would stress cracks affect popcorn expansion rate?

1.2.11.7   Grain Weight

1. How do insect and mold damage affect thousand kernel weight?

2. How does malting affect thousand kernel weights of a given lot of barley? Why do they differ?

3. Why is the thousand kernel weight of wheat closely related to milling yields?

4. How does fertilization affect 1000 kernel weights of wheat?

1.2.11.8   Dockage and Foreign Material

1. Explain why grain dockage and foreign material is penalized by grain inspection agencies.

2. How does dockage and foreign material affect the storability of a given lot of grain?

3. Describe commercial processes to remove dockage and foreign material before storage.

4. Explain how grain breakage susceptibility and handling affect dockage.

5. How does dockage and foreign material affect susceptibility to grain explosions and fires? Why?

6. Compare grain turning or rotation and grain aeration or ventilation in terms of producing grain dust and dockage.

1.2.11.9   Damaged Kernels

1. What are the main factors affecting heat-damaged kernels? Why is this category of damaged kernels the most relevant for grain inspectors?

2. How can you identify heat-, insect-, mold-, frost-damaged, and sprouted kernels?

3. Which category of kernel damage affects the most diastatic activity and color of refined wheat flour? Why?

4. Explain the principle of the tetrazolium test and how it relates to the quality of malting barleys.

5. What are the main indicators of chemical damages in the fat, protein, and starch fractions of damaged kernels?

6. What are differences in diastatic activities between sound and mold-damaged wheat? How does mold damage or sprouting affect the rheological properties of wheat dough and texture (stickiness)?

7. What are the differences in nixtamalization (cooking time and tortilla chip quality) between sound and mold-damaged maize? How does mold damage affect cooking time, dry matter losses, *masa* texture, color, and tortilla chip texture (stickiness)?

1.3   DETERMINATION OF GRADE AND CLASS

Grain quality standardization is an essential marketing function which facilitates the movement and transactions of grains through the marketing channel. Standardized grain is easier to move and results in reduced transaction costs. The developmental stage of an economic system affects the structure and sophistication of grain standards and grades. As a result, there are several grain classification systems that are used for trading and quality purposes in several countries around the globe. These systems vary in the number of tests applied to classify and grade the grain but have the same philosophy. The basic purposes of grain standards are to characterize the physical and biological properties of grain at the time of inspection. The six goals of the U.S. Grain Standard Act are to (a) define uniform and accepted descriptive terms to facilitate trade, (2) provide information to aid in determining storability, (3) offer end-users the best possible information from which to determine finished product yield and quality, (4) to create a tool for the market to establish quality improvement incentives, (5) to reflect the economic value-based characteristics in the end uses of grains, and (6) to accommodate scientific advances in testing new knowledge concerning factors related to end use performance of grain (Kiser 1991).

In the United States and other grain-exporting countries around the globe, grain standards are legally mandated, and the systems employed are more elaborate compared with the classification systems of developing countries. In some underdeveloped countries, the systems simply consist of determining grain moisture accompanied by a visual inspection. The U.S. grain grading and classification system (USDA-GIPSA 1999) is one of the most recognized around the world. Most classification systems determine grade and class. Grade is aimed toward the determination of grain condition, soundness, or health, and class is related to industrial use or functionality.

1.3.1   Evaluation of Grade

The determination of grade of any lot of grain is based on the ratings of quality factors associated to the grain. Most grade assignation systems use specific standard tables for the inspected grain. These tables specify important objective and subjective factors such as test weight, amount of foreign material, and damaged kernels. Many tables also include shrunken and broken kernels. There are several grain classification systems that are used in several countries around the globe. However, the grain grading and classification system in the United States (USDA-GIPSA 1999) is one of the most recognized because this country is one of the main grain exporters and trades practically with all countries around the globe. Grade is aimed toward the determination of grain condition, soundness, or health. Buyers want to acquire dry, insect-free, and sound grain that will store well and processors' grain that will yield a high percentage of finished products with good quality. Several tests are applied for the determination of grade; the main ones are moisture, test weight, damaged and broken kernels, and amount of foreign material associated with the lot of grain (refer to procedures listed in Section 1.2). After analyzing these factors, inspectors input quality parameters into the tables described in Chapter 2 of the textbook (refer to Tables 2.2–2.13) to assign a specific grade. The maximum grade value will correspond to the minimum individual test value.

1.3.1.1 Determination of Maize Grade

Six grades of maize are recognized by U.S. Grades and Grade Requirements. Moisture content is also determined and reported but is not a part of the grade (Rooney 2007). Heat-damaged and moldy maize caused by improper drying, inadequate aeration during storage, and heating should not be used for food purposes. Corn that is not viable or does not germinate should also be rejected.

A. *Samples, Ingredients, and Reagents*
   • Different lots of maize kernels
B. *Materials and Equipment*
   • Winchester bushel meter
   • Round-holed sieve (12/64 in. or 0.1875 cm)
   • Carter dockage test meter
C. *Procedure*
   1. Determine test weight of the lot of maize (refer to procedure in Section 1.2.1.1), broken kernels, and foreign material (refer to procedure in Section 1.2.8.2), heat-damaged and total damaged kernels (refer to procedure in Section 1.2.9.1). In addition, determine the moisture content of the lot of maize (refer to procedure in Section 2.2.1.1).
   2. Input obtained values in the maize grade table (see Table 2.2 of the textbook) and assign grade according to the lowest rated factor.

1.3.1.2 Determination of Wheat Grade
   A. *Samples, Ingredients, and Reagents*
      • Different lots of wheats
   B. *Materials and Equipment*
      • Winchester bushel meter
      • Carter dockage test meter

C. *Procedure*
   1. Determine the class of wheat according to the procedure.
   2. Determine test weight of the lot of wheat (refer to procedure in Section 1.2.1.1), foreign material (refer to procedure in Section 1.2.8.1), heat-damaged and total damaged kernels (refer to procedure in Section 1.2.9.1) shrunken and broken kernels, and the amount or percentage of contrasting wheat classes. In addition, determine the moisture content of wheat (refer to procedure in Section 2.2.1.1).
   3. Input obtained values in the wheat grade table (see Table 2.6 of the textbook) and assign grade according to the lowest rated factor.

1.3.1.3 Determination of Grade of Rough, Brown, or White Polished Rice

Rice is the only cereal that could be graded as rough, brown (naked caryopsis), or white polished (see Tables 2.3–2.5). The criteria used for grading are damaged kernels, percentage of chalky kernels, and color. The grading system is more elaborate because the properties affect quality, milling yields, and performance during cooking. In the United States, rice is marketed according to size, form, and condition. These properties are related to milling performance, cooking time, and organoleptic properties of the cooked rice (Webb 1985; USDA 1983). The test weight, although not considered in the official U.S. grading, is an important selection parameter because it relates to milling yields and decreases when the lot has higher amounts of dockage, immature, shriveled, and empty kernels. The average test weight of long, medium, and short rough rices is 56, 58.5, and 60 kg/hL, respectively.

Another important rice grading criteria is the amount of kernels with chalky endosperm or white bellies. This factor is not desirable because these kernels are more susceptible to breakage during handling and milling and, on milling, yield lower amounts of products. In addition, these soft textured kernels tend to overcook and produce undesirable texture in the prepared rice. The incidence of white belly caryopses is associated with the variety and increases when the kernels mature under harsh conditions or is harvested at high moisture contents.

Color is another critical quality factor. It is subjectively evaluated by inspectors in a representative rice sample that has been previously milled using laboratory equipment. The color varies from desirable white to undesirable dark gray (see Table 2.5 of the textbook). One of the most common off-colors is pink or rosy which results from the contamination of rice with red wild rice. The red pigments present in the aleurone contaminate the white kernels which acquire a pink coloration. Parboiled rice is classified according to color as light- or dark-colored. The hydrothermal process enhances color formation.

A. *Samples, Ingredients, and Reagents*
   • Different lots of rough (paddy) rice, brown rice, or white polished rice

B. *Materials and Equipment*
- Carter dockage test meter

C. *Procedure*
1. Determine the class of rice according to procedure in Section 1.3.2.3.
2. For rough rice, determine heat-damaged, red-colored, total damaged kernels (procedure in Section 1.2.9.1), foreign material (refer to procedure in Section 1.2.8.1), chalky kernels, and kernels belonging to a different class. For brown rice, determine the amount of paddy kernels, heat-damaged, red-colored, total damaged kernels (refer to procedure in Section 1.2.9.1), chalky kernels, broken kernels, and kernels belonging to a different class. For white polished rice, determine the amount of paddy and brown kernels, heat-damaged, red-colored, total damaged kernels (refer to procedure in Section 1.2.9.1), chalky kernels, milling grade, color, broken kernels, and kernels belonging to a different class. In addition, determine the moisture content of the rice kernels (refer to procedure in Section 2.2.1.1).
3. Input the obtained values in the rough, brown, or white polished rice grade table (see Tables 2.3, 2.4, or 2.5 of the textbook, respectively) and assign grade according to the lowest rated factor.

1.3.1.4 Determination of Barley Grade
Barley is graded following the same tests used for other cereals. Tables 2.10 and 2.11 of the textbook depict different criteria used to assign grade.

A. *Samples, Ingredients, and Reagents*
- Different lots of husked barley

B. *Materials and Equipment*
- Winchester bushel meter
- Carter dockage test meter

C. *Procedure*
1. Determine test weight of the husked barley (refer to procedure in Section 1.2.1.1), foreign material (refer to procedure in Section 1.2.8.1), heat-damaged and total damaged kernels (refer to procedure in Section 1.2.9.1), and shrunken and broken kernels. In addition, determine the moisture content of the barley sample (refer to procedure in Section 2.2.1.1).
2. Input obtained values in the barley grade table (see Table 2.10 of the textbook) and assign grade according to the lowest rated factor.

1.3.1.5 Determination of Sorghum Grade
A. *Samples, Ingredients, and Reagents*
- Different lots of sorghum kernels

B. *Materials and Equipment*
- Winchester bushel meter
- Triangular-holed sieve (5/64 in. or 0.0781 cm)
- Carter dockage test meter

C. *Procedure*
1. Determine the test weight of the lot of sorghum (refer to procedure in Section 1.2.1.1), broken and foreign material (refer to procedure in Section 1.2.8.1), heat-damaged and total damaged kernels (refer to procedure in Section 1.2.9.1). In addition, determine the moisture content of the sorghum kernels (refer to procedure in Section 2.2.1.1).
2. Input obtained values in the sorghum grade table (see Table 2.12 of the textbook) and assign grade according to the lowest rated factor.

1.3.1.6 Determination of Oats Grade
Oats are husked caryopsis that are graded according to test weight, dockage, and damaged kernels. An important consideration in oats grading is contamination with wild oats (*Avena fatua*). Wild oats generally contaminate commercial oat plantations during mechanical harvesting. The main difference between commercial oats and wild oats is that wild oats produce twisted awns and has pubescence in the basal or germinal part.

A. *Samples, Ingredients, and Reagents*
- Different lots of husked oats

B. *Materials and Equipment*
- Winchester bushel meter
- Carter dockage test meter

C. *Procedure*
1. Determine test weight of the husked oats (refer to procedure in Section 1.2.1.1), foreign material (refer to procedure in Section 1.2.8.1), heat-damaged (refer to procedure in Section 1.2.9.1), and wild oats. Wild oats are recognized by their twisted awns and pubescence in the basal or germinal part. In addition, determine the moisture content of the oat sample (refer to procedure in Section 2.2.1.1).
2. Input obtained values in the oats grade table (see Table 2.15 of the textbook) and assign grade according to the lowest rated factor.

1.3.1.7 Determination of Rye Grade
The U.S. grading system for rye includes four grades and one additional special grade that does not meet the requirements for U.S. grade nos. 1 to 4. The Canadian Grain Commission also grades rye into four main and two special categories (refer to Table 2.14 of the textbook). For the specific case of rye, it is of upmost importance to identify ergot (*Claviceps purpurea*) contaminated kernels because this mold produces a toxin highly toxic to humans.

A. *Samples, Ingredients, and Reagents*
- Different lots of rye kernels

B. *Materials and Equipment*
- Winchester bushel meter
- Carter dockage test meter

C. *Procedure*
1. Determine test weight of the rye sample (refer to procedure in Section 1.2.1.1), foreign material

excluding wheat (refer to procedure in Section 1.2.8.1), heat-damaged, and total damaged kernels (refer to procedure in Section 1.2.9.1). In addition, determine the moisture content of the rye sample (refer to procedure in Section 2.2.1.1).

2. Input obtained values in the rye grade table (see Table 2.13) and assign grade according to the lowest rated factor.

1.3.2 EVALUATION OF CLASS

1.3.2.1 Determination of Maize Class

Maize is classed according to the form of the caryopses into dent or flint and is subclassed according to color as either white or yellow. Three classes are recognized in U.S. Grades and Grade Requirements. If a given lot of maize exceeds 10% from another color, it is classified as mixed maize (USDA-GIPSA 1999; Paulsen et al. 2003). Dent and yellow maize is the most popular class. This particular class is widely used as animal feed, starch production, and for fuel ethanol production. The characteristic dent or indentation is observed on top of the kernel. Flint maize does not have the characteristic dent and has an oval or tear-shaped form (i.e., popcorn). These kernels usually have a hard or vitreous endosperm texture. In practice, food grade maize should have reduced levels of broken and chipped kernels and requires guarantees that the aflatoxin and fumonisin levels should be lower than 20 ppb and 2000 ppb (2 ppm), respectively (Rooney 2007).

1.3.2.2 Determination of Wheat Class

Wheat is classified into several classes and subclasses and is considered as the most elaborated classing system. Wheat is classed into three categories: hard, soft, and durum. The hard and soft wheat classes are subclassed according to color (red or white) and growth habit (winter or spring; see Table 2.7). Hard wheats are used to produce yeast-leavened breads and related bakery items. The most common class in terms of trade is the hard red winter wheat (HRWW) and the class recognized as the best quality is the hard red spring wheat (HRSW). The white hard wheats are starting to gain popularity because they produce better quality whole wheat products. Soft wheats are mainly used for the production of cookies, cake mixes, and related chemical-leavened products. The most popular soft wheat is classed as soft red winter wheat (SRWW) and the one with the highest market value is the soft white winter (SWW), which is also called club. Durum wheats have a simpler classification system and are divided into hard amber (75% or more of hard and vitreous kernels of amber color), amber (60% or more but less than 75% of hard and vitreous kernels of amber color, and durum (less than 60% of hard and vitreous kernels of amber color).

Winter wheats are generally planted in the late summer or early fall and they stop growing when the first snows fall or when the temperature drops; therefore, they pass dormant all winter and mature and finish their growing cycle after the arrival of the spring season. On the other hand, spring wheats are planted in the early spring and are generally harvested during the fall. These wheats are usually irrigated and fertilized and produce larger kernels with more protein and gluten strength.

The different classes of wheat differ in their physical and chemical properties. Durums have a corneous or vitreous endosperm texture, high test weight and density, and high protein (12.5–16.5%) whereas soft wheats have a soft textured endosperm, lower test weight, and low protein content (8.0–10.5%; Carver 2009).

1.3.2.3 Determination of Rice Class

The majority of rice is directly channeled for human consumption. Because paddy rice is a husked caryopsis, that is the way it is graded, marketed, and stored. Most rough rices are dry-milled into white polished kernels. The milling process is aimed toward the sequential removal of the husks or glumes, pericarp, germ, and aleurone tissues. The last three are commonly removed by abrasion.

Rice is generally classified according to size as large, medium, and short. The dimensions of large paddy rice are 8.9 mm to 9.6 mm length and 2.3 mm to 2.5 mm width with a length/width ratio of 3.8 to 3.9:1. The medium paddy rice has a length, width, and length/width ratio of 7.9 mm to 8.2 mm, 3.0 mm to 3.2 mm, and 2.5 to 2.6:1, respectively, whereas the short paddy rice is 7.4 mm to 7.5 mm length, 3.1 mm to 3.6 mm width, and 2.1 to 2.4:1 length/width ratio. This last measurement is used as one of the most important criteria for classification. The average length and width is calculated after the longitudinal arrangement of 10 caryopses positioned lengthwise or widthwise (Webb 1985).

1.3.2.3.1 Determination of Rice Length, Width, and Length to Width Ratio

A. Samples, Ingredients, and Reagents
- Different types of paddy or rough, brown, or white rices

B. Materials and Equipment
- Ruler with a millimeter scale

C. Procedure
1. Obtain a representative rough rice sample from the lot of grain.
2. Randomly choose 10 caryopses and place them lengthwise. Measure the total length with an accuracy of 1 mm. Place the same caryopses side to side or widthwise and measure the average width with an accuracy of 0.1 mm.
3. Calculate the average length and width and then the length/width ratio.
4. Repeat the same procedure for the brown and white polished rice obtained after experimental dehulling and decortications/polishing procedures (refer to Chapter 5, procedure in Section 5.2.3.1).
5. Classify rough or paddy, brown, and white polished rice according to the length/width depicted in Table 1.1.

TABLE 1.1

Range of Length (L), Width (W), and L/W Ratio for the Different Classes of Rice

Class of Rice	Type of Rice	Length (mm)	Width (mm)	L/W Ratio
Long	Paddy	8.9–9.6	2.3–2.5	3.8:1–3.9:1
	Brown	7.0–7.5	2.0–2.1	3.4:1–3.6:1
	White	6.7–7.0	1.9–2.0	3.4:1–3.6:1
Medium	Paddy	7.9–8.2	3.0–3.2	2.5:1–2.6:1
	Brown	5.9–6.1	2.5–2.8	2.2:1–2.4:1
	White	5.5–5.8	2.4–2.7	2.1:1–2.3:1
Short	Paddy	7.4–7.5	3.1–3.6	2.1:1–2.4:1
	Brown	5.4–5.5	2.8–3.0	1.8:1–2.0:1
	White	5.2–5.4	2.7–3.1	1.7:1–2.0:1

Source: Webb, B. D. In *Rice: Chemistry and Technology*, B. O. Juliano (ed.), 1985. St. Paul, MN: American Association of Cereal Chemists. With permission.

1.3.2.4 Determination of Barley Class

Barley is a husked caryopsis that is mainly used for malting or as a feed for domestic animals. Malting barley is divided in two- and six-rowed varieties. The caryopses of six-rowed barleys are usually smaller or with lower thousand kernel weights compared with counterparts from two-rowed varieties. Malt and feed barleys differ in protein content and diastatic activity. The malting types usually have a lower protein content but higher starch content that upon germination yield more fermentable sugars. Generally, malting barleys contain 9.5% to 12.5% protein. These varieties are selected based on viability, percentage of germination, and germination vigor and uniformity. In addition, they should have low dormancy.

The Canadians market two-rowed and six-rowed malting barleys, hull-less barley, and feed barley. The malting barleys are selected based on germination, protein, varietal purity, plumpness, damaged kernels, and foreign material. The two-rowed barleys have higher thousand kernel weight and more uniform kernel size.

Barley is among the four most used cereals for animal feed. The protein content of feed barley varies from 12.5% to 17%. Barley is suitable for all domestic animals except poultry because birds are negatively affected by the high β-glucan content. There are two specialty types that have enhanced nutritional value for monogastrics: hull-less and high-lysine. The naked or hull-less barleys have a lower fiber content and more digestible energy whereas the Hyproly or high-lysine variety has a better essential amino acid profile due to improved lysine content. The use of Hyproly barley lowers the use of more expensive protein feedstuffs such as soybean without affecting the efficiency of feed conversion (McGregor and Bhatty 1993).

1.3.2.5 Determination of Sorghum Class

The U.S. Federal Grain Inspection Service recognizes four sorghum classes (USDA-GIPSA 1999): brown or high tannin, yellow or red, white, and mixed. Worldwide, the most popular class is the yellow or red. Brown sorghums, also known as bird-resistant or tannin sorghums, possess a testa which contains significant amounts of condensed tannins (Rooney and Serna-Saldivar 1991; Serna-Saldivar and Rooney 1995; Rooney and Miller 1982). These are more resistant to sprouting in the field, bird damage, weathering, molds, and other phytopathogens. However, tannins act as antinutritional compounds decreasing protein digestibility and the overall nutritional value of the grain. This is the reason why these sorghums are usually sold at a discount price in grain markets. White or food-grade sorghums possess a white pericarp without pigmented testa and are widely planted for direct human food uses in India and Africa. The red or yellow sorghums are widely used to substitute maize in the production of animal feedstuffs. These sorghums do not contain significant amounts of condensed tannins. The mixed sorghum class contains more than 10% of other classes and therefore do not meet any of the specifications of the other three main classes. The most practical way to classify brown sorghums is by the careful removal of the pericarp with the objective to expose the testa or outer layer of the endosperm. These high-tannin sorghums have a pigmented testa (brown, purple, or red). The other way to identify these sorghums is by immersing a representative lot of the grain in a Chlorox solution according to the procedure detailed by Waniska et al. (1992). Brown sorghums acquire a characteristic black coloration after bleaching.

1.3.2.5.1 Chlorox Procedure to Identify Brown or High-Tannin Sorghums

This procedure was previously described by Waniska et al. 1992.

A. Samples, Ingredients, and Reagents
- Different sorghums (types I, II, and III)
- Potassium hydroxide (KOH)
- 5.25% sodium hypochlorite (NaOCl)
- Distilled water

B. Materials and Equipment
- Digital scale
- Perforated containers
- Magnetic stirrer
- Stir magnetic bar
- Laboratory clock
- Thermometer
- Beaker (250 mL)
- Aluminum or glass pan
- Graduated cylinder (100 mL)
- Plastic gloves

C. Procedure
1. Obtain a representative sorghum grain sample.
2. Set the heat dial of the magnetic stirrer to maintain a water temperature of 60°C.
3. Fill aluminum or glass pan to a depth of approximately 3 mm and set on heated magnetic stirrer.

4. In a 250 mL beaker, place a stir bar, 7.5 g of KOH, 15 g of the sorghum grain sample, and 70 mL of 5.25% NaOCl (chlorox or bleach solution). Place the beaker in the water pan.
5. Adjust stirrer for maximal agitation and stir for 7 minutes.
6. After the treatment time, remove beaker and discard bleach solution. Then, rinse the sorghum with cold water.
7. Place treated kernels on top of a clear surface for rating.
8. Count the total number of kernels and then those that acquired a black or dark coloration. Express the result as a percentage of high tannin kernels = [(number of dark-colored kernels/total number of kernels) × 100].

1.3.2.6 Determination of Oats Class

Oats are classified according to color as white or yellow, red, gray, black, and mixed oats. White or yellow caryopses are generally obtained from *Avena sativa*, whereas red-colored caryopses are from *Avena byzantina*. Red oats are generally planted during the winter whereas white varieties are planted during the spring. The food industry prefers the top grades of the white and red classes. There is one oat cultivar that yields naked caryopses (*Avena nuda*) that will probably gain a market share soon because of the increased interest in the nutraceutical properties of this cereal grain.

1.3.2.7 Determination of Rye Class

The U.S. Federal Grain Inspection Service does not assign classes or subclasses to rye. Thus, the quality is mainly affected by the assigned grade and the incidence of ergoty rye.

1.3.3 Research Suggestions

1. Determine grade of a given type of cereal before and after cleaning with an air aspirator or sieves (Carter dockage tester).
2. Determine the grade of a given type of cereal subjected to insect and mold damage (refer to Chapter 4).
3. Determine flour milling yields and flour quality of two lots of wheat with different grades (refer to Chapter 5).
4. Determine insect fragments of flours obtained from two lots of wheat with different grades especially in terms of damaged kernels (refer to Chapter 4).
5. Determine diastatic activity of two lots of barley with different grades especially in terms of damaged kernels (refer to Chapter 14).
6. Determine thousand kernel weight and the starch content and composition (percentage of amylose and amylopectin) of typical rices classified as short and long.

7. Determine the protein content and alveograph properties of wheats classified as soft and hard.
8. Determine color of whole wheats and their refined flours classified as white and red (for instance, compare soft winter white wheat vs. soft winter red wheat).
9. Determine the thousand kernel weight of a sample classified as two- and six-rowed barley.
10. Determine the diastatic activity and protein content of two barleys classified as malting and feed.

1.3.4 Research Questions

1. What is the main aim and advantages of grain grading?
2. Calculate the difference in true wheat content of two contrasting lots of wheats weighing 5000 tons each. Lot A, graded as no. 4, contains 15.5% moisture, 5.6% foreign material, and 10% shriveled kernels whereas lot B, graded as no. 1, contains 13.7% moisture, 0.4% foreign material, and 0.1% shriveled kernels. Assume that shriveled wheat will be discarded by cleaning systems. If the buyer paid 210 dollars/ton for lot A and 226 dollars/ton for lot B, which lot of wheat was more convenient to buy? Why? Which lot of wheat will have better storability? Why?
3. Why is test weight one of the most important criteria for grain grading?
4. Why is heat damage considered as one of the most important criteria for assigning grade?
5. Why is ergot-contaminated rye heavily penalized by grading systems? How do grain inspectors recognize ergot-contaminated rye?
6. How do grain inspectors differentiate wild from commercial oats?
7. Investigate how vision computer systems can be used for inspection and grading of cereal grains.
8. What are the main aims and advantages of grain classification systems? What are the main differences between wheat grading/classification between the United States and Canada? Which system includes a class of wheat suited for noodle production?
9. What are the main physicochemical characteristics and main food uses of the three different classes of wheat?
10. Why are hard red spring wheats (HRSW) considered better than hard red winter wheats (HRWW) for bread-baking operations?
11. What are the main physicochemical characteristics of long, medium, and short rices? What are the main criteria used to differentiate these classes of rice?
12. What are main differences between dent and flint maizes in terms of the form of the caryopses and endosperm hardness and texture?

13. What are the major differences between two- and six-rowed barleys and between malting and feed barleys?
14. What are the three major classes or grain sorghum? Which class is the most planted worldwide?
15. Why do brown or type III sorghums have more resistance to sprouting, molds, birds, and other biotic agents? What is the basis of the identification of tannin sorghums using chlorine solution? Why are tannins considered as antinutritional agents?

1.4 MACROMORPHOLOGY AND MICROMORPHOLOGY OF CEREAL GRAINS

1.4.1 Observation of Inflorescences

Different types of cereal plants produce two types of inflorescence: spikes or panicles. In the specific and unique case of maize, the reproductive organs are located in two different parts of the plant and the female flower produces a fused panicle botanically denominated as a central axis. Wheat, barley, rye, and triticale yield spikes, whereas the rest of the commercial cereals have panicles. In spikes, the flowers that eventually produce caryopses are directly positioned along a unique axis. On the other hand, the flowers and caryopses of panicles are arranged or distributed in the inflorescence branches or accessory axes. Rice, sorghum, oats, and all millets produce these types of inflorescences. For the specific case of pearl millet, it produces a compact panicle characterized as containing many small branches that are frequently erroneously confused with a spike. As indicated previously, maize is the only cereal that produces an ear classified as a central axis. However, its parents, *Teosintle* and *Euchlaena mexicana* produce open panicles. Most cytogeneticists hypothesize that the unique architecture of the female inflorescence is due to a genetic mutation or aberration. The accessory axes of the ear of maize fused along the central axis in such a way that the caryopses are positioned in rows. The glumes that cover every single flower or caryopsis in other cereals covers the whole cob and all the styles, commonly called silks, emerge at the ear's top.

1.4.1.1 Observation of Immature Inflorescences

A. *Samples, Ingredients, and Reagents*
- Immature inflorescences, collected postanthesis, of different cereal grains (maize cobs and tassels, wheat spikes, paddy rice panicles, barley spike, sorghum panicle, etc.)

B. *Materials and Equipment*
- Dissection microscope
- Digital scale
- Ruler with millimeter markings
- Tweezers

C. *Procedure*
1. Carefully observe and draw the whole architecture of the inflorescence. Make sure to measure the different parts of the inflorescence and identify the number of branches, male and female flowers, and glumes. For the specific cases of wheat, barley, triticale, and oats, make sure to identify and measure the average length of the awns that are part of the lemma. For the specific case of maize, draw the male tassel and separate and weigh the glumes or husks, silks, and cob. Make sure to identify where the styles or silks originate. In addition, count the number of glumes or shucks and kernel rows.
2. Under a microscope, carefully dissect randomly selected flowers and draw male and female reproductive organs and the glumes (lemma and palea). Make sure to identify and count the number of male stamens (filaments and anthers) with their characteristic color and all the parts of the female flower (stigma, style, and ovary). Observe if the anthers released pollen and if the pollen is attached to the stigma.

1.4.1.2 Observation of Mature Inflorescences

A. *Samples, Ingredients, and Reagents*
- Mature inflorescences of different cereal grains (maize cobs and tassels, wheat spikes, paddy rice panicles, barley spike, sorghum panicle, etc.).

B. *Materials and Equipment*
- Dissection microscope
- Scale
- Tweezers
- Ruler

C. *Procedure*
1. Weigh the inflorescence.
2. Carefully observe and draw the architecture of the inflorescence. Under a microscope, observe the two types of glumes (lemma and palea). For the specific cases of wheat, barley, triticale, and oats, make sure to identify and measure the average length of the awns that are part of the lemma. For maize, count the number of glumes or shucks and record the weight. Count the number of kernel rows and measure the corn cob (width and length). For sorghum and millets, identify the color and size of the glumes.
3. Carefully separate kernels from the mature inflorescence and record the weight and number of kernels, glumes, and other vegetative tissues.
4. Determine the percentage of weight of the kernels, glumes, and other vegetative tissues. Keep kernels for determination of physical and chemical properties.

1.4.2 Observation and Identification of the Anatomical Parts of Cereal Kernels

The cereal caryopsis is divided into three main anatomical parts: pericarp, endosperm, and germ. In general, these constitute 7% to 10%, 82% to 85%, and 3% to 10%, respectively. However, the proportions vary among cereal types. Husked or covered grains retain their glumes after harvesting. The glumes are not considered part of the caryopsis but floral structures in the form of leaves that cover the caryopsis. They protect the kernel during development against external agents such as insects, molds, and moisture. The glumes consist of two structures: the lemma and the palea. Generally, the lemma covers the embryo and has a pointed end or awn in wheat, oat, barley, and rye. The palea generally covers the ventral part of small cereal grains. In the sorghum grain, the lemma differs from the palea in the incision point of the floral structure. The glumes can be short or medium, and in some varieties, they can completely cover the kernel. The glumes constitute approximately 20% of the weight of the covered caryopses of rice, barley, and oats.

The pericarp is the part of the kernel that covers the seed and contains several layers. The main cellular layers are the epicarp, mesocarp, and endocarp. The endocarp is subdivided into intermediate, cross, and tube cells. The epicarp is the outermost layer of the pericarp and contains elongated rectangle-shaped cells. The mesocarp and endocarp vary on thickness and number of layers depending on the type of cereal. The cross cells, located below the intermediate cells, are elongated and cylindrical-shaped in a transversal position. These cells prevent moisture loss when water is transported in the tube cells; therefore, they act as a seal. The tube cells are approximately the same size as the cross cells but with the elongated axis being parallel and transversal to the kernel. These cells are responsible for transporting and distributing the water that is absorbed by the germ during germination. The pericarp constitutes between 5% and 7% of the kernel weight and is high in fiber, minerals, and phenolic compounds.

The endosperm is the major part of any cereal grain. Basically, it is the second and most abundant reserve tissue and is divided in the testa or seed coat, aleurone, and starchy endosperm. The testa is firmly adhered to the ventral part of the tubular cells and consists of one or two layers. The color of some cereal grains depends in part on the presence of pigments in these cells. For instance, the testa of red winter wheat and sorghum can be highly pigmented, substantially affecting the color and appearance of the grains. Sorghums express significant amounts of condensed tannins when the B (presence of pigmented testa) and the spreader S genes are dominant. These sorghums usually have a brown coloration and are classed as type III. The tannins are bitter or astringent; therefore, these seeds are less susceptible to bird attack and damage, molding, and preharvest germination or sprouting.

The aleurone layer consists of a single cellular layer in maize, sorghum, wheat, rye, and millets whereas they are multilayered in barley, rice, and oats. The composition and structure of the aleurone layer is entirely different from the starchy endosperm. The aleurone cells do not contain starch granules and are high in protein concentrated as aleurone grains, fat (20%) stored in spherosomes, and minerals mainly associated with phytic acid stored in phytic bodies. The aleurone cell walls are high in fiber and show fluorescence when observed under UV light. The aleurone layer synthesizes the necessary enzymes to break down the constituents of the endosperm during germination. In the case of pigmented maize, the aleurone layer can be red or blue, giving one of these colors to the mature kernels. In the case of wheat and rice, the aleurone layer is removed during milling, becoming part of the bran fraction when producing refined flours or white polished rice. The aleurone is a rich source of B vitamins and minerals and its mechanical removal during milling significantly lowers these essential nutrients.

The starchy endosperm is divided into peripheral, vitreous, and floury. Independently of the type of starchy endosperm, the mature cells are constituted of cell walls, starch granules, protein matrix, and protein bodies. The fibrous cell walls are thin and encase the rest of the components. The starch granules represent the main proportion of the endosperm; they are surrounded by a protein matrix which acts as a "glue" to hold together the internal cell structure. The protein bodies are round and very small compared with the starch granules. The protein bodies are dispersed in the cells mainly surrounding the starch granules. The outer peripheral endosperm is high in protein and contains starch units that are small, angular, and compact whereas cells of the vitreous endosperm are comprised of angular starch granules covered by the protein matrix. As a result, these cells do not contain air voids or spaces and show the typical vitreous or translucent appearance because light is not diffracted. On the other hand, the floury endosperm is constituted by larger starch granules that are less angular in shape. Thus, the association between the starch granules and the protein matrix is weaker and the starch is less surrounded by protein bodies. The presence of minuscule air spaces gives the typical floury or opaque-chalky appearance. The floury endosperm is located in the innermost part of the kernel and is always surrounded by the vitreous endosperm. The ratio of floury vs. vitreous endosperm determines the hardness and density of the grain; thus affecting the food processing attributes.

The germ consists of the embryonic axis and the *scutellum*. It is adhered to the endosperm by the *scutellum*, which (together with the epithelium) is the only cotyledon of Gramineae caryopses. The cotyledon acts as nutrient storage and communication link between the plant or developing embryo and the nutrient storage of the endosperm. The embryonic axis results from the differentiation of the embryo and it is formed by the root and the *plumulae*, which will form the roots and the vegetative part of the plant, respectively. The germ does not have starch; in contrast, it is high in oil, protein, soluble sugars, and ash. Among cereals, pearl millet, maize, and sorghum contain the highest proportion of germ (Desai et al. 1997).

1.4.2.1 Determination of Relative Amounts of Husks or Glumes, Pericarp, Endosperm, and Germ Tissues

A. *Samples, Ingredients, and Reagents*
- Different types and classes of kernels
- Distilled water

B. *Materials and Equipment*

- Dissection microscope
- Digital scale
- Tweezers
- Carter dockage tester
- Beaker (2 L)
- Convection drier
- Desiccator
- Tweezers
- Boerner divider
- Knife or scalpel
- Winchester bushel meter
- Automatic seed counter
- Aluminum dishes

C. *Procedure*

1. Obtain a representative sample from the lot of grain, preferably by using the Boerner divider. Clean the sample using the Carter dockage tester.
2. Determine original grain moisture content, test weight, and thousand kernel weight of cleaned grain.
3. Weigh 100 g or a known amount of clean grain.
4. If the sample is from husked caryopses (paddy rice, oats, or barley), manually remove the glumes and weigh the glumes and naked caryopses (brown rice, groats, or naked barley). Determine the number of husks in relation to the original sample weight.
5. Immerse 100 g of naked caryopses for 2 minutes in 200 mL of water. Discard the water and manually separate the pericarp and germ from the endosperm. In the specific case of maize, make sure to remove the tip cap from the germ. Place the different anatomical parts in aluminum dishes for drying at 60°C for at least 1 hour.
6. Remove the aluminum dishes from the oven and let the different anatomical parts equilibrate at room temperature.
7. Record the total weight of each anatomical part and determine the residual moisture of a small subsample. The sample should be dehydrated at 100°C for at least 8 hours. Express all weights on dry matter basis and determine the amount of each anatomical part based on the original dry sample weight = (dry weight of the anatomical part/original dry grain weight) × 100.
8. Reserve each anatomical part partially dehydrated at 60°C for further analyses.

1.4.3 Research Suggestions

1. Compare the cob structure of a regular dent vs. popcorn maizes.
2. Compare the spike structures of wheat, rye, and triticale.
3. Compare spikes of two-rowed vs. six-rowed barley inflorescences.
4. Determine the total weight of kernels associated with a mature spike of wheat, paddy rice panicle, or maize cob.
5. Compare the structure of inflorescences of commercial and wild oats.
6. Compare the structure of spikes of regular and hull-less barleys.
7. Compare the structure of an open and compact panicle of sorghums.
8. Compare the microstructure of a soft textured dent maize against a flint type such as popcorn.
9. Compare the microstructure of white and blue maizes.
10. Compare the microstructure of wheat, rye, and triticale kernels.
11. Compare the microstructure of panicles and kernels belonging to the short and large rice classes.
12. Compare the microstructure of regular, waxy, and high-tannin or brown sorghums.
13. Compare the microstructure of wild and commercial oats.

1.4.4 Research Questions

1. Draw the structure of a wheat spike and the flower.
2. Explain the mechanism of fertilization of the ovum and polar nuclei. From which flower structures do the pericarp and glumes develop?
3. How much does a mature field-dried ear of maize weigh? Determine the relative amounts of kernels, corn cob, and shank/husks.
4. How much does a mature spike of wheat weigh? Determine the relative amounts of kernels and vegetative material.
5. How much does a mature panicle of sorghum weigh? Determine the relative amounts of kernels and vegetative material.
6. How much does a mature spike of barley weigh? Determine the relative amounts of kernels, glumes, and other vegetative material.
7. Compare immature and mature spikes of two-rowed and six-rowed barleys.
8. Compare immature and mature spikes of wheat, rye, and triticale.
9. Draw the structure of a mature pearl millet panicle and then determine the relative amount of kernels based on the total panicle weight.
10. Why are cereal grains considered fruits rather than seeds?
11. How can you differentiate waxy vs. regular endosperm maize?
12. Where are the pigments (anthocyanins) of blue corn located?
13. Compare and draw the aleurone layer of wheat and barley? Which type of cereal contains a multilayered aleurone?

14. Construct a table indicating the weight percentage of each of the main anatomical parts of maize, wheat, rough rice, barley, oats, and sorghum.

15. Draw the anatomical parts of the pericarp of wheat or maize.

16. What is a testa? Where is it located? What is its main functionality?

17. Draw the typical microstructure of the aleurone cell and a starchy endosperm cell.

18. What is the major difference between a starchy endosperm cell from the floury or soft part and the vitreous or hard part?

19. Compare the pericarp anatomy of a regular and thick mesocarp sorghum?

20. Where are the condensed tannins of type III sorghum kernels located?

REFERENCES

American Association of Cereal Chemists (AACC). 2000. *AACC Approved Methods of Analysis*. 10th ed. St. Paul, MN: American Association of Cereal Chemists.

Association of Official Seed Analysts (AOSA). 2000. "Tetrazolium Testing Handbook." *Handbook on Seed Testing*. Lincoln, NE: AOSA.

Carver, B. T. 2009. "Overview of Wheat Classification and Trade." In *Wheat Science and Trade*, 439–454. Ames, IO: Wiley Blackwell.

Champagne, E. T. 2004. *Rice Chemistry and Technology*. 3rd ed. St. Paul, MN: American Association of Cereal Chemists.

Desai, B. B., P. M. Kotecha, and D. K. Salunke. 1997. "Seed Morphology and Development." In *Seeds Handbook. Biology Production, Processing and Storage*. New York: Marcel Dekker.

Gunasekaran, S. 1988. "Evaluation and Comparison of Wisconsin and Stein Breakage Testers on Corn." *Cereal Chemistry* 65(4):287–291.

Hoffman, P. C., D. Ngonyamo-Majee, and R. D. Shaver. 2010. "Determination of Corn Hardness In Diverse Corn Germplasm Using Near-Infrared Reflectance Baseline Shift as a Measure of Grinding Resistance." *Journal of Dairy Science* 93:1685.

Kiser, H. L. 1991. "Grading Grain under the U.S. Grain Standards." In *Israel-Cyprus Grain Grading, Storage and Handling Short Course*. Manhattan, KS: International Grains Program, Kansas State University.

Kohlwey, D. E. 1994. "New Methods for the Evaluation of Rice Quality and Related Technology." In *Rice Science and Technology*, edited by W. E. Marshall and J. I. Wadsworth. New York: Marcel Dekker.

Li, P. X.-P., A. K. Hardare, O. H. Camanella, and K. J. Kirkpatrick. 1996. "Determination of Endosperm Characteristics of 38 Corn Hybrids Using the Stenvert Hardness Test." *Cereal Chemistry* 73(4):466–471.

McGregor, A. W., and R. S. Bhatty. 1993. *Barley: Chemistry and Technology*. St. Paul, MN: American Association of Cereal Chemists.

Miller, B. S., J. W. Hughes, R. Rousser, and G. D. Booth. 1981. "Effects of Modification of a Model CK2 Stein Breakage Tester on Corn Breakage Susceptibility." *Cereal Chemistry* 58(3):201–203.

Miller, B. S., J. W. Hughes, R. Rousser, and Y. Pomeranz. 1979. "Measuring the Breakage Susceptibility of Shelled Corn During Handling." *Cereal Foods World* 26:75–80.

Moore, R. P. 1985. *Handbook on Tetrazolium Testing*. Zurich, Switzerland: International Seed Testing Association.

Oomah, B. D., R. D. Reichert, and C. G. Youngs. 1981. "A Novel, Multi-sample Tangential Abrasive Dehulling Device (TADD)." *Cereal Chemistry* 58(5):391–395.

Paulsen, M. R., S. A. Watson, and M. Singh. 2003. "Measurement and Maintenance of Corn Quality." In *Corn Chemistry and Technology*, edited by P. White and L. Johnson. 2nd ed. St. Paul, MN: American Association of Cereal Chemists.

Pomeranz, Y., Z. Czuchajowska, C. R. Martin, and F. S. Lai. 1985. "Determination of Corn Hardness by the Stenvert Hardness Tester." *Cereal Chemistry* 62:108–112.

Pomeranz, Y., Z. Czuchajowska, and F. S. Lai. 1986a. "Gross Composition of Coarse and Fine Fractions of Small Corn Samples Ground on the Stenvert Hardness Tester." *Cereal Chemistry* 63:22.

Pomeranz, Y., Z. Czuchajowska, and F. S. Lai. 1986b. "Comparison of Methods for Determination of Corn Hardness and Breakage Susceptibility of Commercially Dried Corn." *Cereal Chemistry* 63:39.

Rooney, L. W. 2007. *Corn Quality Assurance Manual*. 2nd ed. Arlington, VA: Snack Food Association.

Rooney, L. W., and F. Miller. 1982. "Variation in the Structure and Kernel Characteristics of Sorghum." In *International Symposium on Sorghum Grain Quality*, edited by L. W. Rooney and D. S. Murty. Patancheru, A. P., India: ICRISAT.

Rooney, L. W. and S. O. Serna-Saldivar. 1991. "Sorghum." In *Handbook of Cereal Science and Technology*, edited by K. Lorenz and K. Kulp. New York: Marcel Dekker.

Rooney, L. W., and E. L. Suhendro. 2001. "Food Quality of Corn." In *Snack Foods Processing*, edited by E. Lusas and L. W. Rooney, 39–71. 1st ed. Lancaster, PA: Technomic Publishing.

Serna-Saldivar, S. O., and L. W. Rooney. 1995. "Structure and Chemistry of Sorghum and Millets." In *Sorghum & Millets: Chemistry and Technology*, edited by D. A. V. Dendy. St. Paul, MN: American Association of Cereal Chemists.

Stenvert, N. L. 1974. Grinding resistance, a simple measure of wheat hardness. *Journal of Flour and Animal Feed Milling* 12:24.

Stephens, L. E., and G. H. Foster. 1976. *Breaker Tester Predicts Handling Damage in Corn*. ARS-NC-49. U.S. Department of Agriculture, Agricultural Research Service.

Thompson, R. A., and G. H. Foster. 1963. *Stress Cracks and Breakage Susceptibility of Artificially Dried Corn*. Marketing Research Report No. 631. Washington, DC: USDA, Agricultural Marketing Service.

U.S. Department of Agriculture (USDA). 1983. *United States Standards for Rice*. Washington, DC: Federal Grain Inspection Service, U.S. Department of Agriculture.

U.S. Department of Agriculture (USDA). 1993. *Official Grain Standards of the United States*. Washington, DC: U.S. Government Printing Office.

U.S. Department of Agriculture, Grain Inspection, Packers and Stockyards Administration (USDA-GIPSA). 1999. *Official United States Standards for Grain*. Washington, DC: USDA-GIPSA.

Waniska, R. D., L. F. Hugo, and L. W. Rooney. 1992. "Practical Methods to Determine the Presence of Tannins in Sorghum." *Journal of Applied Poultry Research* 1:122–128.

Watson, S. A., and F. L. Herum. 1986. "Comparison of Eight Devices for Measuring Breakage Susceptibility of Shelled Corn." *Cereal Chemistry* 63:139–142.

Webb, B. D. 1985. "Criteria of Rice Quality in the United States." In *Rice: Chemistry and Technology*, edited by B. O. Juliano. St. Paul, MN: American Association of Cereal Chemists.

2 Determination of Chemical and Nutritional Properties of Cereal Grains and Their Products

2.1 INTRODUCTION

Research and quality control in cereal science and technology require the determination of the composition and characteristics of grains, other raw materials, and finished products. The chemical composition of cereal grains, milled, and finished products are used to determine nutritive value for labeling purposes, functional characteristics, and acceptability of the wide array of cereal-based products. Numerous methods often are available to assay samples for a specific characteristic or chemical component. Methods are chosen based on specificity, precision, accuracy, and reliability. The most common analytical procedures used in the cereal industry are detailed in the American Association of Cereal Chemists-International (AACC 2000) and in the Association of Official Analytical Chemists (AOAC 2005) official methods of analyses. The AACC provides a check sample service in which a subscribing laboratory performs the specific analyses on the samples. The overall objective is to provide the industry check samples so that their own laboratories can evaluate the reliability of the method and their own analytical infrastructures. The AACC recently changed its paper-laboratory methods to a friendlier Internet program. The advantage of this new program is the continuous updating and reviewing of existing methods.

Cereal grains are composed of macronutrients (carbohydrates, protein, and lipids) and micronutrients (vitamins and minerals). The chemical component present in the highest amount is the starch which is composed of hundreds of glucose units that, after digestion, provide most of the calories consumed by humankind. Beside its nutritional attributes, starch plays a key role in the functional properties and processing of cereals. Starch has contrasting properties if is in its native, gelatinized, or retrograde stages. The second most abundant chemical component is protein which is composed of different fractions distributed in the different anatomical parts of the grain. Those associated with the endosperm are commonly denominated as gluten proteins whereas those associated with the germ are albumins and globulins. Only the wheat gluten possesses viscoelastic properties when the dough is hydrated and kneaded. The types and amounts of macronutrients and micronutrients differ among cereals and affect the nutritional, functional, and organoleptic properties of processed products. The interaction between genotype and environment, especially during grain filling and field maturation, affects the chemical composition of all cereal grains.

The proximate composition of cereals is widely practiced because they help to determine class, processing parameters, and nutritional composition. Starch or nonfibrous carbohydrates and protein are the most abundant components. Ash or minerals, fat, and crude fiber are widely determined especially by the milling industries because they are closely related to degree of milling (refer to Chapter 5) and quality of refined products. The milling processes also affect amino acids, fat, minerals, and vitamin concentration and composition. The amino acid profile is usually determined by ion exchange chromatography or high-pressure liquid chromatography (HPLC) systems equipped with UV-fluorescent detectors. The fatty acid composition is, in most instances, analyzed via gas chromatography (GC) coupled with a flame ionization detector (FID). New capillary columns allow the analysis of fatty acid isomers such as *trans* configurated that need to be declared in food labels in many countries around the globe.

Minerals are usually analyzed by the traditional method of atomic absorption spectroscopy (AAS) or with the newer induced coupled plasma analyzers. Most vitamins are analyzed by HPLC systems or colorimetric assays. Many laboratories still quantify folic acid with the use of a microbiological assay. The analysis of dietary and detergent (neutral and acid) fibers are critically important for foods and feeds, respectively. Raw materials and feeds should be examined for rodent contamination, pathogenic bacteria, molds and mycotoxins, and undesirable toxicants such as polychlorinated biphenyl, insecticides, herbicides, and heavy metals. The proper selection of ingredients will assure the production of high-quality foods and feeds that meet sensory properties for humans and are palatable and can meet sensory properties for domestic animals.

Most regulatory agencies around the world have mandatory nutrition labeling regulations applied for almost all processed foods sold in packages or containers. Nutritional labeling differs in countries around the world. However, in most instances, the labeling information includes the amount of food and the number of servings in a package, its common name, the list of ingredients, the address and information of the processors, and the nutritional information that, in some instances, could include health claims. The aim of the nutritional label is to inform the consumers of the raw materials used to manufacture the food item and the most relevant nutrients affecting human health. It is important to inform consumers of the raw materials because segments of the general population have food allergies; some of the most common being to lactose, gluten, sulfites, and monosodium glutamate. Emphasis is made in the relationship between nutrients and dietary concerns. Consumers are aware of the strong relationship between the abuse of some nutrients and the incidence of chronic diseases and cancer (Nielsen and Metzger 2003).

2.2   PROXIMATE COMPOSITION

Many of the methods in use today for the analysis of foods are procedures based on a system initially introduced approximately 125 years ago by the German scientists Henneberg and Stohmann (James 1999). These analytical procedures are commonly known as the proximate analysis of foods. The various assays involve the estimation of the main food components without the use of sophisticated equipments and chemical reagents. The proximate analysis of foods includes the estimation of moisture, ash or minerals, crude fat, crude protein, crude fiber, and nitrogen-free extract that gives an indication of the soluble carbohydrates and starch. The term crude for fat, protein, and fiber components are a reflection of the fact that the estimation made does not necessarily give a true value of the food fraction. Moisture and ash are determined by gravimetric procedures in which the food sample is dehydrated or incinerated in a muffle furnace to a constant weight. Crude protein is determined by the estimation of the total nitrogen content associated with the food. The procedure involves the acid hydrolysis of the sample followed by nitrogen distillation and titration to determine nitrogen. The nitrogen is converted to protein using a conversion factor that ranges from 5.55 to 6.25. Crude fat is determined by a gravimetric method in which the fat associated with the sample is extracted with petroleum ether. Crude fiber is determined by a gravimetric procedure in which the sample is first hydrolyzed with acid and then with alkali to digest nonfibrous constituents and recover the crude fiber residue. Finally, the nitrogen-free extract fraction is obtained after subtracting all these values from 100. The nitrogen-free extract is an indication of soluble or available carbohydrates. In cereal grains, the nitrogen-free extract is closely related to the starch content.

2.2.1   MOISTURE

The moisture content of cereal grains and their foods is an indication of the keeping qualities of raw grains and their products, and greatly influences the texture of finished products such as breads, cookies, tortilla snacks, and breakfast cereals.

2.2.1.1   Determination of Moisture (Gravimetric Method 44-15 A)

Moisture was determined according to the methods of the AACC (2000).

A. *Samples, Ingredients, and Reagents*
- Different cereals or their products
- Desiccant (activated alumina)

B. *Materials and Equipment*
- Boerner grain divider
- Analytical scale
- Desiccator
- Convection oven
- Laboratory or Udy mill
- Aluminum dishes or moisture capsules
- Laboratory tweezers
- Thermometer (200°C)

C. *Procedure*
1. Obtain a representative grain sample using the Boerner divider.
2. Grind the sample with a laboratory or Udy mill. The ground sample should pass a 20-mesh sieve.
3. Place aluminum or moisture dishes in an oven set at 100°C or 135°C for at least 30 minutes. Using the laboratory tweezers, remove dishes from the oven and immediately place them in a desiccator for cooling (20 minutes; Figure 2.1).
4. Weigh the empty dish and then add approximately 2 g of ground sample. Record both the empty dish weight and the dish plus sample weight with an accuracy of 0.0001 g.
5. With tweezers, place dishes in a convection oven set at 100°C or 135°C for 8 or 2 hours, respectively.
6. Remove dishes from the oven and immediately place them for 30 minutes of cooling in a desiccator.
7. In the same analytical scale, weigh the dishes containing the dried sample.
8. Calculate moisture using the following equation:

$$\% \text{ moisture} = [(\text{original sample weight} - \text{dried sample weight})/(\text{original sample weight})] \times 100.$$

2.2.2   MINERALS OR ASH

Ash is determined by a gravimetric method that weighs inorganic residues after incineration of a given sample at 600°C.

2.2.2.1   Analysis of Ash or Minerals (Method 08-12)

Ash and mineral analysis was determined according to the methods of the AACC (2000).

A. *Samples, Ingredients, and Reagents*
- Different cereals or their products
- Desiccant (activated alumina)

B. *Materials and Equipment*
- Analytical scale
- Muffle furnace
- Long crucible tongs
- Desiccator with a vacuum release valve
- Crucibles
- Protective gloves

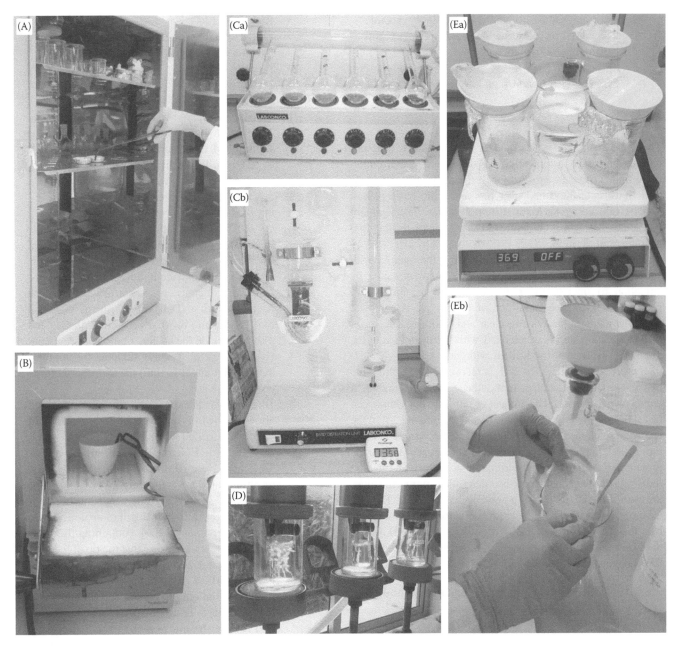

FIGURE 2.1 Proximate analyses of foods. (A) Moisture; (B) ash; (Ca) digestion of crude protein; (Cb) nitrogen distillation of crude protein; (D) crude fat; (Ea) digestion of crude fiber; (Eb) filtration and recovery of crude fiber residue.

C. *Procedure*

1. Turn on the muffle furnace and allow it to reach 600°C.

2. With protective gloves and tweezers, place cleaned crucibles in the muffle furnace for 1 hour. Then, remove crucibles for cooling (30 minutes) in an airtight desiccator. Make sure to leave a small gap on top of the desiccator or use a desiccator with a vacuum release valve, otherwise the high temperature will cause a hermetic seal.

3. Weigh using the analytical scale crucibles and approximately 2 g of ground sample with an accuracy of 0.0001 g.

4. Place crucibles with samples in the muffle furnace set at 600°C for at least 2 hours or until a constant weight is reached (the ash should be free of black coloration which indicates the presence of carbonized organic matter).

5. With protective gloves and long tongs, remove crucibles with ash for cooling (30 minutes) in a desiccator.

6. Weigh crucibles with ash in the analytical balance.

7. Calculate the amount of ash by subtracting the empty crucible weight from the crucible plus ash weight. Express ash content based on the

original sample weight (subtract empty crucible weight from the crucible plus sample weight) using the following equation:

$$\% \text{ ash} = (\text{ash weight/sample weight}) \times 100.$$

2.2.3 PROTEIN

The Kjeldahl method is a method for the quantitative determination of nitrogen in foods that was developed by J. Kjeldahl more than 120 years ago. Although the technique and apparatus have been modified over the years, the basic principles introduced by Kjeldahl still apply today. The Kjeldahl method consists of three sequential steps: acid digestion, distillation, and titration.

The method consists of first digesting the sample with sulfuric acid, which decomposes the organic substance by oxidation to liberate the reduced nitrogen as ammonium sulfate. Chemical decomposition of the sample is complete when the medium has become clear and colorless. The speed of the digestion step is accelerated with the use of catalysts. Then, the hydrolysate is distilled with excess alkali (NaOH) to convert NH_4 to NH_3. The NH_3 is recovered by distilling the reaction product. Titration quantifies the amount of ammonia in the receiving solution. The amount of nitrogen in a sample can be calculated from the quantified amount of ammonia ion in the receiving solution with a color change. The most common is the titration of ammonia with a standard HCl solution (0.1 N) in the presence of a mixed indicator (bromocresol green and methyl red). Because the Kjeldhal method determines nitrogen, values are transformed to protein by a given correction factor. The factor most widely used is 6.25, which is obtained by dividing 100 over the 16% of nitrogen that most proteins contain. However, the factor preferred for wheat is 5.7, indicating that wheat proteins contain an average of 17.5% nitrogen.

2.2.3.1 Crude Protein Analysis (Kjeldahl Method)

A. *Samples, Ingredients, and Reagents*
- Different cereals or their products
- Ethanol
- Sulfuric acid
- Potassium sulfate
- Salicylic acid
- Methyl red indicator
- Distilled water
- Sodium hydroxide
- Boric acid
- Cupric sulfate
- Zinc granules
- Standardized NaOH (0.02–0.1 N) solution

B. *Materials and Equipment*
- Analytical scale
- Digestion unit for Kjeldahl flasks
- Manual or automatic burette
- Graduated cylinder (100 mL)
- Filter paper
- Protective glasses
- Kjeldahl flasks
- Distillation unit for Kjeldahl hydrolysates
- Erlenmeyer flasks (200 mL)
- Agitator
- Protective gloves

C. *Procedure*
1. Prepare the methyl red indicator by dissolving 1 g of methyl red in 200 mL of ethanol and the sodium hydroxide solution by dissolving 450 g of NaOH in 1 L of distilled water.
2. Using a filter paper, weigh the following:
   a. 1.90–2.00 g of potassium sulfate
   b. 0.04–0.05 g cupric sulfate
   c. 0.095–0.105 g sample.
   Register sample weight with an accuracy of 0.0001 g. Wrap the filter paper with the reagents and sample, and place it in a Kjeldahl flask.
3. Add 2 mL of concentrated sulfuric acid to each Kjeldahl flask and place them in the digestion unit. Make sure to wear protective glasses and gloves. Turn on the heaters of the digestion unit.
4. Hydrolyze or acid-digest samples for approximately 45 minutes or until the hydrolysate turns green–turquoise.
5. Turn off the heater of the digestion unit and allow the hydrolysate to cool down. Then add 10 mL of distilled water.
6. In a 100 mL Erlenmeyer flask, mix 5 mL of boric acid with 20 mL of distilled water. The resulting solution should be gray.
7. Connect flask to a digestion bulb on the condenser of the nitrogen distillation unit. Then, place the Erlenmeyer flask containing the boric acid solution making sure that the tip of the condenser is immersed in the acid solution.
8. Place 10 mL of the sodium hydroxide solution in the distillation unit container. Gradually add the solution to the Kjeldahl flask. This reaction will release the nitrogen from the hydrolysate. The nitrogen released will be trapped by the boric acid solution which will turn green.
9. Titrate the green solution with the normalized HCl solution until the color disappears. Then, carefully add more drops until the color first turns light-red salmon. Register the amount and strength of the normalized solution needed to titrate the sample.
10. Calculate the percentage of nitrogen and protein using the following equations:

$$\% \text{ nitrogen} = [(\text{mL HCl}) \, (\text{N HCl}) \, (14.007) \, (100)]/ (\text{mg sample weight})$$

$$\% \text{ crude protein*} = (\% \text{ nitrogen}) \, (\text{correction factor}).$$

---

* The most used correction factor is 5.7 for wheat, and 6.25 for the rest of the cereals.

2.2.4 FAT

This fraction is also called crude fat because ether dissolves lipids and lipid-like compounds. The analysis is conducted by continually washing a sample in ether. This is accomplished by placing the sample in an apparatus in which ether can flow through and collect in a lower spot. The ether is continually evaporated from this location and condensed above the sample so it can flow back over the sample. The sample is then placed in a drying oven to drive off the excess ether and weighed. The difference between the initial weight and the end weight is an estimate of crude fat. The reason the term crude fat is used is that triglycerides and free fatty acids (FFA; i.e., the fat compounds we are most interested in measuring with ether extract) are not the only chemicals dissolved by ether, and therefore, other lipophilic compounds are included in the extract. This is not a large problem when extracting animal foods; however, plants contain a variety of ether-soluble compounds such as pigments, waxes, volatile oils, resins, and sterols.

2.2.4.1 Analysis of Crude Fat

Crude fat is an indication of the lipid fraction associated with the food. Therefore, it determines the triglycerides, phospholipids, waxes, sphingolipid steroids, terpenes, and fat-soluble vitamins. The procedure involves extracting the lipids with petroleum ether or diethyl ether, followed by removal of the solvent and weighing the fatty residue. The degree of fat extraction is mainly dependent on the polarity of the solvent and the amount of fat associated with the food matrix.

A. *Samples, Ingredients, and Reagents*
- Different types of cereals or products
- Desiccant (activated alumina)
- Petroleum ether or diethyl ether

B. *Materials and Equipment*
- Analytical scale
- Whatman paper
- Goldfisch flasks
- Absorbent cotton or glass wool
- Extraction thimbles
- Airtight desiccator
- Tweezers
- Goldfisch extraction apparatus
- Thimbles
- Soxhlet extractor
- Convection oven

C. *Procedure*
1. With tweezers, place cleaned extraction thimbles and Goldfisch flasks in the convection oven set at 100°C for 30 minutes. Then, remove thimbles and flasks for cooling (30 minutes) in a desiccator.
2. With tweezers, weigh in the analytical scale empty flasks with an accuracy of 0.0001 g.
3. With tweezers, first weigh the empty thimbles and then add 2 g to 3 g of sample that has been previously dried. Record empty thimble and sample weights with an accuracy of 0.0001 g. For Goldfisch extraction, place a small amount of cotton or glass wool on top of the thimble.
4. For Goldfisch extraction:
   a. Place thimble with the unextracted sample in the Goldfisch extraction apparatus.
   b. Place 25 mL of ethyl ether in the Goldfisch flask.
   c. Place flask on the heater and immediately seal the system. Make sure to open the water so the solvent gases recondense and extract the fat from the sample.
   d. Turn on heater and adjust heat to obtain five to six drops of recondensed solvent per second. Allow sample to extract for at least 4 hours.
   e. Lower the heating plate temperature and allow residual solvent to evaporate at low temperature from the flask which contains the fat.
   f. With tweezers, place flask in an oven set at 100°C for 30 minutes for drying.
   g. Remove the flask from the oven and place it in a desiccator for 30 minutes for cooling.
   h. Weigh the flask with fat in the analytical balance.
   i. Calculate the fat weight by subtracting the empty flask weight from the flask and fat weight.
   j. Calculate percentage of fat or ether extract as follows:

% crude fat = (fat weight/sample weight) × 100.

5. For Soxhlet extraction:
   a. Place thimble(s) with sample(s) in the Soxhlet extraction apparatus.
   b. Place 25 mL of ethyl ether or petroleum ether in the Soxhlet flask.
   c. Place flask on the heater and immediately seal the system. Make sure to open the water so the solvent gases recondense and extract the fat from the sample.
   d. Turn on heater to evaporate solvent and open the condenser water valve to recondensate the solvent gases. Allow samples to extract for at least 4 hours.
   e. After extraction, remove the solvent flask and thimbles from the apparatus.
   f. Allow thimbles to rest for 30 minutes at room temperature.
   g. Place thimbles with tweezers in a convection oven set at 100°C for 8 hours for drying.

h. Remove thimbles from the oven and place them in a desiccator for 30 minutes for cooling.

i. Weigh thimbles with the fat-free sample in the analytical balance.

j. Calculate the fat weight by subtracting the sample weight from the fat-free sample weight.

k. Calculate the percentage of fat or ether extract as follows:

% crude fat = (fat weight/sample weight) × 100.

2.2.5 Crude Fiber

Crude fiber is still determined by an old laboratory analysis procedure and is mainly composed of lignin and cellulose. The analysis of crude fiber involves the treatment of the ground food sample to sequential acid (sulfuric acid) and alkaline (sodium hydroxide solution) hydrolyses followed by oven-drying. The residue is defined as crude fiber. The amount of crude fiber is, in most instances, lower compared with detergent and dietary fiber values.

2.2.5.1 Analysis of Crude Fiber

A. *Samples, Ingredients, and Reagents*
- Different types of cereals or their processed products
- 1.25% Sulfuric acid solution
- 95% Ethanol
- Desiccant (activated alumina)
- 1.25% Sodium hydroxide solution
- Antifoam solution

B. *Materials and Equipment*
- Analytical scale
- Digestion beakers (600 mL)
- Vacuum convection oven
- Crucibles
- Crude fiber digestion apparatus with condenser
- Buchner funnel for filtration through a 200 mesh screen
- Muffle furnace
- Airtight desiccator

C. *Procedure*
1. Weigh 2 g of ground sample that was previously dried and ether extracted (fat free). If fat content is less than 1%, ether extraction may be omitted. Record sample weight with an accuracy of 0.0001 g.
2. Transfer the sample to a cleaned digestion beaker.
3. Add 200 mL of 1.25% sulfuric acid and one drop of antifoam solution.
4. Place beaker on digestion apparatus and turn on the hot plate of the digestion apparatus to obtain gentle boiling. Digest sample for 30 minutes. During digestion, make sure to rotate beaker periodically to keep solids from adhering to the sides.
5. Vacuum-filter the acid hydrolysate through the Buchner filter device. Without breaking suction, add 50 mL to 75 mL of boiling water at least three times.
6. Return the solids from the filter to the beaker for alkaline hydrolysis. Add 200 mL of 1.25 NaOH solution and place beaker on the digestion apparatus and turn on the hot plate to obtain gentle boiling. Digest sample for an additional 30 minutes. During digestion, make sure to rotate the beaker periodically to keep the solids from adhering to the sides.
7. Vacuum-filter the alkaline hydrolysate through the Buchner filter device. Without breaking suction, first add 25 mL of boiling 1.25% H_2SO_4, three additional washes with 50 mL of boiling water, and a wash with 25 mL of alcohol.
8. Remove solids from the filter and place it in a tared crucible for drying and ashing.
9. Place tared crucible with residue in an oven set at 100°C for 8 hours or until a constant weight could be achieved.
10. Remove the crucible from the oven and place it in a desiccator for 30 minutes for cooling.
11. Weigh crucible with fiber residue in the analytical balance. Calculate the residue weight by subtracting the empty crucible weight from the crucible and sample weight.
12. Place the crucible with the dried residue in a muffle furnace set at 600°C for 4 hours for ashing.
13. Remove the crucible from the muffle furnace and place it in a desiccator for 30 minutes for cooling.
14. Weigh the crucible with the ash residue in the analytical balance. Calculate the ash weight by subtracting the empty crucible weight from the crucible and ash weight.
15. Calculate the percentage of crude fiber as follows:

% crude fiber = [(dried residue weight − ash weight)/ sample weight] × 100.

Make sure to correct values if fat was previously removed from the sample.

2.2.6 Nitrogen-Free Extract

The proximate analysis detailed in the previous sections determines a variety of food constituents; however, it does not measure the most abundant chemical constituents of cereal grains and their products (starch). The nitrogen-free extract (NFE) is estimated by adding up ash, crude fiber, crude protein, and ether extract, and subtracting from 100. This value is calculated after performing all the proximate analyses described above and is only a crude indication of starch and soluble sugars including soluble fiber components that were not estimated in the crude fiber analysis. Any mistake in the various proximate analyses ends up affecting the NFE fraction.

2.2.6.1 Calculation of Nitrogen-Free Extract

A. *Procedure*

1. Determine the moisture content, crude protein, crude fat, ash, and crude fiber following the procedures described previously. Make sure to express values either on a dry matter basis or at a given moisture content.
2. The nitrogen-free extract or NFE, expressed on a dry matter basis, is calculated using the following equation: NFE = 100 − (crude protein + crude fat + ash + crude fiber). Make sure all values are expressed on a dry matter basis.
3. Convert the NFE expressed on a dry matter basis to a fixed moisture-based value using the following equation: NFE (dry matter basis) × (100 − % moisture content).

2.2.7 RESEARCH SUGGESTIONS

1. Determine the proximate composition of soft and hard whole wheats and their respective flours. What can you conclude about the proximate composition of these products?
2. Determine the proximate composition of a rough, brown, and white polished rice. What can you conclude about the proximate composition of these products?
3. Determine and compare the nitrogen-free extract and starch content of a given sample of wheat flour. What can you conclude about the values?
4. Determine the crude fiber, detergent fiber, and dietary fiber of a sample of whole wheat. In your opinion, which assay underestimates fiber? Why?

2.2.8 RESEARCH QUESTIONS

1. What are the principles behind the determination of the following components of proximate analyses?
   a. Ash
   b. Ether extract or fat
   c. Crude fiber
2. Which of the components of the proximate analysis are usually required on a nutrition label?
3. What are the main constituents of crude fiber? Why does crude fiber underestimate the amount of dietary fiber?
4. What are the conversion factors of nitrogen to protein and the average nitrogen content of the following cereals:
   a. Wheat
   b. Maize
   c. Rice

5. Determine the amount of NFE as is and expressed on dry matter basis in a corn snack which contains 2% moisture, 1.2% crude fiber, 2.3% ash, 5.6% crude protein, and 24% crude fat or ether extract. What is the major component of the NFE?

2.3 METHODS FOR MOISTURE ANALYSIS

Moisture is one of the most frequently applied tests to cereal grains and their products. It is widely determined in grain elevators because it is closely related to keeping properties or resistance to deterioration of cereal grains throughout storage. It is also frequently tested in milling operations because most cereals are tempered before milling. Furthermore, moisture content plays an important role in baking, breakfast cereal, and snack food operations because it affects the rheological properties of intermediate products and textural properties of finished products. Determination of moisture is also necessary to calculate the dry matter of a given cereal, food, or ingredient. The moisture content of cereals and their products can be determined by a variety of methods, each having their advantages and disadvantages. Table 2.1 summarizes the methods commonly used to determine moisture content of cereals and their products.

2.3.1 RESEARCH SUGGESTIONS

1. Determine the moisture content of table bread or flour tortillas using the official gravimetric technique, microwave oven, thermogravimetric balance, and NIRA. Compare values with the official gravimetric technique.
2. Investigate the best method to determine moisture in a high-fructose corn syrup which contains approximately 68% solids.
3. Dehydrate and temper a given grain to obtain a series of samples with contrasting moisture contents (i.e., 1%, 3%, 5%, 8%, 10%, 12%, 14%, 16%, 18%, 20%, 22%, 24%, and 26% moisture). After overnight equilibration, determine the A_w of each sample and graph moisture vs. A_w.

2.3.2 RESEARCH QUESTIONS

1. What are the principles behind the following moisture assays?
   a. Microwave
   b. Near-infrared
   c. Electric conductivity
2. What are the advantages and disadvantages of the Karl Fischer moisture determination?
3. What are three factors that you would consider when choosing a moisture analysis for a specific cereal-based food product?
4. What are the potential advantages of using a vacuum oven rather than an air-forced oven?

TABLE 2.1
Principles and Advantages and Disadvantages of the Most Commonly Used Analytical Methods for Moisture or Solid Analyses

Method	Principle	Advantages and Disadvantages
Air-forced oven (AACC 2000, Method 44-15 A)	The moisture content of the product is evaporated until a constant weight is achieved. The moisture is gravimetrically determined by difference.	Official method. It is accurate but it usually takes several hours.
Vacuum oven	The moisture content of the product is evaporated in a vacuum oven until a constant weight is achieved. The moisture is gravimetrically determined by difference.	Official method, it is accurate but takes several hours. The main advantage is that samples are dehydrated at a relatively lower temperature (60°C).
Karl Fischer	The moisture associated with a given food is titrated with the Karl Fischer reagent (iodine and sulfur dioxide). The volume of the reagent required to reach the endpoint of the titration (visual, conductometric, or coulometric) is directly related to the amount of moisture (Bradley 2003; Nielsen 2003).	Use of potentially hazardous reagents such as the Karl Fischer reagent and methanol. Need to conduct test under a hood with the use of appropriate eye and skin protection.
Microwave drying	The moisture content of the product is evaporated in a microwave oven. The moisture is gravimetrically determined by difference.	Sample weight and preparation are important to decrease experimental error. It is considered as a fast method (approximately 10 minutes).
Moisture balances (thermogravimetric tester)	The ground sample is placed on a digital scale under controlled high-heat conditions. The moisture content of the ground product is rapidly evaporated with an infrared radiator for a fixed period (constant weight). The moisture is gravimetrically determined by difference.	Sample weight and preparation and dehydration time are important to decrease experimental error. It is easy to overheat or burn the sample. It is considered as a fast method (approximately 10 minutes).
Electric conductivity testers	Predicts moisture content according to electric conductivity after a few seconds (AACC 2000, Method 44-10).	These moisture meters are developed to test whole grains and therefore are widely used by producers, elevators, and government agencies and has a proven history of both durability and reliability. Current testers are provided with digital scales and a thermometer to adjust moisture values. The moisture values are automatically obtained or manually calculated by imputing values in a chart for each specific cereal grain.
NIRA	The moisture content of the product is determined by scanning in the infrared spectra. Specific frequencies are absorbed by the functional groups characteristic of water. The water concentration is determined by measuring the energy that is reflected or transmitted by the sample (Nielsen 2003).	The moisture can be determined in whole or ground grain samples in a matter of seconds. Samples are not destroyed. The instrument should be calibrated for each type of product. Sample preparation and standardization play an important role in accuracy.

5. Describe the way you would put into operation a new method for moisture analysis using the near-infrared apparatus. What are the most important considerations to decrease the experimental error and obtain accurate results?

2.4 METHODS FOR MINERAL ANALYSIS

The mineral composition of foods is, in most instances, determined in wet or dry ash samples that are diluted with acid in preparation for analysis in either the AAS or inductively coupled plasma (ICP; Figure 2.2). These instruments are very accurate and widely used to analyze almost all minerals that can act as nutrients or toxicants. Atomic absorption has played a major role in mineral analysis since the 1960s whereas ICP has enhanced the ability to measure the overall mineral composition of foods rapidly and accurately. These two instruments have largely replaced traditional wet-chemistry methods for mineral analysis of foods, although traditional wet-chemistry methods for sodium, calcium, and phosphorus remain in wide use today. In theory, all the mineral elements may be determined by AAS or ICP (Miller and Rutzke 2003).

2.4.1 WET AND DRY ASHING

Wet ashing or oxidation is primarily used to prepare samples for mineral analyses. The advantage of the wet ashing procedure is that minerals usually stay in the acid solution, free of organic compounds. The disadvantage is that it requires corrosive acid reagents and the digestion should be performed in a special hood that traps fumes with a water curtain. Nitric, sulfuric, or percholoric acids are used in varying

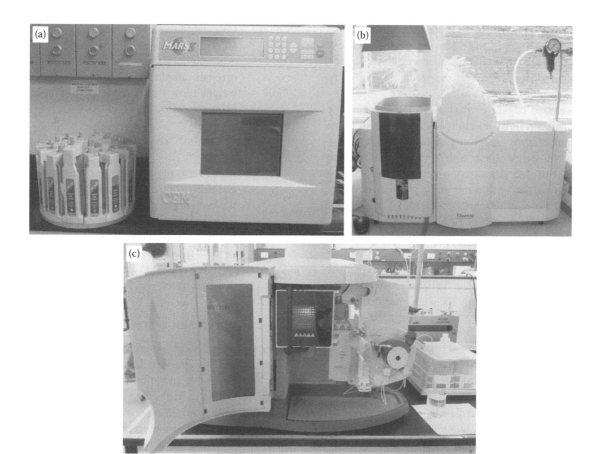

FIGURE 2.2 Atomic absorption and ICP instruments widely used for the analysis of minerals. (a) Microwave oven for rapid wet-ashing hydrolysis; (b) AAS apparatus; (c) ICP apparatus.

combinations. The nitric-perchloric combination is the most commonly used because it is the fastest. Unfortunately, perchloric acid has a tendency to explode so digestion should be performed in acid hoods equipped with wash-down capabilities.

Dry-ashing refers to the procedure in which water and organic substances associated with food are incinerated in the presence of air; therefore, obtaining the ash or minerals. The material is burned in a muffle furnace at temperatures around 600°C (refer to procedure in Section 2.2.2). During dry-ashing, most minerals are converted to oxides, sulfates, phosphates chlorides, and silicates. The main advantage of this method is that it is relatively safer compared with wet ashing. However, the main limitation of dry ashing is the loss of volatile elements such as arsenic, chromium, copper, lead, nickel, phosphorus, and zinc.

2.4.1.1 Wet-Ashing Procedure

A. *Samples, Ingredients, and Reagents*
- Different types of cereal or cereal based foods
- 60% Perchloric acid
- Distilled deionized water
- Nitric acid
- 50% Hydrochloric acid

B. *Materials and Equipment*
- Acid hood with wash-down capabilities
- Hot plate or digestion unit
- Safety glasses
- Pipettes (5 mL and 10 mL)
- Volumetric flasks (50 mL)
- Analytical scale
- Long tongs
- Beakers or micro-Kjeldhal flasks
- Watch glasses
- Glass funnel

C. *Procedure*
1. Weigh 1 g of ground sample that was previously dried. Record sample weight with an accuracy of 0.0001 g.
2. Transfer the sample to a cleaned digestion beaker or a micro-Kjeldhal flask. Make sure to acid-wash beakers or flasks before use.
3. Add 10 mL of concentrated nitric acid and 3 mL of 60% perchloric acid to each beaker or flask.
4. Turn on hot plate or Kjeldhal digestion unit and slowly heat the sample until frothing stops and the nitric acid is almost evaporated. Continue boiling until perchloric acid generates copious

fumes. If beakers are used, then place a glass watch on top of the container. Continue digestion until the solution becomes the color of light straw. Do not let the solution completely evaporate.

5. Remove beaker or flask from the hot plate or digestion unit and allow to cool down to room temperature under the hood. Upon cooling, wash watch glass with a minimum amount of distilled deionized water, making sure to recover the wash water in the respective beaker and then add 10% mL of 50% HCl. For Kjeldhal flasks, add 10 mL of 50% HCl.

6. Carefully transfer contents to 50-mL volumetric flasks using a glass funnel. Add more distilled deionized water to the beaker or flask to recover the leftovers. Transfer the wash waters to the volumetric flask and then add more distilled water to the volume mark.

2.4.1.2 Dry-Ashing Procedure

A. Samples, Ingredients, and Reagents
- 50% Hydrochloric acid
- Desiccant (activated alumina)
- Distilled deionized water

B. Materials and Equipment
- Analytical scale
- Airtight desiccator with a vacuum release valve
- Laboratory tongs
- Pipettes (5 mL and 10 mL)
- Glass funnels
- Muffle furnace
- Crucibles
- Protective glove
- Volumetric flasks (50 mL)

C. Procedure
1. Turn on the muffle furnace and allow it to reach 550°C to 600°C.
2. With protective gloves and tongs, place cleaned crucibles in the muffle furnace for 1 hour. Then, remove crucibles for cooling (30 minutes) in a desiccator. Make sure to leave a small gap on top of the desiccator or use a desiccator with a vacuum release valve; otherwise, the high temperature will cause a hermetic seal.
3. Weigh the analytical scale crucibles and 5 g to 10 g of sample.
4. Place crucibles with samples in a cool muffle furnace. Then, turn on the furnace and ignite samples for 12 to 18 hours at approximately 550°C to 600°C.
5. Turn off furnace and allow the interior temperature to drop to approximately 250°C. With protective gloves and tweezers, remove crucibles with ash for cooling (30 minutes) in a desiccator.
6. Weigh crucibles with ash in the analytical balance.

7. Calculate the amount of ash by subtracting the empty crucible weight from the crucible plus ash weight. Express ash content based on the original sample weight (subtract empty crucible weight from the crucible plus sample weight) using the following equation:

$$\% \text{ ash} = (\text{ash weight/sample weight}) \times 100.$$

8. Add 10 mL of 50% HCl to crucible.
9. Carefully transfer contents to 50 mL volumetric flasks using a glass funnel. Add 5 mL of distilled deionized water to the crucible to recover leftovers. Repeat the washing operation at least twice. Transfer the wash waters to the volumetric flask and then bring to volume with more distilled water.

2.4.2 Atomic Absorption Spectroscopy

AAS is an analytical technique that has been traditionally used for mineral analysis. It is based on the absorption of UV light or visible radiation by free atoms in the gaseous state. According to Miller and Rutzke (2003), this analytical tool is relatively simple to perform. The instrument is widely being replaced by the more versatile ICP spectroscopy. The instrument consists of a beam source produced by a lamp that passes through a flame produced by a nebulizer–burner system, a UV-vis monochromator, a detector, and a computer system that reads out the signals. The wet or dry ash sample is nebulized, mixed with fuel and an oxidant, and burnt into an atomic vapor. Once the sample is atomized in the air-acetylene or nitrous oxide-acetylene flame, its quantity is measured by determining the attenuation of the beam passing through the flame. For the measurement of a specific mineral, the radiation source is selected so that the emitted radiation contains an emission line that corresponds to one of the most intensive lines in the atomic spectrum of the element being measured. This is accomplished by selecting specific hallow lamps in which the mineral to be determined serves as a cathode. Therefore, the radiation emitted from the lamp is the emission spectrum of the element (Miller and Rutzke 2003; Haswell 1991).

2.4.2.1 Analysis of Minerals with AAS

A. Samples, Ingredients, and Reagents
- Dry or wet ash samples (refer to procedures in Sections 2.4.1.1 or 2.4.1.2)
- Distilled deionized water
- Mineral standards (1000 mg/L) or commercially available standard solutions
- HCl concentrate
- Lanthanum chloride

B. Materials and Equipment
- AAS apparatus
- Acetylene cylinder
- Test tubes

- Pipettes (5 mL and 10 mL)
- Air gas tank
- Diluter or automatic dispensing system
- Test tube shaker
- Volumetric flasks (50 mL)

C. Procedure

1. Preparation of reagents
   a. For calcium analysis, prepare a lanthanum chloride solution by dissolving 29 g in 250 mL concentrated HCl (caution: reaction is violent) and dilute to 500 mL with distilled deionized water.
2. Obtain the wet- or dry-ashed stock solution (refer to procedures in Sections 2.4.1.1 or 2.4.1.2).
3. Dilute the test sample with distilled deionized water using preferably the automatic diluter. Then with the test tube shaker agitate contents. Make sure to use test tubes that were previously acid washed. Prepare the mineral standard by making at least six dilutions which produce an absorbance of 0.0 to 0.7. Calibration standards can be prepared by diluting the stock metal solutions in the same acids and acid concentrations as the samples (refer to procedures in Sections 2.4.1.1 or 2.4.1.2). Label each test tube with the dilution rate. Note: the dilution factor will depend on the mineral to analyze and the concentration of the minerals used to construct the standard curve. For the specific case of calcium analysis, the test solution should contain lanthanum chloride that avoids interference produced by oxyanions.
4. Install the recommended hollow cathode lamp for the specific mineral. In general, after choosing the proper hollow cathode lamp for the analysis, the lamp should be allowed to warm up for a minimum of 15 minutes. During this period, align the instrument, position the monochromator at the correct wavelength, select the proper monochromator slit width, and adjust the hollow cathode current according to the manufacturer's recommendation. Subsequently, light the acetylene-air flame and regulate the flow of fuel and oxidant; adjust the burner and nebulizer flow rate for maximum percentage of absorption and stability, and balance the photometer. The air and acetylene output gas pressures should be 50 to 65 psi and 12 to 14 psi, respectively.
5. Run a series of standards of the element under analysis and construct a calibration curve by plotting the concentrations of the standards against the absorbance. The curve should have an $r^2 > .99$. Then, calculate the slope of the calibration curve. For those instruments which read directly in concentration, set the curve corrector to read out the proper concentration. Aspirate the samples and determine the concentrations either directly or from the calibration curve.

Standards must be run each time a sample or series of samples are run.

6. Read the mineral concentration value from the calibration curve or directly from the readout system of the instrument. Then, adjust values first according to the dilution factor and then according to the original sample weight.

2.4.3 ICP Spectroscopy

The ICP spectrometry is a relatively new analytical technique used for the analysis of major and trace minerals. It is a type of emission spectroscopy that uses the ICP to produce excited atoms and ions that emit electromagnetic radiation at wavelengths characteristic of a particular element. The intensity of this emission is indicative of the concentration of the element within the sample. The ICP is based in the production of a plasma or a gaseous mixture containing cations and electrons produced by an argon torch which generates temperatures of 5000 K to 10,000 K resulting in a very effective atomization. The ICP-AES is composed of three fundamental parts: the ICP, the optical spectrometer, and a computer for data collection and treatment. The heart of the ICP is the plasma torch consisting of two or three quartz glass tubes centered in a copper coil. Argon gas is typically used to create the plasma. Wet or dry-ash diluted solutions are almost always introduced as aerosols carried by a stream of argon in the injector tube. The temperature in the zone of the load coil ranges from 1000 to 3000 K. The plasma is heated to a temperature ranging from 1000 K to 5000 K to excite the atoms and produce an emission light that is read by a spectrometer. All minerals can be quantified in the same run because the equipment is equipped with monochromators or polychromators capable of scanning over a wavelength range. When the torch is turned on, an intense electromagnetic field is created within the coil by the high-power radio frequency signal flowing in the coil. This radio frequency signal is created by the radio frequency generator which is, effectively, a high-power radio transmitter driving the "work coil" the same way a typical radio transmitter drives a transmitting antenna. The argon gas flowing through the torch is ignited with a Tesla unit that creates a brief discharge arc through the argon flow to initiate the ionization process. Once the plasma is "ignited," the Tesla unit is turned off. The argon gas is ionized in the intense electromagnetic field and flows in a particular rotationally symmetrical pattern toward the magnetic field of the radio frequency coil. A stable, high-temperature plasma of approximately 7000 K is then generated as a result of the inelastic collisions created between the neutral argon atoms and the charged particles.

2.4.3.1 Analysis of Minerals with ICP Spectroscopy

A. Samples, Ingredients, and Reagents

- Dry or wet ash samples (refer to procedures in Sections 2.4.1.1 or 2.4.1.2)
- Distilled deionized water
- Mineral standards (1000 mg/L) or commercially available standard solutions

B. *Materials and Equipment*
- ICP analyzer
- Diluter or automatic dispensing system
- Test tube shaker or vortex
- Volumetric flasks (50 mL)
- Argon gas tank (high purity grade)
- Test tubes
- Pipettes (5 mL and 10 mL)

C. *Procedure*
1. Obtain the wet or dry ash stock solution (refer to procedures in Sections 2.4.1.1 or 2.4.1.2).
2. Dilute the test sample with distilled deionized water preferably using the automatic diluter. Then, with the test tube shaker, agitate the contents. Make sure to use test tubes that were previously acid-washed. Prepare at least five different dilutions of the mineral standard.
3. Turn on at least 45 minutes before the test and set up operating conditions of the ICP and initiate configuration of instrument computer. Make sure to set up the peristaltic pump tubing on the pump.
4. When the instrument is operating at steady state, nebulize calibration standards to obtain a reliable calibration curve covering the appropriate calibration range. The sample is nebulized and the resulting aerosol transported by argon gas into the plasma torch. The ions produced by high temperatures are entrained in the plasma gas and extracted through a differentially pumped vacuum interface and separated on the basis of their mass-to-charge ratio by a mass spectrometer.
5. Nebulize the test samples and determine concentrations of the different minerals by a channel electron multiplier or Faraday detector and the instrument's data-handling system.
6. First, adjust values according to the dilution factor and then according to the original sample weight.

2.4.4 Phosphorus Analysis

Phosphorus is the mineral found in highest concentrations in all cereal grains. Most of this essential mineral is bound to phytic acid and its salts. Phytic acid has several relevant physiological functions such as antioxidant protection during dormancy, storage of phosphorus and cations, and precursor of cell walls. In addition, phytic acid plays an important and critical role during germination. Approximately 80% of the total phosphorus is bound to phytates in maize, rice, and wheat. Most phytic acid is found in the aleurone cells, although in the special case of maize, 80% of the phytic acid is located in the germ. The phosphorus bound to phytate has a low bioavailability (40–80%) and binds other minerals, such as calcium, magnesium, zinc, copper, and iron, lowering their availability. The availability of phosphorus and other minerals improves after germination or mating and fermentation due to the production of phytases.

Most phosphorus is analyzed by the molybdate tests. The original acid molybdate method was developed by Osmond in 1887 and became more widely used after the modifications suggested by Murphy and Riley (1962). The principle of this test is that phosphate reacts with ammonium molybdate to form the compound $(NH_4)_3PO_4 \cdot 12MoO_4$ which, after it is reduced with aminonaptholsulfonic acid, forms a blue-colored complex that is measured in a spectrophotometer. Free (unbound) molybdates will not reduce under these conditions so only the molybdate that is bound with phosphate will form the blue compound. This blue color has a maximum absorption of light at a wavelength of 690 nm or 710 nm. The other test is known as vanadate–molybdate. In this similar assay, the vanadate–molybdate yields an orange complex that is measured in the colorimeter at 420 nm (James 1995).

2.4.4.1 Analysis of Phosphorus with the Blue Molybdate Colorimetric Analysis

Phosphorus has been traditionally analyzed with the blue molybdate colorimetric assay, in which the phosphorus present as orthophosphate reacts with ammonium molybdate yielding a purple complex commonly known as molybdenum blue. The absorbance at 710 nm of the solution is directly related to the phosphorus concentration.

2.4.4.1.1 *Molybdenum Blue Colorimetric Assay*

A. *Samples, Ingredients, and Reagents*
- Dry or wet ashed samples (refer to procedures in Sections 2.4.1.1 or 2.4.1.2)
- Distilled deionized water
- Ammonia
- Sulfuric acid
- Phenolphthalein indicator
- Phosphorus standard (0.1 mg/mL)
- Ammonium molybdate
- Tin chloride

B. *Materials and Equipment*
- Spectrophotometer
- Spectrophotometer cuvettes
- Test tube shaker or vortex
- Volumetric flasks (100 mL)
- Graduated cylinders (100 mL and 500 mL)
- Dropper bottle
- Diluter or automatic dispensing system
- Test tubes (10 mL capacity)
- Pipettes (1 mL, 5 mL, and 10 mL)
- Thermometer
- Volumetric flask (100 mL)

C. *Procedure*
1. Prepare a 1:4 ammonia solution, a 4% ammonium molybdate in sulfuric acid solution, and a 2% tin chloride solution. Use distilled deionized water for the preparation of the various solutions.

2. Prepare the standard phosphorus solution by adding 0, 0.25, 0.5, 1.0, and 2 mL of the standard phosphorus solution containing 0.1 mg/mL to 100 mL volumetric flasks. Add one drop of phenolphthalein, neutralize with 1:4 ammonia and make up to approximately 85 mL with distilled deionized water. Add 4 mL of ammonium molybdate reagent and shake well. Then, add 0.7 mL of the 2% tin chloride solution and add water to the 100 mL mark.

3. Dilute the wet ash test sample with distilled deionized water, preferably using the automatic diluter. The dilution factor will vary according to the phosphorus concentration and calibration standard curve. For instance, pipette 5 mL of the wet ash solution into a 100 mL volumetric flask. Next, add distilled deionized water to the 100 mL mark and shake contents. Then, obtain exactly 10 mL of the diluted test sample and place it in a 100 mL volumetric flask. Add one drop of phenolphthalein, neutralize with 1:4 ammonia and make up to approximately 85 mL with distilled deionized water. Add 4 mL of ammonium molybdate reagent and shake well. Then, add 0.7 mL of the 2% tin chloride solution and add distilled water to the 100 mL mark.

4. Turn on the spectrophotometer at least 15 minutes before the test and set up the wavelength to 710 nm.

5. Read the absorbance of the standard solutions to construct the calibration curve. The standard solutions contain 0, 0.25, 0.5, 0.75, and 1 mg of phosphorus/100 mL. Determine the slope of the curve and the r^2 factor (should be >.99). Then, read the absorbance of the test solution. If the color of the obtained solution is greater or inferior compared with the highest and smallest standard, repeat the procedure adjusting the dilution factor.

6. Calculate the % phosphorus = (absorbance × 10)/sample weight (g) × volume of ash solution diluted to 100 mL.

2.4.4.1.2 Analysis of Phosphorus with the Molybdate– Vanadate Colorimetric Method

Phosphorus is, in most cases, analyzed by the vanadium phosphomolybdate colorimetric method in which the phosphorus present as the orthophosphate reacts with a vanadate–molybdate reagent to produce a yellow–orange complex. The absorbance at 420 nm of the solution is directly related to the phosphorus concentration (James 1995).

A. Samples, Ingredients, and Reagents
- Dry or wet ash samples (refer to procedure in Section 2.4.1)
- Phosphorus standard (1000 mg/L)
- Nitric acid
- Distilled deionized water
- Vanadate–molybdate reagent

B. Materials and Equipment
- Spectrophotometer
- Spectrophotometer cuvettes
- Test tube shaker or vortex
- Volumetric flasks (100 mL)
- Graduated cylinders (100 mL and 500 mL)
- Diluter or automatic dispensing system
- Test tubes (10 mL capacity)
- Pipettes (1 mL, 5 mL, and 10 mL)
- Thermometer
- Volumetric flask (1 L)

C. Procedure
1. Prepare the vanadate–molybdate reagent by dissolving 20 g of ammonium molybdate in 400 mL of water at approximately 50°C. Dissolve 1 g of ammonium vanadate in 300 mL of boiling distilled water, cool and gradually add 140 mL of concentrated nitric acid. Obtain the wet or dry ash stock solution (refer to procedures in Sections 2.4.1.1 or 2.4.1.2). Add the vanadate–molybdate solution to the acid vanadate solution and dilute to exactly 1 L with distilled water.

2. Prepare the standard phosphorus solution by dissolving 4.39 g of potassium dihydrogen phosphate (KH_2PO_4) in 1 L of distilled water. Dilute 1 to 10 with distilled water to give a solution containing 0.1 mg phosphorus/mL.

3. Prepare the series of phosphorus standards by adding 0, 2.5, 5, 7.5, and 10 mL of the standard phosphorus solution of step 2 to 100 mL volumetric flasks and dilute with 30 mL of distilled deionized water. Then, add 25 mL of the vanadate–molybdate reagent and mix contents and then add distilled deionized water to the 100 mL mark. Label each of the standard solutions.

4. Dilute the wet ash test sample with distilled deionized water, preferably using the automatic diluter. The dilution factor will vary according to the phosphorus concentration and calibration standard curve. For instance, pipette 2 mL of the wet ash solution into a 100 mL volumetric flask. Next, add 25 mL of the vanadate–molybdate reagent and mix contents and then add distilled deionized water to the 100 mL mark. Allow the solution to stand 10 minutes before measuring absorbance.

5. Turn on the spectrophotometer at least 15 minutes before the test and set up the wavelength at 420 nm.

6. Read the absorbance of the standard solution to construct the calibration curve. The standard solutions contain 0, 0.25, 0.5, 0.75, and 1 mg of phosphorus/100 mL. Determine the slope of the curve and the r^2 factor (should be >.99). Then, read the absorbance of the test solution.

If the color of the solution obtained is greater or inferior compared with the highest and smallest standard, repeat the procedure adjusting the dilution factor.

7. Calculate the % phosphorus = (absorbance × 10)/sample weight (g) × volume of ash solution diluted to 100 mL.

2.4.5 SODIUM CHLORIDE ANALYSIS

Sodium chloride is widely used to prepare a wide range of cereal-based food items. Almost all wheat-based foods (breads, cookies, pasta, and tortillas), breakfast cereals, and snack foods contain significant amounts of sodium chloride that is added to enhance gluten formation, as a preservative, and as a seasoning agent. In addition, the sodium of the sodium chloride molecule should be declared in the nutritional label because it has negative health implications (i.e., hypertension). There are many analytical procedures to determine the sodium and sodium chloride present in foods. The most popular methods are the Mohr and Volhard titration tests, the Dicromat analyzer, and the Quantab chloride strip tests. The Dicromat analyzer is a fast method in which soluble salt is read directly from a digital readout whereas the Quantab chloride titrator is ideal for quickly and quantitatively determining salt.

2.4.5.1 Mohr Titration Method

The Mohr method uses chromate ions as an indicator in the titration of chloride ions with 0.1 M silver nitrate standard solution. After the precipitation of the whole amount of chloride (usually as white silver chloride), the first excess of titrant results in the production of a silver chromate precipitate, which indicates the endpoint. When the stoichiometry and moles consumed at the endpoint are identified, the amount of chloride in the experimental sample can be determined.

A. Samples, Ingredients, and Reagents
- Samples of cereal-based products
- 5% Silver nitrate solution
- Distilled and deionized water
- 5% Potassium chromate solution
- Silver nitrate (0.1 N)

B. Materials and Equipment
- Analytical scale
- Volumetric flasks (0.1 L, 0.5 L, and 1 L)
- Graduated cylinders (25 mL)
- 250 mL and 500 mL Erlenmeyer flasks
- 125 mL Erlenmeyer flask
- Filter paper
- Chronometer
- Laboratory or coffee mill
- 10 mL pipette
- Stirring rod
- Burette with 0.1 mL divisions
- 125 and 250 mL funnels
- 500 mL graduated cylinder

C. Procedure
1. Prepare the following reagents:
   a. 5% K_2CrO_4 indicator solution by dissolving 5 g K_2CrO_4 in 100 mL of distilled deionized water.
   b. Standard $AgNO_3$ solution. Dissolve 8.49 g of $AgNO_3$ in a 500 mL volumetric flask and make up to volume with distilled water. The resulting solution is approximately 0.1 M.
2. Mill the test sample using a laboratory or coffee mill. For fat-rich products, the material can be crushed by hand.
3. Weigh 25 g of the test sample. Transfer sample to 500 mL beaker or Erlenmeyer flask and add 250 mL of distilled deionized water from a graduated cylinder.
4. Stir and let stand at least 5 minutes (make sure the entire sample is covered by water).
5. Stir again and filter into a beaker.
6. Pipette 10 mL of the clear filtrate into a clean 250 mL Erlenmeyer flask.
7. Add 25 mL of distilled water and stir.
8. Add six to seven drops of potassium chromate indicator and stir.
9. Fill burette with 0.1 M of silver nitrate and titrate the salt solution with indicator until the solution changes to a faint brick-red color.
10. Register the volume (in mL) of 0.1 N silver nitrate solution dispensed by the burette.
11. Determine the percentage of chloride and sodium chloride in the sample using the following equations:
    a. % Chloride = (mL of $AgNO_3$/g of sample weight) × (Mol $AgNO_3$/L) × 35.5 × 2.5
    b. % Sodium chloride = (mL of $AgNO_3$/g of sample weight) × (Mol $AgNO_3$/L) × 58.5 × 2.5

2.4.5.2 Volhard Titration Method

Chloride ions can also be determined by the Volhard procedure. Briefly, the protocol starts when the food sample is boiled in diluted nitric acid, and then the addition of excess silver nitrate and back-titration with potassium thiocyanate. The addition of excess silver nitrate to a solution containing chloride ions results in the precipitation of silver chloride. The concentration of chloride can then be analyzed by back-titrating of the excess silver ions with a thiocyanate solution to create a silver thiocyanate precipitate. Ferric ion (Fe^{3+}) is usually used as an indicator for the titration because as soon as all the silver ions have reacted, the minimum excess of thiocyanate will react with the indicator to yield a bright-red complex.

A. Samples, Ingredients, and Reagents
- Samples of cereal-based products
- HNO_3
- $KMnO_4$
- Ferric ammonium sulfate [$Fe_2NH_4(SO_4)_2$]

- Distilled and deionized water
- $AgNO_3$
- Dietyl ether
- NH_4SCN
- NaCl (reagent grade)

B. *Materials and Equipment*
- Analytical scale
- Erlenmeyer flasks (300 mL)
- Magnetic stirrer
- Volumetric flasks (1 L)
- Graduated cylinders (25 mL)
- Laboratory or coffee mill
- Hot stirring plate
- Burette
- 5 mL and 20 mL pipettes
- Brown glass bottles (1 L)

C. *Procedure*
1. Prepare the following reagents:
   a. Standard silver nitrate solution (0.5 M). In a 1-L volumetric flask, dissolve 84.94 g of $AgNO_3$ in distilled deionized water. Bring volume to 1 L and store in a brown bottle.
   b. In a 100 mL volumetric flask, dissolve 7.42 g of $KMnO_4$ in 100 mL of distilled deionized water and store in a brown bottle.
   c. In a 100 mL flask, dissolve 22.4 g of ferric ammonium sulfate [$FeNH_4(SO_4)_2$] in 100 mL of distilled deionized water and store in brown bottle.
   d. Dissolve 29.2 g of reagent grade NaCl in distilled deionized water and bring volume to exactly 1 L (0.5 M solution).
   e. Dissolve 38.06 g of NH_4SCN in distilled deionized water, bring volume to exactly 1 L and store in a brown glass bottle (0.5 M).
2. Mill the sample using a laboratory or coffee mill.
3. In an analytical scale, weigh 2.5 g of the sample and carefully place it in an Erlenmeyer flask (250 mL).
4. Add 29 mL of the 0.5 M $AgNO_3$ and mix. Then, carefully add 15 mL of HNO_3 and place on a hot plate inside a laboratory hood. Boil the resulting acid solution for 10 minutes. Add 2 mL of the $KMnO_4$ and continue boiling until the blue–purple color disappears or until the sample has a slight yellowish coloration.
5. Add 25 mL of distilled deionized water and keep boiling for 5 minutes. Remove the Erlenmeyer flask from the hot plate and allow contents to cool down. After cooling, add distilled deionized water to a volume of 150 mL.
6. Add 25 mL of diethyl ether and mix contents.
7. Add 5 mL of the ferric ammonium sulfate indicator right before titration. Place a magnetic stirrer in the Erlenmeyer flask and titrate with 0.5 M of NH_4SCN until the solution turns light

brown–orange in color. Register the volume (in mL) of NH_4SCN dispensed by the burette.
8. Calculate the percentage of NaCl with the following formula:

$$\{[(Mol\ AgNO_3)\ (mL\ AgNO_3)/100] - [(Mol\ NH_4SCN/100) \times 58.5 \times 100]\}/sample\ weight.$$

2.4.5.3 Analysis of Salt Content with the Dicromat Analyzer

This method was previously described by Rooney (2007).

A. *Samples, Ingredients, and Reagents*
- Samples of cereal-based products
- Distilled and deionized water

B. *Materials and Equipment*
- Digital scale
- Dicromat salt analyzer (Noramar Co., Chagrin Falls, OH)
- Beaker (250 mL)
- Coffee filters
- Laboratory or coffee mill
- Electric blender
- Large funnel
- Chronometer

C. *Procedure*
1. Mill the sample using a laboratory or coffee mill.
2. Weigh 50 g of the sample and place it in the electric blender bowl.
3. Add exactly 150 mL of distilled deionized water.
4. Grind the sample in the electric blender to obtain a slurry.
5. After 10 minutes of resting, filter the slurry through a coffee filter. Obtain 100 to 120 mL of the filtrate.
6. Determine salt content of the filtrate by pouring the filtrate through the dicromat cylinder which has been calibrated following instructions from the manufacturer.
7. Salt content is read directly from the digital readout.

2.4.5.4 Analysis of Chloride (Salt) with the Quantab Strip Test

The Quantab chloride titrator is ideal for quickly and quantitatively determining salt. The test simply consists of dipping the chloride strip in the sample. When test strips are placed on a solution, the fluid reacts with the strip. The height of the column is proportional to the total chloride or salt concentration. A calibration table converts the strip value to parts per million of chloride ion. The approximate titration range is 0.005% to 1% NaCl equivalent to 30 ppm to 6000 ppm, respectively.

A. *Samples, Ingredients, and Reagents*
- Samples of cereal-based products
- Distilled and deionized water

- Quantab chloride titrator strips
- 2.5% Salt solution

B. *Materials and Equipment*
- Analytical scale
- Erlenmeyer flasks (300 mL)
- Volumetric flasks (1 L)
- Graduated cylinders (100 mL)
- Laboratory or coffee mill
- Conical funnel
- Whatman no. 1 filter paper
- Chronometer

C. *Procedure*
1. Obtain a representative sample of the food and grind it in a coffee or laboratory mill. If the sample is rich in fat (i.e., snacks), crush sample by hand.
2. Weigh 10 g of finely blended sample and add 90 mL of boiling distilled water and blend for 30 seconds. Allow to sit for 1 minute then blend again. Cool to room temperature. Filter at least 5 mL through a Whatman no. 1 filter paper folded into a cone as specified and supported in a conical funnel.
3. Place lower end of Quantab chloride titrator in the solution. Allow test solution to saturate the column. This is accomplished when the yellow signal across the top of the column turns completely dark. This usually takes approximately 12 minutes.
4. Determine the height of the white column in Quantab units within the time specified (2–30 minutes). Samples should be diluted so that results are within a readable range for the selected strip.
5. Convert reading to percentage of sodium chloride using the calibration chart which accompanies the titrator. If the sample was diluted, multiply the result by the dilution factor.

2.4.6 RESEARCH SUGGESTIONS

1. Determine the sodium and sodium chloride contents of a given processed sample of tortilla chips or pretzels using atomic absorption, Mohr, Dicromat, and Quantab techniques.
2. Investigate the best method to determine iron in a sample of table bread which was produced with enriched flour.
3. Determine the phosphorus, zinc, and iron composition of whole wheat processed into refined flour. Determine the amounts of these minerals in the whole grain, refined flour, bran, and shorts (refer to procedure in Section 5.2.2.1).
4. Determine the sodium composition of tortilla chips before and after the addition of seasonings.
5. Determine total phosphorus and phytates of barley before and after sprouting or malting.

2.4.7 RESEARCH QUESTIONS

1. What are advantages and disadvantages of wet and dry ash procedures?
2. What are the principles, components, and advantages and disadvantages of an AAS?
3. Why is lanthanum chloride recommended for use in atomic absorption calcium analysis?
4. What are the principles, components, and advantages and disadvantages of an ICP spectrometer?
5. Explain the importance of mineral standards and elaboration of calibration curves before mineral analysis.
6. Describe and investigate procedures to determine total phosphorus and phosphorus associated with phytates in a given grain sample.
7. What are the differences and similarities between the phosphorus blue molybdate and vanadate molybdate assays?
8. Compare the quantification of sodium via atomic absorption, Mohr, Volhard, Dicromat, and Quantab methods. How can you convert sodium to sodium chloride?
9. Describe the recommended procedure to determine the mineral composition of bones obtained from laboratory animals. What is the typical mineral composition of bones?

2.5 METHODS FOR NITROGENOUS COMPOUND ANALYSIS

Protein or nitrogenous compounds are the second most abundant chemical compounds associated with cereal grains. The concentration present in cereal grains differs according to species and even within the same type of grain due to genetics and environmental conditions during kernel development and maturation in the field. The factors that affect protein concentration the most are nitrogen fertilization and water availability during grain filling. Oats and rice are the cereals with the highest and lowest protein contents, respectively. Among the different wheat classes, the soft wheats have been bred to contain the lowest protein; therefore, they contain the weakest gluten. Hard and durum wheats usually contain 10.5% to 14% protein. The gluten of durum wheat is usually stronger but less extensible compared with the gluten of hard wheats. As in other cereals, the protein is distributed in the different anatomical parts of the grain. The germ and aleurone layers contain the highest concentration; however, because the starchy endosperm is the largest anatomical part, it contains approximately 70% to 80% of the total protein.

The total protein concentration is usually evaluated with the Kjeldhal procedure described previously. However, the cereal proteins are classified according to solubility into albumins, globulins, prolamins, and glutelins. The water- and weak salt solution–soluble fractions are called albumins and globulins, respectively. These two fractions are mainly concentrated in the germ and are composed of enzymes, nucleoproteins, and glycoproteins. These proteins are considered biologically active and play an important role during grain germination and nutritionally contain the best amino acid balance and quality (contain high amounts of lysine and other essential amino acids). Approximately 80% of the cereal proteins are considered as reserves. In most cereals, the most abundant protein fraction is the prolamin synthesized in the protoplastids during grain development. The environmental conditions and soil fertility affect the amount of prolamins. In general, a high nitrogen fertilization level increases the amount of these proteins that are stored in protein bodies distributed throughout the endosperm cells. They are water-insoluble but have good solubility in alcohol. This protein fraction has different denominations according to the cereal grain: maize, zein; rice, oryzin; wheat, gliadin; sorghum, kafirin; rye, secalin; and barley, hordein. From the nutritional viewpoint, prolamins are the poorest in terms of essential amino acid composition. These are rich in nonessential amino acids such as glycine, glutamic acid, and aspartic acid and very poor in lysine and tryptophan. In some cereals such as sorghum, the prolamins are highly crosslinked because of disulfide bonds; therefore, reducing agents such as mercaptoethanol are required to improve the extraction rate. The glutelins are more difficult to extract because of their high molecular weight and the presence of disulfide bonds. These proteins are extracted with detergents, alkaline compounds, or mercaptoethanol. The glutelins are the main structural endosperm proteins. They are basically located in the protein matrix. The nutritional quality of glutelins is better than prolamins. In quality protein maize, the proportion of glutelins and albumins/globulins are higher, and consequently, the amount of prolamins is significantly reduced.

When proteins are completely digested or hydrolyzed, they yield their building blocks or amino acids. Cereals contain high quantities of leucine, proline, aspartic acid, and glutamic acid. Among these amino acids are lysine, tryptophan, phenylalanine, leucine, isoleucine, threonine, valine, and methionine, which are considered essentials for humans. The two most important in cereals grains are lysine and tryptophan. The lysine structure contains two amino groups. This amino acid is highly reactive and is required for the synthesis of other amino acids, enzymes, peptide hormones, antibodies, and muscle mass. On the other hand, tryptophan is a precursor of the neurotransmitter serotonin, the B vitamin niacin, and of the nicotinamide containing coenzymes nicotidamide adenine dinucleotide (NAD) and nicotidamide adenine dinucleotide phosphate (NADP). The amino acid profile of cereal grains and other foods is usually determined with ion exchange chromatography or with an HPLC system. For both analytical techniques, the sample is hydrolyzed with acid to obtain most of the individual amino acids. Unfortunately, tryptophan is lost during acid hydrolysis and, if analyzed, the sample has to be hydrolyzed following alternative protocols. The amino acid composition is critically important for the prediction of protein quality for humans and domestic animals.

2.5.1 Determination of Protein Fractions

Cereal grains and their products contain four major protein fractions: albumins, globulins, prolamins, and glutelins. The combination of the last two is commonly known as gluten. These protein factions vary in molecular weight, electrophoretic patterns, structure, functionality, and amino acid composition. The determination of protein fractions is critically important especially in wheat. The first scientists that fractionated cereal proteins were Osborn and Mendel back in 1924. Later on, Landry and Moureaux (1970) devised a fractionation scheme which is currently used or is the base for other related methods. The sequential extraction of protein according to the Mendel and Osborne method was based on the solubility of protein in different solvents: water, salt, alcohol, and alkali-soluble and residual proteins. The residues remaining after these successive extractions were determined by the Kjeldhal procedure (refer to procedure in Section 2.2.3.1). In 1970, Landry and Moureaux (1970, 1980) reported a procedure that allowed five protein fractions to be isolated from maize kernels by sequential extraction. Fraction I, corresponding to albumins and globulins, was extracted from defatted meal with NaCl 0.5 M. Fraction II composed of prolamins was extracted with 55% (w/w) isopropanol after the removal of albumins, globulins, and salt whereas fraction III was isolated in the presence of 55% isopropanol and 0.6% (w/v) 2-mercaptoethanol (cross-linked prolamins). Mercaptoethanol was included because it has the capacity to break the disulfide bonds responsible for cross-linking. Fraction IV, called salt-soluble glutelins, was isolated in the presence of 0.5 M NaCl and 0.6% mercaptoethanol buffered at pH 10, whereas fraction V, known as true glutelins, was isolated in the presence of 0.5% (w/v) sodium dodecyl sulfate and 0.6% mercaptoethanol buffered at pH 10. Other fractionation schemes consist of the sequential extraction of soluble protein with 0.5 M NaCl solution (fraction I albumins and globulins), 60% tert-butyl alcohol (fraction II corresponding to prolamins), 60% tert-butyl alcohol containing 2% mercaptoethanol (fraction III corresponding to cross-linked prolamins), and a mixture of 2% sodium dodecylsulfate (SDS), 5% mercaptoethanol and 0.0625 M tris buffer adjusted to pH 6.8 (fraction IV glutelins; Paulis and Wall 1975, 1979; Vivas Rodriguez et al. 1987).

2.5.1.1 Protein Fractionation Scheme

This method was described by Paulis and Wall (1975, 1979) and Vivas Rodriguez et al. (1987).

A. *Samples, Ingredients, and Reagents*
- Test samples
- Tert-butyl alcohol
- Mercaptoethanol
- HCl
- NaCl (reagent type)
- Sodium dodecyl sulfate
- Tris buffer

B. *Materials and Methods*
- Analytical scale
- Micro-Kjeldhal flasks
- Glass beads
- Water bath shaker
- Centrifuge
- pH meter
- Thermometer
- Laboratory mill (Udy mill)
- Kjeldhal equipment (procedure in Section 2.2.3.1)
- Test tubes (centrifuge)
- Erlenmeyer flasks (25 mL)
- Pipettes (5 mL and 10 mL)
- Volumetric flasks (1 L)
- Chronometer

C. *Procedure*

1. Weigh exactly 1.5 g of the finely ground test material. The moisture and total protein contents of the test material should be determined beforehand (refer to procedures in Sections 2.2.1.1 and 2.2.3.1).
2. Place sample in a test tube, add 3 g of glass beads and 9 mL of 0.5 M NaCl solution and place tube in a shaker at 4°C. After 2 hours, centrifuge at $10,000 \times g$ for 20 minutes. Carefully remove the supernatant and place it in a 25 mL flask. Repeat the addition of the 0.5 M NaCl and extract this a second time for 1 hour. Mix the two supernatants and determine protein content of an aliquot using the Kjeldhal procedure. This extract will yield albumins and globulins.
3. Add 9 mL of 60% tert-butyl alcohol to the test tube containing the albumin/globulin-free sample and glass beads, and place tube in a shaker at room temperature. After 2 hours, centrifuge at $10,000 \times g$ for 20 minutes. Remove the supernatant cautiously and place it in a 25 mL flask labeled as fraction II. Repeat the addition of the tert-butyl alcohol and extract this a second time for 1 hour. Mix the two supernatants and determine the protein content of an aliquot using the Kjeldhal procedure. This extract will yield the prolamins.
4. Add 9 mL of 60% tert-butyl alcohol with 2% mercaptoethanol to the test tube containing the extracted sample from step 3 and place the tube in a shaker at room temperature. After 2 hours, centrifuge at $10,000 \times g$ for 20 minutes. Carefully remove the supernatant and place it in a 25 mL flask labeled as fraction III. Repeat the addition of the tert-butyl alcohol and 2% mercaptoethanol and extract this a second time for 1 hour. Mix the two supernatants and determine the protein content of the aliquot using the Kjeldhal procedure. This extract will yield the prolamin-like fraction or alcohol-soluble reduced glutenins.
5. Add 9 mL of buffer containing 2% SDS, 5% mercaptoethanol, and 0.0625 M tris buffer adjusted to pH 6.8 to the test tube containing the extracted sample from step 4 and place the tube in a water bath shaker adjusted to 50°C. After 2 hours, centrifuge at $10,000 \times g$ for 20 minutes. Carefully remove the supernatant and place it in a 25 mL flask labeled as fraction IV. Repeat the addition of the buffer and extract this a second time for 1 hour. Mix the two supernatants and determine the protein content of the aliquot using the Kjeldhal procedure. This extract will yield the glutelin fraction.
6. After protein determinations of the four different supernatants, convert the aliquot protein to the total volume (18 mL). Divide the protein extracted in each fraction by the total protein content to express values as a percentage of the original protein. Subtract from 100 the percentage protein of fractions I to IV and express this value as the percentage of residual protein.

2.5.2 Determination of Free Amino Nitrogen

Free amino nitrogen is an essential component of yeast nutrition in brewing and ethanol production because it promotes proper yeast growth and fermentation efficiency. In addition, free amino nitrogen is highly related to the degree of protein hydrolysis. The amino nitrogen groups of free amino acids in the sample react with N-acetyl-L-cysteine and o-phthaldialdehyde to form isoindole derivatives (Wilson 2008). The amount of isoindole derivative formed in this reaction is stoichiometric with the amount of free amino nitrogen. It is the isoindole derivative that is measured by the increase in absorbance at 570 nm.

2.5.2.1 Determination of Free Amino Nitrogen (Ninhydrin Reaction)

A. *Samples, Ingredients, and Reagents*
- Test samples
- Sodium dibasic phosphate ($Na_2HPO4\cdot12H_2O$)
- Ninhydrin (2,2-dihydroxyindane-1,3-dione)
- Potassium iodate (KIO_3)
- Glycine (reagent grade)
- Distilled water
- Potassium phosphate (KH_2PO_4)
- Fructose
- Ethanol

B. *Materials and Equipment*
- Analytical scale
- pH meter
- Volumetric flask (100 mL)
- Pipettes (1 mL)
- Hot plate
- Chronometer
- Spectrophotometer UV-vis

- Dark bottle
- Beaker (1 L)
- Test tubes with caps
- Cuvettes

C. Procedure

1. Prepare the following reagents:
   a. Wearing protective gloves, in a 100 mL volumetric flask, prepare the ninhydrin reagent by mixing 10 g of $Na_2HPO4\cdot12H_2O$, 6 g KH_2PO_4, 0.5 g ninhydrin, and 0.3 g fructose with distilled water. The pH should be in the range of 6.6 to 6.8. Store the ninhydrin reagent in a brown or dark bottle under refrigeration (5°C). The solution is stable for 2 weeks under these storage conditions. Prepare the dilution solution by mixing 2 g of KIO_3, 400 mL of ethanol, and 600 mL of distilled water. Keep the dilution solution in a closed container under refrigeration.
   b. Prepare the glycine standard solution by placing 107.2 mg of glycine in a volumetric flask and then adding distilled water to the 100 mL mark. After shaking the resulting solution, store the glycine stock standard at 0°C. The working glycine standard is prepared by diluting 1 mL of the stock glycine standard solution with water to a 100 mL volume.

2. For solid samples, a known amount of ground solids should be diluted in a known amount of distilled deionized water for extraction of soluble proteins. Samples should be extracted under stirring for at least 2 hours. Then, allow insoluble solids to precipitate and take an aliquot of the supernatant. Liquid samples (i.e., wort, beer, and hydrolysates) should be diluted according to the original soluble protein content.

3. Take a 2 mL aliquot of the test sample and place it in a test tube. Then add 1 mL of the ninhydrin reagent solution. Place sealed test tubes in a boiling water bath for 16 minutes.

4. After heating, immediately cool the test tubes by immersing for 20 minutes in a water bath (20°C).

5. Add 5 mL of the dilution solution, manually mix contents and then place solution in a cuvette. Read absorbance in the spectrophotometer set at 570 nm.

6. Run a distilled water blank and a diluted glycine standard following steps 3 to 5.

7. Calculate the free amino nitrogen using the following equation:

Free amino nitrogen (mg/L) = (test sample absorbance × 2 × dilution)/(average absorbance glycine standard).*

---

* Correct values according to the dilution factor used in step 2.

2.5.3 Determination of Amino Acid Profile

Hydrolysis of protein samples is necessary for amino acid analysis. The digestion of 6 N HCl is the most common method for hydrolyzing a protein sample because it recovers most of the amino acids. However, tryptophan is destroyed and methionine might undergo oxidation. To prevent oxidation of sulfur amino acid, the acid hydrolysis is done under an atmosphere rich in nitrogen. Tryptophan is usually obtained after an alkaline-separated hydrolysis. Microwave acid hydrolysis has been used and is rapid but requires special equipment as well as special precautions. The sample is hydrolyzed in a microwave oven for approximately 5 to 30 minutes with temperatures up to 200°C. During this method of hydrolysis, the hydrochloric acid vaporizes, comes into contact with the protein samples and hydrolyzes them.

Spackman et al. (1958) developed an ion exchange chromatography method for the analysis of amino acids which has been used for many decades. The amino acids are detected after postcolumn reaction with ninhydrin with a colorimeter set at two different wavelengths. In this instrumental method, the protein is first acid-hydrolyzed to yield a mixture of amino acids. These are then separated from one another by applying the mixture to the top of a column of ion exchange resin and then eluting the column with a series of buffer solutions of progressively changing acidity. The amino acids emerge separately from the column and can be identified by their rate of emergence. The quantity of each amino acid is measured by the intensity of the blue color after reaction with ninhydrin. In the 1980s, a reverse phase HPLC chromatography technique was developed with precolumn derivatization commonly known as the pico tag method (Bidlingmeyer et al. 1984). The method is based on the formation of a phenylthiocarbamyl derivative of the amino acids. The derivatization method is rapid, efficient, sensitive, and specific for the analysis of primary and secondary amino acids in protein hydrolysates. The liquid chromatographic system allows for the rapid, bonded-phase separation with UV detection of the common amino acids within 12 minutes of analysis and a 1 pmol sensitivity. The ground sample is hydrolyzed with 6 N HCl under vacuum for 65 minutes at 150°C. After hydrolysis, the sample is dissolved in distilled water containing EDTA in preparation for derivatization. Derivatization is performed automatically on the amino acid analyzer by reacting the free amino acids, under basic conditions, with phenylisothiocyanate to produce phenylthiocarbamyl amino acid derivatives. A standard solution containing a known amount of common free amino acids is also derivatized. This will be used to generate a calibration file that can be used to determine the amino acid content of the sample. The phenylthiocarbamyl amino acids are separated on a reverse phase C18 silica column and the phenylthiocarbamyl chromophore is detected at 254 nm. All of the amino acids will elute in approximately 25 minutes. The buffer system used for separation is 50 mM sodium acetate (pH 5.45) as buffer A and 70% acetonitrile/32 mM sodium acetate (pH 6.1) as buffer B. The program is run using a gradient of buffer A and buffer B with an initial 7% buffer B concentration and ending with a 60% buffer B concentration at the end of the gradient. Finally, the computer automatically calculates chromatographic peak areas to calculate the amount of amino acid (in picomoles) present in the sample. These two analytical techniques are the most commonly used to analyze the amino acid profile (except tryptophan) of food proteins.

Several analytical methods have been developed to assay tryptophan. However, most protocols are time-consuming and unreliable. Friedman and Finley (1971) reviewed methods of tryptophan analysis using ion exchange chromatography. The sample preparation includes acid hydrolysis, alkaline hydrolysis, biological and enzymatic assays, and the combination of these. Anderson and Clydesdale (1978) proposed a methodology for tryptophan analysis using α-ketoglutaric acid in which a yellow chromophore is read at 358 nm. Nurit et al. (2009) developed an accurate, reliable, and inexpensive method for tryptophan analysis in whole-grain maize flour. In this method, tryptophan reacts with glyoxylic acid in the presence of sulfuric acid and ferric chloride, producing a colored compound that absorbs at 560 nm. A series of experiments varying the reagent concentrations, hydrolysis time, and length of the colorimetric reaction resulted in an optimized protocol which uses 0.1 M glyoxylic acid in 7 N sulfuric acid and 1.8 mM of ferric chloride, and 30 minutes reaction time. This method produced stable and reproducible results for tryptophan concentration in whole-grain maize flour and was validated by comparison with data obtained using an acetic acid-based colorimetric procedure ($r^2 = .80$) and HPLC ($r^2 = .71$). This procedure was used to identify the most promising quality protein maize lines in breeding programs.

2.5.3.1 Acid Hydrolysis Procedure for Determination of Amino Acids

A. *Samples, Ingredients, and Reagents*
- Test samples
- HCl
- Nitrogen gas
- Distilled water
- Sodium citrate
- Glass fiber filter paper

B. *Materials and Equipment*
- Analytical scale
- Hydrolysate flask (500 mL)
- Vacuum pump
- Graduated cylinder (200 mL)
- Flat burner with temperature controls
- Thermometer
- Laboratory mill or grinder
- Rotary evaporator
- Glass beads
- Coil glass condensers
- Volumetric flasks
- Buchner-type filtration unit

C. *Procedure*
1. Weigh approximately 0.5 g of ground sample and place it in a 500 mL hydrolysate flask.
2. Add five or six glass beads and 200 mL of 6 N HCl.
3. Place flasks on distillation set up with coil-type condensers (be sure that water to condensers is on and traps are empty). Adjust flasks so they are resting flat on the burners and all fittings are tight. Turn on heat and evaporate approximately 100 mL of HCl.
4. Move flasks to preheated burners under reflux condensers.
5. Turn on water to reflux condensers and open nitrogen valve. Check water traps for bubbles to insure that nitrogen is going into condensers in use.
6. Continue refluxing under nitrogen pressure until 24 hours after sample initially started boiling.
7. Cool hydrolysates and evaporate to dryness using a rotary evaporator. Establish vacuum gradually on cool sample to prevent excess boiling and sample loss. After maximum vacuum (15 psi) is reached, lower sample into heated water bath adjusted to 37°C.
8. Wash with 50 mL of deionized water and evaporate to dryness twice to remove all HCl.
9. Bring to desired volume (100 mL) with pH 2.2 sodium citrate-HCl buffer.
10. Filter through glass fiber filter paper.
11. The hydrolysate is ready for amino acid analysis. Make sure to write the volume used of sodium citrate-HCl buffer. If samples are not immediately used, they should be placed in a freezer.

2.5.3.2 Determination of Tryptophan with a Colorimetric Procedure

Nurit et al. (2009) recently developed an accurate, reliable, and inexpensive method for tryptophan analysis in whole-grain maize flour. The procedure is based on the reaction of tryptophan with glyoxylic acid in the presence of sulfuric acid and ferric chloride to produce a colored compound that absorbs at 560 nm. A series of experiments varying the reagent concentrations, hydrolysis time, and length of the colorimetric reaction resulted in an optimized protocol which uses 0.1 M glyoxylic acid in 7 N sulfuric acid and 1.8 mM ferric chloride, and 30 minutes reaction time. This method produced stable and reproducible results for tryptophan concentration in whole-grain maize flour and was validated by comparison with data obtained using an acetic acid-based colorimetric procedure ($r^2 = .80$) developed by Villegas et al. (1984) and HPLC ($r^2 = .71$).

A. *Samples, Ingredients, and Reagents*
- Test samples
- Glyoxylic acid
- $FeCl_3 \cdot 6H_2O$
- DL-tryptophan (reagent grade)

- Distilled water
- Sulfuric acid
- Papain
- Sodium acetate

B. *Materials and Equipment*

- Analytical scale
- Graduated cylinder (100 mL and 200 mL)
- Brown or dark bottles
- Cuvettes
- Water bath
- Pipettes (1 mL, 5 mL, and 10 mL)
- Centrifuge
- Chronometer
- Laboratory mill or grinder
- Volumetric flasks
- Spectrophotometer
- Test tubes
- Test tube stirrer
- pH meter
- Thermometer

C. *Procedure*

1. Prepare the following reagents:
   a. Reagent A. Prepare 0.1 M glyoxylic acid in 7 N sulfuric acid (mix 35 mL of 30 N sulfuric acid with 115 mL of distilled water and adding distilled water, if necessary, to complete 150 mL volume).
   b. Reagent B (colorimetric reagent). Prepare 1.8 mM $FeCl_3 \cdot 6H_2O$ solution and mix with an equal volume of 30 N sulfuric acid. Store in a brown bottle.
   c. Stock standard solution. Prepare a stock solution of 100 µg/mL of DL-tryptophan in 0.165 M sodium acetate at pH 7 and store at 4°C.
2. Grind the sample using a laboratory mill. Then, determine the moisture content (refer to procedure in Section 2.2.1.1), protein (refer to procedure in Section 2.2.3.1), and extract the fat with hexane in a Soxhlet-type continuous extractor for 6 hours (refer to procedure in Section 2.2.4.1). Register the percentages of moisture and fat to correct values.
3. After hexane evaporation, weigh 80 mg of sample and place it in a test tube for protein digestion.
4. Add 3 mL of 4 mg/mL of papain. Include a blank with only papain solution as a control. Prepare a set of tryptophan calibration samples ranging from 0.5 µg to 30 µg of tryptophan/mL.
5. Place test tubes in a water bath adjusted to 65°C for 16 hours (shaken at least twice in the first hour of incubation).
6. Allow sample to cool to room temperature, and centrifuge at 3600 *g* for 10 minutes.
7. Take 1 mL aliquot of the hydrolysate (supernatant) and transfer to a clean test tube. Add 3 mL of reagent B (colorimetric reagent) and

stir contents (vortexed) and then incubate for 30 minutes at 65°C.
8. Allow samples to cool to room temperature before reading their optical density (OD) at 560 nm in a UV-vis spectrophotometer.
9. Prepare the working calibration samples by diluting the stock standard solution to obtain 0, 10, 15, 20, 25, and 30 µg of tryptophan/mL in the same sodium acetate to develop the standard curve. Read the OD at 560 nm in a spectrophotometer and construct the standard curve. Calculate the slope of the curve.
10. Calculate the percentage of tryptophan by multiplying the corrected OD (OD 560 nm sample — OD 560 nm average of papain blank) by the factor [hydrolysate volume/(slope of standard curve × sample weight)]. Correct values according to moisture and original fat content removed before the assay. Express tryptophan value in grams per 100 g of protein or grams per 16 g of nitrogen.

2.5.4 RESEARCH SUGGESTIONS

1. Determine the protein fractions of whole maize and its anatomical parts (germ, bran, and endosperm) derived from the dry-milling process described in procedure in Section 5.2.1.1.
2. Determine and compare protein fractions of wheat, maize, rice, and oats.
3. Determine the amino acid composition expressed on percentage of grain weight and grams of amino acid per 100 g of protein and chemical scores of a quality protein and regular maize samples.
4. Investigate the quickest method to determine tryptophan in a sample of table bread.
5. Determine the protein content and protein fractions of whole wheat processed into refined flour.
6. Determine the free amino nitrogen of barley and sorghum beer mashes (refer to Chapter 14) and explain why the free amino nitrogen contents are quite different.
7. Determine the protein content, free amino nitrogen, and protein fractions of barley before and after sprouting or malting?

2.5.5 RESEARCH QUESTIONS

1. Why is tryptophan partially lost during acid hydrolysis?
2. What are the main amino acids found associated with albumins, globulins, prolamins, and glutelins? Rank these protein fractions in terms of essential amino acid balance.
3. Why is the free amino nitrogen critically important during yeast fermentation for the production of beer, distilled spirits, and fuel ethanol? During

yeast fermentation, what kinds of metabolites are produced from the free amino nitrogen?

4. Explain how the free amino nitrogen assay can be used to estimate mold damage or deterioration of stored cereal grains.

5. Why is flushing with nitrogen recommended during acid hydrolysis of samples for amino acid analysis?

6. Compare the principles, advantages, and disadvantages of ion exchange and HPLC amino acid analyses?

7. Explain the importance of amino acid standards and elaboration of calibration curves before analysis.

8. Convert the percentage of amino acid composition to grams of amino acid per 100 g of protein and then calculate the limiting amino acid and chemical scores of the two following maize samples. Which sample has a better chemical score and protein quality? Why?

	Regular Maize	Quality Protein Maize	Requirement[a]	
	g/100 g protein	g/100 g protein	g/100 g protein	Chemical Score
Protein content	9.4	9.2		
Amino Acids				
Histidine	0.21	0.22	1.9	
Isoleucine	0.33	0.35	2.8	
Leucine	1.25	1.27	6.6	
Lysine	0.23	0.41	5.8	
Methionine + cysteine	0.41	0.40	2.5	
Phenylalanine + tyrosine	1.10	1.20	6.3	
Threonine	0.31	0.33	3.4	
Valine	0.45	0.45	3.5	
Tryptophan	0.04	0.09	1.1	

[a] Food and Agriculture Organization/World Health Organization requirement for children aged 2 to 5 years old.

9. What are differences and similarities between the Landry-Moreaux and Paulis-Wall protein fractionation schemes?

10. Explain the rationale of using mercaptoethanol during fractionation of prolamins and glutelins.

11. Describe the recommended procedure to determine tryptophan in quality protein maize breeding programs. Why is this amino acid essential for humans?

12. What are the main factors that affect protein quality of cereal-based products? In your opinion, which of these factors affect the most protein quality for humans?

2.6   METHODS FOR FATS AND OILS ANALYSIS

The quality control of refined fats and oils consists of more determinations because these products are fit for human consumption or further processed via fractionation, hydrogenation, or esterification. The fatty acid profile of refined oils is usually tested via GC-FID. The test consists of the hydrolysis of the triglycerides to yield FFAs that are methylated or derivatized with the aim of making these compounds nonpolar. The sample is injected and the fatty acids elute according to their molecular weight and degree of insaturation. The fatty acid profile is used to calculate the ratio of saturated/monounsaturated/polyunsaturated fatty acids required for food labeling purposes. A similar chromatography method is used to determine the amount of *cis* and *trans* fatty acids. The major modification of the procedure is the use of other gas carriers such as helium, long capillary columns, and *trans* fatty acid standards. This is important because several countries around the world are enforcing the declaration of *trans* fatty acids in food labels (Serna-Saldivar 2008c).

The stability or susceptibility of refined oils to oxidation is the most significant functionality test associated with the organoleptic properties of snacks and other cereal-based and fat-rich products. The peroxide value is the test traditionally used to determine the susceptibility to rancidity and shelf life of snacks and other related products, whereas the active oxygen method (AOM) is the quick accelerated stability test most commonly used by the industry to assess the properties of frying oils and their products. The AOM predicts the resistance of the heated oil to oxidation by bubbling air into the sample via quantification of peroxide values after several tests. The aim of the AOM method is to determine the induction period at which the oil starts forming peroxides at a constant rate or the number of hours required to reach 100 mEq peroxides per kilogram of oil. Other important tests for refined oils are fat acidity, color, iodine value, and the smoke/ignition/fire points, although the latter tests are usually for testing the quality of used oils.

The iodine value and refractive index are used to determine the degree of insaturation of oils and to follow fractionation and hydrogenation processes. Both tests are aimed toward the determination of the degree of insaturation of the oil. The main advantage of the refractive index is that it can be performed in a short time and does not destroy the sample and therefore is used for in-plant quick testing. The functionality of oleins, stearines, partially hydrogenated oils, shortening, and esterified shortening are usually tested via the determination of melting point and solid fat index (SFI). The method is based on dilatometry and is ideally suited to test the functionality of plastic shortening and tropical oils used for confectionary purposes. The SFI is used to determine the temperature range in which a fat/oil melts and relates to the fatty acid composition and distribution. The SFI is based on the dilatometry behavior of the fat, which is considered as a fingerprint of these products (Serna-Saldivar 2008a).

The quality control of oils and fats plays a key role in the value of end products and dictates processing adjustments. The quality control of crude oil, especially those associated with germ-rich by-products from various maize milling industries, is important because it greatly affects processing conditions during refining. The Official Methods and Recommended Practices of the American Oil Chemists' Society (AOCS) are the analytical methods most commonly used (AOCS 2009). The most important test for oil refiners is the total refining loss because it correlates very highly with refined oil yield. Mechanically extracted or solvent-extracted crude oil is generally tested for FFAs or acidity to determine the amount and strength of alkali used during neutralization. The color of crude oil is also an important parameter because it affects the amount of bleaching earths required to achieve a certain color value in refined oils.

Today, it is common practice to indirectly calculate the iodine and saponification values from the fatty acid composition of a given fat or oil. The calculated iodine value is obtained using the following equation: IV = (% hexadecenoic acid × 0.95) + (% octadecenoic acid × 0.86) + (% octadecadienoic acid × 1.732) + (% octadecatrienoic acid × 2.616) + (% eicosenoic acid × 0.785) + (% docosenoic acid × 0.723), whereas the saponification value after the analysis of the fatty acid profile is shown using Method Cd3a-94 in AOCS (2009).

During the frying of foods, the oil or fat is kept at elevated temperatures (175–195°C) and exposed to air, water, and chemical compounds associated with the food being processed. These conditions lead to thermal, oxidative, and hydrolytic breakdown of the oil (Serna-Saldivar 2008b). The frying oil gradually oxidizes, polymerizes, smokes, and produces volatiles that negatively affect the sensory properties of the snacks. Some of the breakdown products have been implicated in producing adverse health effects. Many criteria have been proposed to determine the state or condition of the frying oils but none have been entirely satisfactory (Stevenson et al. 1984).

To maintain the high quality of fried snack foods, processors must choose efficient equipment, select an oil with desirable flavor and durability, and monitor oil quality throughout its usage and frying performance (Jacobson 1991). A good and sound quality control program should assure good flavor, appearance, and texture of the snack food and minimize fluctuations on these important parameters. The most common defect in frying operations is an excessive oil uptake that can be caused by a low setting of the temperature of the frying oil and the use of an oil high in FFAs. To protect the frying oil from a high acidic value, the oil should be regularly filtered to remove food particles and the oil temperature lowered when the fryer in not in use. The use of a bad quality or degraded oil can also yield darker colorations in the fried products. To avoid this common defect, the oil should be replaced or the frying temperature decreased. Foaming and smoking are a result of the use of degraded oils and high operational temperatures. These factors also increase the chances of polymerization.

The quality control of frying oil operations generally consists of rapid in-plant determinations. Undoubtedly, the most common assay is the FFA content or acid value because the frying oil gradually increases its value as it is heated and used. The percentage of FFA in fresh oil is generally less than 0.05%, and abused oils may contain levels higher than 1.5%. There are many strip tests used to check the condition of the frying oil and spot tests that monitor FFAs by a colorimetric procedure. A high FFA or acid value increases the dielectric constant, oil color values, foaming, smoking, production of polar compounds, and also decreases oil stability. As the oil degrades and forms polar compounds, the dielectric constant increases. The advantage of the dielectric value is that it is quick and easy to perform but one of its disadvantages is that the reading is influenced by many outside and uncontrollable factors such as water and oil type. There are also strips that can give rough indications of the quality of the oil from the peroxide value viewpoint. The quick Oxifrit (oxidized fatty acid) or RAU test consists of a colorimetric kit that contains redox indicators that react with the total amount of oxidized compounds in a frying oil. The condition of the oil is determined by comparing the color developed to a four-color scale (Serna-Saldivar 2008b).

2.6.1 Analysis of FFAs

The FFAs or fat acidity values reflect the amount of FFAs no longer associated with the triglycerides. The fat acidic value is defined as the milligrams of potassium hydroxide (KOH) necessary to neutralize the FFAs present in 1 g of fat, whereas the FFA value is the percentage by weight of unesterified fatty acids (usually expressed as oleic equivalents; Nielsen 1998).

This test is very relevant because it gives an indication of the fat condition in grains, milled and processed products, and when used for frying purposes. The FFAs are liberated because of lipases or heat treatments. The fat acidity is an excellent indicator of grain quality or condition during storage.

A. *Samples, Ingredients, and Reagents*
- Test fat or oil
- Phenolphthalein
- Distilled water
- Ethyl alcohol
- NaOH

B. *Materials and Equipment*
- Scale
- Burette
- Hot plate
- Dropper
- Beaker (250 mL)
- Graduated cylinder (50 mL)
- Stirring bar
- Chronometer

C. *Procedure (Method 58-15)*
  This method was described in AACC (2000).
  1. Extract the oil from the food sample using the petroleum ether procedure described previously.

2. Weigh approximately 28 g of the oil or fat and place it in a 250 mL beaker.
3. Add 50 mL of ethyl alcohol and a stirring bar.
4. Place beaker on a heated stirring plate and heat until the fat melts and is uniformly dispersed.
5. Add three drops of phenolphthalein indicator.
6. Titrate with 0.1 N sodium hydroxide while stirring until a pale pink color remains for 30 seconds.
7. Calculate the FFA as oleic acid (18:1) using the following formula: % FFA = (mL NaOH) (normality of NaOH) (28.2)/sample weight.

2.6.2 PEROXIDE VALUE AND ACTIVE OXYGEN

The peroxide value is widely used to predict fat deterioration. Peroxides are considered intermediates in the lipid oxidation reaction scheme. Peroxides form after the generation of free radicals in the fatty acid insaturations. These react with iodide ions to form iodine which is titrated with thiosulfate. Peroxide values are expressed in milliequivalents (mEq) of iodine per kilogram of fat. A peroxide value greater than 100 mEq/kg indicates that the fat will have reduced stability in the finished product.

2.6.2.1 Determination of Peroxide Value (Cd 8-53 Method)

This method was described in AOCS (2009).

A. *Samples, Ingredients, and Reagents*
- Test fat or oil
- Iso-octane
- Phenolphthalein
- Distilled water
- Acetic acid
- Saturated potassium iodide solution
- Starch solution

B. *Materials and Equipment*
- Scale
- Burette
- 1 mL graduated pipette
- Dropper
- 250 mL flask
- 50 mL graduated cylinder
- Stirring bar
- Chronometer

C. *Procedure*
1. Extract the fat or oil from the food sample using the petroleum ether procedure described previously.
2. Weigh approximately 10 g of the oil or fat and place it in a 250 mL flask. Add 30 mL of 3:1 acetic acid/iso-octane solution. Then, add 0.5 mL of saturated potassium iodide solution.
3. Swirl contents and allow the solution to stand for exactly 60 seconds. After this 1-minute period, if the solution is very yellow, titrate to a pale yellow before adding the starch solution.

Add 30 mL of distilled water and then 0.5 mL of starch solution.
4. While stirring, titrate with 0.1 N sodium thiosulfate solution until a clear endpoint is reached.
5. Calculate the peroxide value in milliequivalents per kilogram using the following formula: PV = (mL sodium thiosulfate for sample) − (mL sodium thiosulfate for blank) (normality of sodium thiosulfate) (1000)/sample weight.

2.6.2.2 Active Oxygen Stability Method (Procedure Cd 12-57)

The AOM method is an accelerated method of measuring the stability of oils and fats or an indicator of a primary stage of oil oxidation (AOCS 2009). The method consists of bubbling air through the material at a temperature of $97.8°C \pm 0.2°C$ and measuring the peroxide value at intervals or done automatically. The time required for the sample to attain a predetermined peroxide value, usually 100 mEq/kg, is measured. A higher AOM value indicates better quality and stability in a given oil. The test is widely used to determine stability or the induction period of frying oils. It is also known as the Swift stability test.

A. *Samples, Ingredients, and Reagents*
- Different types of oils, shortening, or fats
- Petroleum ether
- Potassium dichromate ($K_2Cr_2O_7$)
- Acetone (reagent grade)
- Reagents of peroxide value (method 2.6.2.1)
- Distilled water
- Sulfuric acid
- Glass wool
- Detergent for cleaning glassware

B. *Materials and Equipment*
- AOM apparatus*
- Pipette (25 mL)
- Hot plate
- Chronometer

C. *Procedure*
1. Place 20 mL of the test oil or fat on the sample tubes. It is recommended to run at least duplicates. For fats, the sample should be melted at a temperature no higher than 10°C above its melting point. Carefully pour the liquid fat or

---

* Consists of a constant temperature bath or heater which will maintain all samples at a temperature of $97.8°C \pm 0.2°C$, an air-distributing manifold calibrated to permit the same flow through each outlet when the total flow is adjusted to 2.33 mL per tube per second, an air purification train consisting of an air inlet tube, air-washing column containing distilled water, an air-washing column consisting of a hydrometer cylinder containing 2% potassium dichromate ($K_2Cr_2O_7$) in 1% sulfuric acid (H_2SO_4), water-cooled condenser, and a wide mouth trap (500 mL bottle containing glass wool), pressure-regulating columns, manifold for air distribution, a source of low-pressure, oil-free compressed air, and a thermometer (temperature to within ±0.1°C in the range of 95–110°C), a gas flow meter, test tubes (25 × 200 mm) provided with a two-hole neoprene stopper, and aeration tube and test tube handling tongs.

oil into the center of the tube to avoid contact with the top of the tube and stopper.

2. Insert the aeration tube and adjust it so that the end of the air delivery tube is 5 cm below the surface of the test sample.

3. Place the tube with sample in a container with boiling water for 5 minutes. After heating, remove the tube from the boiling water, wipe dry, and transfer immediately to the constant temperature heater maintained at $97.8°C \pm 0.2°C$. Connect the aeration tube to the capillary on the manifold, having previously adjusted the air flow rate, and immediately record the starting time.

4. Record the time (to the nearest hour) required for the sample to attain a peroxide value of 100 mEq. The peroxide value is determined according to AOCS Official Method Cd 8-53, with the exception that the sample weight is 1 g instead of 5 g. If this determination indicates that the peroxide value is between 75 mEq and 175 mEq, another peroxide value determination should be made immediately, using a 5-g sample. It is recommended to plot peroxide values at different aeration times because the AOM stability value is the time (in hours) at which a straight line connecting these two points crosses the 100 mEq coordinate. Repeat this procedure on the duplicate sample and report the average of the two observations.

2.6.3 SAPONIFICATION VALUE

The saponification value is defined as the amount of alkali necessary to saponify a given quantity of fat. It is expressed in milligrams of KOH required to saponify 1 g of fat. During this reaction, the neutral fat (mainly triglycerides) breaks down into the FFAs and glycerol; the fatty acids form potassium salts. The saponification value is an index of the average molecular weight of the triglycerides in the sample. The average molecular weight of the fatty acids associated with the triglycerides is obtained by dividing by three. The smaller the saponification value, the longer the fatty acid chain length.

A. Samples, Ingredients, and Reagents
- Different types of fats and oils
- 0.5 M alcoholic KOH
- Phenolphthalein
- Distilled water
- 0.5 M HCl

B. Materials and Equipment
- Analytical scale
- Reflux condenser
- Dispenser or 25 mL pipette
- Chronometer
- Distillation flask
- Burette
- Pipette (5 mL)
- Graduated cylinder (100 mL)

C. Procedure
1. Obtain the fat or oil associated with the food matrix following the crude fat or other related procedure.
2. Weigh 0.75 to 1.25 g of the fat or oil in a distillation flask and add 25 mL of 0.5 M alcoholic KOH. Prepare a blank adding the same solutions but omitting the fat or oil.
3. Heat blank and sample flasks under reflux for 30 minutes.
4. Remove flasks and allow for cooling and equilibration at room temperature.
5. Titrate the remaining KOH with 0.5 M hydrochloric acid using several drops of phenolphthalein as an indicator. Make sure to continuously shake the flask while titrating.
6. Calculate the saponification value using the following equation: $SV = (B - S) \, mL \times 0.5$ or M of $HCl \times 56.1/fat$ weight (g), where B = blank titer and S = sample titer.

2.6.4 IODINE VALUE

The iodine value or number is defined as the amount (in grams) of iodine absorbed by 100 g of the fat or oil and represents the amount of iodine that would react directly with the double bonds of the fat molecules. Thus, it is the most practiced assay to determine the degree of fat instauration. Animal fats rich in saturated fatty acids tend to have low iodine values (26–38 g of iodine/100 g of oil), whereas vegetable oils rich in unsaturated and polyunsaturated fatty acids have iodine values of 129 to 136 g of iodine/100 g of oil. The iodine value is commonly used to follow the hydrogenation process and is closely related to lipid oxidation. The iodine value test consists of first treating the oil or fat with an excess of Wij's solution, which contains iodine monochloride that reacts with the double bonds of the oil molecule. Then, the iodine is liberated from the unreacted Wij's solution by the addition of potassium iodide. Finally, the free iodine is determined by titration with standard sodium thiosulfate.

A. Samples, Ingredients, and Reagents
- Different samples of fats and oils
- Wij's solution (iodine monochloride)
- Carbon tetrachloride
- Starch indicator solution
- Distilled water
- 10% Potassium iodide solution
- 0.25 M sodium thiosulfate

B. Materials and Equipment
- Analytical scale
- Burette
- Pipette (5 mL)
- Graduated cylinder (100 mL)

- Conical flask
- Dispenser or 25 mL pipette
- Chronometer

C. *Procedure*

1. Obtain the fat or oil associated with the food matrix following the crude fat or other related procedure.
2. Weigh 0.2 g to 0.3 g of the fat or oil in a conical flask.
3. Add 10 mL of carbon tetrachloride to the conical flask and dissolve the fat. Then, add 25 mL of Wij's solution. Prepare a blank adding the same solutions but omitting the fat or oil.
4. Mix well and allow samples to stand in the dark for 30 minutes.
5. Add to each flask (sample and blank) 20 mL of potassium iodide solution and 100 mL of distilled water.
6. Titrate the liberated iodine with 0.25 M sodium thiosulfate solution to a pale yellow color, then add 2 mL of the starch solution and continue titration until it is colorless. Make sure to continuously shake the flask while titrating.
7. Calculate the iodine number or value using the following equation: IV = $(B - S) \times 0.03175 \times 100$/fat weight (g), where B = blank titer and S = sample titer.
   Note: 1 mL 0.25 M sodium thiosulfate = 0.03175 g iodine.

2.6.5 Smoke Point

The smoke point is related to the FFA content and the amount of impurities in the oil. A lower smoke point value may indicate reduced oil stability. This is also undesirable in frying and can result in a fire in the fryer.

A. *Samples, Ingredients, and Reagents*
Test fat or oil

B. *Materials and Equipment*
- Metal smoke tin
- Ring stand
- Ruler
- Protective gloves
- 250°C thermometer
- Clamp for thermometer
- Chronometer
- Protective eye lenses

C. *Procedure (Method 58-82)*
This procedure was described in AACC (2000).

1. Place a sufficient amount of the test fat or oil into a clean metal smoke tin. Place tin or cup in a ring stand at a height that allows sufficient room to place the Bunsen burner and its flame.
2. Fasten a thermometer with a clamp so that the bulb is suspended in the fat or oil. Make sure to leave at least a 0.7-cm space between the bottom of the metal tin and the lower end of the thermometer.
3. Wearing protective gloves and lenses, turn on the Bunsen burner and adjust flame and height of the ring stand with the tin so that the temperature increases at a rate of 5°C to 7°C/min. Immediately turn off the burner as soon as you detect a continuous smoke to avoid fire.
4. Register the temperature when the sample gives off a continuous stream of bluish smoke. If you observe a slight puff before the sample begins to smoke continuously, disregard the temperature reading.

2.6.6 Solid Fat Index

The SFI is an empirical value that is derived from the expansion of a fat as a chilled sample is gradually warmed. In the process of melting, previously crystallized parts of the sample become liquefied. Because the fat molecules in a liquid state are less efficiently arranged in space compared with closely packed crystalline regions, liquid fat takes up more volume. Therefore, the degree of expansion is related to the change in the solid content. The SFI indicates a measure of solid fraction in the shortening or margarine at the specific temperatures listed. The 10°C SFI is important for frozen foods whereas the 40°C index is critical for baked goods. SFI results are expressed as melting dilation in milliliters per kilogram of fat. Besides the dilatometry assay, the SFI can be alternatively determined with nuclear magnetic resonance, infrared spectroscopy, and differential scanning calorimetry (Walker and Bosin 1971; Van de Voort et al. 1996).

A. *Samples, Ingredients, and Reagents*
- Different fats and oils
- High vacuum grease (silicone)
- Cement or equivalent
- Potassium dichromate
- Petroleum ether
- Mercury

B. *Materials and Equipment*
- Analytical scale
- Volumetric flask (500 mL)
- Fat dilatometer*
- Springs for dilatometer stoppers
- Thermometers
- Capillary two-way stopcock (2 mm ID)
- Chronometer
- Beakers (50 mL)
- Pipettes (1 mL and 2 mL)
- Dilatometer stopper
- Thermometer clamps

---

* Bulb connected to a precision bore capillary tube (1.400 mL, graduated in 0.005 mL divisions and a 14/20 joint). The C19514/20 stopper is equipped with hooks. Units are numbered serially. Complete with springs (AOCS 2009, method Cd 10-57).

- Several water baths (thermoadjustable)
- Vacuum pump

C. Procedure (Method Cd 10-57 or Method 58-25)

These methods were previously described in AOCS (2009) and AACC (2000).

1. Prepare a 1% potassium dichromate indicator solution. Securely clamp cleaned dilatometer in inverted position and then clamp capillary stopcock in the corresponding place at the end of the dilatometer stem and seal with cement.
2. Immerse tip of stopcock into reservoir of cleaned mercury at room temperature. Using a vacuum pump, draw mercury into the dilatometer stem until calibrated portion is full.
3. Successively withdraw 0.2-mL portions of mercury into tared beaker and record weights.
4. Calculate the true volume in milliliters using the following equation [weight of mercury/(final —initial scale reading)] × specific volume of mercury at room temperature × 1000.
5. Before filling the dilatometer,
   a. Deaerate 50 mL of dichromate indicator solution for 3 minutes at more than 24 mm.
   b. Heat sample to 80°C and deaerate for at least 2 minutes or until no more gas bubbles are observed.
   c. Pipette 2 mL of deaerated indicator into dilatometer bulb. Lubricate stopper lightly with silicone grease and weigh the assembled dilatometer to the nearest 0.01 g.
   d. Carefully overlay indicator with sample and fill until overflowing. Insert stopper so that indicator solution rises to approximately the 1200 mark of the stem. Reading should be 1200 ± 100 at 60°C, if not, repeat procedure.
   e. Wash fat from outer surface of dilatometer with petroleum ether. Attach retaining springs and reweigh dilatometer when solvent has evaporated. Record the fat weight.
6. To standardize thermal expansion, immerse dilatometer to the 300 mark in a water bath adjusted to 60°C and record reading after 15 minutes and then at 5-minute intervals until change is less than two units in 5 minutes. Then, transfer dilatometer to a 37.8°C bath and immerse to the 300 mark. Read level of indicator at 5-minute intervals until change is less than two units in 5 minutes. Record reading.
7. For sample conditioning, transfer dilatometer to 0°C bath and immerse to the 300 mark and hold for 15 minutes. Then, transfer to a 26.7°C bath and hold for 30 minutes and transfer back to 0°C bath and hold for 15 minutes.
8. For measuring sample dilatation, transfer dilatometer from the 0°C batch to a bath at the lowest desired temperature. Immerse to the 300 mark and record reading after 30 minutes. Repeat procedure at the next highest temperature and so on until readings have been obtained at all temperatures.
9. Calculate the SFI at a given temperature using the following equation:

SFI at a given temperature = [total dilation − (thermal expansion) × (60 − observed temperature)].

2.6.7 RESEARCH SUGGESTIONS

1. Evaluate the iodine value, SFI, peroxide value, and active oxygen value of a frying cottonseed oil and a hydrogenated plastic shortening obtained from cottonseed.
2. Evaluate the smoke point, color, fat acidity, peroxide, and active oxygen values of a new deep fat frying oil and after 1, 5, 10, and 15 hours of use.
3. Compare smoke point, fat acidity, peroxide, and active oxygen values of a frying oil with high and low iodine values after 1, 5, 10, and 15 hours of use.
4. Prepare two kinds of groats using the milling procedure described in Chapter 5; the first type obtained after conventional steaming and heat treatment, and the other skipping the heat treatment steps. Compare fat acidity, peroxide, and active oxygen values of the oils associated with the two types of groats.
5. Prepare two kinds of corn chips following the production procedure described in Chapter 12. One lot of *masa* will be fried at 175°C for 1 minute with a high iodine value oil, whereas the other will be fried with a plastic shortening (low iodine value hydrogenated shortening). Compare the organoleptic properties of the resulting chips and fat acidity, peroxide, and active oxygen values after 1 month of storage at room temperature.
6. Compare SFIs of an oil that has been partially and fully hydrogenated into a vegetable shortening. How do the SFI indexes relate to iodine values?

2.6.8 RESEARCH QUESTIONS

1. What does a high vs. a low saponification value tell you about a given oil or fat sample?
2. What does a high vs. a low iodine value tell you about a given oil or fat sample? What is the effect of iodine value to oxidative rancidity?
3. What are the best methods to follow degree of hydrogenation during elaboration of plastic shortenings?
4. Define SFI and explain the practical usefulness of this test. How does it relate to slipping point and iodine values?
5. What is the usefulness of the fat acidity test in snack-frying operations?

6. What methods would be useful in determining the effectiveness of tocopherol and other antioxidants added to an oil?

7. What are the similarities and differences among peroxide value, thiobarbituric or TBA, and hexanal content used to characterize fats/oils content?

8. What methods are useful in determining the effectiveness of antioxidants added to oils?

9. How are saturated, monounsaturated, and polyunsaturated fatty acids determined in a given food sample for nutrition labeling purposes?

10. How are *cis* and *trans* fatty acids determined in a given food sample? Which types of fatty acids are produced during hydrogenation? What are their negative effects on human health?

11. What are the most common methods to determine the efficiency of degumming, neutralization, bleaching, and deodorization of crude oils?

12. What are the most common methods to determine the quality of frying oils in snack food operations?

13. Describe a method used to test rancidity in headspace of packaged snacks.

2.7 METHODS FOR FIBER ANALYSIS

Whole cereal grains are considered as a good source of dietary fiber. From the nutritional and health viewpoints, the importance of dietary fiber and consumption of whole grains has greatly increased during the past decades. Dietary fiber is viewed as therapeutic for people with diabetes, high cholesterol, metabolic syndrome, and gastrointestinal problems. Both insoluble and soluble dietary fibers have positive health benefits. Insoluble fiber increases the peristaltic movement or transit of digested food throughout the gastrointestinal tract, increases fecal bulk, and prevents constipation, hemorrhoids, diverticulosis, and colon cancer. On the other hand, soluble fiber has recently received more attention because it reduces blood cholesterol and lowers any sudden increases in blood glucose levels. Both types of fibers have the ability to bind bile acids decreasing cholesterol. However, it has been documented that insoluble dietary fiber reduces mineral bioavailability. Oats is the cereal that has received more attention because of the quality of its dietary fiber. It is the only cereal grain that has a good ratio between insoluble and soluble fiber. The soluble fiber is particularly rich in β-glucans and arabinoxylans.

The chemical composition of insoluble and soluble dietary fibers differs. The insoluble fiber is mainly formed from cellulose and lignin mainly located in the glumes or husks, pericarp, and endosperm cell walls. Cellulose is the major building block of the cell wall and is usually associated with other structural components such as hemicelluloses and pectin. The cellulose may contain up to 10,000 β1,4-linked glucopyranose units. Unlike the other fibrous components, lignin is not a carbohydrate. It is formed from cinnamyl alcohols which first form phenyl-propane units that by a complex further polymerization form lignin. Lignin is viewed as a three dimensional molecule formed by the aromatic hydroxyohenyl, guaiacyl and springlyl moieties. As cellulose, lignin is the main structural component of plant tissues. It is considered as one of the most resistant molecules found in nature because is extremely resistant to both chemical and enzymatic degradation. The soluble fiber associated with cereals is mainly formed of hemicellulose, arabinoxylans and β-glucans. Hemicellulose is a branched polymer constituted by different sugar moieties (xylose, arabinose, galactose, gluconic acid, and glucose). β-Glucans are glucopyranosil polymers joined by β1–4 or 1–3 bonds. β-Glucans occur in larger amounts in barley and oats. The β-glucans composed entirely of glucose units have an affinity for water and are within the soluble dietary fiber fraction. β-Glucans readily ferment in the hindgut and are considered hypocholesterolemic. On the other hand, the arabinoxylans are heteropolysaccharides consisting predominantly of arabinose and xylose residues. The D-xylopyranose molecules are generally linked by β1–4 bonds, whereas the bonds with L-arabinofuran to carbon 3 or less frequently than carbon 2. They are commonly called pentosans because the polysaccharides are mainly constituted of five-carbon monosaccharides. β-Glucans and pentosans have high affinity for water, therefore, they are commonly known as gums. These are considered as prebiotics (because they readily ferment in the hindgut) and nutraceuticals (because they prevent colon cancer and diabetes). In addition, the hydrolysis of soluble fibers yields organic acids and short-chain volatile fatty acids that are known to inhibit HMG-CoA reductase, which is considered the key hepatic enzyme for endogenous cholesterol synthesis. That is the main reason why soluble dietary fibers are also considered as hypocholesterolemic.

Soluble dietary fiber is not measured in the proximate analysis because crude fiber is the residue obtained after the food sample is subjected to a sequential hydrolyses with acid and alkali (refer to procedure in Section 2.2.5.1). Crude fiber clearly underestimates values when compared with other methods of analysis such as dietary fiber and detergent fiber. The acid and neutral detergent fiber analyses were developed to estimate hemicellulose, cellulose, and lignin of forages (Goering and Van Soest 1970; Van Soest et al. 1991; Undersander et al. 1993; Mertens 1992; Mongeau and Brassard 1979).

The official method of fiber analysis for labeling purposes is the dietary fiber which consists of emulating the passage of the food through the human gastrointestinal tract. Ground samples are treated with proteases and amylases, and washed with solvents to remove protein, starch, and fat-soluble compounds. The residue obtained after filtration is the insoluble fiber, whereas the recovered filtrate that contains the soluble fiber is treated with warm alcohol (Asp and Johansson 1981, 1984; Asp et al. 1983; Asp 2001; Englyst 1981). The alcohol precipitates soluble fibers that are recovered by filtration and gravimetrically measured after oven-drying.

2.7.1 ANALYSIS OF DETERGENT FIBER

The detergent fiber analysis is divided into two assays: acid and neutral detergent fibers. These methods are mainly used to characterize forage and feedstuff. The main advantage is that fiber residues are further analyzed into cellulose, hemicellulose, and lignin. Generally speaking, the detergent fiber analysis is lower than most types of total dietary fiber determinations and significantly higher compared with crude fiber (Goering and Van Soest 1970; Van Soest et al. 1991; Undersander et al. 1993; Mertens 1992; Mongeau and Brassard 1979).

A. Samples, Ingredients, and Reagents
- Sodium lauryl sulfate
- Sodium borate ($Na_2B_4O_7 \cdot 10H_2O$)
- Triethylene glycol, reagent grade
- H_2SO_4 (concentrated)
- Thermoresistant α-amylase
- Silver sulfate
- Silver nitrate
- Cetyl trimethylammonium bromide (CTAB)
- Ethylene diamine tetraacetic acid (EDTA)
- Dibasic sodium phosphate (Na_2HPO_4)
- Sodium sulfide (Na_2SO_3)
- Distilled water
- Potassium permanganate
- Ferric nitrate monohydrate
- 99.0% *Tert*-butanol

Neutral Detergent Solution

Mix 0.99 L of distilled water with 30 g of SDS (sodium lauryl sulfate), 18.61 g of EDTA, 6.81 g of sodium borate decahydrated ($Na_2B_4O_7 \cdot 10H_2O$), 4.56 g of dibasic sodium phosphate (Na_2HPO_4), and 10 mL of triethylene glycol.

Acid Detergent Solution

Prepare 1 L of 1 N H_2SO_4 and add 20 g of cetyl trimethylammonium bromide or CTAB.

B. Materials and Equipment
- Analytical scale
- Magnetic hot plate
- Vacuum trap
- Hood
- 50 mL Gooch equipped with coarse filters
- Manifold
- Vacuum pump
- Air-forced convection oven
- Berzelius beakers (600 mL)
- Tongs

C. Procedure
Neutral Detergent Fiber
1. Place filter gooch in a convection oven set at 100°C for drying until constant weight is achieved. Allow filter gooch to cool down for approximately 30 minutes in a desiccator. Then, record the filter weight with an accuracy of 0.0001 g.
2. Weigh approximately 1 g of dried and ground sample with an accuracy of 0.0001 g and transfer to a beaker.

3. Add 5 mL of α-amylase solution, 75 mL of distilled water, and 20 mL of neutral detergent solution.
4. Set the beaker on a hot plate and adjust heater to a gentle boiling. Allow the solution to hydrolyze for 1 hour.
5. Using protective gloves and goggles or protective lenses, remove the beaker from the hot plate and allow contents to settle for approximately 60 seconds.
6. Place the filter gooch into the filter apparatus equipped with vacuum (Figure 2.3). Then, pour the contents of the beaker into the filter with minimal transfer of the settled material. With hot water, transfer the remaining particles. Apply vacuum only when necessary.
7. Rinse the filter with two consecutive washes of approximately 50 mL of hot water. Apply vacuum if necessary.
8. With the vacuum disconnected, rinse the rim of the funnel with acetone to wash any sample adhering to the sides of the filtering device. Let the acetone stand for approximately 30 seconds and then apply vacuum.
9. With tongs, remove the filtering device and place it in an oven set at 100°C until a constant weight is achieved.
10. Remove the filtering device from the oven, cool it in a desiccator and then weigh with an accuracy of 0.0001 g.
11. Calculate NDF as follows: NDF = [(filter weight with dry fiber residue − empty filter weight)/original sample weight] × 100.

Acid Detergent Fiber
1. Place filter gooch in a convection oven set at 100°C for drying until constant weight is achieved. Allow filter gooch to cool down for approximately 30 minutes in a desiccator. Then, record the filter weight with an accuracy of 0.0001 g.
2. Weigh approximately 1 g of dried and ground sample with an accuracy of 0.0001 g and transfer to a beaker.
3. Add 100 mL of acid detergent fiber solution and place a reflux head on the beaker.
4. Set the beaker on a hot plate and adjust heater to a gentle boiling. Allow the solution to hydrolyze for 1 hour.
5. Using protective gloves and goggles or protective lenses, remove the beaker from the hot plate and allow contents to settle for approximately 60 seconds.
6. Place the filter gooch into the filter apparatus equipped with a vacuum. Then, pour the contents of the beaker into the filter with minimal transfer of the settled material. With hot water, transfer the remaining particles. Apply vacuum only when necessary.

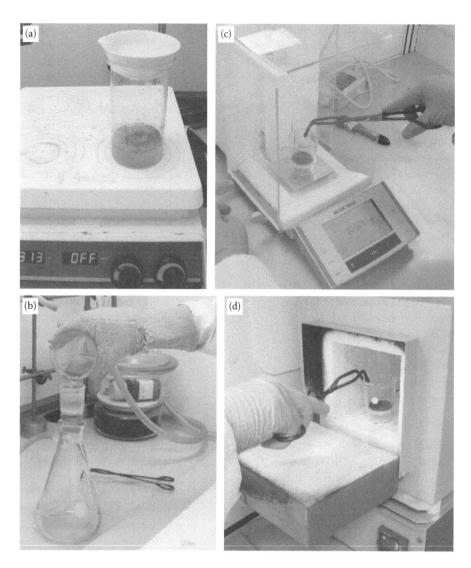

FIGURE 2.3 Detergent fiber analysis of foods. (a) Digestion with detergent solution; (b) filtration of detergent fiber; (c) gravimetric determination of detergent fiber residue; (d) incineration of detergent fiber for ash correction.

7. Rinse the filter with two consecutive washes of approximately 50 mL of hot water. Apply vacuum if necessary.
8. With the vacuum disconnected, rinse the rim of the funnel with acetone to wash any sample adhering to the sides of the filtering device. Let the acetone stand for approximately 30 seconds and then apply vacuum.
9. With tongs, remove the filtering device and place it in an oven set at 100°C until constant weight is achieved.
10. Remove the filtering device from the oven, cool it in a desiccator, and then weigh with an accuracy of 0.0001 g.
11. Calculate ADF as follows:

ADF = [(filter weight with dry fiber residue − empty filter weight)/original sample weight] × 100.

The ADF value may be corrected according to bound protein. The ADF residue is recovered and analyzed for protein content. The protein-corrected ADF value is calculated as follows: corrected ADF = [(% ADF − (protein content of residue/100)].

2.7.2 Dietary Fiber

The standard enzymatic–gravimetric method for the measurement of total dietary fiber (method 985.29, AOAC 2005) includes enzymatic treatments for starch and protein removal, isolation and weighing of the dietary fiber residue. In cereals, the enzymatic removal of starch with α-amylase and amyloglucosidase is an essential step. The method is designed to simulate the digestive process of the small intestine. Protein and ash are determined on the residue and values are corrected. This is the official analytical technique for the estimation of total dietary fiber for labeling purposes.

2.7.2.1 Determination of Total Dietary Fiber

A. *Samples, Ingredients, and Reagents*

- Test samples
- Protease
- NaOH
- Celite (acid washed)
- Acetone
- Aluminum foil
- Desiccant
- Heat-resistant α-amylase (Termamyl)
- Amyloglucosidase
- HCl
- Ethanol
- Phosphate buffer
- Distilled water

B. *Materials and Equipment*

- Analytical scale
- Graduated cylinder (1 L)
- Manifold filtration unit for crucibles
- Air-forced convection oven
- Muffle furnace
- Water bath
- Beakers (400 mL)
- Laboratory mill
- Volumetric flasks (1 L)
- Vacuum pump
- Tongs
- Desiccator
- Thermometer
- Fritted crucibles (coarse porosity)

C. *Procedure*

1. Prepare the following reagents:
   a. 78% and 95% ethanol solutions.
   b. Phosphate buffer. In a volumetric flask, dissolve 1.4 g of anhydrous dibasic sodium phosphate and 9.68 g of monobasic and monohydrated sodium phosphate in approximately 700 mL of distilled water. Then, adjust volume to exactly 1 L with distilled water. The pH should be 6 ± 0.2.
   c. Sodium hydroxide solution (0.275 N). In a 1-L volumetric flask, dissolve 11 g of NaOH in approximately 700 mL of distilled water. Then, adjust volume to exactly 1 L with distilled water.
   d. Hydrochloric acid solution (0.325). Prepare a 1 M HCl acid solution by adding 83.3 mL of concentrated HCl in distilled water to a 1-L volume. Then, in a volumetric flask, mix 325 mL of 1 M HCl with distilled water to exactly 1 L.
2. Place cleaned fritted crucibles for 1 hour in a muffle furnace set at 525°C and after cooling in a desiccator, add 0.5 g celite and dry at 130°C for at least 1 hour. Allow fritted crucible with celite to cool down for approximately 30 minutes in a desiccator. Then, record the filter weight with an accuracy of 0.0001 g. It is recommended that two or three repetitions should be run for each test sample. One will be used to obtain a residue for protein content and the other for ash content.
3. Weigh approximately 1 g of dried and finely ground sample (through a 0.5-mm mesh) with an accuracy of 0.0001 g and transfer to a 400 mL beaker (Figure 2.4). If the sample is rich in fat (contains >10% fat), remove the fat with petroleum ether before milling (refer to procedure in Section 2.2.4.1). Record loss of fat weight and make appropriate corrections to final dietary fiber found after the analysis. Run blank through the entire process.
4. Add 50 mL of phosphate buffer (pH 6) to each beaker and then add 0.1 mL of heat-resistant α-amylase (Termamyl). Cover beaker with aluminum foil and place it in a boiling water bath at 95°C to 100°C. Shake contents at 5-minute intervals for 30 minutes.
5. Cool solution to room temperature, adjust the pH to 7.5 by adding 10 mL of 0.275 N NaOH. Add 5 mg of protease that was previously diluted in phosphate buffer (0.1 mL of a 50 mg protease in 1 mL phosphate buffer). Cover beaker with aluminum foil and incubate for 30 minutes at 60°C with continuous agitation. Cool, and then add 10 mL of 0.325 M HCl. The final pH should be adjusted to 4 to 4.6. Add 0.3 mL of amyloglucosidase and incubate for 30 minutes at 60°C with continuous agitation.
6. Add 280 mL of 95% ethanol preheated to 60°C. After the addition of alcohol, allow contents to cool down for 1 hour at room temperature to enhance the precipitation of the residue.
7. Filter contents through the previously weighed crucible containing the celite. Apply suction until all of the solution passes the filter. Then, wash the residue successively three times with 20 mL of 78% ethanol, twice with 10 mL 95% ethanol, and twice with 10 mL acetone. Apply vacuum during the whole filtering procedure.
8. Dry crucibles with the residue until constant weight is achieved or dry overnight at 105°C. Cool crucibles in a desiccator for 20 to 30 minutes and then weigh to nearest 0.1 mg. Subtract crucible and celite weight of step 1 to calculate the weight of the residue (Figure 2.4).
9. Analyze protein of the residue contained in one of the crucibles and incinerate the other to calculate ash. The protein and ash contents of the residue will be used to correct dietary fiber values. Subtract the protein and ash contents from the residue weight to obtain the dietary fiber weight. Express dietary fiber as a percentage

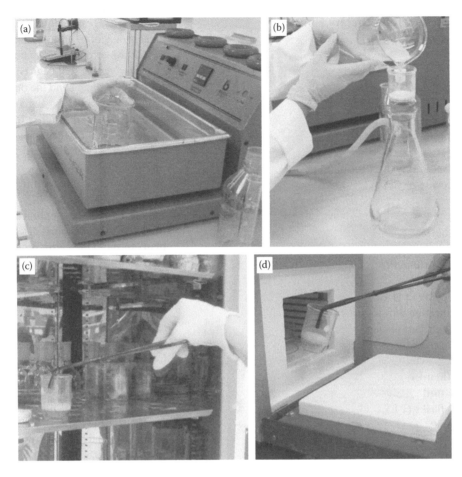

FIGURE 2.4 Dietary fiber analysis of foods. (a) Enzyme hydrolysis; (b) filtration of dietary fiber residue; (c) dehydration of dietary fiber residue; (d) incineration of dietary fiber for ash correction.

using the following equation: % total dietary fiber = (dietary fiber weight/sample weight) × 100. If sample was previously defatted, make sure to correct values according to the original fat content.

2.7.2.2 Determination of Insoluble and Soluble Dietary Fiber

This method was previously described by Asp et al. (1983).

A. *Samples, Ingredients, and Reagents*
- Test samples
- Protease
- NaOH
- Celite (acid washed)
- Acetone
- Aluminum foil
- Desiccant
- Heat-resistant α-amylase (Termamyl)
- Amyloglucosidase
- HCl
- Ethanol
- Phosphate buffer
- Distilled water

B. *Materials and Equipment*
- Analytical scale
- Graduated cylinder (1 L)
- Manifold filtration unit for crucibles
- Air-forced convection oven
- Muffle furnace
- Water bath
- Beakers (400 mL)
- Laboratory mill
- Volumetric flasks (1 L)
- Vacuum pump
- Tongs
- Desiccator
- Thermometer
- Fritted crucibles (coarse porosity)

C. *Procedure*
1. Prepare the following reagents:
   a. 78% and 95% ethanol solutions.
   b. Phosphate buffer. In a volumetric flask, dissolve 1.4 g of anhydrous dibasic sodium phosphate and 9.68 g of monobasic and monohydrated sodium phosphate in approximately 700 mL of distilled water. Then,

adjust volume to exactly 1 L with distilled water. The pH should be 6 ± 0.2.

c. Sodium hydroxide solution (0.275 N). In a 1 L volumetric flask, dissolve 11 g of NaOH in approximately 700 mL of distilled water. Then, adjust volume to exactly 1 L with distilled water.

d. Hydrochloric acid solution (0.325 M). Prepare a 1 M HCl acid solution by adding 83.3 mL of concentrated HCl in distilled water to a 1 L volume. Then, in a 1 L volumetric flask, mix 325 mL of 1 M HCl with distilled water to exactly 1 L.

2. Place cleaned fritted crucibles for 1 hour in a muffle furnace set at 525°C and, after cooling in a desiccator, add 0.5 g celite and dry at 130°C for at least 1 hour. Allow fritted crucible with celite to cool down for approximately 30 minutes in a desiccator. Then, record the filter weight with an accuracy of 0.0001 g. It is recommended that two or three repetitions should be run per test sample. One will be used to obtain a residue for protein content and the other for ash content.

3. Weigh approximately 1 g of dried and finely ground sample (through a 0.5-mm mesh) with an accuracy of 0.0001 g and transfer to a 400 mL beaker. If the sample is rich in fat (contains >10% fat), remove the fat with petroleum ether before milling (refer to procedure in Section 2.2.4.1). Record loss of fat weight and make appropriate corrections to final dietary fiber found after the analysis. Run blank through the entire process.

4. Add 25 mL of phosphate buffer (pH 6) to each beaker and then add 0.1 mL of heat-resistant α-amylase (Termamyl). Cover beaker with aluminum foil and place it in a boiling water bath at 95°C to 100°C for 14 minutes. Make sure to shake contents every 3 to 4 minutes.

5. Cool solution to room temperature, add 20 mL of distilled water and adjust pH to 1.5 with 0.1 N HCl. Then, add 100 mg of pepsin. Cover beaker with aluminum foil and incubate for 60 minutes at 40°C with continuous agitation.

6. Cool and then add 20 mL of distilled water and adjust pH to 6.8 with 0.1 N NaOH. Add 100 mg of pancreatin. Cover beaker with aluminum foil and incubate for 60 minutes at 40°C with continuous agitation.

7. Adjust pH to 4.5 with 0.1 M HCl.

8. Filter contents through the previously weighed crucible containing the celite. Apply suction until all the solution passes the filter. Wash twice with 10 mL distilled water. Make sure to recover all the filtrate for soluble fiber analysis.

9. Then, wash the residue retained by the crucible twice with 10 mL of 95% ethanol and twice with 10 mL acetone. Apply vacuum during the whole filtering procedure.

10. Dry crucibles with the residue until constant weight is achieved or dry overnight at 105°C. Cool crucibles in a desiccator for 20 to 30 minutes and then weigh to the nearest 0.1 mg. Subtract crucible and celite weight to calculate the weight of the insoluble residue.

11. Incinerate the crucible to calculate the ash associated with the residue. Subtract the ash content from the insoluble residue weight to obtain the insoluble dietary fiber weight. Express insoluble dietary fiber as a percentage using the following equation: % insoluble dietary fiber = (dietary fiber weight/sample weight) × 100. If sample was previously defatted, make sure to correct values according to the original fat content.

12. To recover the soluble fiber, the total volume of the filtrate and wash waters of step 8 should be adjusted to exactly 100 mL. Then add 400 mL of warm (60°C) 95% ethanol.

13. Allow soluble fiber to precipitate for 1 hour and then filter the solution through a dried and weighed crucible containing celite. Then, wash the soluble fiber retained by the crucible twice with 10 mL of 78% ethanol, twice with 10 mL of 95% ethanol, and twice with 10 mL of acetone. Apply vacuum during the whole filtering procedure.

14. Dry crucibles with the soluble fiber until constant weight is achieved or dry overnight at 105°C. Cool dry crucibles in a desiccator for 20 to 30 minutes and then weigh to nearest 0.1 mg. Subtract crucible and celite weight to calculate the weight of the soluble residue. Incinerate the crucible to calculate the ash associated with the soluble residue. Subtract the ash content from the soluble residue weight to obtain the soluble dietary fiber weight. Express soluble dietary fiber as a percentage using the following equation: % soluble dietary fiber = (soluble dietary fiber weight/sample weight) × 100. If the sample was previously defatted, make sure to correct values according to the original fat content.

2.7.3 Research Suggestions

1. Determine and compare crude fiber, detergent fiber, and dietary fiber values of a whole wheat bread sample.

2. Determine the acid and neutral detergent fiber and dietary fiber of regular barley and hull-less barley.

3. Determine and compare dietary fiber values of wheat, white-polished rice, and oats.

4. Determine the insoluble and soluble dietary fiber of whole wheat processed into refined flour.

5. Investigate the Englyst-Cummings procedure to determine dietary fiber and compare the method with the official AOAC (2005) dietary fiber procedure.
6. Determine the insoluble and soluble dietary of barley before and after sprouting or malting.

2.7.4 RESEARCH QUESTIONS

1. What are the principles behind fiber determination using the detergent fiber and official dietary fiber procedures?
2. What are the main fiber components associated with crude fiber, acid-detergent fiber, neutral detergent fiber, insoluble dietary fiber, and soluble dietary fiber?
3. Explain the purpose(s) of each of the following steps of the official AOAC (2005) dietary fiber method:
    a. Heating sample with thermoresistant α-amylase
    b. Treating sample with protease
    c. Adding warm ethanol
    d. Washing with acetone
4. Why is resistant starch associated with cereal-based foods considered as part of dietary fiber?
5. Explain the rationale of using bromidic acid in the acid-detergent fiber analysis.
6. What are the positive health effects of the insoluble and soluble fiber components?
7. What are the main chemical components of the soluble dietary fiber of oats or groats? How do these components affect blood cholesterol?

2.8 METHODS FOR NONFIBROUS CARBOHYDRATE ANALYSIS

Nonfibrous carbohydrates are the most abundant components of cereal grains and their products. Approximately 75% of naked caryopses are composed of these carbohydrates. Most of the carbohydrates are constituted by starch considered as an energy reserve or depot. The starch is a polymer of glucose units joined by α1–4 and 1–6 glycosidic bonds stored in granules located within the endosperm. The granules are packed with amylose and amylopectin molecules. Amylose is a linear chain devoid of α1–6 glycosidic bonds. The amylose contains approximately 1500 glucose molecules, and has an average molecular weight of 2.5×10^5. The glucose molecules conforming to amylopectin or branched starch are mainly linked by α1–4 glycosidic bonds but also contain branches that occur when α1–6 bonds forms. Only approximately 4% to 5% of the total glycosidic bonds are α1–6. These glucose polymers have a molecular weight of 10^8 (600,000 glucose units/amylopectin molecule) and are structurally divided into type A, B, and C chains.

Amylose and amylopectin are packed inside the starch granule in such a way that this structure shows crystallinity and concentric circles when viewed under the microscope. The crystallinity is clearly observed when native starch granules are viewed under the microscope equipped with polarized filters

(refer to Chapter 6). The presence of a Maltese cross or birefringence indicates that the granule is native or undamaged. When the starch granules gelatinize due to heat treatment or undergoes mechanical or enzymatic damage, it loses birefringence and is considered gelatinized. The gelatinization phenomena is critically important for most processes because it affects processing, product quality, water absorption, and shelf life.

The starch of most cereals contain 75% amylopectin and 25% amylose. However, some cereals such as maize, wheat, rice, barley, and sorghum can contain from 95% up to 100% amylopectin and therefore are almost amylose-free. These prototypes are termed waxy because their endosperm acquires this appearance when viewed with the naked eye. Waxy cereals and their starches have special industrial uses because they are less prone to retrogradation. When starch is enzymatically degraded during beer mashing, syrup or alcohol production yields several types of simpler sugars such as glucose, maltose, maltotriose, and dextrins. The further conversion of glucose into fructose is also widely used by the industry to produce an array of fructose-containing syrups. The presence and relative amounts of these carbohydrates affect viscosity and sweetness of syrups.

Mature cereal grains contain less than 2% of monosaccharides, disaccharides, and oligosaccharides. Most of these soluble sugars are located in the germ tissue. Fructose, glucose, and sucrose are the soluble carbohydrates present in the highest amounts. The quantities of these sugars significantly increase when the grain is malted or germinated due to the enzymatic hydrolysis of starch and even some fiber components. The main soluble sugars present in malted cereals are maltose, glucose, maltotriose, and linear and branched dextrins.

The most common analytical techniques to estimate the amount of nonfibrous carbohydrates are total starch, glucose, and various assays aimed toward the estimation of reducing sugars. The analysis of the amount of specific carbohydrates is usually performed in an HPLC system equipped with a refractive index detector.

2.8.1 DETERMINATION OF TOTAL STARCH

Starch is the most important polysaccharide in cereals. It is composed of amylose and amylopectin, molecules that are tightly organized within starch granules. Most starches are quantified by analytical techniques that hydrolyze starch components into simple sugars. There are basically two ways to hydrolyze the molecules—with amylolytic enzymes or with chemical reagents. The resulting sugars (generally glucose) are, in most instances, colorimetrically assayed.

The anthrone starch assay consists of first treating the ground sample with 80% alcohol to remove sugars and then starch is extracted with perchloric acid. Under these hot, acidic conditions, the starch is hydrolyzed to glucose and dehydrated to hydroxymethyl furfural. This compound forms a green-colored product with anthrone that is read in the spectrophotometer.

Most starch is determined with the enzymatic method in which the sample is hydrolyzed with amylase and amyloglucosidase to completely hydrolyze into glucose. The resulting glucose is colorimetrically assayed and converted to starch.

2.8.1.1 Determination of Total Starch with the Anthrone Assay

A. Samples, Ingredients, and Reagent
- Test samples
- Anthrone
- Ethanol
- Glucose (reagent grade)
- Distilled water
- Sulfuric acid
- Perchloric acid

B. Materials and Equipment
- Analytical scale
- Water bath (100°C)
- Pipettes (0.1 mL and 1 mL)
- Stirrer
- Thermometer
- Spectrophotometer
- Volumetric flask (100 mL)
- Test tubes
- Cuvettes
- Chronometer

C. Procedure
1. Reagent preparation:
   a. Anthrone reagent: dissolve 200 mg anthrone in 100 mL of ice-cold 95% sulfuric acid.
   b. Standard stock glucose solution: dissolve 100 mg of glucose in 100 mL of water.
2. Weigh 0.1 g to 0.5 g of the sample and place sample in 5 mL hot 80% ethanol to remove sugars. Centrifuge and retain the residue. Wash the residue repeatedly with hot 80% ethanol until the washings do not give color with the anthrone reagent. Dry the residue well over a water bath at 100°C.
3. To the residue, add 5.0 mL of water and 6.5 mL of 52% perchloric acid and allow contents to react for 20 minutes at 0°C. Centrifuge and decant and save the supernatant.
4. Repeat the extraction using fresh perchloric acid. Centrifuge and pool the supernatants and make up to 100 mL in a volumetric flask.
5. Pipette out 0.1 mL or 0.2 mL of the supernatant and make up the volume to 1 mL with water.
6. Prepare the working standard by diluting 10 mL of the stock glucose solution to 100 mL of distilled water. Prepare the standards by taking 0.2, 0.4, 0.6, 0.8, and 1 mL of the working standard and make up the volume to 1 mL in each tube with distilled water.
7. Add 4 mL of anthrone reagent to each tube, stir and heat content for 8 minutes in a boiling water bath.

8. Cool rapidly, place sample in a cuvette and read the intensity of green coloration in a spectrophotometer set at 630 nm.
9. Find out the glucose content in the sample using the standard graph. Multiply the value by a factor 0.9 to arrive at the starch content.

2.8.1.2 Determination of Total Starch with the Enzymatic Method (Method 76-11)

This method was previously described by AACC (2000).

A. Samples, Ingredients, and Reagents
- Test samples
- Glucoamylase (30 IU/mL)
- Anhydrous sodium acetate
- Trihydroxymethylaminomethane
- Phosphoric acid
- Peroxidase (type I)
- Sulfuric acid
- Distilled water
- Glacial acetic acid
- Glucose (reagent grade)
- $NaH_2PO_4 \cdot H_2O$
- Glucose oxidase (type II)
- *o*-Dianisidine dihydrochloride
- Filter paper

B. Materials and Equipment
- Analytical scale
- Autoclave
- Cuvettes
- Water bath with shaker
- Pipettes (1 mL, 5 mL, and 25 mL)
- Volumetric flasks (1 L)
- Funnel
- Thermometer
- Laboratory mill
- Spectrophotometer
- pH meter
- Erlenmeyer flasks (100 mL and 250 mL)
- Test tubes
- Graduated cylinders
- Test tube shaker
- Chronometer

C. Procedure
1. Prepare the following reagents:
   a. Acetate buffer 4 M (pH 4.8). In a volumetric flask, place 120 mL of glacial acetic acid and 164 g of anhydrous sodium acetate and dissolve with distilled water to exactly 1 L.
   b. Tris phosphate buffer. Dissolve 36.3 g of trihydroxymethylaminomethane (Tris) and 50 g of $NaH_2PO_4 \cdot H_2O$ in 500 mL of water. Adjust pH to 7 with phosphoric acid at 37°C before bringing to 1 L with distilled water.
   c. Enzyme buffer chromogen mixture. In 100 mL of tris phosphate buffer, dissolve 30 mg of glucose oxidase (type II), 3 mg of peroxidase (type I), and 10 mg of *o*-dianisidine

dihydrochloride. Disperse the *o*-dianisidine dihydrochloride completely in a small amount of buffer before combining with the rest of the enzyme buffer mixture.

    d. 18 N H_2SO_4 solution. Carefully add 50 mL of concentrated H_2SO_4 to a volumetric flask containing 50 mL of distilled water. If necessary, adjust volume to the 100 mL mark.

    e. Standard glucose solution. Dissolve 400 mg of anhydrous reagent grade glucose in 1 L of distilled water.

2. Determine the moisture content of the test sample. Then, weigh approximately 0.5 g of finely ground sample (through a 0.5-mm mesh) with an accuracy of 0.0001 g and transfer to a dried and tared Erlenmeyer flask.

3. Add 25 mL of distilled water with stirring to disperse the sample and, if necessary, adjust pH between 5 and 7.

4. Heat the suspension to 100°C for 3 minutes with gentle stirring. Then, place sample in an autoclave for pressure-heating at 135°C for 1 hour.

5. Remove flask from autoclave and, when the temperature drops to 55°C, add 2.5 mL of acetate buffer and sufficient water to adjust total weight to 45 g ± 1 g.

6. Place flask in water bath adjusted to 55°C and add 5 mL of the glucoamylase solution.

7. Hydrolyze for 2 hours under continuous shaking.

8. Filter through folded filter paper into a 250 mL flask and, with distilled water, bring to the 250 mL mark.

9. Transfer 1 mL aliquots to test tubes and add 2 mL of enzyme buffer chromogen mixture, shake tubes and place in the dark at 37°C for exactly 30 minutes to develop color.

10. Stop reaction with 2 mL of 18 N H_2SO_4 and measure absorbance in a spectrophotometer set at 540 nm.

11. Prepare the standard glucose curve from 0 (blank) to 60 µg/mL for each series of analysis.

12. Calculate the percentage of starch using the following equation:

$$\% \text{ starch} = 2.25 \times \frac{\text{(weight in micrograms of glucose obtained from standard curve)}}{\text{(volume of aliquot from 250 mL flask} \times \text{sample weight in g} \times \% \text{ dry matter of test sample)}}.$$

2.8.1.3 Determination of Enzyme-Susceptible Starch

The enzyme-susceptible starch assay gives an indication of the susceptibility of the starch to amyloglucosidase and is closely related to the degree of starch gelatinization. High values indicate a higher susceptibility of the starch to amyloglucosidase. This assay is used to estimate the degree of cooking and gelatinization.

A. *Samples, Ingredients, and Reagents*
- Test samples
- Glucoamylase (30 IU/mL)
- Anhydrous sodium acetate
- Trihydroxymethylaminomethane
- Phosphoric acid
- Peroxidase (type I)
- Sulfuric acid
- Distilled water
- Glacial acetic acid
- Glucose (reagent grade)
- $NaH_2PO_4 \cdot H_2O$
- Glucose oxidase (type II)
- *o*-Dianisidine dihydrochloride
- Filter paper

B. *Materials and Equipment*
- Analytical scale
- Spectrophotometer
- Cuvettes
- Water bath with shaker
- Pipettes (1 mL, 5 mL, and 25 mL)
- Volumetric flasks (1 L)
- Funnel
- Chronometer
- Laboratory mill
- Thermometer
- pH meter
- Erlenmeyer flasks (100 mL and 250 mL)
- Test tubes
- Graduated cylinders
- Test tube shaker

C. *Procedure*
1. Prepare the following reagents:

    a. Acetate buffer 4 M (pH 4.8). In a volumetric flask, place 120 mL of glacial acetic acid and 164 g of anhydrous sodium acetate and dissolve with distilled water to exactly 1 L.

    b. Tris phosphate buffer. Dissolve 36.3 g of trihydroxymethylaminomethane (Tris) and 50 g of $NaH_2PO_4 \cdot H_2O$ in 500 mL of water. Adjust pH to 7 with phosphoric acid at 37°C before bringing to 1 L with distilled water.

    c. Enzyme buffer chromogen mixture. In 100 mL of tris phosphate buffer, dissolve 30 mg glucose oxidase (type II) 3 mg peroxidase (type I) and 10 mg of *o*-dianisidine dihydrochloride. Disperse the *o*-dianisidine dihydrochloride completely in a small amount of buffer before combining with the rest of the enzyme buffer mixture.

    d. 18 N H_2SO_4 solution. Carefully add 50 mL of concentrated H_2SO_4 to a volumetric flask containing 50 mL of distilled water. If necessary, adjust volume to the 100 mL mark.

    e. Standard glucose solution. Dissolve 400 mg of anhydrous reagent grade glucose in 1 L of distilled water.

2. Determine the moisture content of the test sample. Then, weigh approximately 0.5 g of finely ground sample (through a 0.5-mm mesh) with an accuracy of 0.0001 g and transfer to a dried and tared Erlenmeyer flask.

3. Add 25 mL of distilled water, with stirring, to disperse the sample and, if necessary, adjust pH between 5 and 7. Then, add 2.5 mL of acetate buffer and sufficient water to adjust total weight to 45 g ± 1 g.

4. Place flask in water bath adjusted to 55°C and add 5 mL of the glucoamylase solution.

5. Hydrolyze for 2 hours under continuous shaking.

6. Filter through folded filter paper into a 250 mL flask and, with distilled water, bring to the 250 mL mark.

7. Transfer 1 mL aliquots to test tubes and add 2 mL of enzyme buffer chromogen mixture, shake tubes and place in the dark at 37°C for exactly 30 minutes to develop color.

8. Stop reaction with 2 mL 18 N H_2SO_4 and measure absorbance in a spectrophotometer set at 540 nm.

9. Prepare the standard glucose curve from 0 (blank) to 60 μg/mL for each series of analysis.

10. Express enzyme-susceptible starch values as milligrams of glucose per gram of starch (refer to procedure in Section 2.8.1.2).

2.8.1.4 Determination of Damaged Starch (Method 76-30A)

This method determines the percentage of starch granules in flour or starch preparations that are susceptible to hydrolysis with α-amylase (AACC 2000). The percentage of starch damage is directly related to the amount of reducing sugars after enzymatic hydrolysis.

A. Samples, Ingredients, and Reagents
- Test samples
- α-Amylase (*Asp. oryzeae* 50–100 U/mg)
- Anhydrous sodium acetate
- Whatman filter paper no. 4
- Sulfuric acid
- Distilled water
- Glacial acetic acid
- Coarse filter paper
- Sodium tungstate ($Na_2WO_4 \cdot 2\,H_2O$)

B. Materials and Equipment
- Analytical scale
- Spectrophotometer
- Cuvettes
- Water bath with shaker
- Pipettes (1 mL, 5 mL, and 25 mL)
- Volumetric flasks (1 L)
- Funnels
- Glass rod with rubber policeman
- Chronometer
- Laboratory mill
- Thermometer
- pH meter
- Erlenmeyer flasks (100 mL and 250 mL)
- Test tubes
- Graduated cylinders
- Coarse filter paper
- Test tubes

C. Procedure
1. Prepare the following reagents:
   a. Acetate buffer (pH 4.6–4.8). In a volumetric flask, place 4.1 g of anhydrous sodium acetate and 3 mL to 1 L with distilled deionized water.
   b. Sodium tungstate solution. Dissolve 12 g of $Na_2WO_4 \cdot 2H_2O$ in 100 mL water.
   c. H_2SO_4 solution (3.68 N). Carefully add 100 mL of concentrated H_2SO_4 to a 1 L volumetric flask containing 700 mL of distilled water. Then, dilute with distilled water to the 1-L mark.
   d. α-Amylase solution. Dissolve 125,000 units of enzyme in 450 mL of acetate buffer (refer to step 1a). Filter the solution through coarse filter paper.

2. Determine the moisture content of the test sample. Then, weigh approximately 1 g of finely ground sample (through a 0.5-mm mesh) with an accuracy of 0.0001 g and transfer to a 125 mL Erlenmeyer flask. Add exactly 45 mL of the α-amylase solution tempered to 5°C to 30°C. With the glass rod, obtain a uniform suspension and then incubate contents in a water bath set at 30°C for exactly 15 minutes.

3. Add 3 mL of the 3.68 N sulfuric acid solution of step 1c and 2 mL of the sodium tungstate solution (step 1b). Immediately mix contents and let stand for 2 minutes and filter through a no. 4 Whatman filter paper. Discard the first 10 drops of the filtrate.

4. Prepare a blank following the same procedure except for the addition of the sample.

5. Pipette 5 mL of the filtrate into a test tube and determine the amount of reducing sugars (refer to procedures in Sections 2.8.5.1 or 2.8.5.2).

6. Subtract the blank from the sample and multiply by 5 to obtain the amount (in milligrams) of maltose per 10 g of sample because a 1.50 dilution was used in this procedure. Convert the amount of maltose to the amount of starch (in milligrams) hydrolyzed per 10 g by multiplication of 1.64.

2.8.2 Determination of Amylose

Starch is composed of two components, that is, amylose and amylopectin. Amylose is a linear or nonbranched polymer of glucose. The glucose units are joined by $\alpha 1$–4 glucosidic linkages. Amylose exists in coiled form and each coil contains six glucose residues. The iodine is adsorbed within the helical coils of amylose to produce a blue-colored complex which is measured colorimetrically in a spectrophotometer.

2.8.2.1 Determination of Amylose and Amylopectin

A. *Samples, Ingredients, and Reagents*
- Test samples
- Sodium hydroxide
- Ethanol
- Iodine
- Amylose (reagent grade)
- Distilled water
- Hydrochloric acid (HCl)
- 0.1% Phenolphthalein
- Potassium iodide (KI)

B. *Materials and Equipment*
- Analytical scale
- Water bath (100°C)
- Pipettes (0.1 mL and 1 mL)
- Stirrer
- Thermometer
- Spectrophotometer
- Volumetric flask (100 mL)
- Test tubes
- Cuvettes
- Chronometer

C. *Procedure*
1. Prepare the following reagents:
   a. Iodine reagent. Dissolve 1 g of iodine and 10 g of potassium iodide in distilled water and make up to 500 mL.
   b. Standard stock solution. Dissolve 100 mg of amylose in 10 mL 1 N NaOH and make up to 100 mL with distilled water.
2. Weigh 100 mg of the ground sample and add 1 mL of distilled ethanol. Then, add 10 mL of 1 N NaOH and leave it overnight. Alternatively, heat the solution for 10 minutes in a boiling water bath instead of the overnight dissolution.
3. Transfer the solution to a 100 mL flask and make up the volume.
4. Take 2.5 mL of the extract, add 20 mL of distilled water and three drops of 0.1% phenolphthalein.
5. Add 0.1 N HCl drop by drop until the pink color disappears.
6. Add 1 mL of iodine reagent and make up the volume to 50 mL and read the color in a spectrophotometer set at 590 nm.
7. Take 0.2, 0.4, 0.6, 0.8, and 1 mL of the standard amylose solution and develop the color as in the case of the sample.
8. Calculate the amount of amylose present in the sample using the standard graph.
9. Dilute 1 mL of iodine reagent to 50 mL with distilled water for a blank.

10. Absorbance corresponds to 2.5 mL of the test solution: % amylose = x mg amylose/100 mL = $x/2.5 \times 100$ mg amylose.
11. Estimate the amount of amylopectin by subtracting the amylose content from that of total starch.

2.8.3 DETERMINATION OF RESISTANT STARCH

By definition, resistant starch is that portion of the carbohydrate that is not broken down by human enzymes in the small intestine and therefore reaches the hindgut where it is partially or totally fermented. Resistant starch is now considered to be part of dietary fiber. Any method used to measure resistant starch must give values in-line with those obtained from patients with an ileostomy. In recent years, several methods for the measurement of resistant starch have been developed (Englyst et al. 1992; Champ et al. 1999, 2000; Goñi et al. 1996; McCleary and Monaghan 2002; McCleary et al. 2002; AOAC 2005, Method 2002.02). The general steps to obtaining resistant starch are incubation with α-amylase and amyloglucosidase to remove enzyme-prone starch. The resistant starch is recovered and then completely hydrolyzed to glucose that is colorimetrically quantified (Megazyme 2011).

2.8.3.1 Determination of Resistant Starch

The official procedure (AOAC 2005, Method 2002.02; AACC 2000, Method 32-40) for the determination of resistant starch is based on the principle that samples are incubated with pancreatic α-amylase and amyloglucosidase for 16 hours at 37°C. During hydrolysis, the nonresistant starch is solubilized and hydrolyzed into glucose. The reaction is terminated by the addition of an equal volume of ethanol or industrially methylated spirits (IMS, denatured ethanol), and resistant starch is recovered as a pellet after centrifugation. The pellet containing the resistant starch is then washed twice by suspension in aqueous IMS or ethanol (50% v/v), followed by centrifugation. Free liquid is removed by decantation. Resistant starch in the pellet is dissolved in 2 M KOH by vigorously stirring in an ice-water bath over a magnetic stirrer. This solution is neutralized with acetate buffer and the starch is quantitatively hydrolyzed to glucose with amyloglucosidase. Glucose associated with the resistant starch is measured with the glucose oxidase/peroxidase reagent (GOPOD; Megazyme 2011).

A. *Samples, Ingredients, and Reagents*
- Test samples
- Ice
- Megazyme reagents
  a. Pancreatic α-amylase (10 g pancreatin and 3 ceralpha units/mg). Store dry at 4°C. Stable for more than 3 years.
  b. Amyloglucosidase (12 mL, 3300 units/mL). Store at 4°C. Stable for more than 3 years.
  c. GOPOD (for 1 L). Reagent concentrations after dissolution in buffer: glucose oxidase >12,000 U/L, peroxidase >650 U/L, and 0.4

mM 4-aminoantipyrine. The reagent is stable at −20°C for more than 3 years.

d. Glucose reagent buffer (concentrate; 50 mL). Stable at 4°C for more than 3 years. Before use, dilute the entire contents to 1 L with distilled water to yield the GOPOD. Divide the GOPOD reagent into aliquots of desired volume for storage. The stability is 2 to 3 months at 4°C or more than 2 years at −20°C.

e. Glucose standard solution (1 mg/mL in 0.2% benzoic acid). Stable at room temperature for more than 5 years.

f. Resistant starch control (with known level of resistant starch). It is stable for more than 5 years at room temperature.

B. *Materials and Equipment*
- Analytical balance
- Pipette
- Test tubes
- Water bath
- Magnetic stirrer
- pH Meter
- Spectrophotometer
- Positive displacement pipette (2–4 mL)
- Glass test tubes (16 × 100 mm, 14 mL capacity)
- Volumetric flasks (0.1, 0.2, 0.5, 1, and 2 L)
- Laboratory grinding mill
- Centrifuge (test tubes)
- Shaking water bath
- Vortex mixer
- Magnetic stirrer bars
- Stop-clock timer
- Cuvettes
- Culture tubes with screw cap
- Ice chest to hold test-tube rack
- Thermometer

C. *Procedure*
1. Prepare the following reagents:
   a. Sodium maleate buffer (0.1 M, pH 6.0). Dissolve 23.2 g maleic acid in 1600 mL distilled water and adjust the pH to 6.0 with 4 M (160 g/l L) sodium hydroxide. Add 0.6 g of calcium chloride ($CaCl_2 \cdot 2H_2O$) and 0.4 g of sodium azide and adjust the volume to 2 L. Stable at 4°C for 12 months.
   b. Sodium acetate buffer (1.2 M, pH 3.8). Add 69.6 mL of glacial acetic acid to 800 mL of distilled water and adjust to pH 3.8 using 4 M sodium hydroxide. Adjust the volume to 1 L with distilled water. Stable at room temperature for 12 months.
   c. Sodium acetate buffer (100 mM, pH 4.5). Add 5.8 mL of glacial acetic acid to 900 mL of distilled water and adjust to pH 4.5 using 4 M sodium hydroxide. Adjust the volume to 1 L with distilled water. Stable at 4°C for 2 months.

d. Potassium hydroxide (2 M). Add 112.2 g KOH to 900 mL of deionized water and dissolve by stirring. Adjust volume to 1 L.

e. Aqueous IMS. Approximately 50% v/v. Dilute 500 mL of ethanol (95% or 99%) or IMS denatured ethanol (~95% ethanol plus 5% methanol) to 1 L with distilled water.

f. Amyloglucosidase (AMG) stock solution. 12 mL, 3300 U/mL in 50% glycerol. Solution is viscous; thus, for dispensing, use positive displacement dispenser. AMG solution is stable for up to 5 years when stored at 4°C (Note: one unit [U] of enzyme activity is the amount of enzyme required to release 1 μM of glucose from soluble starch per minute at 40°C and pH 4.5).

g. Dilute amyloglucosidase solution (300 U/mL). Dilute 2 mL of concentrated AMG solution to 22 mL with 0.1 M sodium maleate buffer (pH 6.0). Divide into 5-mL aliquots and store frozen in polypropylene containers between uses. Stable to repeated freeze–thaw cycles, and for more than 5 years at −20°C.

h. Pancreatic α-amylase (10 mg/mL) plus AMG (3 U/mL). Immediately before use, suspend 1 g of pancreatic α-amylase in 100 mL of sodium maleate buffer and stir for 5 minutes. Add 1.0 mL of AMG (300 U/mL) and mix well. Centrifuge at 1500 *g* for 10 minutes and carefully decant the supernatant. This solution should be used on the day of preparation.

i. Glucose oxidase–peroxidase–aminoantipyrine reagent (GOPOD). Prepare the GOPOD mixture by diluting 50 mL of buffer concentrate to 1.0 L. Use part of this diluted buffer to dissolve the entire contents of the vial containing the freeze-dried glucose oxidase–peroxidase–aminoantipyrine mixture. Quantitatively transfer the contents of the vial to a 1-L volumetric flask containing diluted buffer. This mixture contains at least 12,000 U/L of glucose oxidase, 650 U/L of peroxidase, and 0.4 mM of 4-aminoantipyrine. The reagent is stable for 2 to 3 months when stored at 4°C and at least 2 years when stored at −20°C.

j. Preparation of additional buffer concentrate. Dissolve 136 g of potassium dihydrogen orthophosphate, 42 g of sodium hydroxide, and 30 g of 4-hydroxybenzoic acid in 900 mL of distilled water. Adjust to pH 7.4 with either 2 M HCl or 2 M NaOH. Dilute the solution to 1 L and add 0.4 g of sodium azide and mix well until dissolved. Buffer concentrate is stable for up to 3 years at 4°C. Check color formation and stability of glucose oxidase–peroxidase–aminoantipyrine buffer mixture by incubating 3.0 mL of the GOPOD mixture with 0.1 mL of glucose standard (1 mg/mL in 0.2% benzoic acid solution) plus 0.1 mL of 0.1 M sodium acetate buffer. Maximum color formation should be achieved within 20 minutes and should be stable for at least 60 minutes.

2. Grind approximately 50 g of the grain or food sample using a laboratory grinding mill to pass a 1.0-mm sieve. Determine moisture content of the sample.

3. Accurately weigh a 100 mg ± 5 mg sample directly into each screw cap tube and gently tap the tube to ensure that the sample falls to the bottom. Add 4.0 mL of pancreatic α-amylase (10 mg/mL) containing AMG (3 U/mL) to each tube. Tightly cap the tubes, mix them on a vortex mixer and attach them horizontally in a shaking water bath aligned to the direction of motion.

4. Incubate tube contents at 37°C with continuous shaking (200 strokes/min) for exactly 16 hours.

5. Remove the tubes from the water bath and remove excess surface water with paper towel. Remove the tube caps and treat the contents with 4.0 mL of ethanol (99%) or IMS (99%) with vigorous stirring on a vortex mixer.

6. Centrifuge the tubes at 1500 g (~3000 rpm) for 10 minutes (noncapped).

7. Carefully decant supernatants and resuspend the pellets in 2 mL of 50% ethanol or IMS with vigorous stirring on a vortex mixer. Add a further 6 mL of 50% IMS, mix the tubes and centrifuge again at 1500 g for 10 minutes. Decant the supernatants and repeat this suspension and centrifugation step once more and then carefully decant the supernatants and invert the tubes on absorbent paper to drain excess liquid.

8. Add a magnetic stirrer bar and 2 mL of 2 M KOH to each tube and resuspend the pellet containing the resistant starch by stirring for approximately 20 minutes in an ice/water bath over a magnetic stirrer.

9. Add 8 mL of 1.2 M sodium acetate buffer (pH 3.8) to each tube with stirring on the magnetic stirrer. Immediately add 0.1 mL of AMG (3300 U/mL), mix well and place the tubes in a water bath at 50°C. Incubate the tubes for 30 minutes with intermittent mixing on a vortex mixer.

10. For samples containing more than 10% resistant starch content, quantitatively transfer the contents of the tube to a 100 mL volumetric flask (using a water wash bottle). Use an external magnet to retain the stirrer bar in the tube while washing the solution from the tube with the water wash bottle. Adjust to 100 mL with water and mix well. Centrifuge an aliquot of the solution at 1500 g for 10 minutes.

11. For samples containing less than 10% resistant starch content directly centrifuge the tubes at 1500 g for 10 minutes (no dilution). For such samples, the final volume in the tube is approximately 10.3 mL.

12. Transfer 0.1 mL aliquots (in duplicate) of either the diluted or undiluted supernatants into glass test tubes (16 mm × 100 mm), treat with 3.0 mL of GOPOD reagent and incubate at 50°C for 20 minutes.

13. Measure the absorbance of each solution at 510 nm against the reagent blank. The reagent blank solution is prepared by mixing 0.1 mL of 0.1 M sodium acetate buffer (pH 4.5) and 3.0 mL of GOPOD reagent. In addition, prepare at least three glucose standards by mixing 0.1 mL of glucose (1 mg/mL) and 3.0 mL of GOPOD reagent.

14. Calculate resistant starch (RS) in test samples as follows:
resistant starch (g/100 g sample) (samples containing >10% RS):

$$= \Delta E \times F \times 100/0.1 \times 1/1000 \times 100/W \times 162/180$$
$$= \Delta E \times F/W \times 90.$$

resistant starch (g/100 g sample) (samples containing <10% RS):

$$= \Delta E \times F \times 10.3/0.1 \times 1/1000 \times 100/W \times 162/180$$
$$= \Delta E \times F/W \times 9.27.$$

where ΔE = absorbance (reaction) read against the reagent blank; F = conversion from absorbance to micrograms (the absorbance obtained for 100 μg of glucose in the GOPOD reaction is determined and F = 100 (μg of glucose) divided by the GOPOD absorbance for 100 μg of glucose; 100/0.1 = volume correction (0.1 mL taken from 100 mL); 1/1000 = conversion from micrograms to milligrams; W = dry weight of sample analyzed = "as is" weight × (100 − moisture content)/100]; 100/W = factor to present resistant starch as a percentage of sample weight; 162/180 = factor to convert from free glucose, as determined, to anhydro-glucose as occurs in starch; 10.3/0.1 = volume correction (0.1 mL taken from 10.3 mL) for samples containing 0% to 10% resistant starch where the incubation solution is not diluted and the final volume is approximately 10.3 mL.

2.8.4 Determination of Total Sugars

It is sometimes necessary to quantify the amount of sugar in a certain medium. Whether the sugar is in the presence of various salts or protein residues, or attached to a polymer, the phenol-sulfuric acid assay can be performed. With the exception of certain deoxysugars, the method is very general, and can be applied for reducing and nonreducing sugars and many other classes of carbohydrates including oligosaccharides. Determination of sugars using phenol-sulfuric acid is based on the absorbance at 490 nm of a colored aromatic complex formed between phenol and the carbohydrate. The amount of sugar present is determined by comparison with a calibration curve using a spectrophotometer. Under the proper conditions, the phenol-sulfuric acid method is accurate to ±2%. If a spectrophotometer is not available, the method can be performed qualitatively by direct visual comparison with colored samples of known concentration. In hot acidic medium, glucose is dehydrated to hydroxymethyl furfural. This forms a green-colored product with phenol and has absorption maximum at 490 nm.

2.8.4.1　Determination of Total Sugars (Phenol Method)

A. *Samples, Ingredients, and Reagents*
- Test samples
- Hydrochloric acid (HCl)
- Sulfuric acid (H_2SO_4 96% reagent grade)
- Sodium carbonate (Na_2CO_3)
- Distilled water
- Phenol (reagent grade)
- Anhydrous sodium sulfate

B. *Materials and Equipment*
- Analytical scale
- Water bath (100°C)
- Volumetric flask (100 mL and 1 L)
- Pipettes (0.1 mL and 1 mL)
- Stirrer
- Incubator (37°C)
- Chronometer
- Spectrophotometer
- Centrifuge
- Beaker (1 L)
- Test tubes
- Cuvettes
- Thermometer

C. *Procedure*
1. Reagent preparation
   a. Prepare the 5% phenol solution by mixing 50 g of reagent-grade phenol dissolved in water and diluted to 1 L.
   b. Prepare the stock standard glucose solution by mixing 100 mg of glucose in 100 mL of distilled water. Then prepare the working standard solution by diluting 10 mL of stock to 100 mL of distilled water (100 μg/mL).
2. Weigh 100 mg of the sample into a boiling tube.
3. Place tube with sample in a boiling water bath for 3 hours with 5 mL of 2.5 N HCl and cool to room temperature.
4. Neutralize solution with solid sodium carbonate until the effervescence ceases. Make up the volume to 100 mL and centrifuge.
5. Pipette out 0.2, 0.4, 0.6, 0.8, and 1 mL of the working standard into a series of test tubes.

6. Pipette out 0.1 mL and 0.2 mL of the sample solution in two separate test tubes. Make up the volume in each tube to 1 mL with water.
7. Set a blank with 1 mL of water.
8. Add 1 mL of phenol solution to each tube.
9. Add 5 mL of 96% sulfuric acid to each tube and shake well.
10. After 10 minutes, shake the contents in the tubes and place in a water bath at 25°C to 30°C for 20 minutes.
11. Transfer the solutions from the test tubes to the cuvettes and measure the absorbance at 490 nm of the sugar standards and unknown solutions.
12. Calculate the amount of total carbohydrate present in the sample solution using the standard graph. To calculate the concentration of sugar present in the sample, make a graph plotting absorbance vs. sugar weight (μg) of the sugar calibration standards. The intercept of the absorbance of the unknown sample with the calibration line represents the amount (g) of sugar present in the sample.
13. Calculate the unknown sample concentration using the following equations: where x is the mass (g) of sugar sample deduced from the graph, mol. wt. represents the molecular weight of the monosaccharide or polysaccharide in the sample, and w is the weight (g) of the sample.

Absorbance corresponds to 0.1 mL of the test = x mg of glucose

100 mL of the sample solution contains = $0.1/x \times 100$ mg of glucose = % of total carbohydrate present.

2.8.5　Determination of Total Reducing Sugars

Reducing sugars have an aldehyde group that can give up electrons to an oxidizing agent yielding a carboxylic acid group. The most often used methods to determine the amounts of reducing sugars are the Somogyi-Nelson and dinitrosalicylic acid (DNS) assays. The first is based on the ability of reducing sugars, when heated with alkaline copper tartrate, to reduce the copper from the cupric to cuprous state and thus cuprous oxide is formed. The Cu^{1+} then reduces molybdic acid to molybdenum, yielding a blue solution that is measured spectrophotometrically at 620 nm. The blue color developed is compared with a set of glucose standards also read in a colorimeter set at 620 nm.

2.8.5.1　Determination of Reducing Sugars with the Somogyi–Nelson Procedure

A. *Samples, Ingredients, and Reagents*
- Test samples
- Anhydrous sodium carbonate
- Potassium sodium tartrate
- Copper sulfate
- Ammonium molybdate

- Glucose reagent grade
- Aluminum foil
- Distilled water
- Sodium bicarbonate
- Anhydrous sodium sulfate
- Sulfuric acid
- Disodium hydrogen arsenate
- Ethanol

B. *Materials and Equipment*
- Analytical scale
- Water bath (100°C)
- Volumetric flask (100 mL and 1 L)
- Pipettes (0.1 mL and 1 mL)
- Stirrer
- Incubator (37°C)
- Chronometer
- Spectrophotometer
- Brown or dark bottles
- Beaker (1 L)
- Test tubes
- Cuvettes
- Thermometer

C. *Procedure*
1. Prepare the following reagents:
   a. Somogyi reagent (Solution A). In a 1-L volumetric flask, prepare solution A by mixing 25 g of anhydrous sodium carbonate, 20 g of sodium bicarbonate, 25 g of potassium sodium tartrate, and 20 g of anhydrous sodium sulfate in 80 mL of water. Then, add distilled water to the 1-L mark. Transfer contents to a brown or dark bottle.
   b. Solution B. In a 1-L volumetric flask, dissolve 150 g of copper sulfate in a small volume of distilled water. Add one drop of sulfuric acid and make up to 1000 mL. Mix 40 mL of solution B and 960 mL of solution A before use.
   c. Nelson reagent. In a 1-L volumetric flask, dissolve 25 g ammonium molybdate in 450 mL of water. Add 25 mL of sulfuric acid and mix well. Then, add 3 g disodium hydrogen arsenate dissolved in 250 mL of water. Mix well, transfer Nelson reagent to a brown or dark bottle and incubate at 37°C for 24 to 48 hours.
   d. Stock standard glucose solution. Prepare the solution by mixing 100 mg of glucose in 100 mL of distilled water. Then, prepare the working standard solution by diluting 10 mL of stock to 100 mL of distilled water (100 μg/mL).
2. Weigh 100 mg of the sample and extract the sugars with hot 80% ethanol twice (5 mL each time). Collect the supernatant and evaporate it by keeping it on a water bath at 80°C. Then, add 10 mL of distilled water and dissolve the sugars. For sugar solutions, weigh 100 mg and then make up a volume of 10 mL with distilled water.
3. Pipette out aliquots of 0.1 mL or 0.2 mL of the test solution to separate test tubes and pipette out 0.2, 0.4, 0.6, 0.8, and 1 mL of the working standard glucose solution into a series of test tubes. Make up the volume in both sample and standard tubes to exactly 2 mL with distilled water.
4. Add 1 mL of the Somogyi reagent to each tube and stir contents. Cover the tubes with aluminum foil and heat for 10 minutes in a boiling water bath at 100°C. Remove test tubes from the hot water bath and allow contents to cool at ambient temperature. Then, add 1 mL of the Nelson reagent and stir contents. Make up the volume in each tube to 10 mL with distilled water, stir contents, wait 10 minutes, and read the absorbance at 620 nm.
5. Construct the standard curve with the spectrophotometer reading of glucose samples (0.2, 0.4, 0.6, 0.8, and 1 mL) and then calculate the amount of reducing sugars present in the sample. Calculation: absorbance corresponds to 0.1 mL of test = x mg of glucose

$$\% \text{ reducing sugars} = 10 \text{ mL contains} = (x/0.1) \times 10 \text{ mg of glucose}.$$

2.8.5.2 Determination of Reducing Sugars with the DNS Procedure

A. *Samples, Ingredients, and Reagents*
- Test samples
- DNS reagent
- Potassium sodium tartrate
- Ethanol
- Distilled water
- Sodium hydroxide
- Glucose reagent grade
- Aluminum foil

B. *Materials and Equipment*
- Analytical scale
- Water bath (100°C)
- Volumetric flask (100 mL and 1 L)
- Pipettes (0.1 mL and 1 mL)
- Stirrer
- Incubator (37°C)
- Chronometer
- Spectrophotometer
- Brown or dark bottles
- Beaker (1 L)
- Test tubes
- Cuvettes
- Thermometer

C. *Procedure*
1. Reagent preparation
   a. DNS reagent. Prepare the reagent by dissolving 10 g of DNS, 2 g of crystalline

phenol, and 0.5 g of sodium sulfite in 1 L of 1% NaOH. Store the resulting solution under refrigeration (4°C).

b. Rochelle salt solution. Prepare a 40% Rochelle salt solution by mixing 40 g of potassium sodium tartrate in 100 mL of distilled water.

c. Stock standard glucose solution. Prepare the solution by mixing 100 mg of glucose in 100 mL of distilled water. Then, prepare the working standard solution by diluting 10 mL of stock to 100 mL of distilled water (100 µg/mL).

2. Weigh 100 mg of the sample and extract the sugars with hot 80% ethanol twice (5 mL each time). Collect the supernatant and evaporate it by keeping it in a water bath set to 80°C. Then, add 10 mL of distilled water and dissolve the sugars. For sugar solutions, weigh 100 mg and then make up a volume of 10 mL with distilled water.

3. Pipette out 0.5 mL to 3 mL of the extract in test tubes and equalize the volume to 3 mL with distilled water. Then, add 3 mL of the DNS reagent. Cover the tubes with aluminum foil and heat for 5 minutes in a boiling water bath set to 100°C. While the contents of the tubes are still warm, add 1 mL of the 40% potassium sodium tartrate (Rochelle salt) solution.

4. Let cool and read the intensity of dark-red color and read absorbance at 510 nm.

5. Plot the standard curve with a series of glucose standards containing 0, 25, 50, 100, 200, 400, and 500 µg of glucose and then calculate the amount of reducing sugars present in the test sample.

2.8.6 Determination of Glucose

Glucose is a widely distributed simple sugar with an active aldehyde group. Estimation of glucose by glucose oxidase gives the true glucose concentration, eliminating the interference by other reducing sugars. The glucose oxidase enzyme catalyzes the oxidation of α-D-glucose to D-glucono-1,5 lactone (gluconic acid) with the formation of hydrogen peroxide. The oxygen liberated from hydrogen peroxide by peroxidase reacts with the o-dianisidine and oxidizes it to a red chromophore solution that is measured in a spectrophotometer.

A. Samples, Ingredients, and Reagents
- Test samples
- Glucose reagent grade
- Glucose oxidase
- Phosphate buffer
- Aluminum foil
- Distilled water
- Peroxidase
- Ethanol
- Hydrochloric acid (HCl)

B. Materials and Equipment
- Analytical scale
- Water bath (100°C)
- Volumetric flask (100 mL and 1 L)
- Pipettes (0.1 mL and 1 mL)
- Stirrer
- Incubator (37°C)
- Thermometer
- Spectrophotometer
- Brown or dark bottles
- Beaker (1 L)
- Test tubes
- Cuvettes
- pH meter
- Chronometer

C. Procedure
1. Prepare the following reagents:
   a. Glucose oxidase reagent. Prepare reagent by dissolving 25 mg o-dianisidine completely in 1 mL of methanol. Add 49 mL of 0.1 M phosphate buffer (pH 6.5). Then add 5 mg of peroxidase and 5 mg of glucose oxidase to the solution.
   b. Standard glucose solution. Prepare the stock solution by mixing 100 mg glucose in 100 mL distilled water. Then prepare the working standard solution by diluting 10 mL of stock to 100 mL distilled water (100 µg/mL).

2. Place 0.5 mL of the test sample solution and mix it with 0.5 mL distilled water and 1 mL of the glucose oxidase reagent.

3. Into a series of test tubes, pipette out 0 (blank), 0.2, 0.4, 0.6, 0.8, and 1 mL of working standard glucose solution and make up the volume to 1.0 mL with distilled water. Then, add 1 mL of glucose oxidase-peroxidase reagent.

4. Incubate all the tubes at 35°C for 40 minutes.

5. Terminate the reaction by the addition of 2 mL of 6 N HCl.

6. Cool and read the intensity of dark red color and read absorbance at 540 nm.

7. Plot the standard curve with a series of glucose standards containing 0, 25, 50, 100, 200, 400, and 500 µg glucose and then calculate the amount of glucose present in the test sample.

2.8.7 Research Suggestions

1. Determine and compare total starch, enzyme-susceptible starch, total sugars, and reducing sugars of wheat bread sample.

2. Prepare corn tortillas from white maize and determine resistant starch in the masa and processed tortillas at 0, 1, 2, 5, and 7 days of storage at room temperature.

3. Determine the amount of reducing sugars generated throughout the hydrolysis time of maize

starch hydrolyzed with heat-resistant α-amylase (refer to procedure in Section 13.3.1.2). Then, determine the amount of glucose generated throughout the hydrolysis time with amyloglucosidase of the liquefied starch suspension (refer to procedure in Section 13.3.1.1).

4. Determine the total starch and damaged starch of whole wheat processed into refined flour (refer to procedure in Section 5.2.1.1).
5. Determine the amount of reducing sugars and glucose in whole corn and its dry-milled fractions (fiber, germ, and grits).
6. Determine the amount of reducing sugars, glucose, and sugar composition of regular and sugar-coated corn flakes.
7. Determine the kinetics of reducing sugars, maltose, and glucose use during yeast fermentation of wort.
8. Investigate the detailed HPLC procedure to determine the soluble sugar profile including dextrins of a barley mash.
9. Determine the total starch and reducing sugars of barley before and after sprouting or malting.
10. Propose analytical methods to determine the relative amounts of glucose, fructose, and maltose in corn syrups.
11. Investigate the use of a polarimeter to analyze sugars and compare results with chemical methods.

2.8.8 Research Questions

1. What are the principles of total starch determination using the enzymatic method?
2. Discuss at least three ways to damage starch.
3. What are the main types of resistant starches? Which type of resistant starch is more common in cereal-based processed products?
4. Which method is the most commonly used to determine total sugars for food labeling purposes?
5. What are the principles behind total carbohydrate determination using the phenol sulfuric acid method?
6. What are the principles behind the determination of reducing sugars using the Somogyi-Nelson method?
7. Explain the purpose(s) of each of the following steps of total starch enzymatic method:
   a. Heating sample with thermoresistant α-amylase
   b. Treating sample with amyloglucosidase
   c. Reaction with glucose oxidase and peroxidase
8. How can soluble sugars be analyzed with HPLC and GC methods? What kinds of detectors are recommended for these two instruments?
9. What are the main types of sugars found in beer mashes or worts obtained with barley malt? Which of these sugars is fermentable?
10. What are potential advantages of using a polarimeter to analyze sugars in syrups?

2.9 VITAMIN ANALYSIS

Cereals are considered as an adequate source of certain vitamins. The aleurone and germ are the anatomical parts that contain the highest concentrations of these nutrients. The various types of milling systems yield refined products that contain lower amounts of these micronutrients. This is the main reason why refined dry-milled fractions are generally enriched with vitamins B_1, B_2, niacin, and folic acid. Cereals are considered as one of the best sources of B vitamins—thiamine, riboflavin, niacin, pyridoxine, and folates—but a poor source of fat-soluble vitamins and vitamin B_{12}. Most B vitamins are associated with the aleurone. The niacin associated with cereals is found in free and bound forms. Bound niacin is not well used by the human system. Interestingly, the alkaline treatment of maize for the production of tortillas and other traditional food products increases niacin bioavailability because the alkali and heat treatment breaks the glycosidic bond that binds free niacin with the other components.

Analysis of the various types of vitamins has played a critical role in the estimation of the nutritional attributes of foods and feeds because their deficiencies could result in diseases. Furthermore, food-labeling regulation mandates the declaration of certain vitamins (vitamins A, C, and some of the B complexes). Thus, accurate composition information is required to determine dietary intakes to assess their adequacy. Vitamin assays can be classified as microbiological and physicochemical assays. The microbiological assays are used for the analysis of niacin and folates, whereas the physicochemical assays could practically analyze all vitamins. The physicochemical assays mainly include HPLC, GC, spectrophotometric, fluorometric, and enzymatic methods.

2.9.1 Analysis of Liposoluble Vitamins

2.9.1.1 Analysis of Vitamin A and Carotenes (Method 86-05)

The active form of vitamin A or retinol could be synthesized from β-carotenes (AACC 2000). Cereals do not contain retinol but some contain significant quantities of carotenes. These carotenes are efficiently converted to retinol in the intestinal mucosa and liver. One molecule of β-carotene is transformed into two identical retinol units because of the hydrolysis of the carotene by diooxygenase to yield two retinoaldehyde molecules with the later transformation to retinol with a liver reductase. Fat-soluble retinol units are transported from the intestinal epithelial cells in chylomicrons to the liver and then to the rest of the body bound to retinol-binding protein. The vitamin A is stored in the liver and gradually used by the body.

Most nutritionists agree that the second most prevalent global deficiency of micronutrients is vitamin A. Recent statistics indicate that, annually, more than half a million children become partially or totally blind due to chronic deficiency of vitamin A, whereas 13 million preschool children are affected by xerophthalmia (Onuma Okezie 1998). Vitamin A deficiency occurs more frequently among people in developing countries such as Asia, Africa, and Latin

America. Approximately one-fourth to one-half of preschool children show symptoms of vitamin A deficiency in these countries. As with most nutrient deficiencies, the lack of vitamin A is more prevalent among children between 1 and 5 years of age that live in poverty. Humans require vitamin A to sustain normal growth, resist infectious diseases, and to have normal vision. More specifically, the lack of vitamin A is observed in the eyes and condition of epithelial tissues associated with skin, gastrointestinal tract, respiratory, and urogenital systems which leads to dry skin, diarrhea, and pneumonia. Its deficiency also affects bone development, exacerbates anemia, and depresses the immune and nervous systems. The most common symptoms are xerophthalmia, hyperkeratinization, and keratomalacia characterized by the irreversible drying of the eye which leads to cornea degeneration and permanent blindness (Hoffmann 1972; Mason et al. 2001; Van dan Briel and Webb 2003).

The typical vitamin A deficiency starts when newborns rapidly deplete the stored hepatic vitamin A reserves that usually last 4 to 6 months. In developing countries, most infants are weaned with cereal-based gruels that, unfortunately, lack sufficient amounts of carotenes. The chronic deficiency of vitamin A leads to night blindness and a higher susceptibility to infectious diseases. The vitamin A requirement increases in infants that present episodes of diseases such as measles, chicken pox, intestinal parasites, and calorie and protein malnutrition.

Both carotenes and vitamin A or retinol are frequently determined because they should be declared in nutritional food labels. These compounds are usually extracted with solvents and then quantified in a spectrophotometer or using HPLC systems.

A. Samples, Ingredients, and Reagents
- Test samples
- Aluminum oxide
- Chloroform (reagent grade)
- Ethanol
- Potassium hydroxide (KOH reagent grade)
- Acetic anhydride
- Vitamin A reference solution
- Cotton
- Phenolphthalein
- Distilled water
- Sulfuric acid (H_2SO_4)
- Hexane
- Acetone (reagent grade)
- Antimony trichloride ($SbCl_3$)
- Anhydrous sodium sulfate (Na_2SO_4)
- Carotene reference crystals
- Cottonseed oil

B. Materials and Equipment
- Analytical scale
- UV spectrophotometer
- Thermoregulated water bath
- Muffle furnace
- Dispenser
- Stopcock or extraction apparatus

- Glass tube
- Delivery pipette (10 mL)
- Stirrer
- UV light
- Separator
- Chronometer
- Laboratory grinder
- Eluate receiver*
- Saponification reflux apparatus[†]
- Desiccator
- Extraction apparatus (500 mL)
- Glass rod
- Volumetric flask (100 mL and 1 L)
- Chromatographic tubes (18 mm × 200 mm)
- Cuvettes
- Amber bottles
- Thermometer

C. Procedure
1. Prepare de following reagents:
   a. Aluminum oxide adsorbant. Hydrate to 5% water by pouring measured amount of water into small glass-stoppered bottle. Distribute over walls, then add alumina and mix by shaking bottle until no lumps are observed. Let stand to cool at least 2 hours before use and store in tightly closed bottle. Do not expose to air. Heat in muffle furnace at 750°C, cool, spread in thin layers over flat dishes in desiccators at 200 mL H_2SO_4 (specific gravity of 1.35) for 48 hours equilibration, and place adsorbant in tightly closed jars. Moisture content must be 4.5% to 5%.
   b. Acetone in hexane solution (4% and 15%). Dilute acetone with hexane.
   c. Potassium hydroxide solution. Dissolve 50 g of reagent-grade KOH in water and dilute to 100 mL with water in a volumetric flask.
   d. Antimony trichloride. Add $CHCl_3$ to 200 g of $SbCl_3$ to make 1 L. Warm and shake to dissolve and then cool. Add 30 mL of acetic anhydride. If solution is not clear, filter, centrifuge, or let settle, and decant. Store in stoppered amber bottles. The translucent solution should be stable for several months.
   e. Vitamin A reference solution (obtained from USP Reference Standards, 12601 Twinbrook Pkwy, Rockville, MD).
   f. Carotene reference crystals (from General Biochemicals). Crystals are 10% α-carotene, and 90% β-carotene in sealed 100 mg or 200 mg vials. Crystals should dissolve in hexane

---

* A lipless graduated cylinder (100 mL) fitted with a two-hole stopper. Insert chromatographic tube through one hole and glass tube to vacuum through the other. A water aspirator is satisfactory for vacuum.
† Any refluxing apparatus with ground-glass joint water-cooled condenser, and amber flask of 300 mL to 500 mL heated with boiling water or steam.

without residue and have a characteristic spectrophotometric curve.

2. Prepare the adsorption column as follows:

   a. Place a small amount of cotton at the bottom of the chromatographic tube and pack with alumina adsorbent mixture, adding in several portions, tamping each lightly with a blunt rod, to a depth of 7 cm. Keep column under suction during packing. Add a 0.5-cm layer of powdered anhydrous Na_2SO_4 on top of the column, level and pack lightly.

   b. Check for recovery of vitamin A as follows: saponify 0.1 g of USP vitamin A reference solution plus 2 g of fresh cottonseed oil. Extract with hexane. Mix solution of 50 µg to 100 µg of carotene and 100 USP units of saponified vitamin A. Dilute to 15 mL. Wash column with 20 mL of hexane and adjust elution rate to two drops per second. Before the top of the column runs dry, add vitamin A with 15% acetone in hexane (30 mL should be enough). Inspect last few milliliters of this eluate that is suitable for vitamin A fluorescence and continue until no fluorescence is observed. Evaporate suitable aliquot to dryness under nitrogen, add 1 mL of $CHCl_3$ and determine vitamin A levels. Compare results with aliquot of saponified vitamin A in hexane that was not chromatographed.

3. Determination

   a. Mill or grind the test sample to pass a 20-mesh screen. Accurately weigh sample containing approximately 400 to 800 units of vitamin A. Add 1 g of fresh cottonseed oil to premixes or concentrates with low fat contents. Add a volume of ethanol that is three times the sample weight (in grams), and swirl until particles are wet. Then, add a volume of 50% KOH equal to the sample weight and mix.

   b. Reflux 30 minutes at a rate of two drops per second. Swirl occasionally during saponification to prevent lumping. Cool to room temperature under running water. Add a volume of distilled water that is twice the sample weight.

   c. Extract three times with hexane, first using a volume of hexane that is two to three times the sample weight and two thirds as much for subsequent extractions.

   d. Combine all hexane extracts into one separator. Pour 100 mL of cool water into the separator and drain when the layers separate, retaining any emulsion in the hexane layer. Repeat washings with 100-mL portions of water, with shaking, until solution is

colorless to phenolphthalein. If emulsions cause difficulty, use 10% ethanol-water wash containing 0.1% HCl on the third wash. After the final wash, separate water as completely as possible. Swirl separator, let solution stand for 5 minutes and drain any water collected in the bottom. Add 10 g of Na_2SO_4 to the separator and shake to dry the hexane solution. Pour solution carefully from the top of the separator through a small piece of cotton into the appropriate volume flask. Rinse separator and cotton with hexane and make to volume with hexane.

4. Chromatography

   a. Chromatograph aliquot of 10 mL to 15 mL hexane extract containing approximately 100 units of vitamin A (preferably not less than 60 units). If necessary, concentrate portion of hexane extract under vacuum to obtain a sufficient concentration of vitamin A. In no case should more than 25 mL of the solution be chromatographed.

   b. Pack column as explained above, wash with 20 mL of hexane and add extract containing vitamin A just before the top of the column runs dry. Eluate at a rate of two drops per second. Elute carotene and then vitamin A as above.

   c. Dilute carotene and vitamin elutes to volume for colorimetry. For vitamin A, 50 mL is convenient. An aliquot of 10 mL may be taken for carotene determinations.

5. Preparation of standard curves

   a. Vitamin A standard curve. Accurately weigh 100 mg of vitamin A reference solution and transfer to a volumetric flask. Dilute to volume with $CHCl_3$. Use solution as soon as possible (within 8 hours). Use amber glassware. Make a series of dilutions of the vitamin A solution with $CHCl_3$ so that 1-mL aliquots treated similar to the samples give transmissions of 20% to 85%. Plot absorbance against units of vitamin A. Determine the slope of the line.

   b. Carotene standard curve. Prepare series of dilutions of α- and β-carotene reference crystals in hexane. Plot absorbance against the amount (in micrograms) of carotene and determine the slope of the line.

   c. Determination of correction factor for yellow pigment in vitamin A eluate. Correct for pigment if present in more than mere trace amounts. Make correction by saponification and extraction of sample from yellow maize. Chromatograph and save the 15% acetone-in-hexane fraction. Determine concentration of the yellow pigment in this fraction by comparison with carotene calibration. Transfer pigment to $CHCl_3$ and make a series of dilutions covering the range of concentrations of yellow pigment in sample solutions in the 1 mL $CHCl_3$ on which the vitamin A color is read. Obtain correction factor for reaction of this pigment in vitamin A determination.

6. Colorimetry
    a. Carotene. Prepare standard curve as directed previously. Determine the concentration of carotene using a 440 nm filter or wavelength in a spectrophotometer.
    b. Vitamin A. Transfer 10 mL of vitamin A eluate to spectrophotometer cuvette and read yellow color as carotene. If this is present in more than trace amounts, make corrections as directed in the next section. Evaporate solvent under vacuum and heat (60–65°C) in a hot water bath. Dissolve residue in 1 mL of $CHCl_3$ solution. Adjust spectrophotometer to 620 nm and 100% transmittance, using 1 mL $CHCl_3$ and 10 mL $SbCl_3$ solution. Place tube containing 1 mL of $CHCl_3$ solution of vitamin A in the colorimeter and add $SbCl_3$ reagent rapidly. Take maximum reading within 3 to 5 seconds. Convert readings to units of vitamin A by referring to previously prepared standard curves. Correct value for vitamin A lost in analysis by adding a known amount of vitamin A to the sample or to the blank.

7. Calculate the amount of vitamin A or carotenes using the following equations:

Vitamin A, USP units/g = (units of vitamin A per milliliter/recovery factor) × (dilution factor/sample weight, in grams).

β-carotene, μg/g = (μg carotene per milliliter × dilution factor)/(sample weight, in grams).

2.9.2 ANALYSIS OF B-COMPLEX VITAMINS

Historically, humans have traditionally experienced deficiencies of B vitamins. Cereal grains are considered an adequate source of these B vitamins, except B_{12} or cyanocobalamin. The most common deficiencies are due to the lack of thiamine (B_1), niacin (B_3), folic acid, and cyanocobalamin (B_{12}). Thiamine or B_1 has been historically recognized as the main cause of beriberi. Thiamine exists in free and bound forms (thiamine diphosphate and protein-phosphate-thiamine complex). The bound forms are split in the gastrointestinal tract. The absorbed thiamine acts as a coenzyme in energy metabolism mainly in the conversion of glucose to fats. In addition, it has high implications in the functioning of peripheral nerves, brain, and muscles. Thiamine deficiency causes weakness,

lack of appetite, constipation, depression, and in severe cases, cardiac insufficiency. It is one of the major causes of death among Asian babies.

Riboflavin or B_2 functions as part of the enzymes called flavoproteins (FMN and FAD), which are critically important in respiration and cell metabolism. They play a major role with thiamine and niacin in oxidation-reduction reactions. The deficiency of this vitamin is characterized by photophobia, angular lip stomatitis, dermatitis, and swelling of the tongue.

The discovery of the role of niacin was the result of humanities' struggle against pellagra (pelle = skin and agra = sour). Pellagra spread with the dissemination and cultivation of maize and its use in human diet. Pellagra was endemic in Europe and Africa, and reached epidemic proportions in the United States during the Civil War. Today, pellagra is less prevalent thanks to the cereal-enrichment programs enacted in many nations. Africa is the only continent is which pellagra is still a public health problem. The symptoms of pellagra known as the 3D disease, are diarrhea, dermatitis, dementia, and in severe cases, death. In addition, pellagra causes apathy, confusion, anorexia, glossitis, and gastritis. Metabolically, this vitamin is a constituent of two important coenzymes (NAD and NADP) which are necessary for cell respiration and carbohydrate, protein, and fat metabolism. These enzymes are involved in the release of metabolic energy.

Folic acid (pteroylmonoglutamic acid or PGA) exists in different forms in nature. These forms are changed to at least five active coenzymes that are critically important for the formation of purines and pyrimidines needed for the synthesis of DNA and RNA, the formation of hemoglobin, the interconversion of amino acids such as homocysteine to methionine, and the synthesis of choline from ethanolamine. Vitamins B_{12}, B_6, and C are essential for the activity of folacin as coenzymes in many metabolic processes. In practical terms, folic acid is required for cell division and reproduction and prevents neural tube defects in newborns and cardiovascular diseases in adults. Folacin and vitamin B_{12} lower the levels of homocysteine, resulting in a cardiovascular protective role.

2.9.2.1 Analysis of Thiamine (Fluorometric Method 957.17)

This analysis was previously described in AOAC (2005).

A. *Samples, Ingredients, and Reagents*
- Test samples
- Mylase 100
- α-Amylase
- Hydrochloric acid (HCl)
- Sodium hydroxide (NaOH)
- Isobutanol
- Ash-free filter paper
- Distilled water
- Takadiastase
- Thiamine hydrochloride (reagent grade)
- Potassium ferricyanide [$K_3Fe(CN)_6$]
- Sodium acetate (NaOAc)
- Sodium chloride

B. *Materials and Equipment*
- Analytical scale
- Volumetric flasks (200 mL and 1 L)
- Boiling water bath
- pH meter
- Automatic pipette
- Funnel
- Chronometer
- Photofluorometer
- Digestion flasks (250 mL)
- Thermometer
- Stirring rod
- Pipettes (5 mL)
- Test tubes

C. *Procedure*
1. Prepare the following reagents:
   a. Enzyme solution. Prepare a 10% aqueous solution potent in diastatic (amylase) and phospholytic activity by adding Mylase 100 (U.S. Biochemical Corp., Cleveland, OH), takadiastase, and α-amylase (Miles Lab. Inc., Elkhart, IN).
   b. Thiamine hydrochloride solution (1 μg/mL). Add 20 mL of thiamine-HCl solution into a 200 mL volumetric flask and dilute to volume with 0.1 N HCl.
   c. Test standard solution. Add 40 mL of the thiamine hydrochloride solution into a digestion flask and dilute to 150 mL with 0.1 N HCl and run with test samples.
   d. Direct standard solution. Add 40 mL of thiamine hydrochloride solution into a 200 mL flask and add 16 mL of distilled water and dilute to volume with 0.1 N HCl.
   e. Oxidizing reagent. Mix 4 mL of 1% potassium ferricyanide solution with 15% NaOH solution to make 100 mL. The solution has to be prepared less than 4 hours before analysis.
2. Weigh a sufficient amount of the air-dried sample with an accuracy of 0.0001 g containing approximately 40 μg of thiamine and place it in a 250 mL digestion flask.
3. Add 150 mL of 0.1 N HCl and stir. Add half of the acid and use the remainder to wash down the sides of the digestion flask.
4. Digest for 30 minutes in a boiling water bath. Stir contents to prevent lumping. After digestion, cool contents to room temperature and adjust pH to 4.5 by adding 2 N NaOAc.
5. Add 5 mL of enzyme solution rich in diastatic and phospholytic activities, mix and digest in a water bath for 60 minutes at 45°C to 50°C.
6. Remove flasks from water bath for cooling to room temperature. Transfer contents to a 200 mL volumetric flask and dilute to volume with 0.1 N HCl.

7. Mix and filter though ash-free filter paper. Check pH of filtrate with a pH meter. The pH should be 3.5.
8. Pipette duplicate 5-mL aliquots of direct standard solution and duplicate 5 mL aliquots of test sample solution into 40 mL tubes. Add 1.5 g of NaCl and 5 mL of the test standard solution.
9. With an automatic pipette, add 3 mL of oxidizing reagent in 1 to 2 seconds. Gently swirl tube to ensure adequate mixing. Immediately add 13 mL of isobutanol and shake tube vigorously for at least 15 seconds, and then again after 2 minutes.
10. To similar tubes, add 5 mL of the test sample solution and treat similarly as the tubes containing the test sample.
11. Centrifuge tubes at low speed until clear supernatant can be obtained. Pipette 10 mL of the upper layer (isobutanol) and place aliquot into cell for thiochrome fluorescence measurement.
12. The thiochrome fluorescence is obtained after readings in a photofluorometer (input filter at 365 nm and output filter at 435 nm) of the isobutanol extract from oxidized test sample solution (*I*) and the extract from the test sample solution treated with 3 mL of 15% NaOH solution (*B*).
13. Calculate the amount of thiamine (in milligrams) using the following equation: mg thiamine − HCl/kg = (*I/B*) × [40 × 1000 × Wt (g) × 1000].
    Correct values according to the original moisture content of the sample.

2.9.2.2 Analysis of Riboflavin (Fluorometric Method 960.65)

This analysis was previously described in AOAC (2005).

A. *Samples, Ingredients, and Reagents*
- Test samples
- Toluene
- Sodium hydrosulfite
- Hydrochloric acid (HCl)
- Potassium permanganate ($KMnO_4$)
- Hydrogen peroxide (H_2O_2)
- Ash-free filter paper
- Distilled water
- Acetic acid
- Riboflavin (reagent grade)
- Methanol
- Sodium hydrosulfite ($Na_2S_2O_4$)
- Pyridine

B. *Materials and Equipment*
- Analytical scale
- Volumetric flasks (500 mL and 1 L)
- Autoclave
- pH meter
- Automatic pipette

- Funnel
- Chronometer
- Photofluorometer
- Digestion flasks (250 mL)
- Thermometer
- Stirring rod
- 5 mL pipettes
- Test tubes

C. *Procedure*

1. Prepare the following reagents:
   a. Riboflavin standard stock solution (100 μg/mL). Dissolve 50 mg of dried riboflavin in 0.02 N acetic acid to make 500 mL. To ensure dissolution, warm the vitamin with part of the acetic acid on a steam bath with constant stirring and then make up to 500 mL.
   b. Riboflavin intermediate and working solutions (10 μg/mL and 1 μg/mL, respectively). The intermediate solution is prepared by diluting 100 mL of riboflavin stock solution to 1 L with 0.02 N acetic acid, whereas the working solution is prepared by diluting 10 mL of the intermediate solution to 1 L with distilled water.

2. Add at least 10 times the amount of 0.1 N HCl in relation to the sample weight (sample weight should be weighed with an accuracy of 0.0001 g). The resulting solution should contain less than 1 mg of riboflavin per milliliter.

3. After dissolving the sample, heat contents in an autoclave for 30 minutes at 121°C to 123°C. After cooling to room temperature, shake and adjust the pH to 6 to 6.5 with NaOH solution. Then immediately add 0.1 N HCl until no further precipitation occurs (pH 4.5).

4. Dilute mixture to a known volume containing more than 0.1 μg of riboflavin/mL and filter through ash-free filter paper.

5. Take an aliquot of the clear filtrate and check for dissolved protein by adding, dropwise at first, diluted HCl and then, if no precipitation forms while shaking, add NaOH solution to pH 6.8 to a known volume. If precipitation occurs, adjust solution to the point of maximum precipitation, dilute to a measured volume containing more than 0.1 μg of riboflavin/mL and then filter. Then, take an aliquot of the clear filtrate and proceed by adding, dropwise at first, diluted HCl and then, if no precipitation forms while shaking, add NaOH solution to pH 6.8 to a known volume.

6. Add 10 mL of the sample solution to at least two different test tubes, 1 mL of the standard riboflavin to another tube, and 1 mL of distilled water to a blank tube. Then, to each tube, add 1 mL of acetic acid and 0.5 mL of 4% $KMnO_4$

solution and let stand for 2 minutes. Then, add 0.5 mL 3% H_2O_2 solution. The permanganate color must be removed within 10 seconds. Shake vigorously until excess oxygen is expelled.

7. Measure the fluorescence (X) of test samples containing 1 mL of additional standard riboflavin working solution. Next, measure the fluorescence of samples containing 1 mL of distilled water (B). Next, mix in 20 mg of powdered $Na_2S_2O_4$ to the test tubes and measure the minimum fluorescence within 5 seconds (C).

8. Calculate the amount of riboflavin (milligrams per milliliter) using the following equation = $[(B - C)/(X - B)] \times 0.10 \times 0.001$. The value $[(B - C)/(X - B)]$ must be higher than 0.66 and lower than 1.5.

   Correct values according to the adjusted final volume and original moisture content of the sample.

2.9.2.3 Analysis of Niacin (Method 961.14)

This analysis was previously described in AOAC (2005).

A. *Samples, Ingredients, and Reagents*

- Test samples
- Niacin (reagent grade)
- Sodium phosphate ($Na_2HPO_4 \cdot 7H_2O$)
- Hydrochloric acid (HCl)
- Sulfanilic acid
- Calcium hydroxide
- Whatman no. 12 filter paper
- Distilled water
- Ammonium hydroxide (NH_4OH)
- Potassium phosphate (KH_2PO_4)
- Cyanogen bromide (CNBr)
- Bromocresol green indicator
- Ammonium sulfate [$(NH_4)_2SO_4$]
- Crushed ice

B. *Materials and Equipment*

- Analytical scale
- Colorimeter
- Volumetric flasks (0.1, 0.25, 0.5, and 1 L)
- Autoclave
- Thermometer
- pH meter
- Automatic pipette
- Funnel
- Chronometer
- Hood
- Centrifuge
- Digestion flasks (250 mL)
- Water bath with temperature controls
- Refrigerator
- Vortex
- Pipettes (1, 2, 5, 10, and 20 mL)
- Test tubes

C. *Procedure*

1. Prepare the following reagents:
   a. Niacin standard stock solution (100 μg/mL). Dissolve 50 mg of dried niacin in 25% ethanol to make 500 mL.
   b. Working solution (10 μg/mL). The working standard solution is prepared by diluting 10 mL of the niacin standard stock solution to 100 mL of distilled water.
   c. Ammonium hydroxide solution. Dilute 5 mL of NH_4OH to 250 mL with distilled water.
   d. Phosphate buffer solution (pH 8). Dissolve 60 g of $Na_2HPO_4 \cdot 7H_2O$ and 10 g of KH_2PO_4 in warm water and dilute to 200 mL.
   e. Cyanogen bromide solution (10%). Under the hood, warm 370 mL of water to 40°C and add 40 g of CNBr. Shake until dissolved, cool and dilute to 400 mL. Store reagent in refrigerator.
   f. Sulfanilic acid solution (10%). Add NH_4OH in 1-mL portions to a mixture of 20 g of sulfanilic acid and 170 mL of distilled water until acid dissolves. Adjust pH to 4.5 with HCl using bromocresol green indicator (1 + 1). Dilute to 200 mL. Note that the resulting solution should be almost colorless.

2. Accurately weigh 2.5 g of sample (the sample should contain approximately 100 μg of niacin). Run at least one reagent blank and five concentrations of working standard solutions (0, 5, 10, 15, 20, and 25 mL).

3. Place 1.5 g calcium hydroxide into each flask and add 90 mL of distilled water. Shake contents well and place flasks in an autoclave. Hydrolyze samples for 2 hours at 15 psi.

4. After mixing thoroughly, allow contents to cool down to 40°C and transfer to 100 mL of volumetric flasks and dilute to volume.

5. Transfer approximately 50 mL of the supernatant to centrifuge tubes and place it in an ice bath for 15 minutes or in a refrigerator for 2 hours. Centrifuge for 15 minutes and pipette 20 mL of the supernatant from each tube into separated centrifuge tubes containing 8 g of $(NH_4)_2SO_4$ and 2 mL of phosphate buffer solution. Shake to dissolve and warm contents to 55°C to 60°C. Centrifuge for 5 minutes and then filter through Whatman no. 12 paper.

6. In each of two tubes, place 5 mL of standard solution, and in each of two additional tubes, place 5 mL of the sample solution. Prepare one additional tube with 5 mL of distilled water as blank. In one standard tube and in one sample tube to be used as blanks, add 10 mL of distilled water. Let all tubes stand for 30 minutes in an ice bath. In the remaining standard, sample, and reagent blank tubes, first add 10 mL of cold CNBr, followed 30 seconds later by 1 mL of 55% sulfanilic acid solution. Mix immediately and replace ice-cold tubes. Add 1 mL of sulfanilic acid solution to the replaced tubes. Register the time when the sulfanilic acid solution was added to each tube.

7. Set colorimeter to zero absorbance at 470 nm with standard blank and read absorbance of other tubes after the addition of sulfanilic acid. Wipe the exterior of the tubes dry before reading absorbances.

8. Plot the standard curve of absorbances of the set of standards minus that of the reagent blank against the niacin concentration in micrograms of niacin per milliliter. Calculate the slope of the best-fit line and read the concentration of test samples.

9. Calculate the concentration of niacin using the following equation:

mg niacin/g sample = niacin concentration of test sample/ (10 × g sample weight)

Correct values according to the original moisture content of the sample.

2.9.3 RESEARCH SUGGESTIONS

1. Determine the amounts of thiamine, riboflavin, niacin, and other B vitamins of whole wheat processed into refined flour and a commercial enriched flour.
2. Determine β-carotenes of white and yellow maize transformed into tortillas.
3. Compare the amounts of thiamine, riboflavin, and niacin of durum wheat semolina transformed into raw and cooked pasta.
4. Determine the amounts of thiamine, riboflavin, niacin and other B vitamins of maize transformed into tortillas.

2.9.4 RESEARCH QUESTIONS

1. What are the vitamins that must be listed on the nutritional label? Why?
2. What are the B-complex vitamins that are usually added to refined flour enrichment programs? What is the main reason of the addition of each of these vitamins?
3. What are the most common methods to extract vitamin C, B-complex vitamins, and fat-soluble vitamins from foods?
4. What are the principles, advantages, and disadvantages of using microbiological assays for the quantification of niacin and folates?
5. What are the advantages and disadvantages of using HPLC for vitamin analysis?

6. Explain why β-carotenes are considered as provitamin A. What is necessary to transform β-carotenes into retinol?
7. Why do most refined milled fractions contain lower amounts of vitamins and minerals compared with their respective whole grains?
8. Which of the B vitamins is not found in cereal grains?
9. In which anatomical cereal grain part do you find most tocopherols?
10. What happens to niacin during lime-cooking or nixtamalization? Does this process favor or disfavor niacin availability?

2.10 METHODS FOR pH AND ACIDITY ANALYSIS

Acidity in foods is generally determined with the pH or titratable acidity assays. The first quantifies the free hydronium ions (H_3O) in a range of 14 orders of magnitude with a pH meter or chemical pH indicators, whereas the second deals with a measurement of the total acidic concentration contained within a food matrix. pH is defined as the logarithm of the reciprocal of the hydrogen ion concentration or as the negative logarithm of the molar concentration of hydrogen ions. Total acidity is determined by titration of intrinsic acids with a standard base. Titratable acidity is a better predictor of an acid's impact on flavor compared with pH (Sadler and Murphy 1998).

In different segments of the cereal industry, both pH and titratable acidity are widely used. In grain elevators, acidity is related to grain condition, whereas in the milling industry, acidity is related to the quality of flours and the effectiveness of chlorination; in the baking and brewing industries, acidity is related to the fermentation procedures used and yeast activity, and in the rest of the industries, acidity is associated with flavor, color, and other important organoleptic properties. In addition, organic acids and alkaline compounds are purposely added to many formulations to affect acidity and microbial shelf life.

pH is, in most instances, determined with a potentiometer or pH meter. The device consists of an electrolic cell composed of two electrodes dipped in a test solution which measures voltage. The voltage is related to the ionic concentration of the solution. For maximum accuracy, the potentiometer should be standardized using two buffers with pH values approximately 3 pH units apart. For instance, for acidic foods, pH 4 and pH 7 buffers are recommended, whereas for alkaline foods, counterparts having pH values of 7 and 9 should be used.

2.10.1 ANALYSIS OF ACIDITY

One of the more important properties associated with the chemistry of cereal-based foods is the intensity of the acidity measured with the titratable acidity method. Titratable acidity is measured by the potentiometric or colorimetric assays.

Independently of the assay, it measures ionizable hydrogen that is neutralized by a standard base solution. Colorimetric titration is performed with the presence of an indicator. The equivalence point or titration point is when the number of acid equivalents is exactly the same as the number of base equivalents. Phenolphthalein is the most common indicator. It changes from clear to red in the pH region of 8 to 9.6. Titratable acidity should not be confused with the amount of acid present in the substance. The amount of acid is expressed as a percentage of the total composition. Acids are either intentionally added to cereal-based products to lower the pH for preservation purposes or produced by fermenting yeast or lactic acid bacteria. These microorganisms lower the pH to a point where pathogenic bacteria cannot grow. Titratable acidity is defined as the percentage of acidity determined by titrating with a standard NaOH solution. The value is usually expressed in terms of lactic acid, citric acid, or malic acid equivalents. In fermented cereal products, the most recommended way of expression is by using lactic acid equivalents.

2.10.1.1 Determination of pH

A. *Samples, Ingredients, and Reagents*
- Distilled water
- pH standard buffer solutions

B. *Materials and Equipment*
- Top load scale
- 100 mL graduated cylinder
- 25 mL pipette
- Chronometer
- pH meter
- Blender
- Beaker

C. *Procedure*
1. Weigh 10 g of sample and place it in a blender bowl.
2. Add 100 mL of distilled and deionized water.
3. Blend contents for 2 minutes.
4. Allow contents to settle and stand for 5 minutes.
5. Pipette approximately 25 mL of the supernatant and place it in a beaker.
6. Measure the pH with a potentiometer previously calibrated with two buffers. Make sure to rinse the electrode with distilled water after each pH measurement (Figure 2.5).

2.10.1.2 Titratable Acidity

A. *Samples, Ingredients, and Reagents*
- Test samples
- Phenolphthalein
- NaOH
- Distilled water
- Potassium hydrogen phthalate

B. *Materials and Equipment*
- Analytical or top load balance
- Biuret
- Hot plate
- Thermometer

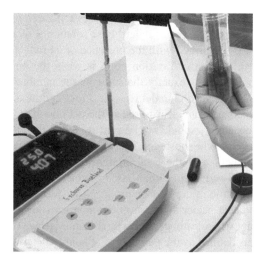

FIGURE 2.5   Potentiometer used to determine pH.

- Volumetric flask (1 L)
- Graduated cylinder (100 mL)
- Beakers

C. *Procedure*

1. Prepare a 0.1 N NaOH solution by adding exactly 4 g of NaOH to 1 L of hot (~95°C) distilled water.
2. Standardize the 0.1 N NaOH solution by weighing three 0.7- to 0.9-g samples of dried potassium phthalate and dissolve each in 60 mL of distilled water. Add a few drops of phenolphthalein indicator and titrate to a faint pink endpoint. Calculate the normality of the NaOH solution using the following equation:

$$\text{N of NaOH} = \text{g dried potassium phthalate}/(\text{mL NaOH}) \\ (0.0204226).$$

3. Add 10 g of the sample (i.e., bread, dough, or cracker) to a mixing bowl and then 100 mL of distilled water. Mix contents until the sample is blended well with the water. Allow contents to settle or filter.
4. Take a known aliquot of the sample solution and add three drops of phenolphthalein. Titrate with the standardized NaOH solution (0.1 N) to a pink endpoint (Figure 2.6). Calculate titratable acidity using the following equation:

$$\% \text{ titratable acidity} = [(\text{mL NaOH}) \times (\text{N}) \times (0.064)]/(\text{mL} \\ \text{of sample solution}).$$

2.10.2   Research Suggestions

1. Determine the pH and acidity of a sample of wheat that has undergone intrinsic and extrinsic deterioration due to faulty storage (refer to procedure in Section 4.2.1.2).
2. Determine the pH and acidity of a lager beer wort during yeast fermentation.

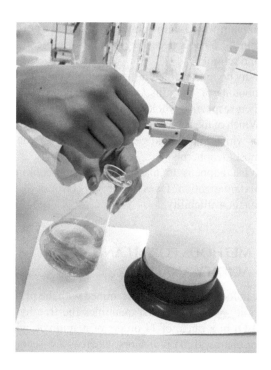

FIGURE 2.6   Determination of titratable acidity.

3. Graph the pH and acidity vs. fermentation time of the typical sponge used for the elaboration of crackers and saltines.
4. Prepare a nixtamalized masa or dough using procedure in Section 7.2.3.1. Then, determine its pH and acidity and add 0.2% of calcium propionate. Determine the amount of fumaric acid necessary to drop the pH to 6.2, 5.8, and 5.2. Prepare the control and acidified tortillas and determine the average shelf life and sensory properties of each type of tortilla.

2.10.3   Research Questions

1. For each of the cereal-based products listed below, what acid should be used to express titratable acidity
   a. Table bread
   b. Sour bread
   c. Lager beer
   d. Opaque or kaffir beer
2. What is the pH of a wheat flour dough suited for French bread right after mixing, during fermentation or proofing, and after bread baking? Which acid is mainly produced during dough fermentation?
3. What is the pH and titratable acidity of a chlorinated soft wheat flour? How does it compare with the regular soft wheat flour?
4. Why is an acidulant almost always used along with antimold agents such as calcium propionate or potassium sorbate in flour or corn tortillas? What are the levels of these additives commonly used?

2.11 METHODS FOR NUTRACEUTICAL COMPOUNDS ANALYSIS

The new trend in the cereal processing industry is the development of nutraceutical or functional foods that exert positive effects on human health. These chemicals are not considered nutrients that have been traditionally associated with deficiencies. The main nutraceuticals are those with proven positive effects to combat oxidative stress, chronic diseases, metabolic syndrome, and cancer. In some instances, the scientific evidence of the positive effects is solid and overwhelming so that regulatory agencies allow processors to claim them on the nutritional label. In most instances, the nutraceuticals are intrinsic to foods such as oats rich in soluble fiber or β-glucans, or maize germ rich in phytosterols, tocopherols, and policosanols. Folic acid has received special attention lately because its deficiency can cause abortion or miscarriage and neural tube defects. In addition, folic acid is related to brain health and prevents cardiovascular disease in adults.

Nutraceutical compounds are classified according to their chemistry and biological activity. Modern humans are more prone to oxidative stress because they are exposed to many oxidative agents such as air contamination, stress, cigarette smoke, and others. In addition, the human body constantly produces free radicals that can cause cell membrane oxidation and DNA damage that exacerbates mutations of protooncogenes, aging, and increases the probability of cancer and chronic diseases.

Phenolic compounds are the most widely distributed secondary metabolites present in the plant kingdom (Dicko et al. 2006). They can be divided into three major categories: simple phenolics, flavonoids, and tannins. Simple phenolics are usually derived from benzoic or cinnamic acids. On the other hand, flavonoids and anthocyanins are built from two units: a C6-C3 unit from cinnamic and a C6 fragment from malonyl-CoA. Tannins are polymers of five to seven units or more of flavan-3-ol or catechins. Most phenolics associated with cereal grains are present in the pericarp, *testa* or seed coat, aleurone, and glumes or husks. Ferulic acid in its free, conjugated, and bound forms is the most important simple phenolic compound present in cereal grains. It is a hydroxycinnamic acid associated with cell walls. In cereals, most ferulic acid is found in bound or conjugated forms. The insoluble-bound ferulic forms (diferulic) are covalently linked to polysaccharides, mainly in the pericarp and aleurone layers. The function of these compounds is to cross-link and strengthen cell walls, therefore, playing an important role in the lignification process that influences the physical and textural attributes of plants and foods. Regardless of the ferulic acid form, it is considered a potent antioxidant and a nutraceutical that prevents inflammation, cancer, low density lipoprotein (LDL) oxidation, and neuron degeneration (Kanski et al. 2002). Among cereals, sorghum and maize have higher antioxidant activity compared with wheat, oats, and rice. Sorghum is known to contain the highest content of phenolic compounds, reaching up to 6% in some varieties (Dicko et al. 2006). The wide array of sorghum genotypes may contain all classes of phenolic compounds including condensed tannins (Awika and Rooney 2004). According

to Sosulski et al. (1982) and Adom and Liu (2002), maize, in some instances, contains up to three times more phenolics compared with wheat, rice, and oats. Milling and nixtamalization greatly affect the amount of phenolics and antioxidant capacity of cereal grains. The physical removal of the fiber-rich outer layers takes away most phenolics, and consequently, greatly affects the nutraceutical potential.

Cereals may contain significant amounts of flavonoids such as flavanols, flavanones, flavones, and anthocyanins. Red, blue, and purple-pigmented maize kernels are rich in anthocyanins and several reports indicate that these are similar to the ones found in red wine. The cumulative results of epidemiological, in vitro, and in vivo research suggest an inverse relationship between anthocyanin consumption and the incidence of various chronic and degenerative diseases. Their health benefits have been related to their high antioxidant and antiradical activities.

Sorghum is the most promising cereal grain in terms of flavonoids and nutraceutical potential. For instance, sorghum may contain flavan-3-ols, flavan-4-ols, and anthocyanins such as apigeninidin and luteolinidin (Dicko et al. 2006). The main type of flavonoid from sorghum is flavanes. The flavanes 3-en 3-ols with double bonds between C3 and C4 and hydroxylated in position C3 are called anthocyanins. Among flavonols, the flavan-4-ols have particular therapeutic interest because of their antitumor activity (Ferreira and Slade 2002) and enhancement of immune response. Sorghums with a black pericarp, such as Shawaya, contain higher levels of flavan-4-ols and anthocyanins compared with other varieties (Dykes et al. 2005).

Among commercial cereals, sorghum is the only one that may contain significant amounts of condensed tannins. Deprez et al. (2001) reported that procyanidins could be absorbed through the intestinal cell monolayer (Caco-2 cells) but only up to trimers. The tannins have nutraceutical benefits because of their strong antioxidant capacity. Experimental animal studies have demonstrated that some high-tannin sorghums decrease the incidence of colon and mammary cancers in induced animals.

The whole rice bran contains significant amounts of oryzanol, although it is also present in other cereals such as barley and maize. Oryzanol is effective in promoting cardiovascular health (Hoffpauer 2005) and decreasing oxidative stress, cholesterol levels, inflammation, anxiety, and menopause. The rice bran obtained from dry-milling is further stabilized to denature lipases that cause oxidative rancidity and to protect the intrinsic nutraceuticals compounds. The stabilization is usually done by applying heat in an extruder.

The lipid fraction of cereals contains significant amounts of phospholipids such as phosphatidyl choline, inositol, ethanolamine, and serine. These polar lipids are considered nutraceuticals because they form part of the cell membranes and keep their integrity. Phosphatidyl choline or lecithin helps to keep the proper functioning of the liver and to transport lipids and its deficiency is related to increased susceptibility to hepatic cancer. Lecithin and choline lower the risk of cardiovascular disease and positively affect brain and mental development of both the fetus and infants, and their chronic inadequacy may be related to Alzheimer's disease. Choline is considered as one of the most important neurotransmitters and is supplemented to geriatrics to maintain proper brain function (Canty 2001; Canty and Zeisel 1994; Signore et al. 2008). Phosphatidyl inositol and serine are lipotropic and reduce blood triglycerides. One of the most relevant effects is the reduction of fatty liver and the prevention of bipolar disorders and Alzheimer disease. The deficiency of these phospholipids is related to increased susceptibility to hepatic cancer (Majumder and Biswas 2006; Phillippy 2003). Inositol, from phosphatidyl inositol or from the enzymatic hydrolysis of phytates by phytases, is known as a potent nutraceutical because it is essential for brain functioning and prevents liver damage and fatty infiltrations. It is especially recommended for newborn babies and geriatrics. Inositol is considered a potent biologically active compound and by some nutritionists as part of the B vitamin complex (vitamin B_8) because it helps to maintain cell membrane integrity and other important metabolic functions, such as the role of phosphatidyl inositol that is required for the proper functioning of the brain and heart. In addition, it helps in the synthesis of RNA and to transport lipids and cholesterol. Thus, inositol is considered to be hypocholesterolemic, cardioprotective, and anticarcinogenic (Holub 1982; Phillippy 2003; Vucenik and Shamsuddin 2006).

There has been much interest in the health benefits of consuming phytosterols especially because the Food and Drug Administration (FDA) issued a health claim for their use. These phytochemicals inhibit the absorption of cholesterol from the small intestine, thus effectively lowering total blood cholesterol and LDL. An amount of only 1 g/day to 3 g/day reduces cholesterol by 5% to 20%. A typical dietary intake of phytosterols varies from 200 mg/day to 400 mg/day. The main sterol present in the whole kernel and extracted oil is β-sitosterol followed by campesterol and stigmasterol. The second dominant sterol in oats is avenasterol (Chung and Ohm 2000). Research on maize fiber (Moreau et al. 1996) has shown that oil associated with the fiber fraction is different in composition compared with regular oil obtained from the germ. The fiber oil contains important amounts of ferulate phytosterol esters, free phytosterols, and fatty acid phytosterol esters that lower serum cholesterol in laboratory animals. The most common class is ferulate phytosterol esters dominated by sitostanol, which is considered more efficient in lowering cholesterol. Phytosterols, such as ergosterol, campesterol, β-sitosterol, and stigmasterol, compete for cholesterol absorption and therefore are considered hypocholesterolemic and preventive against cardiovascular disease. According to Raicht et al. (1980) and Fiala et al. (1985), the supplementation of 0.2% β-sitosterol decreases the occurrence of chemically induced colon tumors.

Another important group of antioxidants are the carotenoids and xantophylls. Carotenoids are polyisoprenoids containing 40 carbons that provide color to plants, microorganisms, fish, and birds but they cannot be synthesized in animals. Carotenoid hydrocarbons are known as carotenes and are the biosynthetic plant precursors of the oxygenated derivatives called xantophylls. The absorption of these compounds is not regulated, therefore, their concentration in blood and peripheral tissues reflect ingestion. Carotenoids are constituted by a conjugated polyene chain which accounts for the color and sensibility to light.

Carotenoids are very minor constituents of cereal grains. They are most abundant in yellow maize, yellow sorghum, and durum wheat. The consumption of these yellow endosperm cereal grains can potentially benefit the at least 1 million children who die every year due to weakness and deficiency of vitamin A, and the 350,000 more that become completely blind. The main nutraceutical role of carotenoids in humans is molecular protection against free radicals. From the nutritional viewpoint, the most important metabolite is β-carotene because one molecule is converted into two of the active form of vitamin A or retinol in a normal human system. In addition, β-carotenes can regenerate the activity of vitamin E and possibly other oxidized antioxidants. β-Carotenes could also act as an antioxidant that scavenges free radicals in human LDL and high density lipoprotein (HDL) as well as in cell membranes. As explained previously, vitamin A is considered the most important liposoluble vitamin for human nutrition and health. The supplementation of vitamin A or β-carotenes prevents partial and complete blindness, xerophthalmia, cancer, cardiovascular disease, and strengthens the immune system. Lutein, zeaxanthin, and cryptoxanthin are xantophylls that have received special attention because they prevent macular degeneration that is highly associated with blindness in geriatric patients (Fullmer and Shao 2001).

Tocol derivatives such as tocopherols and tocotrienols are responsible for the vitamin E activity of plant tissues. Various combinations of all eight tocols are found among cereals. The most predominant forms are α-tocopherol, γ-tocopherol, and α-tocotrienol. Among the structural parts of cereal grains, tocol derivatives are most abundant in the germ of barley, wheat, and maize (Chung and Ohm 2000). Tocols, tocotrienols, and vitamin E are potent antioxidants that reduce the risk of cancers and cardiovascular diseases because they act as potent antioxidants that block the formation of free radicals in cell membranes. As a result, they prevent cardiovascular diseases, LDL oxidation and the oxidation of polyunsaturated fatty acids, and strengthen the immune system by T-lymphocytes (Bender 1992).

A considerable amount of wax-like material that contains significant amounts of policosanols can be extracted from maize kernels. The wax is mainly associated with the outer pericarp layers or epicarp and germ. Policosanols are a mixture of long-chained alcohols containing mostly hexacosanol (26:0), octacosanol (28:0), triacontanol (30:0), and docatriacontanol (32:0). They are commercially obtained from cereal germs that are by-products of the milling industries. Policosanols reportedly exert physiological activities such as reducing serum lipid levels and platelet aggregation (Arruzazabala et al. 1994, 1996; Gouni-Berthold and Berthold 2002; Hargrove et al. 2004).

There are many existing methods to quantify the nutraceutical compounds and antioxidant capacity associated with cereal grains and their products. The most common methods to analyze these compounds are summarized in Tables 2.2 and 2.3.

TABLE 2.2
Methods More Commonly Used to Analyze Phytochemical Compounds Associated with Cereal Grains and Their Products

Compounds	Method	Description	References
Phenolic	Total phenolics assay	Colorimetric assay based on the oxidation of phenolic compounds by the Folin-Ciocalteu reagent (composed of phosphomolybdate and phosphotungstate). The oxidized phenolic compounds are detected and quantified by spectrophotometric readings at 725 nm.	Swain and Hillis (1959)
	Free and bound phenolics	Free phenolic compounds are extracted by blending the ground sample with 80% chilled ethanol whereas bound phenolics by extracting the residue with 2 M sodium hydroxide at room temperature. The mixture is neutralized with hydrochloric acid and extracted with hexane to remove lipids. The final solution is extracted several times with ethyl acetate. Phenolics are quantified with the Folin-Ciocalteu method described previously.	Adom et al. (2002)
	Free and bound ferulic	Free, conjugated, and bound ferulic are analyzed from free, conjugated, and bound phenolic extracts. An aliquot of the extracts is analyzed for ferulic using an HPLC system equipped with a UV detector at 280 nm. Peak identification of ferulic acid in sample extracts is based on retention time and chromatography of a ferulic acid standard.	
	Total anthocyanins	Spectrophotometric assay that measures total anthocyanins in an ethanolic extract. Anthocyanins are extracted with an ethanolic solvent (0.225 N HCl in 95% ethanol). Spectrophotometric readings at 535 nm are taken, subtracting absorbance at 700 nm. Total anthocyanin content is expressed as milligrams of cyanidin 3-glucoside equivalents using a molar extinction coefficient of 25,965 M^{-1} cm^{-1} and a molecular weight of 449 g/mol.	Fuleki and Francis (1968)
	Condensed tannins	Tannins are determined on ground samples treated with acidic methanol (1% HCl). The acidic methanol extracts are dissolved in water and an aliquot of vanillin reagent is added. Absorbance is measured at 500 nm using a spectrophotometer. Tannin content is expressed as milligrams of catechin equivalents per gram of sample.	Price et al. (1978)
	HPLC phenolic profiles	Chromatographic method applied for the detection and quantification of individual phenolic compounds present in an extract. Phenolic compounds are separated though a C-18 reverse phase column and identified with a photodiode array (PDA) detector. Two mobile phases are commonly used: Phase A, water/formic acid 1% (99:1, v/v); and Phase B, acetonitrile. The gradient solvent system varies depending on the phenolic compounds being separated.	
Carotenoids	Total carotenoids	Colorimetric assay that determines the concentration of carotenoids in an extract (i.e., acetone/ethanol; 50:50). Spectrophotometric readings are taken at 470 nm and the concentration of total carotenoids is calculated with the Lambert-Beer law. An extinction coefficient specific for the solvent is used for the calculation of concentrations (2500 M^{-1} cm^{-1} in the case of carotenoids extracted with acetone/ethanol; 50:50).	Gross (1991); Howard et al. (1996)
	HPLC carotenoid profile	Chromatographic method applied for the detection and quantification of individual carotenoids present in an extract. Carotenoids are separated though a C-30 reverse phase column and identified with a PDA detector. Two mobile phases are commonly used: Phase A, methanol/methyl tert-butyl ether (MTBE)/water (81:15:4, v/v); and Phase B, TBE/methanol/water (90:6:5:, v/v). The gradient solvent system varies depending on the carotenoids being separated.	
Phytosterols	Gas–liquid chromatography (GLC) and HPLC	Phytosterols are extracted with chloroform and methanol. Saponification may be used as a purification step, especially when GLC is used because it removes triglycerides, fatty acids, and phospholipids. Phytosterols are converted to trimethylsilyl or acetate derivatives before injection into capillary columns in a GLC equipped with a FID. Reverse-phase HPLC-UV has also been used for the analysis of phytosterols. The advantage of this method is that does not require an intensive sample preparation compared with the GLC technique.	Lampi et al. (2005)

(Continued)

TABLE 2.2 (Continued)

Methods More Commonly Used to Analyze Phytochemical Compounds Associated with Cereal Grains and Their Products

Compounds	Method	Description	References
Tocopherols and tocotrienols	GLC and HPLC	Chromatography methods for the analysis of tocopherols and tocotrienols involve the extraction of the sample with solvents. The analysis of these analytes with HPLC can be performed with UV, fluorescence, or evaporative light-scattering detectors (ELSD). GLC has been used and separates only the mono-, di-, and trimethylated tocopherols but methods are now available which provide separation of all the tocopherols. These developments were made possible by better columns and the use of derivatives of tocopherols. In addition to good separation, GLC is the most sensitive method available for the quantitation of the tocopherols.	Sacchetti and Bruni (2007); Bunnell (1971)
Policosanols	GLC and HPLC	Policosanols are usually extracted with hot hexane and identified and quantified by TLC, HPLC, or GLC. Policosanols are determined with a HPLC equipped with an ELSD operated at 40°C with nitrogen pressure of 3.5 bar or with GLC-FID. The GLC sample is derivatized to trimethylsilyl ethers before injection.	Adhikari et al. (2006); Hwang et al. (2002, 2004)

TABLE 2.3

Methods More Commonly Used to Determine the Antioxidant Capacity Associated with Cereal Grains and Their Products

Antioxidant Activity Assay	Description	References
Oxygen radical absorbance capacity (ORAC)	Fluorescent assay that measures the ability of an antioxidant to inhibit peroxyl radical–induced oxidation. The peroxyl radical [2,2′-azobis (2-amidinopropane)-dihydrochloride (AAPH)] reacts with a fluorescent probe (fluorescein sodium salt) to form a nonfluorescent product. The ORAC value of the antioxidant is determined by a decreased rate on fluorescence decay over time. Trolox (a vitamin E analogue) is used as a positive control.	Wu et al. (2004); Pior et al. (2005)
Hydrophilic and lipophilic antioxidant capacities	Hydrophilic and lipophilic antioxidant capacities are measured with the rapid peroxyl radical scavenging capacity (PSC) assay based on the degree of inhibition of dichlorofluorescein oxidation by antioxidants that scavenge peroxyl radicals, generated from thermal degradation of 2,2′-azobis(amidinopropane). The fluorescence is measured at 485 nm excitation and 538 nm emission. The areas under the average fluorescence–reaction time kinetic curve for control and samples are integrated and used for calculating antioxidant activity. The lipophilic PSC capacity assay is measured in extracts obtained after extraction of compounds with 50% acetone in water. Results obtained for lipophilic antioxidant activity are expressed as micromoles of vitamin E/100 g sample.	Adom and Liu (2005)
2,2′-Azinobis(3-ethylbenzothiazoline-6-sulfonic acid) (ABTS) assay	Colorimetric assay that measures ABTS$^+$ radical cation formation induced by metmyoglobin and hydrogen peroxide. In the presence of an antioxidant, ABTS$^+$ radical is neutralized by electron donation. ABTS$^+$ radical can be spectrophotometrically detected by absorbance at 405 nm. The antioxidant capacity is inversely proportional to the absorbance value. Trolox is used as a positive control.	Bartosz et al. (1998)
β-Carotene bleaching	Spectrophotometric assay that determines antioxidant inhibition of linoleic acid peroxide (LOO*) induced β-carotene oxidation in an emulsion phase. Oxidation of β-carotene emulsion is monitored spectrophotometrically by measuring absorbance at 470 nm.	Taga et al. (1959)

2.11.1 RESEARCH SUGGESTIONS

1. Compare the total phenolics, ferulic, and antioxidant capacity of white corn processed into tortillas.
2. Determine the antioxidant capacity of pasta produced from durum wheat using the methods described in Table 2.3.
3. Compare the total phenolics, ferulic, and antioxidant capacity of whole wheat bread and refined white bread obtained from the same wheat.
4. Compare the β-carotenes, lutein, and zeaxanthin of white and yellow endosperm corns.
5. Compare the tocopherols and tocotrienes of a corn germ samples analyzed via GLC or HPLC.

6. Determine the amounts of policosanols and phytosterols of whole corn and its dry-milled fractions (germ, bran, and grits).
7. Determine the amounts of oryzanol and tocopherols of rough, brown, and white polished rice.
8. Determine the amounts of avenathramides associated with oats, groats, oat bran, and oat endosperm.

2.11.2 Research Questions

1. How can you determine bound, free, and conjugated ferulic acid?
2. Investigate at least three different methods to assess the antioxidant capacity of cereal grains.
3. What is the difference between hydrophilic and lipophilic antioxidant capacities? Which assay is more relevant for cereal grains and their products?
4. What are the differences and similarities between phytosterols and cholesterol? What is the preferred instrumental method to determine the types of phytosterols associated with cereal grains?
5. What is oryzanol? What are the proven health benefits of this particular compound?
6. What are avenathramides? What are the proven health benefits of these particular compounds?
7. What are policosanols? What are the proven health benefits of these particular compounds?
8. For the nutraceuticals listed in the following table, indicate the most common analytical assay to quantify them and their major human health benefits.

Nutraceutical	Analytical Method	Health Benefits
Ferulic acid		
β-Carotenes		
Zeaxanthin		
Lutein		
Phytosterols		
Anthocyanins		
Tannins		
Policosanols		

2.12 INSTRUMENTAL ANALYSIS

2.12.1 Chromatography

Chromatography is defined as the separation of chemical compounds in a mixture. It involves passing a mixture dissolved in a *mobile phase* through a *stationary phase*, which separates the analyte to be measured from other molecules in the mixture based on differential partitioning between the mobile and stationary phases. Most chromatography techniques are analytical and some are aimed toward the predictive separation of analytes of interest. This last technique is commonly known as preparative. The most common and widely used chromatographic techniques include HPLC, GLC, thin-layer chromatography (TLC), and preparative. All these have use or are applied in the various segments of the cereal industry. Practically all organic compounds can be analyzed using one or several of these chromatographic methods.

2.12.1.1 Thin-Layer Chromatography

TLC is a relatively old technique that is used to separate mixtures on a sheet of glass, plastic, or aluminum foil, which is then coated with a thin layer or stationary phase of adsorbent material, usually silica gel, aluminum oxide, or paper (cellulose). A small sample of the extract is applied approximately 1.5 cm from the bottom edge of the TLC plate. Then, the appropriate solvent or eluant is poured into a container to a depth of approximately 1 cm. After the sample has been applied on the plate, a solvent or solvent mixture or is drawn up the plate via capillary action. The different analytes ascend the stationary phase at different rates. The length or distance at which the analyte stays is known as relative mobility or Rf. This factor is characteristic for different organic compounds when separated with a known solvent mixture at a fixed temperature. Authentic standards are frequently run to ensure that the chromatographic conditions remain unchanged. After chromatography, the plate is dried and sprayed with chemical developers to color the spots. By cutting the spots, the analysts can recover separated compounds. TLC is still used to follow the progress of chemical reactions, identify compounds present in a given extract, and determine the purity of a substance. In cereals, it is used to separate mycotoxins such as the different types of aflatoxins, pesticides (organophosphates and carbamates), carotenoids, sugars, lipids, phenolics, flavonoids, and other related compounds (Figure 2.7).

2.12.1.2 High-Performance Liquid Chromatography

Many chemical compounds or contaminants can be detected and quantified in HPLC systems equipped with either UV-vis, refractive index (RI), fluorescence, photodiode array (PDA), light-scattering detector (LSD), or other types of detectors (Table 2.4; Figure 2.7). The HPLC assays can be divided into four major categories: partition, absorption, ion exchange, and size exclusion. The HPLC partition chromatography is the most popular because it can effectively separate both polar and nonpolar compounds in a normal or reverse phase fashion. Separation in ion exchange columns depends on the reversible absorption of charged molecules to immobilized ion exchange groups of opposite charge. Subsequently, analytes are removed from the column by changing the elution conditions (pH) or the ionic strength of the buffer (Anonymous 2011). Size exclusion chromatography is used for the separation of large molecular weight compounds such as proteins. The size exclusion principle is to separate compounds by sieving where larger molecules are not retained and therefore elute first. The column contains

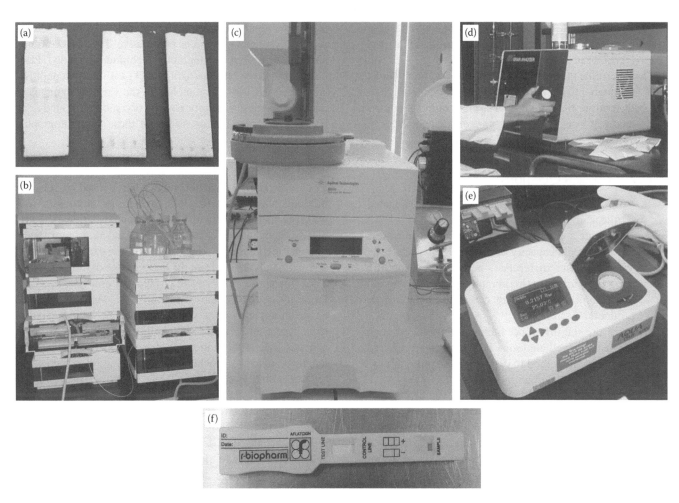

FIGURE 2.7 Instrumental equipments commonly used to analyze cereal-based foods. (a) TLC; (b) HPLC; (c) GLC; (d) NIRA; (e) water activity apparatus; (f) immunoassay (ELISA) for aflatoxins.

a stationary phase generally packaged with porous silica or polymer particles.

2.12.1.3 Gas-Liquid Chromatography

GC is a type of chromatography used for separation and analysis of compounds that can be vaporized (Figure 2.7). In this technique, the mobile phase is a carrier gas such as nitrogen or helium, whereas the stationary phase is a tubular or capillary column with a solid support. GCs can be equipped with FID, thermal conductivity, electron capture (ECD), flame photometric (FPD), and atomic emission (AED) detectors used for the analysis of a wide array of organic components (Table 2.5).

2.12.2 Near-Infrared Analysis

The near-infrared reflectance analyzers (NIRA) have been used for many years for rapid analysis of the chemical composition of a wide range of cereals, dry-milled fractions, and industrially processed products. The main advantage of this technology is that once the spectroscopy instrument has been properly calibrated, several constituents in a sample can be simultaneously measured without destroying the sample.

Thus, the instrument is ideally suited for quick, quality control determinations (Figure 2.7). Most commercial NIRA are used to measure moisture, protein and ash of grains, flours, meals, and ground finished products. Fat or oil and fiber contents may be analyzed in some products. The most sophisticated NIRA are capable of measuring flour absorption, starch damage, and grain hardness.

The NIRA measurements are made in the spectral region of 700 nm to 2500 nm. During the spectral scanning, specific chemical compounds absorb energy at specific wavelengths. The computer analysis of standard samples (i.e., wheat flour, ground whole wheat, specific cereal grain) varying in their chemical composition, will determine the best fit for the specific chemical compound. Most NIRA are equipped with a monochromator, tungsten-halogen lamp with a quartz envelope, and a filter system used to select the wavelength of energy to be directed onto the sample. Samples are generally packed into a cell containing a quartz window.

The key for the generation of reproducible results is the proper chemical analyses of the set of standard samples and sample preparation. The standard set of samples should have chemical compositions in the upper and lower expected range

TABLE 2.4

Main Uses of HPLC Detectors and Their Major Applications in Food and Toxin Analyses

HPLC Detector	Analytes
UV-vis	Organic acids, carotenoids, pesticides, amino acids (ion exchange column with ninhydrin)
Refractive index (RI)	Sugars
Fluorescence	Amino acids, B vitamins, mycotoxins, pesticides
Light-scattering detector (LSD)	Fatty acids, lipids and carbohydrates
Photodiode array (PDA)	Phenolics, flavonoids, carotenoids

of the desired chemical compound. The calibration samples should be analyzed by classical and official methods. For instance, if the NIRA is standardized for the analysis of protein of refined wheat flour, the set of standards should have samples varying from 6.5% to 14.5% protein. The higher the number of standard samples, the more reliable is the prediction of the given chemical compound. In terms of sample preparation, the most important variable is the consistency of the grind. It is very important that standard and test samples are ground with the same type of grinder and grinder procedure. This is because the particle size or granulation influences how light reflects.

2.12.2.1 Analysis via NIRA

A. Samples, Ingredients, and Reagents
- Test samples
- Calibration samples

B. Materials and Equipment
- Laboratory mill
- Sample cups
- NIRA
- Brush

C. Procedure
1. Turn on NIRA at least 30 minutes before testing.
2. Make sure to prepare the test sample using the same procedure previously used to obtain the set of calibration samples. The most important factor to control is the type of grinder and grinding procedure. Allow samples to equilibrate at room temperature if they were kept under refrigeration or frozen storage.
3. Select several calibration samples ranging in composition of the desired chemical compound. Place the sample in the NIRA sample cup and

run the analysis. If the composition of the calibration sample(s) are correct, then run the test samples. If the NIRA is not predicting the composition of the calibration samples, the apparatus has to be recalibrated.
4. Make sure to properly clean the cup after the analysis. Use a brush and avoid scratching the cup window.

2.12.3 Water Activity

The moisture content of foods is often less satisfactory as a measure of the keeping qualities of the foods compared with water activity or A_w. The moisture content alone is not a reliable indicator of stability because foods with the same moisture content differ in their perishability (Bradley 2003). The main reason for the observed differences is in the way that the water associates with other food constituents. Water activity is a better indicator of shelf life because it measures the partial pressure of the water associated with the food in relation to the vapor pressure of pure water. In other words, A_w measures the amount of water tightly bound to chemical compounds. The A_w values range from 0 to 1. Typical water activity values for 14% moisture cereal grains and their refined flours range from 0.65 to 0.75, dehydrated products such as cookies, crackers, breakfast cereals, and snacks have values lower than 0.5, and high-moisture products such as breads and tortillas have values higher than 0.96. Interestingly, high-sugar products such as sweeteners or syrups containing 30% water have a relatively lower A_w (0.7).

2.12.3.1 Determination of Water Activity (A_w)

There is no device that can be put into a product to directly measure water activity. However, the water activity of a

TABLE 2.5

Main Uses of GLC Detectors and Their Major Applications in Food and Toxin Analyses

GC Detector	Analytes
Flame ionization (FID)	Fatty acids (cis and trans), cholesterol, phytosterols, antioxidants, and alcohols
Thermal conductivity	Gases and volatile compounds
Electron capture	Pesticide residues
Flame photometric	Organophosphorous pesticides and volatile sulfur compounds
Atomic emission	Methyl bromide

product can be determined from the relative humidity of the air surrounding the sample when the air and the sample are at equilibrium. Therefore, the sample must be in an enclosed space where this equilibrium can take place. Once this occurs, the water activity of the sample and the relative humidity of the air are equal. The measurement taken at equilibrium is called an equilibrium relative humidity.

Two different types of water activity instruments are commercially available. One uses chilled-mirror dewpoint technology whereas the other measures relative humidity with sensors that change electrical resistance or capacitance. Each has advantages and disadvantages. The methods vary in accuracy, repeatability, speed of measurement, stability in calibration, linearity, and convenience of use. The major advantages of the chilled-mirror dewpoint method are accuracy, speed (<5 minutes), ease of use, and precision. Capacitance sensors have the advantage of being inexpensive, but are not typically as accurate or as fast as the chilled-mirror dewpoint method.

A. *Samples, Ingredients, and Reagents*
- Test samples
- Calibration samples

B. *Materials and Equipment*
- Laboratory mill
- AquaLab

C. *Procedure (AquaLab)*
1. Turn on the AquaLab instrument (Figure 2.7) at least 15 minutes before the test. Make sure the AquaLab is positioned on a level surface and the environmental or room temperature is stable.
2. Adjust equipment with distilled water and calibration samples with known A_w.
3. Calibrate the equipment by pressing the Menu icon on the main screen and then pressing Enter twice to start calibration.
4. Place test sample to at least cover the bottom of the sample cup and preferably to half of the cup (do not overfill). Ensure that the rim and outside of the sample cup are cleaned and that the sample temperature is not more than 4°C above the chamber temperature.
5. Place sample cup in sample chamber. Close lid carefully to avoid spillage. Move latch to the left to start measurement. The instrument will beep when starting A_w measurements. The first A_w will be displayed within a minute or two, and after another beep, the final A_w reading and temperature will be displayed.
6. Record A_w reading.

2.12.4 IMMUNOASSAYS

Enzyme-linked immunosorbent assay (ELISA) is a novel diagnostic technique used to detect the presence of proteins expressed in genetically modified organisms such as maize, mycotoxins, drug residues, or specific allergenic proteins such as gliadin which is responsible for celiac disease. The principle of ELISA is the fixing of a certain amount of antigen to a column or surface (Figure 2.7). After the antigen is immobilized, the detection antibody is added, forming a complex with the antigen. The antibody is usually linked to an enzyme. The plate is developed by adding an enzymatic substrate to produce a visible signal (color or fluorescence) which is directly related to the amount of antigen in the sample. Immunoassays commonly involve chromogenic changes usually quantified with a fluorescence detector. The main advantages of ELISA techniques are the remarkably specific and strong binding of antibodies to antigens and the detection of very small amounts of the analyte of interest. For instance, aflatoxins are usually detected in parts per billion whereas gliadin is detected in micrograms. The other main advantage is that assays are usually quick, easy to perform, and many samples can be analyzed daily. This is the reason regulatory agencies rely on ELISA techniques as a simple and quick method to determine mycotoxins and food allergens.

2.12.5 RESEARCH SUGGESTIONS

1. Determine the water activity of a given lot of maize that contains 14% moisture and has been dried to 4%, 8%, and 10% moisture and tempered to increase its moisture to 16%, 18%, 20%, and 22% moisture. Graph the moisture (*y* axis) vs. A_w (*x* axis) and determine the grain stability of the different lots of maize throughout 1 month storage in sealed plastic bags (refer to procedure in Section 4.2.1.2).
2. Prepare corn tortillas that have been supplemented with 0%, 1%, 2%, and 3% glycerol and then determine their water activities, moisture contents, and microbial stabilities (observation of the days required for tortillas to develop molds). The tortillas should be packaged in polyethylene bags (refer to procedure in Section 7.2.3.1).
3. Determine the amount of aflatoxins in a given lot of contaminated maize using ELISA and chromatographic techniques.

2.12.6 RESEARCH QUESTIONS

1. What are the principles, advantages, and disadvantages of TLC? Investigate the method and solvents used to separate carotenes and xantophylls using TLC.
2. Suggest analytical techniques to quantify organochlorine, organophosphorus, methyl bromide, and phosphine pesticides associated with stored cereal grain.
3. What is an internal standard? Why it is very useful in HPLC and GLC analyses?
4. What are the main components of an HPLC system?
5. Describe three types of HPLC detectors and the principles of operation and one common analytical use for each.

6. What is size exclusion chromatography? What are the main analytical uses of this technique?

7. What is preparative HPLC chromatography? What are the main uses of this technique?

8. What are the differences between normal and reverse phase chromatography?

9. What is the main use of mass spectrometry? Describe at least three different types of mass spectrometers. What are the advantages of each system?

10. What are the main components of a GLC system?

11. Why must fatty acids be derivatized before GLC analysis?

12. What are the advantages of using capillary columns when performing GLC analysis?

13. What are the differences among FID, electron capture, thermal conductivity, and flame photometric detectors used in GC in terms of sensitivity, specificity, and sample destruction?

14. What are the principles, advantages, and disadvantages of near-infrared spectroscopy?

15. What are the steps involved in the calibration of a NIRA for protein or fiber analysis?

16. How can you decrease the water activity of a wheat flour tortilla? What kind of additives can you use?

17. In a table, describe the minimum water activity required by pathogenic bacteria, salt-tolerant bacteria, yeast, and molds. Which type of microorganism is more resistant to water activity?

18. What are the principles, advantages, and disadvantages of ELISA techniques used for mycotoxin analyses?

19. Investigate the use of immunoassays for determination of gluten in foods. What are the principles and accuracy of these techniques?

2.13   NUTRITION LABELING

One of the chief reasons for analyzing the chemical components of cereal-based foods is to meet nutrition labeling regulations. Nutritional labeling differs in countries around the world. However, in most instances, the labeling information includes the amount of food and number of servings in a package, its common name, the list of ingredients, the address and information of the processors, and the nutritional information that, in some instances, could include health claims. The nutrient composition is usually expressed both in concentration/serving and as a percentage of the recommended daily allowance. The aim is to provide consumers with key information regarding food and nutrient composition with current dietary and health concerns. In the specific case of cereal-based industries, the most recent concerns are in terms of gluten-containing ingredients related to celiac disease and the presence of genetically modified grains.

The aim of the nutritional label is to inform consumers of the raw materials used to manufacture the food item and the most relevant nutrients affecting human health.

It is important to inform consumers of the raw materials because segments of the general population have food allergies, some of the most common being to lactose, gluten, sulfites, and monosodium glutamate. Emphasis is made in the relationship between nutrients and dietary concerns. Consumers are aware of the strong relationship between the abuse of some nutrients and the incidence of chronic diseases such as cardiovascular disease, hypertension, hypercholesterolemia, diabetes, and cancer. Table 2.6 summarizes the mandatory nutrients with their corresponding recommended daily allowance considering a 2000 kcal diet and the relationship with human health and chronic diseases.

These nutrient claims are mainly aimed toward health-conscious consumers and people with obesity or chronic diseases. The FDA allows the labeling of health claims for the following nutrients: calcium and osteoporosis, sodium and hypertension, dietary fat and cancer, dietary saturated fat and cardiovascular risk, cholesterol and cardiovascular diseases, fiber and cancer, soluble fiber and cardiovascular diseases, folate and neural tube defects, and sugar alcohol and dental caries (Nielsen and Metzger 2003; Serna-Saldivar 2008c).

2.13.1   Research Suggestions

1. Determine nutrition labels of breads produced (refer to procedure in Section 9.2.6.2) using enriched or unenriched refined hard wheat flours. Labels should include list of ingredients, serving size, nutrients per serving, and percentage daily values.

2. Determine nutrition labels of table bread produced (refer to procedure in Section 9.6.2.2) using refined hard wheat flour and whole wheat flour. Labels should include list of ingredients, serving size, nutrients per serving, and percentage daily values.

3. Determine nutrition labels of flour tortillas produced (refer to procedure in Section 10.5.1.1) using hydrogenated shortening or fractionated stearin from palm oil or a trans-free shortening. Labels should include list of ingredients, serving size, nutrients per serving, and percentage daily values.

2.13.2   Research Questions

1. Estimate the total calories and calories from fat for nutrition labeling purposes of the following cereal-based food.

Wheat Flour Tortilla	Amount
Moisture	30.2
Crude protein	8.3
Crude fiber	1.1
Ash	1.9
Crude fat	7.8
NFE	50.7
Total	100

TABLE 2.6
Food Labeling, Mandatory Nutrients with Their Reference Daily Intake Values and Relationships with Human Health

Nutrient	RDI	Health Implications
Total calories	2000 kcal	The total calorie intake is closely related with being overweight and obesity.
Calories from fat	<585 kcal	The calories from fat should be limited especially in overweight, obese, and superobese people and people with chronic diseases such as cardiovascular disease and arteriosclerosis.
Fat	<65 g	Fat intake should be limited in obese people and those with chronic diseases. Fats should provide less than 30% of the total caloric intake.
Saturated fat	<20 g	High intake of saturated fats is one of the main factors that increase cardiovascular disease.
Trans fats	0	Trans fatty acids have detrimental effects on human health because they increase the risk of cardiovascular disease, hypercholesterolemia, and cancer. Most new food labeling regulations mandate processors to declare the amount of trans fats.
Cholesterol	<300 mg	A high intake of cholesterol from animal sources is associated with a higher risk of cardiovascular disease and hypercholesterolemia.
Total carbohydrate	300 g	The total carbohydrate content is constituted by complex and simple carbohydrates. Complex (starch) are digested more slowly than simple carbohydrates and have lower glycemic index. These carbohydrates provide 4 kcal/g.
Sugar	<50 g	The consumption of high amounts of sugars increases the risk of diabetes and caries or tooth decay. Modern human diets tend to abuse the consumption of simple sugars considered as empty foods.
Dietary fiber	>25 g	The consumption of insoluble and soluble dietary fibers lowers the caloric density of foods and helps to prevent cardiovascular disease, colon cancer, constipation, and hemorrhoids and lowers the glycemic index of foods. Soluble dietary fiber lowers blood cholesterol. Most dietary fibers contain important amounts of nutraceutical compounds that have positive health implications.
Protein	50 g	Protein is especially important to sustain growth in infants, children, and adolescents or teenagers. It also helps to prevent diseases via production of antibodies.
Sodium	<2400 mg	Sodium is the nutrient that is most abused by humans. The high consumption of sodium is related to hypertension.
Vitamin A	5000 IU	The most important liposoluble vitamin in human nutrition. Prevents night blindness, strengthens the immune system, and prevents infectious diseases.
Vitamin C	60 mg	Prevents scurvy.
Calcium	1000 mg	Calcium is the most important macro mineral in human nutrition. Especially required in growing children. Its deficiency is the main cause of osteoporosis, especially among postmenopausal women and geriatric people.
Iron	18 mg	Iron is the most important micro mineral in human nutrition because it is deficient especially among low socioeconomic children and pregnant women. Iron helps to prevent anemia and strengthens the immune system.

Source: Nielsen, S.S., and Metzger, L.E., In *Food Analysis*, 3rd ed., S.S. Nielsen (ed.). Kluwer Academic, New York, NY, 2003; and Serna-Saldivar, S.O., In *Industrial Manufacture of Snack Foods*, Kennedys Publications Ltd., London, UK, 2008. With permission.

Notes: RDI, reference daily intake.

2. How are trans fatty acids analyzed in foods for labeling purposes?

3. Design a food label for wheat flour tortillas according to the composition (g/100 g tortillas) listed below and formulation of procedure in Section 10.5.1.1. The serving is one tortilla that weighs 28 g. List the ingredients, the amount per serving and the % daily values. Do not forget to include calories from fat.

Nutrient (100 g)	Wheat Flour Tortilla
Water, g	30.22
Energy, kcal	312
Protein, g	8.29
Lipids, g	7.75
Saturated, g	1.886
Monounsat., g	3.894
Polyunsat., g	1.584

Cholesterol, g	0
Carbohydrates, g	51.35
Sugars, g	1.92
Dietary fiber, g	3.1
Calcium, mg	129
Iron, mg	3.34
Sodium, mg	636
Vitamin A, IU	10
Vitamin C, mg	0
Thiamine, mg	0.539
Riboflavin, mg	0.267
Niacin, mg	3.572
Folate, μg	104

4. The following table depicts the typical chemical composition of regular tortilla chips.

Nutrient (100 g)	Regular Tortilla Chips
Water, g	1.8
Energy, kcal	501
Protein, g	7.0
Lipids, g	26.2
Saturated, g	5.02
Monounsat., g	15.45
Polyunsat., g	3.63
Carbohydrates, g	62.9
Dietary fiber, g	6.5
Calcium, mg	154
Iron, mg	1.52
Sodium, mg	528

a. If you want to develop light and fat free tortilla chips what is the maximum amount of fat for these products? What are the amounts of calories and calories from fat that you expect on light and fat-free tortilla chips?

b. If you want to label the regular tortilla chips as "reduced sodium" or "light in sodium") items, what are the maximum allowable amounts of sodium in these products?

5. What are the main health reasons of including the following nutrients in food labels?
   a. Calories
   b. Trans-fats
   c. Dietary fiber
   d. Saturated fat
   e. Cholesterol
   f. Vitamin A
   g. Iron
   h. Sodium

6. What are the requirements for labeling a cereal-based product as "gluten free?" What kind of considerations should be made to assure that the product is indeed "gluten free?"

REFERENCES

Adhikari, P., K. T. Hwang, J. N. Park, and C. K. Kim. 2006. "Policosanol Content and Composition in Perilla Seeds." *Journal of Agricultural and Food Chemistry* 54(15): 5359–5362.

Adom, K. K., and R. H. Liu. 2002. "Antioxidant Activity of Grains." *Journal of Agricultural and Food Chemistry* 50:6182–6187.

Adom, K. K., and R. H. Liu. 2005. "Rapid Peroxyl Radical Scavenging Capacity (PSC) Assay for Assessing Both Hydrophilic and Lipophilic Antioxidants." *Journal of Agricultural and Food Chemistry* 53(17):6572–6580.

American Association of Cereal Chemists (AACC). 2000. *AACC Approved Methods of Analysis*. 10th ed. St. Paul, MN: American Association of Cereal Chemists.

American Oil Chemists' Society (AOCS) 2009. *Official Methods and Recommended Practices of the AOCS*. 6th ed. Danvers, MA: The Society.

Anderson, N. E., and F. M. Cleydesdale. 1978. "Analysis of Tryptophan Utilizing its Reaction with Alpha Ketoglutaric acid." *Journal of Food Science* 43(5):1595–1599.

Anonymous. 2011. *Ion Exchange Chromatography. Principles and Methods*. Amersham Biosciences. Edition AA. www.amershambiosciences.com.

Arruzazabala, M. L., D. Carbajal, R. Mas, V. Molina, S. Valdes, and A. Laguna. 1994. "Cholesterol Lowering Effects of Polycosanol on Rabbits." *Biological Research* 27:205–208.

Arruzazabala, M. L., S. Valdes, R. Mas, L. Fernandez, and D. Carbajal. 1996. "Effect of Polycosanol Successive Dose Increase on Platelet Aggregation in Healthy Volunteers." *Pharmacological Research* 34:181–185.

Asp, N. G. 2001. "Development of Dietary Fibre Methodology." In *Advanced Dietary Fiber Technology*, edited by B. V. McCleary and L. Prosky, 77–88. Oxford, England: Blackwell Science Ltd.

Asp, N. G., and C. G. Johansson. 1981. "Techniques for Measuring Dietary Fiber." In *The Analysis of Dietary Fiber in Food*, edited by W. P. T. James and O. Theander, 173–189. New York: Marcel Dekker.

Asp, N. G., and C. G. Johansson. 1984. "Dietary Fiber Analysis." *Nutrition Abstracts and Reviews* 54:735–752.

Asp, N. G., C. G. Johansson, H. Hallmer, and M. Siljestrom. 1983. "Rapid Enzymatic Assay of Insoluble and Soluble Dietary Fiber." *Journal of Agricultural and Food Chemistry* 31(3): 476–482.

Awika, J. M., and L. W. Rooney. 2004. "Sorghum Phytochemicals and Their Potential Aspects on Human Health." *Phytochemistry* 65:1199–1221.

Association of Official Analytical Chemists (AOAC). 2005. *Official Methods of Analysis of AOAC International*, edited by W. Horwitz and G. W. Latimer. 18th ed. Arlington, VA: AOAC.

Bartosz, G., A. Janaszewska, D. Ertel, and M. Bartosz. 1998. Simple Determination of Peroxyl Radical-trapping Capacity." *Biochemistry and Molecular Biology International* 46:519–528.

Bender, D. A. 1992. "Vitamin E: Tocopherols and Tocotrienols." In *Nutritional Biochemistry of the Vitamins*. Cambridge, UK: Cambridge University Press.

Bidlingmeyer, B. A., S. A. Cohen, and T. L. Tarvin. 1984. "Rapid Analysis of Amino Acids Using Pre-column Derivatization." *Journal of Chromatography. B, Biomedical Applications* 336:93–104.

Bradley, R. L. 2003. "Moisture and Total Solids Analysis." In *Food Analysis*, 3rd ed., edited by S. S. Nielsen. New York: Kluwer Academic.

Bunnell, R. H. 1971. "Modern Procedures for the Analysis of Tocopherols." *Lipids* 6(4):245–253.

Canty, D. J. 2001. "Lecithin and Choline: New Roles for Old Nutrients." In *Handbook of Nutraceuticals and Functional Foods*, edited by R. E. C. Wildman. Boca Raton, FL: CRC.

Canty, D. J., and S. H. Zeisel. 1994. "Lecithin and Choline in Human Health and Disease." *Nutrition Reviews* 52(10):327–339.

Champ, M., L. Martin, L. Noah, and M. Gratas. 1999. In *Complex Carbohydrates in Foods*, edited by S. S. Cho, L. Prosky, and M. Dreher, 169–187. New York: Marcel Dekker, Inc.

Champ, M., F. Kozlowski, and G. Lecannu. 2000. In *Advanced Dietary Fiber Technology*, edited by B. V. McCleary and L. Prosky, 106–119. Oxford, UK: Blackwell Science Ltd.

Champ, M., A. M. Langkilde, F. Brouns, B. Kettlitz, and Y. Le-Bail-Collet. 2003. "Advances in Dietary Fiber Characterization. 2. Consumption, Chemistry, Physiology and Measurement of Resistant Starch: Implications for Health and Food Labeling." *Nutrition Research Reviews* 16:143.

Chung, O. K., and J. B. Ohm. 2000. "Cereal Lipids." 2nd ed. In *Handbook of Cereal Science and Technology*, edited by K. Kulp and J. G. Ponte. New York: Marcel Dekker, Inc.

Deprez, S., I. Mila, J. Huneau, D. Tome, and A. Scalbert. 2001. "Transport of Proanthocyanidin Dimer, Timer and Polymer Across Monolayers of Human Intestinal Epithelial Caco 2 Cells." *Antioxidants and Redox Signaling* 3:957–967.

Dicko, M. H., H. Gruppen, A. S. Traore, A. G. J. Voragen, and W. J. H. van Berkel. 2006. "Phenolic Compounds and Related Enzymes as Determinants of Sorghum for Food Use." *Biotechnology and Molecular Biology Review* 1(1):21–38.

Dykes, L., L. W. Rooney, R. D. Waniska, and W. L. Rooney. 2005. "Phenolic Compounds and Antioxidant Activity of Sorghum Grains of Varying Genotypes." *Journal of Agricultural and Food Chemistry* 53:6813–6818.

Englyst, H. N. 1981. "Determination of Carbohydrates and Its Composition in Plant Materials." In: *The Analysis of Dietary Fiber in Food*, edited by W. P. T. James and O. Theander, 173–189. New York: Marcel Dekker.

Englyst, H. N., S. M. Kingman, and J. H. Cummings. 1992. "Classification and Measurement of Nutritionally Important Starch Fractions." *European Journal of Clinical Nutrition* 46(suppl. 2):S33–S50.

Ferreira, D., and D. Slade. 2002. "Oligomeric Proanthocyanidins: naturally Occurring O-heterocycles." *Natural Product Reports* 19:517–541.

Fiala, E. S., B. S. Reddy, and J. H. Weisburger. 1985. "Naturally Occurring Anticarcinogenic Substances in Foodstuffs." *Annual Review of Nutrition* 5:295–321.

Friedman, M., and J. W. Finley. 1971. "Methods of Tryptophan Analysis." *Journal of Agricultural and Food Chemistry* 19:626–630.

Fuleki, T., and F. J. Francis. 1968. "Quantitative Methods for Anthocyanins. 1. Extraction and Determination of Total Anthocyanin in Cranberries." *Journal of Food Science* 33: 72–77.

Fullmer, L. A., and A. Shao. 2001. "The Role of Lutein in Eye Health and Nutrition." *Cereal Foods World* 46(9):408.

Goering, H. K., and P. J. Van Soest. 1970. "Forage Fiber Analysis (Apparatus, Reagents, Procedures, and Some Applications)." USDA Agricultural Research Service. Handbook no. 379 as modified by D. R. Mertens.

Goñi, I., E. Garcia-Diz, E. M. Mañas, and F. Saura-Calixto. 1996. "Analysis of Resistant Starch: A Method for Foods and Food Products." *Food Chemistry* 56:445–449.

Gouni-Berthold, I., and H. K. Berthold. 2002. "Policosanol: Clinical Pharmacology and Therapeutic Significance of a New Lipid Lowering Agent." *American Heart Journal* 143:356–365.

Gross, J. 1991. "Carotenoids." In *Pigments in Vegetables: Chlorophylls and Carotenoids*, edited by J. Gross. New York: Van Nostrand Reinhold.

Hargrove, J. L., P. Greenspan, and D. K. Hartle. 2004. "Nutritional Significance and Metabolism of Very Long Chain Fatty Alcohols and Acids from Dietary Waxes." *Experimental Biology and Medicine* 229:215–226.

Haswell, S. J. 1991. *Atomic Absorption Spectrometry; Theory, Design and Applications*. Amsterdam, Holland: Elsevier.

Hoffmann, F. 1972. *Compendio de Vitaminas. Propiedades de la Vitaminas y su Importancia en Alimentación Humana y Animal*. Basilea, Suiza: La Roche & Cía., S.A.

Hoffpauer, D. W. 2005. "New Applications for Whole Rice Bran." *Cereal Foods World* 50(4):173–174.

Holub, B. J. 1982. "The Nutritional Significance, Metabolism, and Function of Myo-inositol and Phosphatidylinositol in Health and Disease." *Advances in Nutritional Research* 4:107–141.

Howard, L. R., D. D. Braswell, and J. Aselage. 1996. "Chemical Composition and Color of Strained Carrots as Affected by Processing." *Journal of Food Science* 61:327–330.

Hwang, K. T., S. L. Cuppett, C. L. Weller, and M. A. Hanna. 2002. "HPLC of Grain Sorghum Wax Classes Highlighting Separation of Aldehydes from Wax Esters and Steryl Esters." *Journal of Separation Science* 25:619–623.

Hwang, K. T., C. L. Weller, S. L. Cuppett, and M. A. Hanna. 2004. "Policosanol Contents and Composition of Grain Sorghum Kernels and Dried Distillers Grains." *Cereal Chemistry* 81: 345–349.

Jacobson, G. A. 1991. "Quality Control in Deep Fat Frying Operations." *Food Technology* 45(2):72–74.

James, C. S. 1995. *Analytical Chemistry of Foods*. New York: Chapman & Hall.

Kanski, J., M. Aksenova, A. Stoyanova, and D. A. Butterfield. 2002. "Ferulic Acid Antioxidant Protection Against Hydroxyl and Peroxyl Radical Oxidation in Synaptosomal and Neuronal Cell Culture Systems in Vitro: Structure-Activity Studies." *Journal of Nutritional Biochemistry* 13:273–281.

Lampi, A. N., V. Piironen, and J. Toivo. 2005. "Analysis of Phytosterols in Foods." In *Phytosterols as Functional Food Components and Nutraceuticals*, edited by P. C. Dutta, 28–60. New York: Marcel Dekker, Inc.

Landry, J., and T. Moureaux. 1970. "Heterogenicity of the Glutelins of the Grain Core. Selective Extraction and Composition in Amino Acids of the Three Isolated Gractions." *Bulletin de la Société de Chimie Biologique* 52:1021–1037.

Landry, J., and T. Moureaux. 1980. "Distribution and Amino Acid Composition of Protein Groups Located in Different Histological Parts of Maize Grain." *Journal of Agricultural and Food Chemistry* 28:1186–1191.

Majumder, A., and B. Biswas 2006. *Biology of Inositols and Phosphoinositides*. New York: Springer Science & Business Media.

Mason, J. S., M. Lotfi, N. Dalmiya, K. Sethuraman, and M. Deitcher. 2001. *The Micronutrient Report: Current Progress and Trends in the Control of Vitamin A*. Ottawa, Ontario, Canada: Micronutrient Initiative and International Development Research Center.

McCleary, B. V., and D. A. Monaghan. 2002. "Measurement of Resistant Starch." *Journal of AOAC International* 85: 665–675.

McCleary, B. V., M. McNally, and P. Rossiter. 2002. "Measurement of Resistant Starch by Enzymic Digestion in Starch Samples and Selected Plant Materials: Collaborative Study." *Journal of AOAC International* 85:1103–1111.

Megazyme. 2011. Resistant starch. www.megazyme.com/purchase_products/Diagnostic_kits/.

Mertens, D. R. 1992. "Critical Conditions in Determining Detergent Fiber." *Proceedings of NFTA Forage Analysis Workshop. Denver, CO. p C1–C8. Fiber (Acid Detergent) and Lignin in Animal Feed (973.18)*. Official Methods of Analysis, 1990. 15th ed. Association of Official Analytical Chemists.

Miller, D. D., and M. A. Rutzke. 2003. "Atomic Absorption and Emission Spectroscopy." In *Food Analysis*, 3rd ed., edited by S. S. Nielsen, 401–421. New York: Kluwer Academic.

Mongeau, R., and R. Brassard. 1979. "Determination of Neutral Detergent Fiber, Hemicellulose, Cellulose, Lignin in Breads." *Cereal Chemistry* 56(5):437–441.

Moreau, R. A., M. J. Powell, and K. B. Hicks. 1996. "Extraction and Quantitative Analysis of Oil from Commercial Corn." *Journal of Agricultural and Food Chemistry* 44:2149–2154.

Murphy, J., and J. P. Riley. 1962. "A Modified Single Solution Method for the Determination of Phosphate in Natural Waters." *Analytica Chimica Acta* 27:31–36.

Nielsen, S. S. 2003. "Determination of Moisture Content." In *Food Analysis Laboratory Manual*. New York: Kluwer Academic.

Nielsen, S. S., and L. E. Metzger. 2003. "Nutrition Labeling." In *Food Analysis*, 3rd ed., edited by S. S. Nielsen. New York: Kluwer Academic.

Nurit, E., A. Tiessen, K. V. Pixley, and N. Palacios-Rojas. 2009. "Reliable and Inexpensive Colorimetric Method for Determining Protein-Bound Tryptophan in Maize Kernels." *Journal of Agricultural and Food Chemistry* 57(16):7233–7238.

Onuma Okezie, B. 1998. "World Food Security. The Role of Postharvest Technology." *Food Technology* 52(1):64–69.

Paulis, L. W., and J. S. Wall. 1975. "Protein Quality in Cereals Evaluated by Rapid Estimation of Specific Protein Fractions." In *Protein Nutritional Quality of Foods and Feeds*, edited by M. Friedman, 381. New York: Marcel Dekker.

Paulis, L. W., and J. S. Wall. 1979. "Distribution and Electrophoretic Properties of Alcohol Soluble Proteins in Normal and High Lysine Sorghum." *Cereal Chemistry* 56:20–23.

Phillippy, B. 2003. "Inositol Phosphates in Foods." *Advances in Food and Nutrition Research* 45:1–60.

Price, M. L., S. V. Scoyoc, and L. G. Butler. 1978. "A Critical Evaluation of the Vanillin Reaction as an Assay for Tannin in Sorghum Grain." *Journal of Agricultural and Food Chemistry* 26(5):1214–1218.

Prior, R. L., X. Wu, and K. Schaich. 2005. "Standardized Methods for the Determination of Antioxidant Capacity of Phenolics in Foods and Dietary Supplements." *Journal of Agricultural and Food Chemistry* 53:4290–4302.

Raicht, R. F., B. I. Cohen, E. P. Fazzini, A. N. Sarwal, and M. Takahashi. 1980. "Protective Effect of Plant Sterols Against Chemically Induced Colon Tumors in Rats." *Cancer Research* 40:403–405.

Rooney, L. W. 2007. *Corn Quality Assurance Manual*. 2nd ed. Arlington, VA: Snack Food Association.

Sacchetti, G., and R. Bruni. 2007. "Efficiency of Extracting Vitamin E from Plant Sources." In *The Encyclopedia of Vitamin E*, edited by V. R. Preddy and R. R. Watson. Cambridge, MA: CABI Publishing.

Sadler, G. D., and P. A. Murphy. 1998. "pH and Titratable Acidity." In *Food Analysis*, 2nd ed., edited by S. S. Nielsen, 99–118. Gaithersburg, MD: Aspen Publishers, Inc.

Serna-Saldivar, S. O. 2008a. "Properties and Manufacturing of Oils." In *Industrial Manufacture of Snack Foods*. London, UK: Kennedys Publications Ltd.

Serna-Saldivar, S. O. 2008b. "The Process of Frying and Seasoning." In *Industrial Manufacture of Snack Foods*. London: Kennedys Publications Ltd.

Serna-Saldivar, S. O. 2008c. "Nutritional Value of Snack Foods." In *Industrial Manufacture of Snack Foods*. London: Kennedys Publications Ltd.

Signore, C., P. Ueland, and J. Troendle. 2008. "Choline Concentrations in Human Maternal and Cord Blood and Intelligence at 5 Years of Age." *American Journal of Clinical Nutrition* 87:896–902.

Sommer, A. 1987. "Blinding Malnutrition." *World Health* May:20–24.

Sosulski, F., K. Krygier, and L. Hogge. 1982. "Free, Esterified, and Insoluble-Bound Phenolic Acids. Composition of Phenolic Acids in Cereal and Potato Flours." *Journal of Agricultural and Food Chemistry* 30:337–340.

Spackman, D. H., W. H. Stein, and S. Moore. 1958. "Automatic Recording Apparatus for Use in Chromatography of Amino Acids." *Analytical Chemistry* 30(7):1190–1206.

Stevenson, S. G., M. Vaisey-Genser, and N. A. M. Eskin. 1984. "Quality Control in the Use of Deep Fat Frying Oils." *Journal of the American Oil Chemists' Society* 61:1102.

Swain, T., and W. E. Hillis. 1959. "The Phenolics Constituents of *Prunus Domestica*. I. The Quantitative Analysis of Phenolics Constituents." *Journal of the Science of Food and Agriculture* 10(1):63–68.

Taga, M. S., E. E. Miller, and D. E. Patt. 1984. "Chia Seeds as a Source of Natural Lipid Antioxidants." *Journal of the American Oil Chemists' Society* 61:928–931.

Undersander, D., D. R. Mertens, and N. Thiex. 1993. *Forage Analyses Procedures*. 1–139, Omaha, NE: National Forage Testing Association.

Van dan Briel, T., and P. Webb. 2003. "Fighting World Hunger Through Micronutrient Fortification Programs." *Food Technology* 57(11):44–47.

Van de Voort, F. R., K. P. Memon, J. Sedman, and A. A. Ismail. 1996. "Determination of Solid Fat Index by Fourier Transform Infrared Spectroscopy." *Journal of the American Oil Chemists' Society* 73(4):411–416.

Van Soest, P. J, J. B. Robertson, and B. A. Lewis. 1991. "Methods for Dietary Fiber, Neutral Detergent Fiber and Non-Starch Polysaccharides in Relation to Animal Nutrition." *Journal of Dairy Science* 74:3583–3597.

Villegas, E., E. Ortega, and R. Bauer. 1984. *Chemical Methods Used at CIMMYT for Determining Protein Quality in Cereal Grains*. 100. Mexico, DF: CIMMYT.

Vivas Rodriguez, N., R. D. Waniska, and L. W. Rooney. 1987. "Effect of Tortilla Production on Proteins of Sorghum and Maize." *Cereal Chemistry* 64:390–394.

Vucenik, I. and A. M. Shamsuddin. 2006. "Protection against Cancer by Dietary IP6 and Inositol." *Nutrition and Cancer* 55(2):109–125.

Walker, R. C., and W. A. Bosin. 1971. "Comparison of SFI, DSC and NMR Methods for Determining Solid–Liquid Ratios in Fats." *Journal of the American Oil Chemists' Society* 48(2):50–53.

Wilson, W. 2008. "Determination of Free Amino Nitrogen in Proteins." Baltimore, MD: Laboratory of Physiological Chemistry. Johns Hopkins Medical School. Available from: http://www.jbc.org/cgi/reprint/56/1/191.pdf.

Wu, X., G. R. Beecher, J. M. Holden, D. B. Haytowitz, S. E. Gebhardt, and R. L. Prior. 2004. "Lipophilic and Hydrophilic Antioxidant Capacities of Common Foods in the United States." *Journal of Agricultural and Food Chemistry* 52: 4026–4037.

3 Determination of Color, Texture, and Sensory Properties of Cereal Grain Products

3.1 INTRODUCTION

Whether working in product development, quality control, or process design and scale-up, color, texture, and sensory testing play an integral role in manufacturing the best products. The three major aspects related to the overall acceptability of a certain food are color, texture, and flavor or taste. The color of cereal-based foods is the first contact point with the consumer. This attribute can be objectively or subjectively judged. The rheological and textural properties of foods throughout their expected shelf life also greatly affect acceptance. Textural properties are measured with empirical or fundamental tests or with trained panelists. These physical properties closely relate with the acceptance and preference of foods. Sensory testing with trained or untrained panelists has the advantage of judging the main parameters related to the quality of prepared foods: color, texture, aroma, flavor, and overall acceptability. Sensory testing is also critically important for product development, research, and quality control programs.

3.2 COLOR

Color is an appearance property attributable to the spectral distribution of light. The perception of color by the human eye is important because it is the first quality parameter perceived by the consumer. Color is characteristic of the visible spectrum of light measurable in terms of wavelength, visible spectrum, and intensity. The additive and subtractive effects of color combinations produce all colors perceived by the human eye. When lights of various colors are superimposed, color will be the result of the sum of the different ones present. The three primary colors (blue, green, and red), when combined, produce all the visible colors (Hutchings 1994). The combination of red and blue yields purple colors, red and yellow produces orange, whereas blue and yellow produce green colorations. The combination of the three produces a black color.

When light strikes food, it is reflected, absorbed, transmitted, or refracted. The relationship between absorbance and reflectance is called lightness. When light is absorbed at a specific wavelength, it is perceived as hue, whereas the amount of light reflected is called intensity or chroma. Glossiness of color is due to the geometric way in which light is reflected and transmitted. Transmitted light is of importance in transparent foods such as syrups and beer. Color is perceived as the light that passes through a substance.

The colors associated with cereal grains and their products are due to the interaction of several factors. The main intrinsic factors affecting the color of grains, flours, and other milled fractions are natural pigments such as phenolics, anthocyanins, tannins, carotenoids, and xantophylls. In addition, the color of processed products is affected by purposely supplemented natural or artificial additives given to enhance or modify their attractiveness. Many cereal-based products are treated with approved Food, Drug, and Cosmetic (FD&C) colorants or natural pigments. Several milled products are treated with bleaching or oxidizing agents to improve the white appearance of the flour and their processed products. Another important factor affecting color intensity is the pH. It is well known that phenolics, anthocyanins, and tannins change color and intensity when exposed to different pH or acidities. These compounds tend to produce darker colorations when exposed to alkaline pH. The main processing factors affecting color are Maillard, browning, and caramelization reactions in which reducing sugars and proteins play the most critical role.

The evaluation of the color of flour and other milled products is important because it is related to milling efficiency and extraction rate, and influences the quality of finished products. The whiteness of wheat flours is affected by type of wheat, milling extraction rate, flour aging, and extent of oxidation of carotenoid pigments by bleaching compounds. Color is usually measured by light reflectance within the blue range of the light spectrum. The Kent Jones and Agtron color meters are the most common instruments used by the wheat industry. Hunter Lab colorimeters and near-infrared analyzers have also been used for this determination. The advantage of the Hunter Lab color meter is that it determines L, a, b, and hue parameters (Rasper and Walker 2000).

The color of refined wheat flour (American Association of Cereal Chemists [AACC] 2000, Method 14-30) or semolina is generally performed in an Agtron colorimeter operating in the green mode (546 nm). The sample is mixed with distilled water to enhance color formation. Next, the slurry is read in the colorimeter that was previously calibrated with disc standards. Similar assays (AACC 2000, Methods 14-21 and 14-22) are also used to measure pasta and noodle color. Near-infrared analyzers can also be calibrated to determine color (see Chapter 2).

For durum wheats, the rapid measurement of carotenes is performed using a spectrophotometer or colorimeter (AACC 2000, Method 14-50). Yellow pigmentation can be quantified by overnight extraction in aqueous *n*-butanol followed by measurement of absorbance at 435.8 nm (Dexter and Matsuo 1978). More frequently, the color of semolina is judged visually or with refractive light colorimeters (Allen et al. 1989; Symons and Dexter 1991).

3.2.1 Determination of Color

The well-known role of color in the acceptability of foods is irrefutable. The food industry has long been aware of the important contribution of color to overall acceptability. Consequently, the industry assesses and controls the color of their products. Colorants have been in widespread used to modify the appearance of products so that they are more appealing to the consumer or to prevent the formation of undesirable colors due to processing or storage. The color can be assessed visually during the tasting of the product or by comparison with color atlases, charts, or dictionaries; although, in these cases, a subjective description rather than an objective definition is achieved. In contrast to this, it is possible to objectively define any color by using instruments such as spectrophotometers, colorimeters, and near-infrared analyzers following the recommendations laid down by the *Commission Internationale de L'éclairage* or the International Commission on Illumination (CIE). The CIE recommends a series of standard conditions aimed toward the standardization of the objective measurements and definition of color. Therefore, the objective measurement of color leaves behind the uncertainty stemming from the subjective definitions achieved with visual judgments. Furthermore, the instrumental measurement of color presents quite a few advantages such as flexibility, speediness, automation, nondestructiveness, and convenience that make them more practical for quality control or product development purposes. Practically all color meters have different color standards. The ideal standard for calibration purposes is the one that simulates color and product surface.

3.2.1.1 Hunter Lab Color Meter

The Hunter Lab color meters are widely used by all segments of the food industry because the instruments duplicate how our eyes see color. The instruments measure product color and give numerical values that correlate to what is perceived by the human eye. These objective measurements optimize the confidence of the determinations. The instrument measures the parameters known as L, a, and b where L = lightness or darkness, $+a$ = redness, $-a$ = greenness, $+b$ = yellowness, and $-b$ = blueness. All colors that can be visually perceived can be plotted in this L, a, and b rectangular color space. The ratio a/b is denominated as hue, whereas the square root of the addition of a^2 and b^2 is known as chroma $(a^2 + b^2)^{1/2}$. The color score is calculated by the square root of the addition of $L^2 + a^2 + b^2$ or $(L^2 + a^2 + b^2)^{1/2}$.

A. *Samples, Ingredients, and Reagents*
- Different wheat flours

B. *Materials and Equipment*
- Hunter Lab color meter
- Sample cell
- Cloth
- Standard color plates
- Brush

C. *Procedure*
1. Allow the instrument to warm up at least 30 minutes before color determinations. Make sure to clean the sample cell with lens paper. Avoid scratching the cell.
2. Calibrate the instrument with a color plate which is similar to the sample color to be measured. Set L, a, and b to the correct settings (Figure 3.1).
3. Place sample into the color sample cell and make sure to fill it to at least 3/4 capacity. If the

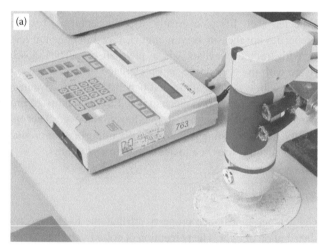

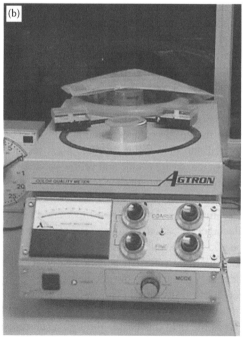

FIGURE 3.1   Color meters; (a) Hunter Lab; (b) Agtron.

sample is liquid or paste, make sure to remove air bubbles by tapping the sample cell on the counter protected with a cloth (avoid damaging or scratching the bottom of the cell).

4. Determine *L, a,* and *b* readings and record on the Hunter Lab color chart.

5. Calculate the hue, chroma, and color score using the following equations.

$$\text{Hue} = a/b; \text{Chroma} = (a^2 + b^2)^{1/2};$$
$$\text{Color score } E = (L^2 + a^2 + b^2)^{1/2}.$$

3.2.1.2 Pekar Color (Method 14-10.01)

One of the most common tests to determine the color of wheat flour is the Pekar or Slick test (AACC 2000). This test is influenced by flour particle size, bran fragments, weed seeds, the presence of carotenoids/xantophylls, and the use of bleaching agents. The Pekar test is used to judge the color of flour and is conducted by pressing one or more flour samples on a paddle with a highly polished slick. The Pekar test is generally used for determining the brightness of flour. In this test, a control sample and a sample of flour that is to be tested are placed side-by-side on a spatula and the surface is smoothed and then the whole sample is moistened.

A. *Samples, Ingredients, and Reagents*
- Flour samples with different extraction rates
- Distilled water
- Control or standard flour sample

B. *Instruments and Equipment*
- Rectangular glass (12 × 8 cm long and wide)
- Chronometer
- Flour slick

C. *Procedure*
1. Place approximately 10 g to 15 g of flour on the rectangular plate. Pack one side in a straight line by using the flour slick. Treat the same quantity of standard flour used by comparison in the same manner. The straight edges of the two flours should be adjacent.

2. Carefully move one of the portions so that it will be in contact with the other and "slick" both with one stroke of the flour slick in such a manner that the thickness of the layer diminishes from approximately 0.5 cm in the middle of plate to a thin film at the edge. The line of demarcation between the two flours should be distinct. Subjectively evaluate the difference in color of the two flours.

3. To emphasize differences in color, cut off edges of layer with flour slick to form a rectangle and carefully immerse plate with flour in cold distilled water for 1 minute. Note color differences of wet samples.

4. Place plate with wet flour in a convection oven set at 100°C and note color differences when completely dried.

3.2.1.3 Agtron Color Meter

The Agtron M45 color meter is a modified spectrophotometer designed to measure specific spectral characteristics for colored homogenous flours, liquids, pastes, and powders. The most important advantage of this analyzer is that all Agtrons read alike and provide accurate and repeated measurements. The small error is due to the homogenous illumination of the sample at a low angle of incidence. The instrument measures the reflected energy of the sample. The color meter is operated by placing a sample cup containing the test material over a 2-in. diameter viewing aperture and measuring the sample's monochromatic reflectance at the desired spectral line. For wheat flours, the green spectral line is used for evaluation. The instrument is calibrated beforehand with calibration standards. Low readings are associated with dark samples whereas high readings are associated with light, bright samples. The instrument is provided with certified calibration disks that are used in standardizing the apparatus before product testing.

A. *Samples, Ingredients, and Reagents*
- Test samples
- Lens paper
- Distilled water

B. *Materials and Equipment*
- Agtron color analyzer
- Standard disks (63 and 85)
- Sample cup
- Brush

C. *Procedure*
1. Turn on Agtron spectrophotometer at least 30 minutes before testing. Clean the sample cup with lens paper. Avoid scratching, especially the base of the cup, because it acts as a lens.

2. Calibrate the instrument with two reflectance calibration disks (Figure 3.1).

3. Fill the sample cup about half full (i.e., 20 g wheat flour). Before placing the cup in the sample well, lightly tap the container three times on the counter with the lens paper. This will remove air tunnels entrapped in the sample.

4. Place the sample cup in the instrument's well and record the reading. Lift the cup and turn it approximately 120-degrees (one-third rotation) and place it again in the well for a second reading.

3.2.1.4 Wheat Flour Color Determination (Method 14-30)

This method determines the color of wheat flours as affected by wheat type, degree of milling, and the addition of oxidizing agents (AACC 2000).

A. *Samples, Ingredients, and Reagents*
- Different wheat flours
- Distilled water

B. *Materials and Equipment*

- Agtron color meter model M40, M-400-A, M-500-A, or Model F2-61. The instrument should be fixed in the green wavelength at 546 nm. The apparatus should be equipped with a metal base that is placed underneath the sample.
- Sample containers
- Pipette (25 mL)
- Cleaning paper
- Scale
- Standard disks (63 and 85)
- Chronometer or laboratory clock
- Glass agitator with plastic terminal tip
- 25 mL graduated cylinder or pipette

C. *Procedure*

1. Turn on the color meter 24 hours before the analysis.
2. Clean the sample containers with cleaning paper. Make sure to avoid scratching the surface.
3. Weigh 20 g of 14% moisture based flour and place it in the sample container.
4. Add exactly 25 mL of distilled water and mix with the flour for 2 minutes using the glass agitator with a plastic terminal tip. The resulting dough should be homogenous, smooth, and lump-free.
5. Allow resulting dough to rest for 5 minutes on a smooth and clean surface.
6. During dough resting, calibrate the Agtron color meter using, first, standard disk 63. Set the reader to zero using the adjustment knob located on the left-hand side. Remove disk 63 and place disk 85 and adjust to 100 using the right-hand side knob (Figure 3.1).
7. Repeat step 6 to make sure the color meter is properly calibrated.
8. Place the 5-minute-rested dough in the sample chamber and register the color score.
9. Make sure to recalibrate the color meter when analyzing new samples.

3.2.2 RESEARCH SUGGESTIONS

1. Prepare pastas with and without whole egg solids and then compare their color scores.
2. Determine the Pekar, Agtron, and Hunter Lab color scores of a wheat flour milled into three different types of refined flours differing in extraction rates.
3. Compare *L*, *a*, *b*, and chroma values of two different types of maize (white and yellow) transformed into tortillas.
4. Compare *L*, *a*, *b*, and chroma values of white nixtamalized white maize transformed into tortillas using a masa adjusted to pH 8 with $Ca(OH)_2$ and pH 5.6 (addition of fumaric acid).
5. Compare flour color score values before and after bleaching with benzoyl peroxide. Then transform the flour into bread and compare color values of the crumb.
6. Compare high fructose corn syrup (HFCS) color values of samples before and after refining through activated carbon and anionic exchange resins.

3.2.3 RESEARCH QUESTIONS

1. What is the meaning of tristimulus colorimetry?
2. Define the CIEXYZ and CIELAB color systems.
3. In a diagrammatic form, relate transmittance, reflectance, absorption, and refraction.
4. Name three factors that affect wheat flour color.
5. What is the principle of the Agtron color meter? What are the main advantages of this apparatus?
6. What is the principle of the Pekar color test that is still used to evaluate refined wheat flours?
7. What Hunter Lab parameters are more critically important for the following cereal-based products? Why?
   a. Tortilla chips
   b. Blue corn tortillas
   c. Pasta from durum wheat
   d. Corn flakes
   e. Dark beer

3.3 TEXTURE

3.3.1 RHEOLOGICAL PROPERTIES

It has been estimated that out of 350 descriptive terms dealing with food quality, approximately 25% are concerned with texture. It is not difficult to visualize the numerousness of these terms such as hardness, softness, brittleness, firmness, ripeness, toughness, tenderness, crustiness, stickiness, gumminess, fibrousness, mealiness, blandness, smoothness, chewiness, juiciness, crispness, flakiness, freshness, flabbiness, lumpiness, oiliness, grittiness, springiness, and others. Texture in foods includes these descriptive terms as well as others such as elasticity, plasticity, and viscosity (Mohsenin 1970). Needless to say, textural properties of foods play an important role during food manufacturing and processing, and in the consumer's response to a particular product. The textural properties deal with the sense of mouth feel. These properties are characterized by compressing, shearing, extending, twisting, cutting, shear pressure, tensile strength, and viscosity.

The textural characteristics of foods are classified as subjective or sensory evaluation and objective or instrumental measurement. The instrumental measurements are subdivided into fundamental or rheological, empirical, and imitative measurements. The instrumental objective methods are particularly useful in evaluating the textural attributes of raw materials, intermediate products, and finished products. The objective methods are intended to eliminate personal factor and human element from measurements. The fundamental or rheological tests are especially used for evaluating the specific functionalities of wheat flour doughs (refer to Chapter 5). The imitative and empirical tests stand between the fundamental rheological tests and service or imitative tests. Its usefulness depends either on the accuracy with which it predicts the behavior of the material under complex conditions or on how accurately it allows the use of fundamental equations for calculation and analysis. Most objective evaluations of foods fall into this category. For example, the tenderometer, puncture tester, texturemeter, maturometer, fibrometer, succolumeter, Kramer shear press, gelometer, Warner Bretzel, farinograph, and other related devices are widely used by the industry (Table 3.1).

There are two basic texture analyzers widely used by various segments of the cereal-based industries: the Instron (Instron Engineering Corporation, Norwood, MA) and the texture analyzer TA.XT2 (Texture Technologies and Stable Micro Systems, Scrasdale, NY). The Instron was first developed in 1946 by Harold Hindman and George Burr, who worked together at Massachusetts Institute of Technology and designed a material-testing machine based on strain gauge load cells and servo-control systems. The Instron (Figure 3.2) was devised to the mechanical properties of materials including prepared foods and raw materials using tension, compression, flexure, fatigue, impact, torsion, and hardness tests. The texture analyzer TA.XT2 (Figure 3.2), in its different versions, is used by the cereal and baking industries throughout the globe. The instrument is easy to use and can be provided with many specific probes, fixtures, and test methods.

The texture profile analysis (TPA) determines a combination of several rheological properties in the same assay. It is widely used to test bread throughout its expected textural shelf life. It generally consists of a two-bite compression test that measures hardness/firmness, adhesiveness, cohesiveness, chewiness, gumminess, springiness, and resilience. A sample preparation procedure is critical to assure acceptable sensitivity of the test to texture characteristics.

The most common are the penetrometers that measure the force required to penetrate the food material or the depth of penetration following impact. The compressimeters measure the resistance of the food material to compression. This instrument is widely used to measure the firmness of bakery goods and the degree of staling.

Chen and Hoseney (1995) developed an objective method to measure dough stickiness using a texture analyzer. The test consists of a probe that is brought into contact with the surface of a dough and then the probe is pulled away. The adhesive force between the surface of the dough and the probe is measured. The procedure is highly reproducible and correlated well with subjective measurements of dough stickiness.

3.3.1.1 Rheological Properties of Wheat Dough

Refer to procedures in Section 5.3.4.

3.3.1.2 Rheological Properties of Masa

Refer to procedures in Sections 7.2.2.4 to 7.2.2.7.

3.3.1.3 Rheological Properties of Tortillas, Pasta, and Breakfast Cereals

Refer to procedures in Sections 7.2.3.2, 11.2.2.3, and 12.2.6.1.

TABLE 3.1
Main Types of Texture Devices Used to Determine Textural Properties of Foods

Type of Device	Principle
Tenderometer	Consists of a grid assembly which simulates jaw action.
Puncture	Uses a needle to penetrate into products.
Texturemeter	Consists of a group of rods which move through the mass of the sample until they pass through matching holes.
Succulometer	Measures the volume of extractable juice under controlled conditions of time and pressure.
Kramer shear press	Consists of a hydraulic drive moving the crosshead of the machine at a given rate. Force is measured by a dynamometer.
Denture tenderometer	Simulate the denture surface and motions of mastication in the mouth. The forces are measured by strain gauges fitted on the arm connecting to the upper jaw.
Gelometer	Measures the rigidity of edible gelatin.
Compression meter	Utilizes a plunger for measuring the firmness of bread in terms of force and deformation.
Warner Bratzler	Shear device that consists of a blade and two shear bars, widely used to determine meat toughness.
Radiused cylinder probe (36 mm)	Allows measurement of bread firmness according to AACC Standard Method 74-09.
Kieffer dough and gluten extensibility rig	A microextension solution for accurate determination of dough and gluten extensibility.
Tortilla/pastry burst rig	Fixture developed to perform extension and elasticity measurements on pastry and tortillas.
SMS/Chen-Hoseney dough stickiness rig	Used to investigate the stickiness of dough with respect to mixing time, water content, enzyme activity, wheat variety, and composition.
Three-point bend rig	Used for assessing the fracturability/break strength of cookies and crackers.
Ottawa cell with watertight base	Used to "Bowl Life" testing of breakfast cereals. The cell is provided with a watertight base plate and liquid catchment tray.
Five-blade Kramer shear cell	Used for the shearing of dry cereal products.

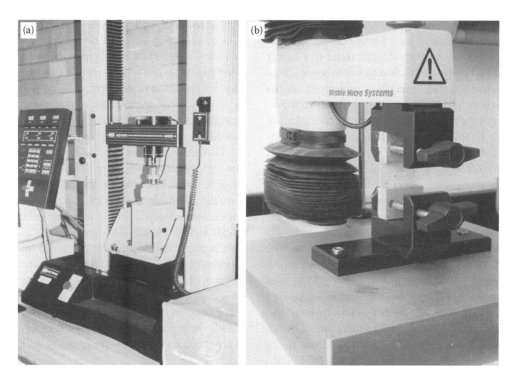

FIGURE 3.2   Texture analyzers; (a) Instron; (b) Texture analyzer TA.XT2.

3.3.2   VISCOSITY MEASUREMENT

The main mode for determining the rheological properties of fluids such as liquid sweeteners or syrups and beer is viscometry. The most widely used instruments are the rotational viscosimeters equipped with concentric cylinders commonly known as bob or cone and plate fixtures. One of the most common rheological devices found in the industry is the Brookfield viscometer. This simple apparatus uses a spring as a torque sensor. The analyst selects a rotational speed (rpm) of the bob which moves through the sample fluid causing the spring to wind. The degree of windup is a direct reflection of the torque magnitude and shear stress (Daubert and Foegeding 2003).

Determination and control of the flow properties of fluid foods is critical for optimizing processing conditions and obtaining the desired beneficial effects for the consumer. Transportation of fluids (pumping) from one location to another requires pumps, piping, and fittings such as valves, elbows, and tees. Proper sizing of this equipment depends on a number of elements but primarily depends on the flow properties of the product. For example, the equipment used to pump a dough mixture would vary differently from that used for milk. Additionally, rheological properties are fundamental to many aspects of food safety. During continuous thermal processing of fluid foods, the amount of time the food is in the system, and therefore, the amount of heating or "thermal dose" received, directly relates to its flow properties.

The rheological properties of a fluid are a function of composition, temperature, and other processing conditions. Identifying how these parameters influence flow properties may be performed using a variety of rheometers.

3.3.2.1   Determination of Viscosity with a Viscometer

A. *Samples, Ingredients, and Reagents*
- Sample (corn syrup, beer, etc.)

B. *Materials and Equipment*
- Brookfield rotational viscometers
- Beakers (250 mL)
- Refrigerator
- Spindles
- Thermometer

C. *Procedure*
1. Before evaluating the samples, make sure the viscometer is level. Use the leveling ball and circle on the viscometer.
2. Fill a beaker with 200 mL of corn syrup (refer to procedures in Sections 13.3.3.1 and 13.3.4.1) and the two remaining beakers with 200 mL of light and dark beers. Allow contents to equilibrate to room temperature.
3. Because rheological properties are strongly dependent on temperature, measure and record fluid temperatures before each measurement.
4. Record the viscometer model number and spindle size, product information (type and brand, etc.) and the sample temperature.
5. Immerse the spindle into the test fluid up to the notch cut in the shaft; the viscometers motor should be turned off (Figure 3.3).
6. Set the digital viscometers to zero if necessary.
7. Set the motor at the lowest speed (revolutions per minute; rpm) setting. Once the digital display shows a stable value, record the

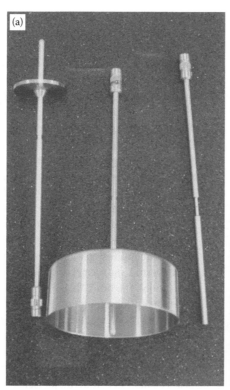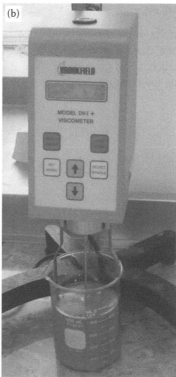

FIGURE 3.3 Brookfield viscosimeter; (a) spindles; (b) viscosimeter.

percentage of full-scale torque reading. Increase the rpm setting to the next speed and again record the percentage of full-scale torque reading. Repeat this procedure until the maximum rpm setting has been reached or 100% (but not higher) of the full-scale torque reading is obtained.

8. Stop the motor and slowly raise the spindle from the sample. Remove the spindle and clean with soap and water, then dry.

9. For every dial reading (percentage of full-scale torque), multiply the display value by the corresponding factor to calculate the viscosity with units of mPa-s.

3.3.3 RESEARCH SUGGESTIONS

1. Determine the average moisture content, viscoamylograph properties, and stickiness of masas that were lime-cooked for 15, 45, and 65 minutes.

2. Determine the rheological properties of a dough from regular soft wheat, chlorinated, and hard wheat flours using the farinograph, extensigraph, alveograph, or mixolab.

3. Compare the rheological properties of a wheat flour treated with 20 ppm and 40 ppm of sodium bisulfite.

4. Determine and compare the TPA of nixtamalized masas obtained from the same type of maize that was purposely undercooked or overcooked.

5. Determine and compare the bending or folding properties of wheat flour tortillas produced with different levels of shortening and emulsifiers throughout 5 days of storage at room temperature.

6. Determine and compare firmness of packaged bread at 0, 1, 2, 3, 5, and 7 days with the universal testing machine or a TA.XT2 texture analyzer.

7. Determine and compare firmness values of packaged corn tortillas stored for 0, 1, 2, 3, and 5 days at refrigeration and at room temperature.

8. Determine and compare the bowl life of corn flakes produced by the traditional and extruded technologies.

9. Determine and compare the viscoamylograph properties of regular and waxy starches (refer to procedures in Sections 6.4.1.1 or 6.4.1.2) and of regular and cross-bonded starches.

10. Determine and compare the viscoamylograph properties (refer to procedures in Sections 6.4.1.1 or 6.4.1.2) of wheat flours obtained from sound and sprouted kernels.

11. Determine and compare the viscosities of dark, regular, and light beer at 5°C and at room temperature.

12. Determine and compare viscosities of maltodextrin, glucose, and fructose syrups (refer to procedures in Sections 13.3.1.2, 13.3.3.1, and 13.3.4.1).

13. Graph the viscosity of a starch slurry (20% solids) during progressive heating to 85°C and then the drop in viscosity after the addition of heat-stable α-amylase (refer to procedure in Section 13.3.1.1).

3.3.4 RESEARCH QUESTIONS

1. What are the principles of the farinograph, extensigraph, and alveograph that are widely used to determine wheat dough rheological properties?
2. Define the following food texture terms:
   a. Hardness
   b. Shear
   c. Compression
   d. Stress
   e. Tensile strength
   f. Cohesiveness
   g. Chewiness
   h. Adhesiveness
   i. Brittleness
3. Compare the textural properties of pan bread, corn tortillas, and hard pretzels.
4. What kind of additives are used to prolong the textural shelf life of bakery products? How do they work?
5. What is the double compression test widely used to determine textural properties of fresh and stored bread? What kinds of parameters are usually evaluated after conducting the double compression test?
6. Define viscosity, Newtonian fluid, and non-Newtonian fluid.
7. What is the effect of temperature on the viscosity of a corn syrup?
8. What are the principles of the full viscoamylograph test? What are the four sequential phases of this test? What sorts of parameters are obtained after analyzing the whole viscoamylograph curve?
9. Define the term "shear thinning" and how this is measured in a viscoamylograph.
10. In which way does the viscoamylograph and falling number instruments relate? What are the advantages of each instrument?
11. Define the terms pseudoplasticity and thixotropic liquids.
12. What are the three most common strategies to prolong the textural shelf life of pan bread or related products?

3.4 SENSORY TESTING

Sensory testing of foods has been conducted for as long as there have been human beings evaluating the goodness and badness of foods. After the Second World War, scientists developed sensory testing in a formalized, structured, and codified methodology and they continue to develop new and improved methods.

Sensory evaluation tests are widely used to determine the consumer preference of finished products and therefore play a key role in the development of new foods. Tests are usually performed in a sensory evaluation laboratory furnished with individual evaluation booths. The more widely practiced tests are the triangular and preference tests. Triangular tests are ideally suited to identifying the consumer's preference between two samples because panelists try to identify the odd and paired samples among the three samples in a set. The triangular test is widely used for product development purposes. In the preference test, trained or untrained panelists evaluate the color, aroma, flavor, texture, and overall acceptability of the products generally using a 9-point hedonic scale, where $4 =$ like extremely, $0 =$ neither like nor dislike, and -4 dislike extremely (Anzaldua-Morales 1994). This test is used for product development purposes, shelf life studies, and to study the functionality of additives/technologies.

The main uses of sensory evaluation techniques are in product development, quality control, and research. When sensory analysts study the relationship between a given physical stimulus and the subject's response is regarded as at least three sequential steps: the stimulus hits the sense organ and is converted into a nerve signal which travels to the brain (sensation), the brain then organizes and integrates the signal into perceptions (perception), and a response is formulated based on the subjects perception (Meilgaard et al. 1999). The steps usually followed to conduct a sensory study are to determine the project and test objectives, screen the samples, design the test, conduct the test, analyze the data, and interpret results. The four major sensory attributes are appearance, odor or aroma, consistency or texture, and flavor. These attributes are mainly sensed by vision, touch, olfaction, and gastation. During testing, most of these attributes overlap and the untrained panelist will not be able to provide an independent evaluation of each. The main factors affecting appearance are color, size and shape, surface texture, and clarity or opacity.

There are basically two types of panelists—untrained and trained. The untrained panelist tests the sample without any previous preparation. In most instances, these individuals get a short instruction about the sensory evaluation procedure and handling of the coded samples [amount of sample to be tested at one time, delivery system, length of time of contact with the product (sip/spit, bite/chew) and the disposition of the product (swallow, expectorate, etc.)] and instructions on how to fill the score sheet.

There are many approaches to determine the sensory properties of a given food. The main categories are difference and discrimination tests. The triangle and duo-trio difference tests are designed to show whether subjects can detect any difference between samples. On the other hand, the "attribute" difference tests concentrates on a single feature (for instance, sweetness), ignoring the rest of the other food traits (color, texture, etc.). The intensity of the selected attribute is measured by ranking, line scaling, or magnitude estimation.

3.4.1 DISCRIMINATORY SENSORY EVALUATION TESTS

The discrimination tests are used to determine if two samples (for instance, your recent product development vs. the leading product in the market) are perceptibly different or sufficiently similar to be used interchangeably.

3.4.1.1 Preparation and Coding

Decide the amount of product to be used and measure by weight or volume using precise equipment, make sure the sample is offered at the same temperature and define the minimum and maximum times that the product can be used for a sensory test.

Make sure to use the same equipment and procedures for product presentation during the test (same glasses, plates, and utensils). Extreme care must be given to regulating the precise amount of product to be given to each subject. After the sample is distributed to each serving container, and just before the test, the product should be inspected to determine if it is at the appropriate temperature.

3.4.1.2 Triangle Test

The triangle test was devised to determine whether a perceptible difference exists between two products. This method is particularly useful for comparing a new product with the benchmark counterpart or in situations in which treatment and processing effects may have produced product changes (i.e., substitution of an additive). The test is based on the evaluation of three coded samples. The panelist is instructed that two samples are identical and the other is different or odd. Generally, 20 to 40 panelists are used to conduct a triangle test. The three coded samples are preferably offered in a partitioned test area in which each panelist can judge samples independently. Control of lighting may be necessary to reduce color variables. The three samples are usually and preferably offered simultaneously and panelists are asked to examine one or several properties (taste, color, aroma, and texture) in the order from left to right, with the option of going back to repeat the evaluation. Panelists are asked to fill a score sheet similar to the one presented in Figure 3.4.

Results of the triangle test are simply analyzed using a two-entry table in which the significance α-level is selected first, followed by the number of correct responses and the

TABLE 3.2

Critical Number of Correct Responses in a Triangle Test with Significance Levels of 0.2, 0.10, 0.05, and 0.01

Number of Total Responses	Minimum Number of Correct Responses			
	α 0.2	α 0.10	α 0.05	α 0.01
10	6	6	7	8
15	8	8	9	10
20	9	10	11	13
25	11	12	13	15
30	13	14	15	17
35	15	16	17	19
60	24	26	27	30
90	35	37	38	42

Source: Meilgaard et al. *Sensory Evaluation Techniques*. 3rd ed., 1999. CRC Press, Boca Raton, FL. With permission.

Note: For values not included in the table, refer to Meilgaard et al. (1999).

number of total responses (Table 3.2). A stricter significance level requires a higher number of corrected responses. For instance, if there were a total of 30 responses or panelists, the correct number of answers for significance levels of 0.1 and 0.01 are 14 and 17, respectively.

3.4.1.3 Duo-Trio Test

The duo-trio test is also used to compare two products that are similar or have small or subtle differences. This test is based on the presentation to panelists of an identified reference sample followed by two coded samples—one that matches the reference sample. The panelists are asked to identify which coded sample matches the reference (Figure 3.5). Because the duo test is statistically inefficient compared

---

Name _____ Date _____

Type of sample _____

Instructions
Taste each three coded samples from left to right. Two are identical and the other different. Select which is the odd sample. If no difference is apparent you must guess. You can comment about the sample in the space provided. If necessary repeat the evaluation procedure.

Sample code	Mark with "X" the odd sample	Comments

FIGURE 3.4 Example of score sheet for the triangle test.

Name _____ Date _____

Type of sample _____

Instructions

Taste the three coded samples from left to right. The left hand sample is a reference. Determine with "X" which of the two coded samples matches the reference. If no difference is apparent between the two unknown samples you must guess. You can comment about the test in the space provided.

Reference   Code _____   Code _____

☐   ☐   ☐

Comments: _____

_____

_____

FIGURE 3.5   Example of score sheet for the duo-trio test.

with the triangle test, as a general rule, a minimum of 16 panelists are required to run the test. Discrimination is much improved if more than 32 subjects are used.

Prepare equal numbers of the possible combinations and allocate a set of samples at random among the panelists. The samples are usually offered simultaneously and results are simply analyzed using a two-entry table in which the significance α-level is selected first, followed by the number of correct responses and total responses. Panelists that responded "no difference" should be discarded.

The results of the duo-trio test are simply analyzed using a two-entry table in which the significance α-level is selected first, followed by the number of correct responses and the number of total responses (Table 3.3). A stricter significance level requires a higher number of corrected responses. For instance, if there were a total of 30 responses or panelists, the correct number of answers for significance levels of 0.1 and 0.01 are 14 and 17, respectively.

3.4.2 Affective Sensory Evaluation Tests

The most common sensory analysis tests are classified as affective. These tests determine the responses of a group of panelists or consumers to a set of questions regarding preference, liking, and sensory attributes (for instance, color, texture, odor, and flavor). These tests are the most commonly practiced because they determine the overall preference for a given product or the consumer response to specific sensory attributes associated with new product developments. The score sheets of these tests contain hedonic or intensity scales. The affective tests are divided into two broad categories: preference and acceptance tests. The first is specifically

designed to compare one product against another (or others) and forces the panelist to pick one over the other(s). The preference tests are subdivided into paired, multiple paired, and ranked preference.

3.4.2.1 Preference Paired Tests

The paired test compares only two samples and the panelist has to make a preference choice of one item over another (Figures 3.6 and 3.7). The multiple paired preference tests also compare three or more samples. The samples are

---

TABLE 3.3

Critical Number of Correct Responses in a Duo-Trio Test with Significance Levels of 0.2, 0.10, 0.05, and 0.01

Number of Total Responses	Minimum Number of Correct Responses			
	α 0.2	α 0.10	α 0.05	α 0.01
10	7	8	9	10
15	10	11	12	13
20	13	14	15	16
25	16	17	18	19
30	18	20	20	22
35	21	22	23	25
40	24	25	26	28
80	45	47	48	51

Source: Meilgaard et al. *Sensory Evaluation Techniques.* 3rd ed., 1999. CRC Press, Boca Raton, FL. With permission.

Note: For values not included in Table 3.3, refer to Meilgaard et al. (1999).

Name _____ Date _____

Type of sample _____

Instructions
Taste each pair of samples from left to right and enter your verdict below. If no difference is apparent enter your best guess, however *"no difference"* verdicts are allowed as a last resort.

Test Pairs   Which sample is more _____

_____ _____   _____

_____ _____   _____

_____ _____   _____

Comments: _____

_____

_____

FIGURE 3.6 Example of score sheet for paired test.

selectively paired with others or paired with all others. The paired samples should be offered simultaneously and the analyst should prepare an equal number of paired combinations and allocate the sets at random among the panelists. Because of the simplicity of the test, it should be conducted with subjects who have received minimum training; however, it requires a fairly large number of panelists because the chance of guessing is 50%.

3.4.2.2 Rank Preference Test

The rank preference test compares three or more samples, and panelists are asked to rank samples using a relative order. This method is used to compare several samples according to a single attribute (preference, color, sweetness). Ranking is particularly useful when items are to be presorted or screened for later analysis. Panelists are simply instructed to rank items according to the attribute of interest. Data is analyzed by assigning ordinal numbers to the first, second, and third places (for instance, 1, 2, and 3). The minimum and recommended number of panelists for this test is 8 and more than 16, respectively. Panelists are usually trained and instructed before the test to familiarize them with the test procedures, product characteristics, and the particular attribute of interest. In this test, the panelists receive coded samples in a random order and they are asked to rearrange them in rank order. In a preference test, subjects are instructed to assign rank 1 to the preferred sample, rank 2 to the next preferred, and so on (Figure 3.8). After tabulating the rank sums for each sample, the data is recommended to

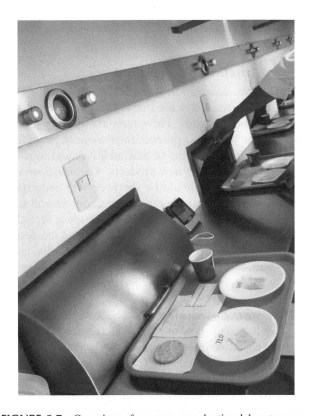

FIGURE 3.7 Overview of a sensory evaluation laboratory prepared for the evaluation of flour tortillas. The tray contains the two different tortilla samples, ballots for declaration of allergies, and score sheet, glass of water, and a cracker to consume as a wash out in-between samples.

Name _____ Date _____

Type of sample _____

Type attribute_____

Instructions
1. Taste the coded five samples from left to right and note the degree of _____ .
   Wait at least 30 seconds between samples and rinse the palate as required.
2. Write "1" in the coded sample which you find with more _____ , "2"
   for the next and so on. If two samples appear the same, make a best guess as to their
   rank order.

Code   _____   _____   _____   _____   _____

Rank   ☐   ☐   ☐   ☐   ☐

Comments: _____

_____

_____

FIGURE 3.8 Example of score sheet for simple ranking test.

be analyzed to detect statistical differences among samples by Friedman's test.

3.4.2.3 Affective or Hedonic Tests

The affective, acceptance, or hedonic tests are the most common and frequently used tests to determine the sensory properties of foods. These tests are used for product development purposes, product improvement, or optimization especially in terms of new additives and to assess the market potential of new products. The questionnaires for affective testing should be short, easy to understand, and simple to follow and contain clear questions and score sheets. Each questionnaire should be tailor-made according to the number of products to be compared and the desired test attributes (appearance, flavor, texture, viscosity, crispness, color, sweetness, odor/aroma, aftertaste, etc.). The questionnaire should avoid asking irrelevant or unnecessary questions.

There are many hedonic scales. The scale should be chosen according to the type of panelist and degree of accuracy. The most common scales are category scales (9, 7, or 5-point), line scale, and facial hedonic. The 9-point scale consists of like extremely, like very much, like moderately, like slightly, neither like nor dislike, dislike slightly, dislike moderately, dislike very much, and dislike extremely (Figure 3.9). There are also score sheets containing 7-point or 5-point scales. The evaluation on the line hedonic scale (Figure 3.10) is done by simply marking the degree of product likeness on the line labeled on each side with two contrasting product attributes,

whereas the facial hedonic scale is generally used to conduct sensory tests for children. The advantage of line scales is that the intensity can be more accurately graded because there are no numbers, whereas the main disadvantage is that the panelist is usually less consistent because sometimes he or she cannot remember the position on the line.

The data generated by hedonic tests is almost always statistically evaluated using t test or analysis of variance (ANOVA) test. The t test is used when comparing two treatments, whereas the ANOVA test is used when comparing more than two treatments. The means of the rank sums are usually compared with least significant differences, Duncan, or Tukey tests at a level of significance of 5% or 1%.

3.4.3 RESEARCH SUGGESTIONS

1. Prepare five loaves of table bread with hydrogenated shortening or fractionated palm stearin (free of trans fatty acids) according to the procedure in Section 9.2.6.1. Slice the bread into 1-in.-thick slices, pack the bread in sealed polyethylene bags and store it at room temperature.
   a. Determine subjective and objective crumb color with the Hunter Lab colorimeter (L, a, b, chroma, hue and color index E).
   b. Determine crumb texture with the universal testing machine or TA.XT2 texture analyzer using the double compression test at days 0, 1, 2, 5, and 7.

Name _____ Date _____ Age _____
Sex: Male_____ Female_____

Evaluate the TEXTURE, COLOR, and FLAVOR of the five coded bread samples marking with an "X" the degree of preference. Please rinse your palate after evaluating each sample.

Sample Code	356	906	488	106	092
TEXTURE					
Like extremely					
Like very much					
Like moderately					
Like slightly					
Neither like nor dislike					
Dislike slightly					
Dislike moderately					
Dislike very much					
Dislike extremely					
COLOR					
Like extremely					
Like very much					
Like moderately					
Like slightly					
Neither like nor dislike					
Dislike slightly					
Dislike moderately					
Dislike very much					
Dislike extremely					
FLAVOR					
Like extremely					
Like very much					
Like moderately					
Like slightly					
Neither like nor dislike					
Dislike slightly					
Dislike moderately					
Dislike very much					
Dislike extremely					

Comments _____
_____
_____

FIGURE 3.9 Example of score sheet for 9-point hedonic test.

c. Design a triangular test to determine if the use of the palm stearin significantly affects the sensory properties of the bread (color, texture, flavor, and aroma).

2. Prepare five different types of corn tortillas following the dry masa flour procedure (procedure in Section 7.2.4.2). The control dry masa will be supplemented with (1) 0.2% fumaric acid/0.2% calcium propionate, (2) 0.5% lecithin/0.1% Sodium Stearoyl Lactylate (SSL), (3) 0.2% carboxymethyl cellulose, (4) 0.2% fumaric acid/0.2% calcium propionate, 0.5% lecithin/0.1% SSL, and 0.2% carboxymethyl cellulose. Pack the resulting tortillas in sealed polyethylene bags and store bags at room temperature.

Name _____ Date _____ Age _____
Sex: Male_____ Female_____

Evaluate the TEXTURE, COLOR, FLAVOR and OVERALL ACCEPTABILITY of the two coded cracker samples by placing a mark on each line below. Please rinse your palate after evaluating each sample.

Texture

Code 732   Hard _____ Soft

Code 175   Hard _____ Soft

Color

Code 732   Light _____ Dark

Code 175   Light _____ Dark

Flavor

Code 732   None _____ Strong

                Like extremely _____ Dislike extremely

Code 175   None _____ Strong

                Like extremely _____ Dislike extremely

Overall Acceptability

Code 732 Like extremely _____ Dislike extremely

Code 175 Like extremely _____ Dislike extremely

Comments: _____

_____

_____

FIGURE 3.10 Example of score sheet with line hedonic scale.

a. Determine the TPA of the different types of masas and the folding and firmness of the tortillas at days 0, 1, 2, and 5.
b. Design a hedonic test to determine if the various types of additives negatively or positively affect the consumer preference of these tortillas (color, texture, flavor, and overall acceptability).
3. Prepare two different types of wheat flour tortillas following the same formulation and the hot-press procedure (procedure in Section 10.5.1.1). One tortilla will be prepared with whole wheat flour whereas the other with whole grain flour. Pack the resulting tortillas in sealed polyethylene bags and store bags at room temperature.
a. Determine and compare the Agtron color of the two different flours.
b. Determine and compare the rheological properties of the two flours using the farinograph.
c. Determine subjectively and objectively the tortilla color with the Hunter Lab colorimeter (L, a, b, chroma, hue, and color index E).

d. Determine and compare tortilla firmness and bending with the TA.XT2 texture analyzer at days 0, 1, 2, 3, and 6.
e. Design a triangular test to determine which of the two tortillas (color, texture, flavor, and overall acceptability) is preferred by panelists.
4. Prepare two different types of lager beers following procedure in Section 14.2.2.1. One beer will be produced using barley malt and refined sorghum grits whereas the other will use sorghum malt and refined sorghum grits.
a. Determine and compare the color of the two different beers.
b. Determine and compare the Brookfield viscosity of the two beers.
c. Determine the alcohol content of the two beers.
d. Design a triangular test with adult panelists to determine which of the two beers (color, body texture, flavor, and aroma) is preferred by panelists.

3.4.4　Research Questions

1. Select the most appropriate test for evaluating the production of beer with a new lot of diastatic malt. The sensory analyst wishes to know if the consumer can distinguish from the control beer.

2. A new lot of pan bread is produced using dry yeast instead of fresh compressed yeast. The sensory analyst wishes to know if breads can be distinguished. A 1% risk factor ($\alpha = 0.01$) is accepted and 20 assessors evaluated the two breads in a triangular test. Fourteen out of the 20 panelists identified the odd sample. What can you conclude from this sensory evaluation test?

3. Design a sensory evaluation test aimed toward the determination of the overall acceptability of two commercially produced beers. One beer was treated with a new hop extract whereas the other was produced with hop pellets. The two lots of beers were held for 1, 2, 4, 6, and 8 weeks under two conditions: refrigeration temperature (1–5°C) and ambient temperature (20°C/70% relative humidity (RH)). Define the minimum number of panelist, score sheets, the sensory evaluation method, and the statistical analysis of the data.

4. What are the advantages and disadvantages of using untrained or trained panelists?

REFERENCES

Allen, H. M., J. R. Oliver, and A. B. Blakeney. 1989. "Use of Tristimulus Color Meter in Wheat Breeding Programme." In *Proceedings 39th Australian Cereal Chemistry Conference*, edited by T. Wescott, Y. Williams, and R. Ryker, 185–189. North Melbourne, Victoria: Royal Australian Chemical Institute.

American Association of Cereal Chemists. 2000. *AACC Approved Methods of Analysis*. 10th ed. St. Paul, MN: AACC.

Anzaldua-Morales, A. 1994. *La Evaluación Sensorial de los Alimentos en la Teoría y la Practica*. Zaragoza, Spain: Editorial Acribia, S.A.

Chen, W. Z., and R. C. Hoseney. 1995. "Development of an Objective Method for Dough Stickiness." *Lebensmittel-Wissenschaft und-Technologie* 28:467–473.

Daubert, C. R., and E. A. Foegeding. 2003. "Rheological Principles for Food Analysis." In *Food Analysis*, edited by F. S. Nielsen. 3rd ed. New York: Springer.

Dexter, J. E., and R. R. Matsuo. 1978. "Effect of Semolina Extraction Rate on Semolina Characteristics and Spaghetti Quality." *Cereal Chemistry* 67:275–281.

Hutchings, J. B. 1994. *Food Color and Appearance*. London: Blackie Academic & Professional.

Meilgaard, M., G. V. Civille, and B. T. Carr. 1999. *Sensory Evaluation Techniques*. 3rd ed. Boca Raton, FL: CRC Press.

Mohsenin, N. N. 1970. *Physical Properties of Plant and Animal Materials. Structure, Physical Characteristics and Mechanical Properties*. New York: Gordon and Breach Science Publishers.

Rasper, V. F., and C. E. Walker. 2000. "Quality Evaluation of Cereals and Cereal Products." In *Handbook of Cereal Science and Technology*, edited by K. Kulp and J. G. Ponte. New York: Marcel Dekker.

Symons, S. J., and J. E. Dexter. 1991. "Computer Analysis of Fluorescence for the Measurement of Flour Refinement as Determined by Flour Ash Content, Flour Grade Color and Tristimulus Color Measurements." *Cereal Chemistry* 68:454–460.

4 Storage of Cereal Grains and Detrimental Effects of Pests

4.1 INTRODUCTION

There are many factors affecting the quality of stored grains. These are broadly divided into intrinsic and extrinsic. Intrinsic deterioration is caused by the grain's metabolic activity resulting from respiration. The grain respiration rate is mainly affected by the kernel moisture content, presence of oxygen in the atmosphere, environmental temperature, and relative humidity (RH). The kernel activates due to its high moisture when environmental conditions, mainly in terms of temperature, are adequate. The grain generates energy or heat, carbon dioxide and metabolic water, and important enzymes that break down lipids, starch, and proteins. Intrinsic grain deterioration is more prevalent than extrinsic deterioration because most pests require water as one of their most important substrates. The RH of air plays an important role in the susceptibility of the grain to deterioration. The grain can surpass its critical moisture content when it is exposed to a high air RH (more than 70%). When the grain exceeds its critical moisture content, it generates heat that catalyzes the respiration process. This is the most common way for properly stored sound grains to lose latency and progressively deteriorate. When the grain exceeds its critical moisture content and is undergoing intrinsic deterioration, it also generates important quantities of free water that could be available for insect and mold growth. Insects and molds generally damage kernels that contain 1.5% and 4% more water, respectively, above the critical moisture (14% for cereal grains). The wheat milling and baking industries are especially susceptible to intrinsically deteriorated grains. Damaged wheat kernels and flours yield sticky doughs that are less functional, yielding bakery items with consistently lower color values, volume, and organoleptic properties.

Extrinsic deterioration is more important in terms of grain losses. It is mainly caused by insects followed by molds and rodents. Insects can proliferate at relatively lower grain moisture contents or water activities compared with molds. These pests cause direct damage and contaminate the lot of grain with insect fragments and feces, rodent hair, and droppings that contaminate a given lot of grain with pathogenic bacteria. Most molds are capable of producing secondary metabolites or mycotoxins that can greatly negatively affect human or animal health. All these biotic agents cause direct and indirect losses.

4.2 EFFECTS OF ENVIRONMENT AND GRAIN MOISTURE CONTENT ON DETERIORATION

The grain moisture content is the most important factor to control in grain elevators because it is the most closely related to respiration rate. Grains tend to equilibrate with environmental moisture and are hydroscopic when exposed to high RHs. The best way to manage grain moisture is through the use and interpretation of isotherm curves. The isotherm curve relates grain moisture and air RH at a given temperature (generally 20°C or 25°C) because grains absorbs or desorbs water according to the surrounding air humidity (Bell and Labuza 2000). In addition, natural temperature fluctuations throughout the day can cause air moisture condensation that enters the grain affecting its storability. Generally speaking, grain elevators located in tropical areas are the most difficult to manage because of the high temperatures and air RH (McFarlane et al. 1995). A high RH also favors the growth of molds that prefer to grow at RHs higher than 65%.

The hydroscopic capacity, equilibrium moisture content or isotherm behavior of different cereal grains kept at 70% RH and 25°C is approximately 14%. Thus, this is the moisture content that is critical for all cereal grains in which the moisture is mostly bound or unavailable for respiration, insects, and molds. Grains stored at higher RH will tend to gradually absorb air moisture, break latency, and increase respiration rate. For instance, cereals with 16% moisture will deteriorate approximately twice as fast compared with counterparts stored at 15% moisture. The understanding and adequate use of the isotherm curve is of upmost importance in the management of cereal grains. Important decisions of when to aerate stored grains could be made based on the results of isotherm graphs (Sauer 1992).

Cereal grains and their products equilibrate with the surrounding moisture content or have the capacity to lose or gain moisture. The moisture gain or loss is related to partial water vapor pressure. The equilibrium grain moisture is achieved when the grain does not lose or gain moisture. This moisture is critically important in stored grain management and greatly affects performance during drying operations. The isotherm curves allow processors to predict grain moisture according to environmental conditions. The environmental conditions that favor intrinsic deterioration or respiration are RH and temperatures higher than 75% and 20°C, respectively. These conditions will enhance grain moisture absorption that eventually surpasses the grain's critical point during which insects and eventually molds will grow. The important decisions to rotate, aerate, or dehydrate grains should take into consideration the environmental conditions and obviously the isotherm behavior of the grain.

4.2.1 Equilibrium Grain Moisture at Different RHs

All cereals, when exposed to air with high RH, will absorb water from the air. When wet cereals are exposed to air with low RH, the kernels will release water to the air. The equilibrium moisture content is the final moisture content of the grain after being stored for some time with surrounding air of a certain temperature and RH. If the grain is not protected against the humidity in the air, particularly during the rainy season when the RH is very high, the grain moisture content will increase and this will lead to intrinsic and extrinsic grain deterioration and loss of quality. If the grain is stored in an enclosed storage environment, such as a bag or silo, the air surrounding the grain, if it is well sealed, is not in free contact with outside air. In this case, the RH of the enclosed air will reach equilibrium with the moisture content in the grain. The final RH of the enclosed air is often expressed as the "equilibrium RH." The higher the grain moisture content of the stored grain, the higher the equilibrium RH, and the higher the chances of insect and mold development or loss of grain viability. Normally, an equilibrium RH inside the facilities of 65% or less is considered a safe prevention against the development of molds.

The isotherm curve relates grain moisture and air RH at a given temperature (usually 20°C or 25°C) because grains absorb or desorb water according to the surrounding air RH.

4.2.1.1 Determination of a Cereal Isotherm Curve

A. *Samples, Ingredients, and Reagents*
- Cereal grains
- Dessicant (activated alumina)
- Distilled water
- Set of salts listed in Table 4.1

B. *Materials and Equipment*
- Airtight dessicators
- Thermometer
- Graduated cylinder
- Hygrometer
- Analytical scale

TABLE 4.1

Relationship between Type of Saturated Salt and Air RH at 25°C

Salt	RH (%) at 25°C
Lithium chloride	11
Magnesium chloride	33
Potassium carbonate	43
Sodium bromide	57
Cupric chlorate	67
Sodium chloride	75
Ammonium sulfate	79
Potassium chloride	86
Potassium chromate	87
Sodium benzoate	88
Potassium sulfate	97

Source: Rockland, B.L. *Anal. Chem.*, 32:1375–1376, 1960. With permission.

- Laboratory tongs
- Plastic bags
- Environmental chamber
- Glass bottles for tempering
- Chronometer
- Water activity apparatus
- Aluminum tins
- Air-forced convection oven

C. *Procedure*
1. Remove dockage or foreign material from the grain (refer to procedure in Section 1.2.8.1). Split the sample into two equal lots.
2. Determine the original grain moisture content (refer to procedure in Section 2.2.1.1).
3. Temper one lot of grain to 25% moisture to conduct the desorption study. Calculate the tempering water requirement using the following equation:

$$\text{tempering water} = \{[(100 - \%\ \text{original moisture})/ (100 - 25\%)] - 1\} \times \text{sample weight}$$

   Place the grain sample in a closed tempering container, add the predetermined tempering water and agitate contents for approximately 5 minutes until all the water has been absorbed by the grain. After a 5-minute rest, reagitate contents for an additional minute. To avoid moisture loss and enhance equilibration, place the conditioned grain inside a sealed plastic bag.
4. Dry the other lot of grain at 68°C for at least 8 hours in an air-forced convection oven to conduct the absorption study. Immediately place the dry grain in a dessicator to avoid environmental moisture uptake (Figure 4.1).
5. Identify aluminum tins for desorption and absorption studies. Then, place containers in a convection oven set at 100°C for at least 30 minutes. Take containers out of the oven and immediately place them in an airtight dessicator for 30 minutes of cooling.
6. Select, prepare, and place at least six different saturated salts that yield different relative humidities (Table 4.1). Place each on the bottom of previously identified dessicators. Make sure to quickly close the dessicator to enhance the fast saturation of the internal atmosphere.
7. Place dessicators with the saturated salt in an environmental chamber set at 25°C. Check the internal RH of each dessicator with a previously calibrated hygrometer.
8. In an analytical balance, weigh 5 g with an accuracy of 0.001 g of dry or conditioned grains placed in tared aluminum tins.
9. Place duplicate samples of dry and conditioned grain in each of the desiccators that were

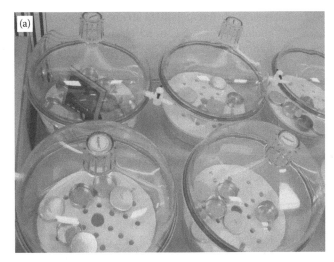

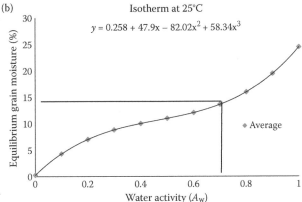

FIGURE 4.1 Determination of a cereal isotherm curve. (a) Dessicators with different saturated salts and RHs; (b) typical isotherm curve for cereal grains.

previously placed in the environmental chamber set at 25°C.

10. Weigh samples every other day with the same analytical balance until the grain achieves constant weight (constant weight is considered when the difference between two consecutive measurements is less than 0.5% of the original sample weight).

11. Determine moisture content and water activity (refer to procedures in Sections 2.2.1.1 and 2.12.3.1) of samples after they achieved constant weight.

12. Graph absorption and desorption curves by relating grain moisture content (y axis) and water activity (x axis) or the RH of the dessicator.

4.2.1.2 Effect of Temperature and Grain Moisture Content on Grain Stability (Figure 4.2)

A. Samples, Ingredients, and Reagents
- 10 kg of sound grain
- Dessicant (activated alumina)
- Adult insects (*Coleopthera* or *Lepidopthera*)

B. Materials and Equipment
- Environmental chamber with temperature and RH controls
- Glass bottles with lids
- Winchester bushel meter
- Digital scale
- Air-convection forced oven
- Dessicator
- Ice pick
- Labels
- Automatic seed counter
- Pipette (10 mL)
- Aluminum tins
- Thermometer
- Sieves and collection pan

C. Procedure
1. Clean the 10 kg grain sample manually, with sieves or with a dockage test meter. Place the extraneous or foreign material in a plastic bag.

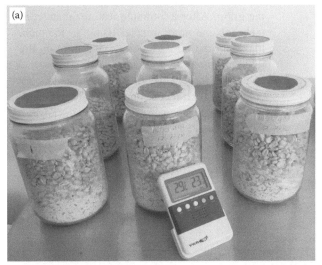

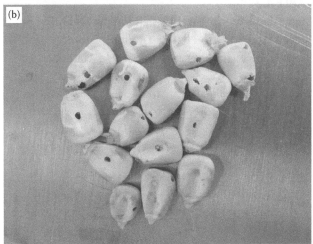

FIGURE 4.2 Effect of temperature and grain moisture content on stored grain stability. (a) Grain samples stored at different moisture contents and conditions; (b) maize kernels with clear evidence of insect damage.

2. Determine the original moisture content of the grain and test thousand kernel weights (refer to procedures in Sections 2.2.1.1 and 1.2.7.1).

3. Weigh 12 identical lots of grains (300–500 g). Identify each glass with the treatment according to Table 4.2 (percentage of moisture, temperature, and whether or not it contains foreign material).

4. Temper four lots of grains to 17% moisture and another set of four samples to 20% moisture. Calculate the tempering requirement using the following equation:

tempering water = {[(100 − % original moisture)/ (100 − % tempering moisture)] − 1} × sample weight

Place the grain sample in a glass bottle and add the predetermined tempering water to achieve the desired moisture content. Place the lid and agitate contents for approximately 5 minutes until all the water has been absorbed by the grain. After a 5-minute rest, reagitate contents for one more minute. Using an ice pick, make at least 20 perforations (1–2 mm) on the lid to ensure air exchange.

5. Add 5% of foreign material to the glasses labeled containing extraneous material. Agitate contents to homogenously distribute the dockage.

6. Add two adult live grain insects per 100 g of sample (10 live insects for 500 g grain) of the *Coleopthera* or *Lepidopthera* order. Make sure insects belong to the same species and are able to damage the test grain.

7. Assign different bottles to the environmental chambers set at 5°C or 25°C.

8. Examine the contents of each bottle every other week in terms of:
   a. Temperature at the geometric center of the lot
   b. Subjective odor and overall grain condition
   c. Total weight
   d. Thousand and test weights
   e. Tnsect-damaged kernels
   f. Live insect count
   g. Evidence of mold growth and damage

9. Return contents to the bottles and place them in the assigned environmental chamber.

10. Repeat steps 6 and 7 for 2 or 3 months.

11. Identify insects and molds according to identification guides of the U.S. Department of Agriculture (USDA 1980), Nelson et al. (1983), Pitt (1979), Dobie et al. (1984), Freeman (1980), and Raper and Fenell (1965).

12. Make biweekly observations of physical grain properties (thousand kernel weight and test weight), dockage, grade, odor, insect counts, grain temperature, and presence of molds. Report dry matter losses during storage and the progressive loss of grade at the end of the experiment. It is recommended to sieve the deteriorated grain to remove fines that count as dry matter loss.

dry matter loss = 1 − [(stored grain weight × % dry matter of stored grain)/(original grain weight × % dry matter)] × 100.

% dry matter = 100 − % moisture content.

4.2.2 RESEARCH SUGGESTIONS

1. Determine equilibrium grain moisture at different RHs of the same grains subjected to 5°C, 15°C, or 35°C and compare absorption and desorption curves to determine the effect of environmental temperature on isotherm behavior.

2. Determine the isotherm curve of corn flakes with an original moisture content of 2% and compare its behavior with that of ground corn meal.

3. Determine falling number values of sound and deteriorated hard wheat kernels subjected to deterioration procedure in Section 6.4.3.4. At the end of the study, roller-mill kernels (procedure in Section 5.2.2.1) and determine yield and quality of the resulting flours in terms of amount of insect fragments, mycotoxins, rheological properties/ dough texture, falling number/starch damage, and color. Then, process flours into pup loaves and compare bread properties (volume, density, crust, and crumb color).

TABLE 4.2
Suggested Experimental Design to Study Stability of Stored Grain as Affected by Grain Moisture, Temperature, and Presence of Foreign Material

Treatment	Grain Moisture (%)	Storage Temperature (°C)	Foreign Material (%)
1	14	5	0
2	14	25	0
3	14	5	5
4	14	25	5
5	17	5	0
6	17	25	0
7	17	5	5
8	17	25	5
9	20	5	0
10	20	25	0
11	20	5	5
12	20	25	5

4.2.3 RESEARCH QUESTIONS

1. Define the following terms:
   a. Adsorption
   b. Desorption
   c. Equilibrium moisture content
   d. Hysteresis
2. Why is grain moisture control the most critical operation in the management of cereal grains?
3. What is the practical use of the isotherm curve for stored grain facilities? What is the effect of environmental temperature on the isotherm of a given cereal grain?
4. What is the equilibrium moisture content of wheat exposed to an environment with 25°C and 70% RH?
5. If you receive from the field 100 kg of green paddy rice with 22.5% moisture, stored at 25°C in an atmosphere containing 60% RH for 2 weeks, what will its equilibrium moisture content and paddy rice weight be after 2 weeks?
6. What would happen to commercial corn flakes with 1.5% moisture when it is taken out of the package and is left for 1 day in a bowl surrounded by air with 85% RH and 20°C?
7. Why is it critically important to thoroughly clean the grain and facilities before storage? What kind of equipments are used to preclean lots of grain in storage facilities?
8. What kind of environmental conditions favor grain deterioration? Describe how sound grains with adequate moisture content can deteriorate throughout prolonged storage.
9. What sorts of chemical changes occur in carbohydrates, protein, and fats when grains have high respiration rates or intrinsic deterioration? What are the most common quality control measurements used to monitor changes in starch, protein, and fats?
10. What are the effects of an atmosphere rich in CO_2 on the respiration rate and deterioration of high-moisture cereal grains kept at environmental temperatures higher than 20°C?

4.3 EXTRINSIC DETERIORATION OF CEREAL GRAINS: INSECTS, MOLDS, AND RODENTS

Globally, insects, molds, and rodents are the main biotic agents responsible for grain losses during storage. Thus, the main goal of managers of storage facilities is to minimize losses in terms of quantity and quality. There are approximately 20 to 30 insect species that damage cereal grains undergoing storage (Baur 1992; Sauer 1992). Besides the direct losses, insects contaminate grains and processed products with fecal material, uric acid, web-like material, cast skins, and body fragments.

Insects are classified as primary or secondary pests according to their habits and characteristics. Primary insects are more harmful because they have the ability to damage sound kernels. They usually perforate the grain for feeding and reproductive purposes. These insects mainly consume the kernel's endosperm and germ tissues and use the grain as an ideal site for laying eggs and the future growth and development of larvae. Secondary insects are also called opportunistic because they attack damaged grains or processed products such as flour, grits, or food products. Both types of insects lower grain viability, food value, and grain quality as raw material for mills and terminal food industries. Insect-damaged kernels will lose 25% to 60% weight and nutrients and leave important contaminants such as bodily parts, cocoons, feces, and eggs. The presence of these contaminants is highly penalized by government agencies because they are closely related to the grain sanitary quality.

The most important indicators of sanitation within milling and processing plants are the analysis of filth, fecal material, insect fragments, rodent hair, and urine. These contaminants indicate a lack of or deficient sanitation procedures in all segments of cereal-based industries (Pedersen 2003).

Aflatoxins and other mycotoxins are sometimes present in cereal grains and must be controlled to avoid problems with animal and human health. Aflatoxins are potent carcinogens produced by the *Aspergillus* species especially in maize maturing during hot drought conditions or other cereals stored under unfavorable conditions. The most popular and practical way to assay mycotoxins in cereal grains is by enzyme-linked immunoassay (ELISA) tests. Confirmation of the levels is usually made with high-performance liquid chromatography (HPLC) or thin-layer chromatography (TLC). For preliminary screening, black light is used to screen maize for the presence of components that absorb UV light and indicate that mycotoxins might be present. If the grain sample glows, the lot of grain should be analyzed for the presence of aflatoxins or other mycotoxins. The fumonisins produced by the *Fusarium* species, which cause ear rot, are widely distributed in maize and have been linked to cancer and neural tube defects in humans and cause important toxicity to equines, swine, and other domestic animals. The Food and Drug Administration has established advisory levels for fumonisins of 4 ppm and 2 ppm in whole maize and dry-milled fractions, respectively (Rooney 2007).

4.3.1 MORPHOLOGY AND IDENTIFICATION OF STORED-GRAIN INSECTS

4.3.1.1 Identification of Stored Grain Insects

The proper identification of insects in grain storage facilities is critical for predicting the development of pest populations and for making important management decisions [U.S. Department of Agriculture-Grain Inspection, Packers and Stockyards Administration (USDA-GIPSA) 2011]. However, many stored grain insect pests, especially beetles, are difficult to identify and can require advanced taxonomic preparation. Thus, the identification of insects is of upmost importance in making pest management decisions. The significance of infestations depends on the species, density, or insect population, and ultimate plans for the grain. Selecting the most appropriate curative or preventative action from among available alternatives is not easily accomplished, especially when the type of insect present is not known. For example, if insects that feed and develop inside the kernels are already present in significant populations, a surface insecticide applied as a dust or spray would not be the best management option. In this situation, the penetrating vapors of a fumigant such as methyl bromide or phosphine are needed to stop further damage. High grain temperatures and moisture, along with excessive grain dockage or broken kernels, provide the necessary conditions for stored-grain insect reproduction and survival. The most favorable grain temperature for these insects is approximately 25°C, whereas the most advantageous grain moisture conditions range from 14% to 18%.

The best preventive measurements for insect infestations are sanitation or removal of leftover grains and dockage from storage facilities as well as any grain handling equipment (conveyors, wagons, trucks, and elevators); treatment using protective residual insecticides on contact surfaces such as bin walls, ceilings, and floors including cracks and crevices; managing grain temperature and aeration; and using chemical insecticides and fumigants (Baur 1992; Sauer 1992).

Insects are the main culprits responsible for grain losses worldwide. Insect pests feed continuously as they develop on a grain. Estimates of the resultant loss vary widely with the type of grain or product, the locality, and the storage practices involved. For grains in the tropics, stored under traditional conditions, a loss in the range of 10% to 30% might be expected over a full storage season. In addition, insects cause loss in grain quality and its market value. Infested grains are contaminated with insect debris, have increased dust content, and are often holed and discolored. Cereal-based foods prepared from infested kernels or flours may have an unpleasant odor or taste. Insects also promote mold development that exacerbates quantity and quality losses, reduced germination because of damage to the embryo, and decreased functionality and nutritional value. Besides the direct losses, insects contaminate grains and processed products with bodily parts, cocoons, feces, eggs, uric acid, and web-like material. Some types also have the ability to attack and damage packaging materials and the structure of grain elevators. The presence of these contaminants is highly penalized by government agencies because they are closely related to the grain sanitary quality (Pedersen 2003).

There are several methods to identify insect infestations including the visual examination of infested kernels, X-ray radiography, and near-infrared analysis (NIRA; Pedersen 2003). Dowell et al. (1999) examined the possibility that NIRA could be used for taxonomic purposes based on the premise that every species may have a unique chemical composition. Tests were conducted with 11 species of beetles commonly associated with stored grain. NIRA spectra from individual insects were collected. The proposed analysis correctly identified 99% of the test insects as primary or secondary pests and correctly identified 95% of test insects to genus. Evidence indicates that the absorption characteristics of cuticular lipids may contribute to the classification of these species.

A. *Samples, Ingredients, and Reagents*
- Grain samples infested with insects
- Ethanol
- Distilled water

B. *Materials and Equipment*
- Digital scale
- Sieves
- Magnifying lens
- Volumetric flask (1 L)
- White tray
- Stereoscopic microscope
- Tweezers
- Light box
- Plastic containers
- Ruler with millimeter markings

C. *Procedure*
1. In a 1-L capacity volumetric flask, prepare a 75% ethanol solution mixing 750 mL of anhydrous ethanol with 250 mL of distilled water.
2. Examine the lot of grain by observing holes, web-like material, live and dead insects, cocoons, and body fragments. Place a sample on a light box and observe holes, burrows, or tunnels and damage to the different anatomical parts. Determine the incidence of insect-damaged kernels.
3. Sample 0.5 kg of infested grain and place it on a sieve that retains the particular grain. Sieve onto a white collection pan to encourage movement of the insects. The grain is placed on the sieve and oscillated a few times before inspecting the collection pan. Any insects in the sample will have fallen through the sieve along with other fine residue.
4. Count the number of insects and place some specimens on a glass container containing 75% ethanol solution. Measure some specimens and observe them with the magnifying lens. Express number and types of insects per 100 g of sample.
5. Identify the insects according to pictures and schematic diagrams of Chapter 6 of the textbook and the USDA (2011) description. In addition, the reader can consult USDA (1980), Dobie et al. (1984), and Freeman (1980). It is recommended to observe adult insects, larvae, and pupae under the stereoscopic microscope.
   - Angoumois grain moth (*Sitotroga cerealella*)
     Length: approximately 8 mm; wing span: approximately 16 mm.

Small buff or yellowish-brown moth. The rear edges of the forewings and hindwings have long fringes. Larvae crawl to the kernel and often spin a small cocoon to assist it in boring into the hard kernel. After entering the grain, it feeds on either the endosperm or the germ until fully grown. It attacks all types of grain, particularly corn and wheat. Badly infested grain has a sickening smell and taste that makes it unpalatable.

- Indian meal moth (*Plodia interpunctella*)
  Length: approximately 17 mm; wing span: approximately 17 mm.

  This insect is easily distinguished from others because of the peculiar markings of its forewings, which are reddish brown with a copper luster on the outer two-thirds but whitish gray on the inner or body ends. Each female lays 100 to 300 eggs. Larvae feed on grains, grain products, dried fruits, nuts, and a rather wide variety of foodstuffs. Fully grown *larvae* leave a silken thread behind wherever it crawls.

- Granary weevil (*Sitophilus granarius*)
  Length: approximately 4 mm.

  The granary weevil is a small, moderately polished, blackish or chestnut-brown beetle. The head extends into a long slender snout with a pair of stout mandibles or jaws at the end. There are no wings under the wing covers, and the thorax is well marked with longitudinal punctures, two characteristics that distinguish this insect from the closely related rice weevil with which it is often found. The adult live an average of 7 to 8 months. Each female lays 50 to 250 eggs during this period. After mass infestation, the grain becomes warm and damp, thus leading to the formation of mold.

- Rice weevil (*Sitophilus oryzae*)
  Length: approximately 3 mm.

  The rice weevil has a small snout and varies from reddish brown to nearly black and is usually marked on the back with four light-reddish or yellowish spots. It has fully developed wings beneath the wing covers. The thorax is densely pitted with somewhat irregularly shaped punctures; except for a smooth narrow strip extending down the middle of the upper (dorsal) side. The adult live an average of 4 to 5 months, and each female lays 300 to 400 eggs during this period. The early life stages are almost identical in habit and appearance to those of the granary weevil.

- Maize weevil (*Sitophilus zeamais*)
  Length: approximately 5 mm.

  The maize weevil has a small snout and varies from dull red-brown to nearly black and is usually marked on the back with four light reddish or yellowish spots. It is slightly larger than the rice weevil and has more distinct colored spots on the forewings. The maize weevil has fully developed wings beneath its wing covers and can fly readily. The thorax is densely pitted with somewhat irregularly shaped punctures, except for a smooth narrow strip extending down the middle of the dorsal (top) side. While developing, the larvae eat the internal contents of the maize; approximately 18 to 23 days.

- Lesser grain borer (*Rhyzopertha dominica*)
  Length: approximately 2.5 mm to 3 mm.

  This small insect is slender and has a cylindrical form with a polished dark brown or black surface that is somewhat roughened. The head is turned down under the thorax and is armed with powerful jaws used for cutting into kernels and wood. Both the beetles and larvae cause serious damage in warm climates by attacking a great variety of grains. The eggs are laid on the outside of the kernels. Badly infested wheat takes on a honey-like odor.

  This insect is capable of infesting all small grain and develops more rapidly in damaged than in sound grain. Adults are dark brown. Females produce between 200 and 400 eggs in their 2- to 3-month lifespan. Eggs are laid on the surface of the grain and larvae burrow into the kernels. Inside the kernel, the larvae completes its growth and pupates. Adults can fly, and also feed on the grain.

- Cadelle (*Tenebroides mauritanicus*)
  Length: approximately 9 mm.

  An elongate, oblong, flattened, black or blackish beetle. Both the larva and adult feed on grain and have the destructive habit of going from kernel to kernel devouring the germs. Found in mills, granaries, and storehouses where it infests flour, meal, and grain. It is one of the longest lived insects that attack stored grain. Many of the adults live for more than 1 year and some of them for nearly 2 years. Both the larvae and adults can live in the woodwork of the bin for a long time after the grain has been removed.

- Saw-toothed grain beetle (*Oryzaephilus surinamensis*)
  Length: approximately 3 mm.

A slender, flat, brown beetle. It gets its name from the peculiar structure of the thorax, which bears six sawtooth-like projections on each side. It attacks in both the larval and adult stages. The adults live average of 6 to 10 months. The female lays 43 to 285 eggs. Infests mainly grain and grain products but also noodles, wafers, nuts, and dried fruits.

- Flat grain beetle (*Cryptolestes pusillus*)

   Length: approximately 2 mm.

   Minute, flattened, oblong, reddish-brown beetle, with elongate antennae about two-thirds as long as the body. One of the smaller beetles commonly found in stored grain. Females deposit small white eggs in crevices in the grain or drop them loosely on farinaceous material. The larvae are fond of the wheat germ, and, in infested grain, many kernels are found uninjured except for the removal of the germ. Larvae also feed on dead insects. Frequently found in enormous numbers with the rice weevil. This insect is a scavenger and often infests grain and meal that are in poor condition.

- Confused flour beetle (*Tribolium confusum*)

   Length: approximately 4 mm.

   Shiny, flattened, oval, reddish-brown beetle. The head and upper parts of the thorax are densely covered with minute punctures. Confused flour beetle antennae gradually enlarge at the tip. The sides of the confused flour beetle head capsule are notched at the eyes so that a visible ridge is present. The eyes of the confused flour beetle are separated by more than three eye diameters. The wing covers are ridged lengthwise and are sparsely punctured between the ridges. Confused flour beetles do not have the ability to fly. The average lifespan is approximately 1 year. Badly infested flour has a sharp odor and turns brown; its baking properties are damaged. This beetle is closely related and almost identical in appearance to the red flour beetle.

- Red flour beetle (*Tribolium castanum*)

   Length: approximately 4 mm.

   Shiny, flattened, oval, reddish-brown beetle. The last three segments of the red flour beetle's antennae abruptly enlarge to form a club-shaped tip. The sides of the red flour beetle head capsule do not have a ridge. When viewed from below, the eyes of the red flour beetle are separated by less than two eye diameters. Red flour beetles fly. The average lifespan is approximately

1 year. Badly infested flour has a sharp odor and turns brown; its baking properties are damaged.

6. Report the incidence of kernel damage, counts, and types of primary and secondary insects and the presence of different stages (larvae, pupae, and adults) of the insects.

4.3.2 Filth, Insect Fragments, and Other Extraneous Materials

4.3.2.1 Determination of Light Filth in Flours (Method 972.32)

This is one of the most common methods used to estimate filth associated with flours. The filth generally consists of insect fragments, rodent hair, and other forms of light filth (Association of Official Analytical Chemists; AOAC 2005). The principle of this assay is that the flour is acid-digested to break down starch, leaving the filth undamaged. Then, mineral oil is added to trap the filth which is later identified and evaluated under a stereoscopic microscope. The current Food and Drug Administration defect action levels for insect fragments and rodent hairs is 75 or more, and 1 or more/50 g flour in six subsamples, respectively.

A. *Samples, Ingredients, and Reagents*
   - Flours
   - Mineral oil-paraffin
   - Distilled water
   - Hydrochloric acid (HCl)
   - Sodium lauryl sulfate

B. *Materials and Equipment*
   - Kilborn funnel or percolator
   - Autoclave
   - Hot plate with magnetic stirrer
   - Graduated cylinder (50 mL)
   - Filter paper
   - Erlenmeyer flask
   - Stirring rod
   - Beakers (1 L and 2.5 L)
   - Ruled filter paper
   - Buchner filter
   - Stereoscopic microscope
   - Chronometer

C. *Procedure*

   These procedures were previously described in Pedersen (2003).

   1. Prepare the following reagents:
      a. 3% HCl solution
      b. 5% Aqueous sodium lauryl detergent solution
   2. Weigh 50 g of flour and place it in a 2.5 L beaker. Then, add 600 mL of 3% HCl acid solution. Stir contents.
   3. Autoclave contents for 5 minutes at 121°C.
   4. Transfer contents to a 1 L beaker and wash walls of the other beaker with 3% HCl.

5. Add 50 mL of mineral oil and stir magnetically for 5 minutes.
6. Transfer the sample to a Kilborn funnel or percolator. Let contents stand for 30 minutes. Stir gently with a glass stirring rod several times during the first 10 minutes. Then, do not disturb the sample (Figure 4.3).
7. Carefully drain the lower layer to approximately 3 cm of interface. Wash sides of the funnel with warm tap water and allow layers to separate for 2 to 3 minutes. Repeat the draining and washing procedure until the bottom phase is clear.
8. After final wash, drain the top oil layer into a clean beaker. Rinse sides of the funnel with 5% detergent solution.
9. Add HCl to approximately 3% volume and heat on a hot plate for 3 to 4 minutes.
10. Filter hot solution through ruled filter paper placed on a Buchner filtering device. Then, thoroughly rinse beaker and funnel with the 5% detergent solution and again filter onto ruled filter paper.
11. Examine microscopically and record light filth composed of insect fragments, rodent hairs, and fragments and feather barbules. Report counts per 50 g of flour.

4.3.2.2 Determination of Insect Fragments in Flours

One of the most important and practiced tests in the milling industry is the determination of insect fragments because it is closely related to the quality of incoming grains and the efficiency of grain-cleaning equipments. This sanitation test determines the number of recognizable insect fragments (antennae, legs, mandibles, exoskeletons or cast skins, and elytras or wing coverings). Generally, the maximum accepted level is 50 insect fragments/50 g or one fragment per gram of flour or milled fraction.

A. *Samples, Ingredients, and Reagents*
- Flours
- Mineral oil
- HCl solution (3%)
- Ethanol

B. *Materials and Equipment*
- Separation funnel or flask
- Petri dishes
- Hot plate
- Pipette (10 mL)
- Filter paper
- Erlenmeyer flask
- Stirring rod
- Beakers (150 mL and 250 mL)
- Magnetic stirrer
- Buchner filter
- Stereoscopic microscope

C. *Procedure*
1. Weigh 7 g of sample and place it in a 150 mL beaker. Then, add 90 mL of 3% HCl acid solution and stir with a magnetic stirrer.
2. Digest or hydrolyze the sample on a hot plate placed under a hood until the hydrolysate turns brown.
3. Remove the beaker from the hot plate and add 7 mL of mineral oil. Agitate contents with a magnetic stirrer (Figure 4.3).
4. Place the sample in a separation flask and bring the solution to 220 mL with distilled water.

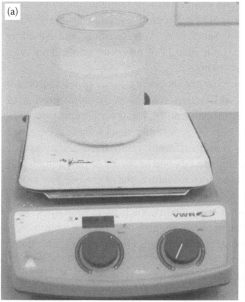
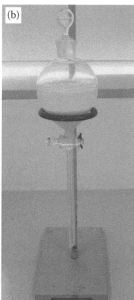
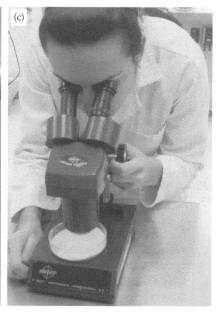

FIGURE 4.3 Determination of light filth or insect fragments in flours. (a) Treatment with HCl acid; (b) separation of the top phase containing insect fragments; (c) identification of insect fragments using the dissection or stereoscopic microscope.

5. Mix the simple with the water with an agitator for 10 minutes. Make sure to clean the agitator after each stirring operation.

6. Allow the resulting solution to rest for 20 minutes.

7. Remove water up to a volume of 170 mL and add more distilled water to the 220 mL mark.

8. Repeat this operation until the wash water is translucent. Make sure the wash water cleans the walls of the separation funnel or flask.

9. Carefully recover the oily phase of the separation funnel and add 3% HCl to double the initial volume. Heat the resulting mixture for 2 minutes or until it starts boiling.

10. When the solution starts to boil, immediately remove it from the hot plate and filter the contents through filter paper placed in a funnel.

11. Pass ethanol through the filter paper.

12. Place the filter paper in a Petri dish and observe it under a stereoscopic microscope.

13. Count and identify the insect fragments observed in the whole field.

4.3.2.3 Determination of Insect Eggs in Flour (Method 940.34)

This method was previously described in AOAC (2005).

A. Samples, Ingredients, and Reagents
- Flours
- Distilled water
- Ethanol
- Sulfuric acid (H_2SO_4)
- Iodine

B. Materials and Equipment
- Digital scale
- Steam bath
- Petri dishes
- Erlenmeyer flask for Buchner filter
- Pipette (5 mL)
- Filter paper
- Sieve (100 mesh) with collection pan
- Buchner filter
- Beakers (250 mL)
- Graduated cylinder (50 mL)
- Chronometer
- Stereoscopic microscope (20×)

C. Procedure
1. Prepare the following reagents:
   a. 1% and 5% H_2SO_4 solutions
   b. 0.1 N iodine solution

2. Weigh 50 g of flour and place it on a 100-mesh sieve with a collection pan. Sift gently until no more flour passes through.

3. Transfer the residue on sieve to a 250 mL beaker and wet with 2 mL to 3 mL of ethanol.

4. Add 30 mL of 5% H_2SO_4, cover the beaker, and heat contents on a steam bath for 10 minutes.

5. Filter through paper on a suction funnel. Keep beaker partially inverted over funnel and rinse with distilled water.

6. Add 15 mL to 20 mL of 0.1 N iodine to paper in funnel. Allow 10 to 15 seconds for iodine to stain contents.

7. Apply gentle suction and then wash with 25 mL to 30 mL of 1% H_2SO_4 followed by several small water washes.

8. Carefully transfer filter paper to Petri dish and examine for the presence of insect eggs under 20× magnification.

9. Register the number of eggs contained in 50 g of flour.

4.3.3 Molds and Mycotoxins

After insects, grain molds are the most important biotic agents affecting grain storage. The most important genus of storage molds are *Fusarium*, *Aspergillus*, and *Penicillum*. Molds reduce seed viability, grain quality, and functionality and therefore its economic value. Molds also cause primary and secondary damages. The first is due to the potent lipolitic, amylolitic, and proteolytic enzymes that degrade stored nutrients, and the second is due to mycotoxins and changes in grain quality (off-colors, odors, and flavors). Storage molds usually infest grains when their moisture is in the range of 16% to 20%, require RHs higher than 70%, and temperatures of at least 25°C. These fungi are more destructive when the air RH and temperatures are 85% and 25°C to 30°C, respectively. The main harmful effects of storage fungi are lower seed viability, grain discoloration, nutrient degradation, mycotoxin production, grain heating, and generation of musty off-odors.

Most mycotoxins have the potential to cause serious diseases and even deaths in humans and domestic animals (Bulla et al. 1977; Krogh 1987; MacFarlane 1995; Mirocha et al. 1980; Sauer 1992; Van Rensburg and Altenkirk 1974). The main toxic effects of mycotoxins are detailed in Table 6.2 of the textbook.

Mycotoxins are secondary metabolites secreted by fungi and molds. Diseases related to the consumption of mycotoxins have been known for several centuries. However, it has been only 50 years since mycotoxicosis became relevant and has greatly affected grain trade. Aflatoxins are currently recognized as one of the most potent naturally occurring carcinogens in nature and therefore are monitored by regulatory government health agencies around the globe. Some other mycotoxins, such as ochratoxins, fumonisins, and zeralenone, have also received attention because of their potent harmful health effects on humans and domestic animals.

Aflatoxins are mainly classified into B_1, B_2, G_1, G_2, M_1, and M_2 (refer to Table 6.2 and Figure 6.3 of the textbook). The B and G aflatoxins could be present in contaminated grains, whereas the M_1 and M_2 counterparts could be present in milk produced by lactating animals or women who have consumed mycotoxin-contaminated grains or products. These metabolites are of upmost importance because they are toxic at very low concentrations (10 ppb). The most common aflatoxins in cereal grains are B₁ and B₂ produced by *Aspergillus flavus*. The presence of the causal mold does not necessarily indicate the existence of toxins. For instance, *A. flavus* does not produce aflatoxins when it grows at relatively low temperatures. The probability of aflatoxin production increases when the mold is stressed because of the lack of water and high ambient temperatures. Almost all mycotoxins fluoresce when exposed to conventional UV light. For instance, aflatoxins fluoresce blue or green at 350 nm.

Undoubtedly, maize is the cereal most susceptible to mold infestation and mycotoxins (Krogh 1987; Mirocha et al. 1980; Sauer 1992). This is because the cob is covered with husks, creating an ideal and protective environment for molds. Research has demonstrated that fungi can penetrate the cob through previous damage caused by ear worms (*Heliothis zea*). The presence of aflatoxins in maize has created lots of problems in grain elevators because, in most countries, the maximum level allowed is 20 ppb for humans and 200 ppb for animals.

Ochratoxins are another important group of mycotoxins, mainly produced by *Aspergillus ochraceus* or in some instances by *Penicillum verbicosum*. Ochratoxicosis produces the Balkan endemic nephropathy first described in Bulgaria. Chemically, ochratoxins are isocoumarin derivatives bound to phenylalanine. The most common and relevant is ochratoxin A or OTA. Most ochratoxicoses are related to field-contaminated maize due to excess rainfall before harvesting or to maize stored at high moisture. Laboratory rats fed with high concentrations of these toxins developed cancer and progeny with teratogenic defects (Krogh 1987; Mirocha et al. 1980; Sauer 1992).

Several species from the genus *Fusarium* produce an array of toxins with important health implications in both humans and domestic animals (Desjardins 2006). The most important are zeralenone, T-2 toxin, trichothecenes, vomitoxin, and fumonisin. Unlike other mycotoxins, fumonisins are highly water-soluble and do not possess an aromatic structure that facilitates analytical detection. In humans, fumonisins have been related to esophageal cancers in China and South Africa, and interference with folic acid metabolism. Therefore, they can exacerbate fetal malformations such as neural tube defects (Hendricks 1999; Marasas et al. 2004). Zeralenone is an acid lactone with a phenolic resorcylic configuration (refer to Figure 6.4 of the textbook). Most cases are related to contaminated maize, although the presence of zeralenone in other cereal grains has been documented. These toxins cause estrogenic syndrome or animal feminization, characterized by vulvovaginitis, prolapsed uterus, and infertility. In swine, zeralenone causes testicular atrophy, infertility, and swelling of the mammary glands. Zeralenone fluoresce greenish-blue when exposed to UV light (260–275 nm; Bulla et al. 1977; Desjardins 2006; Krogh 1987; MacFarlane 1995; Mirocha et al. 1980).

Trichothecenes or T-2s are another type of toxin generally associated with zeralenone and fusarium infestations. Maize is the most common cereal affected by these fungi, especially when it is stored at high moisture levels. Trichothecenes can produce the fatal syndrome known as alimentary toxemia, which is characterized by leucopenia, multiple hemorrhages, loss of bone marrow, and esophageal cancer. In addition, the consumption of these toxins reduces the efficiency of feed conversion in domestic animals and poultry (Desjardins 2006; Krogh 1987; Mirocha et al. 1980; Sauer 1992).

Vomitoxin is a deoxinivalenol or DON derivative also produced by *Fusarium*. It mainly occurs in maize, although it also infests wheat and barley, especially during wet or rainy years. The brewing industry is especially concerned about this toxin because it migrates to the wort and beer when contaminated barley malt is used. Similar to trichothecenes, vomitoxins cause vomiting, lower feed intake, and lower efficiency of feed conversion (Krogh 1987; Mirocha et al. 1980; Sauer 1992).

Ergot produces a couple of alkaloids called ergotamine and ergotine that, on ingestion, produces convulsions, muscle cramps, hallucinations, and gangrene in fingers and toes. In severe cases, affected patients die of suffocation due to paralysis of rib cage muscles (Van Rensburg and Altenkirk 1974). Ergotism, also known as St. Anthony's fire, is the oldest known human toxicosis. Rye is the cereal crop that is most susceptible to this parasitic fungus. The infested kernels turn black and are harder and larger than their normal counterparts (Krogh 1987; Mirocha et al. 1980; Sauer 1992; Van Rensburg and Altenkirk 1974).

There are several laboratory tests to detect the presence of molds and mycotoxins. The simple observation of a representative sample of grain under UV light will indicate the possible presence of mycotoxins (refer to procedure in Section 4.3.3.1). Official tests are based first on the solvent extraction (i.e., ethanol, methanol, chloroform/water), followed by filtration, separation, and detection generally via fluorescence or UV detectors. TLC was extensively used to detect different types of mycotoxins. Nowadays, HPLC systems equipped with fluorescence or UV detectors are commonly used (refer to Chapter 2). However, the most frequent and popular way to quantify mycotoxins are via the use of immune absorbent or ELISA columns. These are accurate and fast so they are widely used as a screening and analytical tool in grain elevators. It consists of first extracting a representative sample of the grain with aqueous solvents, such as aqueous methanol, followed by filtration. The key step is passing an aliquot of the extract through a mini column that contains monoclonal antibodies for the specific toxin. Therefore, the column specifically binds the toxin of interest. Then, the column is washed and the recovered mycotoxins are generally read in a fluorometer. The fluorometer is previously calibrated with standards containing known concentrations of the mycotoxin. These quick and reliable tests have gained popularity because they are accepted by regulatory agencies and are easy to perform.

4.3.3.1 Presumptive Test for Aflatoxins (Method 45-15)

The black-light test is widely used as a presumptive test to identify lots of cereals that may contain aflatoxins, especially in grain elevators (American Association of Cereal Chemists; AACC 2000). The test was devised for maize, although it is also used for other grains. The lot of grain is inspected under UV light to detect the bright greenish-yellow fluorescence associated with *A. flavus* or *Aspergillus parasiticus*. Grains that test positive should be further analyzed to determine the levels of aflatoxins because the growth of these fungi may or may not result in aflatoxin production. This test is the quickest method of detecting kernels that could contain aflatoxins, requires very little equipment, and can easily be done in the field.

A. *Samples, Ingredients, and Reagents*
  - Grain samples
B. *Materials and Equipment*
  - Goggles for UV protection
  - High-intensity black ray lamp B-100 or black-light cabinet
C. *Procedure*
  1. Obtain a 4.5-kg sample of grain by probing or sampling.
  2. Spread a monolayer of approximately 1 kg of the lot of grain underneath a black ray lamp B 100 in a dark room or a smaller sample inside the black-light cabinet. If not using the cabinet, the inspector should wear protective UV goggles.
  3. The presence of one or more fluorescent or glowing particles per kilogram of grain is considered a positive test and should be analyzed for aflatoxins.

4.3.3.2 Determination of Aflatoxins Using the AflaTest

The ELISA technique, AflaTest, is a quantitative method for the detection of aflatoxins in cereal grains and their products (Anonymous 1999). This advanced biotechnology assay allows the measurement of aflatoxins and all the other major mycotoxins in a relatively short time without the use of toxic solvents such as chloroform or methylene chloride. The AflaTest is used in a wide variety of locations from the local farm elevator, food processing quality control laboratories, and government testing laboratories. The main advantages of this easy-to-perform technique are the speed of analysis and accuracy. Aflatoxin, a toxin from a naturally occurring mold, is a group 1 carcinogen proven to cause cancer in humans. Aflatoxin can also cause economic losses in livestock because of disease or reduced efficiency of production. Samples are prepared by mixing with an extraction solution, blending, and then filtering to obtain an extract with the mycotoxins. The extract is then applied to the AflaTest mini column bound with specific antibodies to aflatoxins. At this stage, the aflatoxin binds to the antibody on the column. The column is then washed with water

to rid the immunoaffinity column of impurities. By passing methanol through the column, the aflatoxin is removed from the antibody. This methanol solution can then be measured in a fluorometer for total aflatoxin quantitation or injected into an HPLC system to detect the concentration of each type of aflatoxin. The AflaTest has been validated by the AOAC Research Institute under the *Performance Tested Program* to detect aflatoxin residues in grain and grain products. This quantitative test kit also underwent evaluation by the USDA, Federal Grain Inspection Services for the detection of total aflatoxin for whole maize, germ meal, gluten feed, gluten meal, refined meals, maize/soybean blend, milled rice, popcorn, sorghum, soybeans, and wheat. Under the authority of the U.S. Grain Standards Act, this test kit was found to meet or exceed all design and test performance criteria as defined in the "Design Criteria and Test Performance Specifications for Quantitative Aflatoxin Test kits." This test kit is cited in the AOAC (2005) Official Methods Program, as official method 991.31, applicable for the determination of aflatoxin B_1, B_2, G_1, and G_2 both by fluorometry and HPLC analysis.

Most of the other mycotoxins can be analyzed following similar protocols and procedures used for aflatoxins.

A. *Samples, Ingredients, and Reagents*
  - Cereal grain or product samples
  - Methanol (HPLC grade)
  - AflaTest developer (50 mL)
  - Distilled or deionized water
  - Aflatoxin calibration standards
  - Noniodized sodium chloride (NaCl)
B. *Materials and Equipment*
  - Digital scale
  - AflaTest-P columns
  - Single position pump stand
  - Fluted filter paper (24 cm)
  - KimWipes tissues
  - Beakers
  - Wash bottle (500 mL)
  - Dispenser (500 mL) for methanol–dispenser (50 mL) for developer
  - Fluorometer
  - Filter funnels (65 mm and 105 mm)
  - Blender with stainless steel container
  - Pipettes
  - Microfiber filters (1.5 μm, 11 cm)
  - Disposable cuvettes
  - Graduated cylinders (50 mL and 250 mL)
  - Cuvette rack
  - Vortex mixer
C. *Procedure*
  1. Prepare the following reagents:
     a. Methanol/water (80:20 by volume).
     b. Dilute AflaTest Developer solution. Measure 5.0 mL of AflaTest Developer concentrate solution and place in the 2 oz. amber glass bottle of a 50 mL bottle dispenser for developer.

Add 45.0 mL purified water and mix well. Secure the bottle dispenser top tightly. Keep the dilute developer solution tightly capped when not in use. Do not use dilute developer more than 8 hours after preparation.

2. Calibrate the fluorometer as follows:

   a. Turn on the power and allow fluorometer to warm up for at least 20 to 30 minutes.

   b. Place the green standard in the sample chamber and close the lid. Adjust the zero knob until the digital display reads the desired value.

   c. Remove the green standard from the chamber and then place the red standard in the chamber and close the lid.

   d. Adjust the span knob until the digital display reads the desired value. Remove the red standard from the chamber.

   e. Recheck the calibration of the green standard to make sure that it reads the correct value. Adjust with the zero knob if necessary.

   f. Insert yellow vial. The result of this measurement should be within the range indicated in the procedure. If the result is not within the range specified, recalibrate the fluorometer.

   g. Make sure that the reagent blank (1 mL methanol + 1 mL developer in a cuvette) and 2 mL purified water reads 0 ppb on a calibrated fluorometer.

3. Obtain a representative sample of the lot of grain. Remember that mycotoxins may only occur in a small percentage of the kernels. Because of the wide range in mycotoxin concentrations among individual kernels in a contaminated lot, variation from sample to sample can be large. It is important to obtain a representative sample from a lot. Product should be collected from different locations in a static lot based on a probing pattern. The probe should draw from the top to the bottom of the lot. The samples obtained from the probes should be ground and mixed well and a subsample taken for testing.

4. Weigh 50 g of ground sample with an accuracy of 0.01 g and 5 g noniodized salt (NaCl) and place in blender jar. Add 100 mL of the 80% methanol solution to the jar. Cover blender jar and blend at high speed for 1 minute (Figure 4.4).

5. Pour extract into fluted filter paper. Collect filtrate in a clean vessel.

6. Pipette exactly 10.0 mL of the filtered extract into a clean vessel and dilute extract with 40 mL of distilled deionized water. Mix contents.

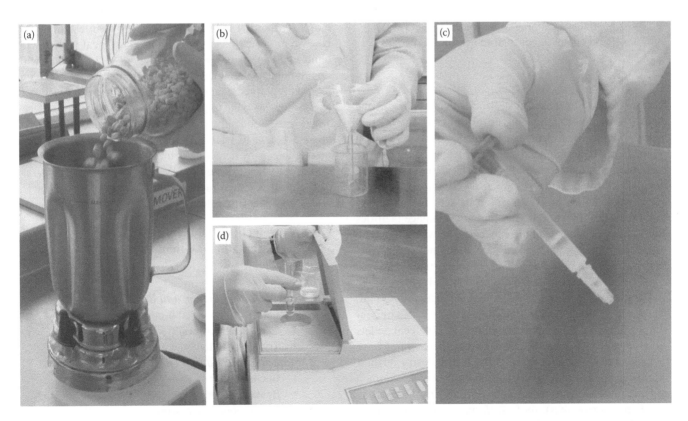

FIGURE 4.4 Determination of aflatoxins using the AflaTest. (a) Grinding of maize sample; (b) filtration of ground maize to obtain the extract; (c) ELISA column which has affinity for aflatoxins; (d) quantification of aflatoxins using a previously calibrated fluorometer.

7. Filter diluted extract through a glass microfiber filter into a glass syringe barrel using markings on barrel to measure exactly 2 mL.

8. Attach AflaTest affinity column to the pump stand (Figure 4.4). The stand has a 10-mL glass syringe barrel that serves as a reservoir for the column. A large plastic syringe with tubing and coupling provides air pressure to manually push liquids through the column. Remove large top cap from column and cut bottom 1/8 in. off the end of the top cap with scissors or a sharp blade. This provides a coupling for attaching the column. Attach column to coupling and place waste collection cup under column outlet. Pass the 2 mL filtered diluted extract (2 mL = 0.2 g sample equivalent) completely through AflaTest-P affinity column at a rate of about one to two drops per second until air comes through column. Then, pass 5 mL of distilled–deionized water through the column at a rate of about two drops per second. Repeat the step of passing 5 mL of distilled water through the column at a rate of about two drops per second.

9. Elute affinity column by passing 1.0 mL of HPLC grade methanol through the column at a rate of one to two drops per second and collecting all of the sample eluate (1 mL) in a glass cuvette.

10. Add 1.0 mL of AflaTest Developer to eluate in the cuvette. Mix well and place cuvette in a previously calibrated fluorometer (Figure 4.4). Read aflatoxin concentration after 60 seconds.

4.3.4 RODENTS

Rats and mice are the most destructive vertebrates in the planet. They consume and harm millions of tons of food yearly. Damage by rodents occurs during all stages of food production, processing, and use. Field losses of cereals are particularly serious, especially in tropical regions around the globe. Postharvest losses are also very important, especially when grains are open-stored or kept in nonrodent-proof facilities. In addition, rats and mice damage facilities and cause secondary damage because they contaminate grains and their products with hair, droppings, and urine. Rodents are highly destructive because they consume approximately 10% of their body weight daily. More grain and grain products are lost due to contamination with hair, feces, and urine. In 1 year, one single rat is capable of consuming 12.25 kg of grain and excreting 25,000 fecal pellets weighing 1 kg to 2 kg. Needless to say, these grains have to be sold at a discount price to the feed industry or thoroughly cleaned to remove contaminants. The most common rodents present in grain storage facilities are the Norway rat (*Rattus norvegicus*), roof rat (*Rattus rattus*), and house mice (*Mus musculus* L). The Norway rat is more common in temperate and urban areas and is considered as a burrowing rodent. Morphologically, they are large (adults weigh 300 g or more), robust, and omnivorous animals with small eyes and ears, a short and blunt nose, and usually dark-colored coats. The most distinctive characteristic is that the tail is shorter than the body (20–25 cm vs. 15–20 cm long). The adults are aggressive, dominant, and consume an average of 28 g of food daily. The adult female or dam has the capacity of producing up to seven litters per year of eight to 12 pups each. Comparatively, the roof rat is smaller but it adapts better to tropical regions and its color varies from black to grayish-white. Two distinctive characteristics are that the ventral or abdominal part is lighter than the rest of the body and that the tail is longer than the body length. Other distinctive features are that these rats have larger eyes and ears and pointed noses. Roof rats can climb and live in overhead areas especially when they coexist with Norway rats. The Norway rat dominates the roof rat especially when they compete for food and space. House mice are small cosmopolitan rodents common to human environment and dwellings. They also have a longer tail compared with the body (7.6–10 vs. 6.3-8.9 cm long). The house mouse only weighs 15 g. The light brown or gray-colored animal has a pointed nose, small eyes, and long ears. Females give birth to up to eight litters per year of nine to 12 pups each. They specialize in consuming cereal grains and the control program should consider that these animals are excellent climbers (Harris and Bauer 1982; Sauer 1992). The best way to detect the presence of these mammals is by looking for nests in double ceilings or walls, fresh fecal pellets, footprints along the walls, and gnawed materials. The size and form of droppings are the best indicators of the type of infestation. The Norway rat excretes larger (1.9 cm long) fecal pellets with blunt ends compared with the roof rat (1.2 cm long with pointed ends). The house mouse droppings average 0.6 cm long with pointed edges A good way to detect footprints is to use flour as a dusting agent and apply it in those places where rats frequently transit, such as corridors and floor areas adjacent to walls. Another way to recognize rodent infestations is by detecting urine using UV light. The urine fluoresces when exposed to UV light (366 nm). This is one of the most common methods used by regulatory agencies to detect rodent infestations.

4.3.4.1 Detection of Rodent Feces by Decantation (Method 28-50)

This method was previously described in AACC (2000).

A. *Samples, Ingredients, and Reagents*
*   Flours or processed products
*   Carbon tetrachloride
*   Trichloromethane

B. *Materials and Equipment*
*   Buchner filter
*   Beaker (250 mL)
*   Stereoscopic microscope
*   Filter paper
*   Graduated cylinder (100 mL)

C. *Procedure*

1. Weigh 50 g of sample in a 250 mL beaker. Fill the beaker with trichloromethane approximately 1 cm before the rim.
2. Mix the contents and allow the solution to rest for 30 minutes.
3. Mix the phases again using an agitator.
4. Separate the trichloromethane and filter the solution in a Buchner filter equipped with filter paper. Make sure the bottom phase is not disturbed.
5. Fill the beaker with carbon tetrachloride to approximately 1 cm before the rim. Mix the phases and allow the solution to rest for 30 minutes.
6. Separate the carbon tetrachloride and filter the solution in a Buchner filter equipped with filter paper. Make sure the bottom phase is not disturbed.
7. Repeat step 6 with equal parts of trichloromethane and carbon tetrachloride. Make sure not to disturb the bottom phase because it contains the fecal material.
8. Wash the bottom phase with carbon tetrachloride and trichloromethane and filter the solution.
9. Examine contents of the filter paper under a stereoscopic microscope.

4.3.4.2 Detection of Urine on Grains (Method 963.28)

The magnesium uranyl acetate test is applied to determine the presence of urine on grains. A sample of the grain is sprayed with magnesium uranyl acetate to cause a greenish fluorescence when viewed under UV light (AOAC 2005). Urea is detected with urease-bromothymol blue paper and is confirmed through its reaction with xanthydrol to form dixanthylurea crystals, which are detected microscopically.

A. *Samples, Ingredients, and Reagents*
- Grain samples
- Magnesium uranyl acetate
- Glacial acetic acid
- Glycerol
- Urease
- Distilled water
- Magnesium acetate [$Mg(C_2H_3O_2)_2 \cdot 4H_2O$]
- Sodium hydroxide (NaOH)
- Bromothymol blue
- Xanthydrol crystals

B. *Materials and Equipment*
- Digital scale
- Sprayer (250 mL)
- Hot plate
- Shallow tray
- Mortar and pestle
- Dark glass bottles
- Microscope slides
- Tweezers
- Laboratory gloves
- UV lamp (253.7 nm)
- Volumetric flasks (10 mL, 50 mL, and 1 L)
- Stereoscopic microscope
- Dropper
- Watch glass
- Chronometer
- Stirring rod
- Spot plate

C. *Procedure*

1. Prepare the following reagents:
   a. Magnesium uranyl acetate solution. Dissolve 100 g of magnesium uranyl in 60 mL of glacial acetic acid and dilute to 500 mL. Dissolve in 330 g of magnesium acetate [$Mg(C_2H_3O_2)_2 \cdot 4H_2O$] in 60 mL of glacial acetic acid and dilute to 200 mL. Heat solution to the boiling point until clear, pour the magnesium solution into the uranyl solution, cool and dilute to 1 L in a volumetric flask. The working magnesium uranyl acetate solution is prepared by mixing the previous solution with the urease solution described next in 1/10 amounts with the posterior addition of 22 mL glycerol. The working solution is mixed and filtered through filter paper.
   b. Urease solution. Wet 0.2 g of urease powder with a small amount of water, stir into a paste and dilute to 10 mL with distilled water.
   c. Bromothymol blue solution. Dissolve 0.15 g bromothymol blue powder in mortar with 2.4 mL 0.1 N NaOH solution. After dissolving, wash mortar and pestle with distilled water and dilute to 50 mL.
   d. Urease-bromothymol blue test paper. Mix 10 mL of the indicator solution c with 10 mL of the urease solution b. Pour mixture onto watch glass and use clean tweezers to dip pieces of filter paper (Whatman no. 5) into the solution. Hang orange paper to dry at room temperature. Store dry paper in well-stoppered dark glass bottle.
2. Weigh 50 g of grain and place it on a shallow tray in a hood or ventilated area.
3. Spray with the magnesium uranyl acetate solution, making several sweeps horizontally and vertically across the sample. Let stand for 1 to 3 minutes and examine under short-wave UV light.
4. Wearing laboratory gloves and with clean tweezers, transfer kernels that showed greenish fluorescence to spot plate.
5. Add one to four drops of distilled water to each suspect kernel on spot plate. Let stand for 3 to 5 minutes.

6. Place strip of urease-bromothymol paper on microscope slide and transfer drop of the aqueous extract of step 5 to paper with stirring rod and cover with a second slide.

7. The development of blue spots within 4 minutes indicate the presence of urea.

8. For a confirmatory test, transfer one to two drops of extract of step 5 to microscope slide and evaporate to dryness. Add drop of a mixture of two parts acetic acid and one part water and a very small amount of xanthydrol crystals.

9. If urea is present, dixanthylurea crystals will quickly form and are visible at 60× or lower with wide-field stereoscopic microscope.

4.3.5 Research Suggestions

1. Compare a sound lot of maize with damaged maize produced according to procedure in Section 4.2.1.2. Treat one lot with the recommended amount of phostoxin or phosphine. After 2 months of storage, determine grain damage in terms of dry matter loss and physical properties (test and 1000 kernel weights) and the number of insects. In addition, mill subsamples into a flour and determine the number of insect fragments.

2. Prepare a lot of the same type of sound maize according to procedure in Section 4.2.1.2 (effect of temperature and grain moisture content on grain stability). Treat one lot with the 0.2% propionic acid that acts as an antimold agent. After 2 months of storage, determine grain damage in terms of physical properties (test and 1000 kernel weights) and aflatoxins using the enzyme immunoadsorbent ELISA assay.

3. Determine the amount of aflatoxins associated with a contaminated lot of maize following the TLC, enzyme immunoadsorbent (AflaTest), and HPLC assays.

4. Determine the presence of mammalian feces by the alkaline phosphatase detection method (AOAC 2005, Method 986.28) and compare results with the AACC method (AACC 2000, Method 28-50).

4.3.6 Research Questions

1. Define the following terms:
   a. Extraneous material
   b. Heavy and light filth
   c. Berlese funnel
   d. Good Manufacturing Practices
   e. Detection action levels
   f. Cast skins
   g. Pheromone

2. List at least three reasons for conducting analysis for extraneous material in cereal-based products and foods.

3. What are the main characteristics of insects belonging to the *Lepidoptera* or *Coleoptera* orders? What environmental factors and intrinsic grain characteristics favor insect growth and infestation?

4. What are the differences between primary and secondary grain insects?

5. How are insects and rodents usually controlled in grain elevators?

6. Besides direct losses, what other sorts of damage do insects usually cause to cereal-based products?

7. Compare environmental minimum and optimum temperature and grain moisture or water activity requirements for insects and molds.

8. Why is a lot of grain with a high amount of dockage or extraneous material more prone to deterioration compared with a clean counterpart?

9. Investigate the use of X-ray and NIRA for the detection of internal insect infestation or insect pests.

10. What is the principle of the insect fragment assay? Why is this test considered as one of the most critical for food trade and an indicator of sanitation?

11. What are the main insecticides used on contact surfaces and to treat stored grains? What are the advantages or disadvantages of these insecticides?

12. What are the main toxic effects to insects and humans of organochloride, organophosphate, and carbamate insecticides?

13. What are the differences between an insecticide and a fumigant? List at least three important insecticides and fumigants applied in grain elevators.

14. Why do most regulatory agencies monitor the amount of residual pesticides in processed grain products? What are the toxic effects of methyl bromide, malathion, and pyrethrines to insects and humans? Which of these insecticides persist more in nature?

15. List at least five types of mycotoxins indicating causal molds, their effects on human and animal health, and the most common way to assess their concentration.

16. What are the effects of lime-cooking and tortilla production on aflatoxins?

17. Investigate methods to commercially detoxify mycotoxin-contaminated kernels.

18. Why do most mycotoxins fluoresce when exposed to UV light?

19. What are the advantages and disadvantages of determining aflatoxins with HPLC and the AflaTest?

20. What are the principles of urine and feces analyses? Why are these tests important for regulatory agencies?

21. What are the morphological differences among the three major rodents that infest grain elevators? How can you detect if the grain elevator or processing industries have rodent infestations?

22. What are the main preventive control measurements for rodents in grain storage facilities or elevators?
23. What are the main toxic effects of methyl bromide, warfarin, fluoroacetamide, and arsenic trioxide?

REFERENCES

American Association of Cereal Chemists (AACC). 1983. *Approved Methods of the AACC.* St. Paul, MN: AACC.

Anonymous. 1999. *AflaTest Instruction Manual GN-MC9508-5.* Watertown, MA: VICAM.

Association of Official Analytical Chemists (AOAC). 2005. *Official Methods of Analysis of AOAC International*, edited by W. Horwitz and G. W. Latimer. 18th ed. Arlington, VA: AOAC.

Baur, F. J. 1992. *Insect Management for Food Storage and Processing.* 4th ed. St. Paul, MN: The American Association of Cereal Chemists.

Bell, L. N., and T. P. Labuza. 2000. *Moisture Sorption. Practical Aspects of Isotherm Measurement and Use.* 2nd ed. St. Paul, MN: Eagan Press.

Bulla, L. A., K. J. Kramer, and R. D. Speirs. 1977. "Insects and Microorganisms in Stored Grain and Their Control." In *Advances in Cereal Science and Technology*, edited by Y. Pomeranz. Vol. II. St. Paul, MN: American Association of Cereal Chemists.

Desjardins, A. E. 2006. *Fusarium Mycotoxins. Chemistry, Genetics and Biology.* St. Paul, MN: American Phytopathological Society.

Dobie, P., C. P. Haines, R. J. Hodges, and P. J. Prevett. 1984. *Insects and Arachnids of Tropical Stored Products: Their Biology and Identification.* London, UK: Storage Department, Tropical Development and Research Institute.

Dowell, F. E., J. E. Throne, D. Wang, and J. E. Baker. 1999. "Identifying Stored-Grain Insects Using Near-Infrared Spectroscopy." *Journal of Economic Entomology* 92(1):165–169.

Freeman, P. 1980. *Common Insect Pests of Stored Food Products. A Guide to Their Identification.* 6th ed. London, UK: Buttler Tanner.

Harris, K. L., and F. J. Bauer. 1982. "Rodents." In *Storage of Cereal Grains and Their Products*, edited by C. Christensen. 3rd ed. St. Paul, MN: American Association of Cereal Chemists.

Krogh, P. 1987. *Mycotoxins in Foods. Food Science and Technology. A Series of Monographs.* San Diego, CA: Academic Press.

McFarlane, J. A., A. E. John, and R. C. Marder. 1995. "Storage of Sorghum and Millets: Including Drying for Storage, with Particular Reference to Tropical Areas and the Mycotoxin Problem." In *Sorghum and Millets: Chemistry and Technology*, edited by D. A. V. Dendy. St. Paul, MN: American Association of Cereal Chemists.

Miller, J. D. and H. L. Trenholm. 1994. *Mycotoxins in Grain. Compounds Other Than Aflatoxins.* St. Paul, MN: Eagan Press.

Mirocha, C. J., S. V. Pathre, and C. M. Christensen. 1980. "Mycotoxins." In *Advances of Cereal Science and Technology*, edited by Y. Pomeranz. Vol. III. St. Paul, MN: American Association of Cereal Chemists.

Nelson, P. E., T. A. Toussoun, and W. F. D. Marasas. 1983. *Fusarium Species. An Illustrated Manual for Identification.* University Park, PA: Pennsylvania State University Press.

Pedersen, J. R. 2003. "Analysis of Extraneous Material." In *Food Analysis*, edited by S. S. Nielsen, 3rd ed., 339–350. New York: Kluwer Academic.

Pitt, J. I. 1979. *The Genus Penicillium and its Teleomorphic States Eupenicillium and Talaromyces.* London, UK: Academic Press.

Raper, K. B. and D. I. Fenell. 1965. *The Genus Aspergillus.* Baltimore, MD: Williams & Wilkins, Co.

Rockland, B. L. 1960. "Saturated Salt Solutions for Static Control of Relative Humidity between 5° and 40°C." *Analytical Chemistry* 32:1375–1376.

Rooney, L. W. 2007. *Corn Quality Assurance Manual.* 2nd ed. Arlington, VA: Snack Food Association.

Sauer, D. B. 1992. *Storage of Cereal Grains and Their Products.* 4th ed. St. Paul, MN: American Association of Cereal Chemists.

U.S. Department of Agriculture (USDA). 1980. *Stored-Grain Insects.* Agriculture Handbook 500. Washington, DC: USDA.

U.S. Department of Agriculture Grain Inspection, Packers and Stockyards Administration (USDA-GIPSA). 2011. *Principal Stored Grain Insects.* Kansas City, MO: USDA-GIPSA, National Grain Center.

Van Rensburg, S. J., and B. Altenkirk. 1974. "*Claviceps purpurea*—Ergotism." In *Mycotoxins*, edited by I. F. H. Purchase, 69–96. Amsterdam, Netherlands: Elsevier.

5 Dry-Milling Processes and Quality of Dry-Milled Products

5.1 INTRODUCTION

The various types of milling systems are aimed toward the production of refined products such as decorticated kernels, grits, semolina, and flours which are further processed into an array of prepared foods. These industries break away the anatomical parts of kernels with the purpose of obtaining the starchy endosperm as whole, grits, or flour. The industry also produces coproducts such as glumes, brans, germ, and low-grade products. In general terms, the dry-milling industry is divided into four major segments: (1) traditional milling systems that yield semirefined products; (2) decortication and polishing for the production of white rice, pearled barley and oats, and decorticated sorghum or millets; (3) roller milling for the production of semolina and an array of wheat and small-grain flours; and (4) degerming-tempering systems for the production of an assortment of maize grits.

Quality control for dry-milling industries is divided into two major types: value of cereals used as raw materials (refer to Chapters 1 and 2) and quality of refined milled fractions such as grits, semolina, and flours. The parameters usually checked in incoming lots of grains are moisture, test weight, dockage or foreign material, broken kernels, damaged kernels, endosperm texture, hardness, thousand kernel weight, and the presence of mycotoxins (Chapter 1). For dry-milled fractions, the most relevant chemical tests are ash, fat, fiber, protein, and starch contents (Chapter 2), whereas the most important physical tests are particle size distribution and color (Chapter 3). Many millers also adopt functional assays. For wheat, protein, starch damage (falling number), and dough rheological properties are usually assessed. For wheat millers, protein content, gluten functionality, and dough rheological properties are of upmost importance.

5.2 LABORATORY DRY-MILLING PROCESSES

The most important objective of the various dry-milling industries is to obtain the maximum yields of refined products that meet quality control expectations and functionality. There are several laboratory and pilot plant milling equipments and procedures that try to imitate commercial processes.

Plant breeders, food technologists, and dry millers have several options available to obtain decorticated kernels, refined grits, flours, or semolina from a relatively small sample of cereal grains. The equipments and protocols are aimed toward the production of similar products as those obtained by commercial milling operations.

5.2.1 DRY-MILLING OF MAIZE—PRODUCTION OF REFINED GRITS AND FLOUR

The most popular dry-milling system for maize is known as tempering–degerming. This milling process involves adding water to the maize kernels to later facilitate the removal of the germ and pericarp tissues. The goal is to produce the maximum percentage of refined grits containing minimum fat, fiber, and specks from the tip cap, and to recover the maximum percentage of clean germ with maximum oil content and largest particle size. Degerming is the most critical step for efficient maize dry-milling. The industry generally uses Beall, impact or entoleter, disc, and other types of impact degerminators. These equipments should release the germ and pericarp from the endosperm to yield grits and finer fractions low in fiber, fat, and ash contents.

Even though there are no commercially specialized maize dry-milling laboratory equipment, some research centers use tempering devices, degerminators, roller mills, and sieves to predict yields of refined products and coproducts. Generally, maize is initially conditioned to 24% moisture before degerming in an experimental horizontal drum equipped with a steel screen with 7.9-mm-diameter round holes. The resulting stock is dried, classified, and air-aspirated to remove fiber and germ. The endosperm pieces are further reduced in particle size by passing through various sets of corrugated rolls and classified/sized with sieves again. The yield of the various dry-milled fractions and by-products is calculated based on the original grain weight (Duensing 2003; Peplinski et al. 1984).

5.2.1.1 Degerming–Tempering Milling of Maize

A. *Samples, Materials, and Reagents*
- Different lots of maize samples
- Distilled water

B. *Materials and Equipment*
- Digital scale
- Spatula
- Clipper or Carter dockage meter
- Graduated cylinder (100 mL)
- Desiccator
- Impact mill
- Drying pans
- Air aspiration system
- Roller mill
- Collection pan for Rotap sieves
- Aluminum dishes
- Udy or laboratory mill

- Tempering device or bottles with lids
- Laboratory tongs
- Experimental horizontal drum degerminator
- Air-forced convection oven
- Chronometer
- Gravity separator
- Rotap (U.S. nos. 6, 10, 40, 60, 80, and 100 sieves)
- Sieve cleaners

C. Procedure

1. Obtain a representative maize sample making sure to determine test weight, 1000 kernel weight, and grain damage (refer to Chapter 1). Clean the grain sample, preferably by using the clipper or Carter dockage test meter. Determine the percentage of extraneous material and moisture content (refer to procedure in Section 2.2.1.1).
2. Weigh the predetermined maize sample. Place sample in the container of the tempering device or in glass or plastic bottles with lids. Calculate the amount of water necessary to increase grain moisture content to 24%.

Amount of tempering water (mL) = [(100 − initial grain moisture)/(100 − 24%)] − 1 × amount of grain (g).

3. Place the maize sample in the tempering device or bottle and add the predetermined amount of tempering water. Place the lid of the container and manually shake contents to promote water distribution. If a tempering device is used, place the container and turn on the apparatus that mechanically shakes the sample. If the tempering is done manually, make sure to shake contents for at least 10 minutes or until no free water is observed. Allow the conditioned maize to temper at room temperature for 3 hours.
4. Remove maize sample from tempering device. Preferably, degerm the tempered maize kernels in an experimental horizontal drum equipped with a steel screen with 7.9 mm diameter round holes. Alternatively, mill sample into coarse fractions to separate the germ and pericarp from the endosperm. Determine the exact weight of the ground sample. After milling, spread ground maize in a container for drying at 60°C. Calculate the milled maize weight adjusted to 14% moisture. For instance, if you are milling 1000 g of 24% moisture grain, the weight of 14% moisture-based maize should be 883.7 g [(1000 − 240)/(100 − 14) × 100]. Dry the sample until the moisture content has decreased to 14%.
5. Allow sample to equilibrate to room temperature for 30 minutes. Then, place sample in an air aspirator and adjust air velocity to remove the pericarp. Record the exact weight of the bran or pericarp and its moisture and chemical composition (mainly ash and fiber contents).

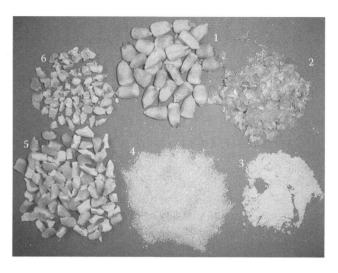

FIGURE 5.1 Dry-milled fractions of maize (clockwise: 1, whole maize; 2, bran; 3, meal; 4, brewing grits; 5, flaking grits; 6, germ).

6. Separate the germ from the endosperm pieces using a gravity separator. If it is not available, then use sieves and visually sort germ pieces. Record the exact weight of the germ and its moisture and chemical composition (mainly fat content).
7. In a rotap furnished with U.S. nos. 6, 10, 40, 60, 80, and 100 sieves and the collection pan, sift the endosperm pieces for at least 5 minutes. Make sure to include at least one sieve cleaner per sieve. After rotaping, collect and weigh each fraction. Determine yields of no. 6 (flaking), no. 10 (coarse), no. 40 (medium brewing), and no. 60 (fine brewing) grits, corn meal (−60 to +80), and corn flour (−80 to −100; Figure 5.1).
8. If finer fractions are desired, reduce, once or in several steps, the particle size of coarse particles with a roller mill. Alternatively, a hammer mill can be used but it will create heat and more starch damage. Sift the resulting particles using the rotap and select the desired particles.
9. Determine the moisture content, chemical composition (protein, starch, ash, fat, and fiber), color, starch damage, and functional properties of the dry-milled fractions (refer to Chapters 2 and 3).

5.2.2 DRY-MILLING OF WHEAT—PRODUCTION OF REFINED FLOURS AND SEMOLINA

Most wheat is commercially milled into flour or semolina using the conditioning-roller milling process. The aim of dry millers is to obtain the maximum flour yield when soft and hard wheats are milled or semolina when durum wheat is milled. The coproducts of these industries are bran, shorts, and germ (Posner and Hibbs 1997). Conventional milling consists of cleaning, tempering, roller milling, and particle separation to obtain refined products and coproducts. Tempering is key because this is needed for a more efficient bran separation, to soften the endosperm enhancing its gradual reduction in particle size, and to improve the sieving efficiency. The different classes of wheat are tempered for different times and final moisture contents. Generally, hard wheats are conditioned to 16.5% moisture for 12 to 24 hours, whereas soft wheats are conditioned to 15% to 15.5% moisture for 5 to 15 hours. On the other hand, durum or pasta wheats require 17% to 17.5% moisture and tempering times of 12 to 24 hours.

Milling is accomplished in two types of roller mills: break and reduction rollers. These mills consist of pairs of horizontal, parallel iron cylinders rotating in opposite directions. They pull the stock down between the rolls into the nip, which is considered the grinding zone. The aim of the break roll system, consisting of corrugated rolls, is to open the wheat kernel and remove the endosperm and germ from the pericarp with the least amount of contamination and obtain a particle size distribution of maximum large middlings with a minimum of flour. The bran should be detached from the kernel in flakes and without any adhered endosperm. The two most common ways to separate stocks from the break and reduction rolls are the plansifter and purifiers. The break material is usually classified into bran (U.S. mesh +35), sizings (U.S. mesh +70), middlings (U.S. mesh +100), and flour (U.S. mesh −100). Sizings and middlings are further milled in reduction rolls consisting of smooth rolls that generally rotate with a small or inexistent speed differential. The objective of these mills is to gradually reduce these fractions into flour, minimizing starch damage. These mills operate with an integrated particle classification system that segregates flours that meet the desired granulation (U.S. mesh −100) and coarser particles that are further milled (Posner and Hibbs 1997). The term extraction rate, commonly used by millers, refers to the amount of flour produced from a given amount of wheat. Generally, the extraction rate varies from 72% to 78%.

Several experimental mills capable of processing from 100 g to 2 kg of wheat are commercially available. These mills are designed to grind tempered wheat with corrugated and smooth rolls, with the subsequent separation of the various mill fractions by sifting. The extraction rate can be obtained after weighing milled fractions and coproducts (bran and shorts). The most common commercial mills are the Quadrumat Jr., Quadrumat Sr. (from Brabender, Co., Duisburg, Germany), and the Chopin Experimental Mill (Villeneuve, France), which are capable of processing wheat samples of 50 g to 100 g, 1 kg or more, and 250 g, respectively. There are larger mills such as the Semiautomatic Experimental Buhler (American Association of Cereal Chemists (AACC), Method 26-20; AACC 2000) and the Allis Chalmers. The refined flours and semolinas obtained can be further analyzed in terms of chemical composition, rheological properties, and functionality (baking and pasta tests, spread factor, etc.). The same equipment with slightly different protocols can be used to mill rye and triticale into flours.

5.2.2.1 Dry-Milling of Wheat for the Production of Refined Flours (Method 26-10)

This method was previously described in AACC (2000).

A. *Samples, Ingredients, and Reagents*
- Different samples of soft and hard wheats
- Distilled water
- Dessicant (activated alumina)

B. *Materials and Equipment*
- Digital scale
- Single-drum tempering device
- Experimental Chopin mill
- Quadrumat Sr. or Jr. Brabender mills
- Buhler mill
- Tempering device or bottles with lids
- Scale
- Airtight dessicator
- Aluminum dishes
- Thongs
- Laboratory Udy mill
- Spatula
- Graduated cylinder (100 mL)
- Air-forced convection oven
- Rotap (U.S. nos. 35, 60, and 100 sieves)
- Rotap collector pan
- Rotating sifter with a U.S. 100-mesh sieve
- Sieve cleaners

C. *Procedure*
1. Obtain a representative grain sample, making sure to determine grade and class (refer to Chapter 1). Clean the grain sample, preferably by using a clipper or Carter dockage test meter. Determine the percentage of foreign material and moisture content (refer to procedure in Section 2.2.1.1).
2. Weigh the predetermined wheat sample with an accuracy of 0.1 g.
3. Temper the grain according to its class:
   a. Soft wheats: 15% to 15.5% moisture for 12 to 15 hours.
   b. Hard wheats: 16% to 16.5% moisture for 16 to 24 hours.
   c. Durum wheats: 16.5% to 17% moisture for 16 to 24 hours.
   Use the following equation:

$$\{[(100 - \% \text{ original moisture})/(100 - \% \text{ desired conditioning moisture})] - 1]\} \times \text{amount of wheat to temper}.$$

4. Place the wheat sample in the tempering device or bottle and add the predetermined amount of conditioning water. Place the lid of the container and manually shake contents to promote water distribution. If a tempering device is used, place the container and turn on the apparatus that mechanically shakes the sample. If the tempering is manually done, make sure to shake contents

for at least 10 minutes or until no free water is observed. Allow the tempered wheat to temper at room temperature for the predetermined time.

Milling Procedure Using the Experimental Chopin Mill

See Figure 5.2.

1. Weigh the predetermined amount of tempered wheat (i.e., 300 g) and gradually grind it through the break rolls. Recuperate the resulting three milling fractions: break flour that passed the U.S. 100-mesh sieve, middlings and shorts that passed the U.S. 35-mesh sieve, and bran that was retained by the U.S. 35-mesh sieve. Alternatively, the bran can be reground and sifted again to recuperate the attached endosperm. Weigh each of the three fractions with an accuracy of 0.1 g.

2. Grind the middlings/shorts fraction at least six times through the reduction rolls. After each pass, make sure to separate the two resulting fractions: reduction flour that passed the U.S. 100-mesh sieve and the reground middlings that did not pass the U.S. 100-mesh sieve. Weigh the two fractions and regrind only the milling fraction that has not achieved the proper granulation. After the sixth pass, weigh and determine yield of shorts/red dog that did not meet granulation. Blend all break and reduction flours and estimate yield or extraction rate with the following equation:

$$\text{Extraction rate} = (\text{refined flour weight/original grain weight}) \times 100.$$

3. Build a table indicating yields of flour as the wheat is progressively milled. Break, first reduction, second reduction, third reduction, etc.

4. Determine the moisture content, chemical composition (protein, starch, ash, fat, and fiber),

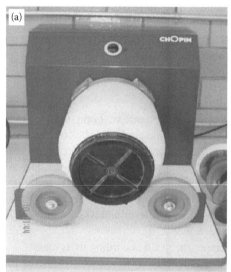
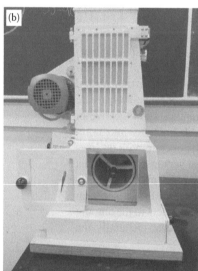
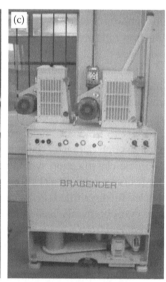
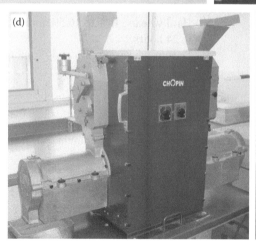
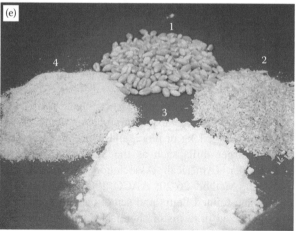

FIGURE 5.2 Laboratory and experimental equipments for the production of refined wheat flour. (a) Tempering device; (b) Quadrumat Jr. Mill; (c) Quadrumat Sr. Mill; (d) Chopin Experimental Mill; (e) wheat dry-milling fractions (clockwise: 1, whole wheat; 2, bran; 3, refined flour; 4, shorts).

color, starch damage, and functional properties (falling number, dough rheological properties, and viscoamylograph) of samples of break, reduction, and straight grade flours.

Milling Procedure Using the Quadrumat Jr. Mill

See Figure 5.2.

1. Weigh the predetermined amount of tempered wheat (i.e., 100 g) and grind it through the Quadrumat Jr. Mill. Recuperate the ground wheat and place it on top of a set of sieves (35, 60, 100, and bottom collection pan) for 5 minutes of rotaping. Separate the milled fractions into bran (+35), middlings (U.S. +60 and 100 mesh), and break flour (U.S. −100 mesh sieve or material collected at the bottom of the pan). Weigh each of the four fractions with an accuracy of 0.1 g. Separate the bran and break flour.
2. Grind the middlings/shorts fraction at least two times through the Quadrumat Jr. reduction rolls and then separate the reduction flour form the shorts/red dog in a rotating U.S. 100-mesh sieve furnished with at least one sieve cleaner. Weigh the two fractions. Blend the break and reduction flours and estimate yield or extraction rate with the following equation:

$$\text{Extraction rate} = (\text{refined flour weight}/\text{original grain weight}) \times 100.$$

3. Determine the moisture content, chemical composition (protein, starch, ash, fat, and fiber), color, starch damage, and functional properties (falling number, dough rheological properties, and viscoamylograph) of samples of break, reduction, and straight grade flours.

Milling Procedure Using the Quadrumat Sr. Mill

See Figure 5.2.

1. Weigh the predetermined amount of tempered wheat (i.e., 1000 g) and grind it through the break and reduction rolls of the Quadrumat Sr. Mill. Make sure to properly adjust wheat feed rate to optimize milling and sifting. The whole milling operation is automated. Recuperate the resulting milling fractions: flour, shorts, and bran. Weigh each of the three fractions with an accuracy of 0.1 g.
2. Calculate extraction rate using the following equation:

$$\text{Extraction rate} = (\text{refined flour weight}/\text{original grain weight}) \times 100.$$

3. Determine the moisture content, chemical composition (protein, starch, ash, fat, and fiber),

color, starch damage, and functional properties (falling number, dough rheological properties, and viscoamylograph) of flours.

Milling Procedure Using the Buhler Roller Mill

1. Weigh the predetermined amount of tempered wheat (i.e., 1–3 kg) and grind it through the break and reduction rolls of the Buhler Roller Mill. Make sure to properly adjust wheat feed rate to optimize milling and sifting. The whole milling operation is automated. Recuperate the resulting milling fractions: flour, shorts, and bran. Weigh each of the three fractions with an accuracy of 0.1 g.
2. Calculate extraction rate using the following equation:

$$\text{Extraction rate} = (\text{refined flour weight}/\text{original grain weight}) \times 100.$$

3. Determine the moisture content, chemical composition (protein, starch, ash, fat, and fiber), color, starch damage, and functional properties (falling number, dough rheological properties, and viscoamylograph) of the refined wheat flour.

5.2.3 Dry-Milling of Rice—Production of Regular and Parboiled White Rice

Rice is the most important staple food for Asians. Most of the crop is dry-milled into white kernels that are free from glumes, pericarp, germ, and aleurone. The milling process that converts paddy into white rice basically consists of six sequential operations: drying, grain cleaning, dehulling, decortication, polishing, and sizing. First, the moist paddy rice is dried in preparation for dehulling. Paddy rice is dehulled to selectively remove the glumes or husks, yielding brown rice. During this operation, approximately 20% of the paddy rice weight is lost. Then, the brown rice is abrasively decorticated to remove pericarp, germ, and the outer endosperm that contains the multilayered aleurone. Finally, the white rice is sized into head, second head, and broken pieces. The yield of head white rice is affected by the grain's physical properties and drying. Vitreous or hard kernels yield higher amounts of head rice. Drying should be aimed at minimizing the formation of stress cracks or fissures. Commercially, the maximum expected yield of head rice is 65% (Juliano 1985).

Approximately 15% of the world rice is parboiled before milling. Parboiling is defined as a hydrothermal process applied to rough rice to improve milling yield especially when low-quality rices are parboiled. There are many types of parboiling methods; however, the key sequential operations are conditioning, heating, and drying. The rough rice is usually tempered to 30% to 35% moisture and then subjected to a thermal treatment for short periods of time (2–5 minutes). During these operations, the starch gelatinizes and acts as glue, sealing microfissures or stress cracks. Finally, the parboiled rough rice is dehydrated to decrease the moisture to approximately 13% to 14%. Parboiling modifies the appearance and culinary properties of the milled rice and its physical, chemical, and nutritional characteristics. Upon parboiling, kernels become somewhat glassy, translucent, and slightly discolored (light yellow or amber). The harder kernels are also less susceptible to insects and more stable during storage. However, parboiled rough rice loses its viability or germination capacity. Parboiled milled rice has different cooking quality and textural properties because of its lower cooking water uptake. Cooked parboiled rice retains its shape, is firmer, fluffier, and less sticky compared with regular rice (Juliano 1985).

Laboratory milling equipment for rice consists of a dehuller and an abrasive decorticator that removes the husks and abrades brown rice to obtain white rice. The white rice, second heads, and broken kernels are removed by sifting. The most broadly used laboratory mills are the shellers and whiteners from McGill and Satake, which only require small samples of rough rice (125–200 g). These laboratory tests highly correlate with commercial milling yields.

5.2.3.1 Milling of Rice

A. *Samples, Ingredients, and Reagents*
- Different samples of short, medium, and long rough or paddy rices

B. *Materials and Equipment*
- Digital scale
- Boerner divider
- Carter dockage test meter or clipper
- McGill dehuller or testing husker (THU 35A)
- McGill rice decorticator or testing mill
- Rice classification system or testing grader

C. *Procedure*
1. Obtain a representative of the rough rice sample. If sample is too big, divide using the Boerner divider. Determine grade and class according to the methods described in Chapter 1.
2. Clean the grain sample using the clipper, Carter dockage tester, or sieves. Record the amount of foreign material expressed on the original sample weight.
3. Place the rough rice sample on the hopper that feeds the dehuller or husker (Figure 5.3). Make sure the aspiration system is properly calibrated. Pass the sample through the dehuller and collect the hulls, brown rice, and rough rice. Manually

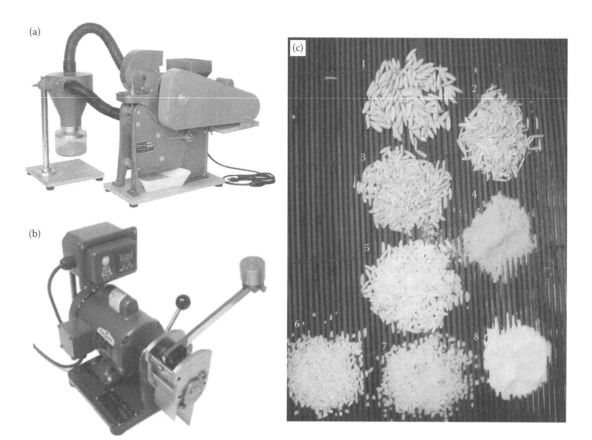

FIGURE 5.3 Laboratory milling equipment for rice. (a) rice sheller; (b) rice miller; (c) rough rice milling fractions (1, rough rice; 2, husks or glumes; 3, brown rice; 4, rice bran; 5, white rice; 6, second head rice; 7, broken rice; 8, rice flour).

sort red or pink-colored kernels. Weigh each fraction with an accuracy of 0.1 g.

4. Pass the unhulled rough rice again through the McGill dehulling device and repeat step 3.

5. Place brown rice, including colored kernels, in the McGill decorticator and polishing machine or testing mill. Decorticate kernels for 30 to 40 seconds. Some experimental milling equipment have adjustment controls that vary according to the physical properties of the brown rice sample. For instance, harder kernels require more pressure compared with their softer counterparts.

6. Collect and weigh milled kernels and bran.

7. Classify and separate the different white rice fractions with a set of sieves (cylindrical testing grader or regular sieves). It is recommended to classify milled rice into head, second head, and broken rice (Figure 5.3). Record the exact weight of each milled sample.

8. Calculate yields of head, second head, brokens, bran, and hulls based on the original cleaned and uncleaned rough rice weight. If colored kernels were present in the rice sample, estimate the amount and also express it in terms of yield.

9. Determine the proximate composition of the paddy, brown, and white rices and the coproducts (glumes or husks and bran). For white rice, determine color, amylose/amylopectin ratio, and functional properties (cooking quality) including the May–Gruenwald dyeing procedure (refer to procedure in Section 5.3.2.1).

5.2.3.2 Dry-Milling of Parboiled Rice

Parboiling is defined as a hydrothermal process applied to rough rice to achieve high milling yields (Amato and Silveira 1991; Battacharya 1985). The advantages of this process were accidentally found many centuries ago in India. Parboiling brings clear benefits in terms of head rice yields especially when low-quality rices are parboiled. However, parboiling is only practiced in approximately 15% of the rice produced worldwide because it demands energy, additional equipment, and labor. There are many types of parboiling methods (Amato and Silveira 1991); however, the operation consists of three basic sequential steps: conditioning, heating, and drying. The rough rice is usually tempered to 30% to 35% moisture to enhance starch gelatinization during the following thermal process. The conditioned and drained kernels are normally subjected to a thermal treatment that could be wet or direct steam (conventional or pressure cooked) or dried (hot air treatment) for short periods of exposure time (2–5 minutes). During these operations, the gelatinized starch acts as a glue, sealing microfissures or stress cracks. Then, the parboiled kernels are dehydrated to decrease the moisture to approximately 13% to 14%. Parboiling modifies the appearance and culinary properties of the milled rice and its physical, chemical, and nutritional characteristics. Milled kernels are slightly shorter and broader than milled raw rice. Upon parboiling, kernels become somewhat glassy, translucent, and slightly discolored (light yellow or amber). One of the most notorious effects of parboiling is grain hardening and the retention of higher amounts of essential minerals and B vitamins. This is due to the leaching of these nutrients located in the aleurone cells to the inner part of the starchy endosperm. The harder kernels are also less susceptible to insects and more stable during storage. Parboiled milled rice has different cooking qualities and textural properties because of its lower cooking water uptake. Cooked parboiled rice retains its shape, is firmer, fluffier, and less sticky compared with regular rice. In addition, parboiled rice loses fewer solids into the cooking water (Battacharya 1985).

A. *Samples, Ingredients, and Reagents*
- Different samples of short, medium and long, rough, or paddy rices
- Distilled water

B. *Materials and Equipment*
- Digital scale
- Boerner divider
- Carter dockage test meter or clipper
- McGill dehuller or testing husker (THU 35A)
- McGill rice decorticator or testing mill
- Rice classification system or testing grader
- Beakers (1 L capacity)
- Graduated cylinder (500 mL)
- Colander
- Hot plate or stove
- Air-forced oven with temperature controls
- Pans for drying
- Thermometer
- Desiccators
- Aluminum dishes
- Laboratory tweezers

C. *Procedure*
1. Obtain a representative rough rice sample. If sample is too big, divide using the Boerner divider. Determine moisture, grade, and class according to the methods described in Chapter 1.

2. Clean the paddy rice sample using the clipper, Carter dockage tester, or sieves. Register the amount of foreign material expressed on original sample weight.

3. Weigh two different lots of exactly 250 g of cleaned rough rice and place it in 1-L beakers. One lot will serve for sampling and the other to determine yield. Add exactly 750 mL of water at room temperature and soak kernels for 3 hours. Determine moisture contents of samples obtained from the sampling beakers after 15, 30, 60, 120, and 180 minutes of soaking.

4. After soaking, remove excess water and obtain wet grains by pouring contents into a colander.

5. Bring to the boil two different beakers containing 750 mL of water. Add soaked rice samples to the beakers for 5 minutes of cooking. Sample

grains from the sampling beakers at exactly 1, 2, 3, 4, and 5 minutes for moisture analysis.

6. Immediately after cooking, remove excess water and obtain parboiled grains by pouring contents into a colander. Pour running water onto the grains for 10 seconds to cool down. Next, allow excess water to drain and place parboiled kernels on pans for drying. Make sure to distribute grains in such a way to promote homogenous drying.

7. Place pans in an air-forced dryer set at 38°C. Sample aliquots of the drying grain of the sampling pan after 10, 20, 60, 120, 180, and 240 minutes for moisture determination. After drying, make sure to place samples inside sealed plastic bags to prevent moisture gain or loss.

8. Determine optimum soaking, cooking, and drying times, considering that soaked and cooked grains should contain 32% to 35% moisture, whereas dried parboiled rice should have a moisture content of 12%. If necessary, repeat the procedure with the optimized parboiling conditions.

9. Allow dry parboiled grains to equilibrate at room temperature for at least 1 hour. Then, weigh a predetermined amount of parboiled rough rice in preparation for milling.

10. Mill the unparboiled and parboiled samples following the steps described previously. Calculate and compare yields of milled white rice, brokens, and by-products. Compare the physical, chemical, and functional properties of the regular and parboiled white rice samples.

5.2.4 DRY-MILLING OF OATS—PRODUCTION OF GROATS, MEALS, AND FLOURS

The main goal of the oats milling process is the removal of glumes or husks to obtain the maximum yield of groats and produce a final product with maximum shelf-life and sensory properties. The end market of groats and derived products has strict tolerance levels in terms of foreign material and husks. Millers have a strict screening process along every step of the milling procedure with regular sampling points for enhanced quality control. There are four basic sequential steps in the milling process: cleaning and grading, steaming, dehulling, and groat classification. Heat treatment can be applied to whole oats before dehulling or to the dehulled groats. Groats are usually rolled or flaked as whole or in large pieces. Steaming is key because it is aimed toward the deactivation of enzymes, mainly lipases that would otherwise produce rancidity. Steamed groats are usually heat-treated to enhance the development of flavors. The oat grain quality greatly affects yields and quality of end products.

The laboratory milling procedure of oats emulates commercial operations. Oats are cleaned, heat-treated, and dehulled to obtain stabilized groats. The groats can be further laminated or reduced into a meal or flour using roller mills.

5.2.4.1 Dry-Milling of Oats

This procedure was previously described in Doehlert and Moore (1997), Doehlert et al. (1999), and Doehlert and McMullen (2000).

A. Samples, Ingredients, and Reagents
- Different lots of whole oats

B. Materials and Equipment
- Digital scale
- Convection oven
- Boerner divider
- Clipper or Carter dockage tester with oat sieves
- Air aspirator system
- Drying pans
- Steamer with a metal wire basket
- Laboratory oat huller
- Roller mill
- 35 Mesh sieve with collection pan
- Groat cutting machine
- Flaking rolls
- Chronometer
- Caliper
- Ruler

C. Procedure
1. Weigh a representative sample of whole oats. If sample is too large, divide it using the Boerner divider. Determine moisture content of the oats before milling and determine grade and class according to the methods described in Chapter 1.

2. Clean the grain sample using the clipper, Carter dockage tester, or sieves. Record the amount of foreign material (dust, stems, other seeds, and broken kernels) that are unsuitable for milling.

3. Place the clean lot of oats in a convection oven set at 75°C to decrease the oat moisture content to 7% to 8.5%. Estimate the required drying time by simply weighing the oats while drying. For instance, if 1000 g of cleaned oats with 13% moisture content (870 g dry weight) is placed in the oven to decrease its moisture to 8%, the sample should weigh 946 g {[870/(100 − 8)] × 100}. Generally, the drying time is between 60 and 90 minutes. After drying, allow the sample to equilibrate to room temperature for at least 30 minutes.

4. Place the sample in the hopper of the dehulling machine (Figure 5.4). Turn on dehuller and slowly pass the sample. If the dehuller has a calibration system, adjust it to minimize the amount of broken groats and maximize the removal of hulls.

5. After dehulling, separate the hulls from the groats by air aspiration. Make sure to calibrate the air speed to aspirate the hulls. Determine the hullability by weighing the amount of groats obtained from the original oat sample. Calculate the yield of hulls and groats.

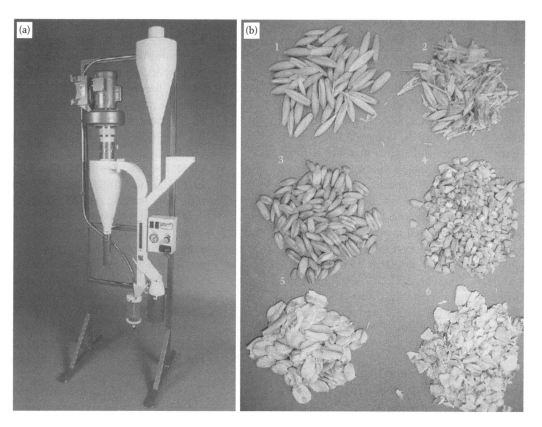

FIGURE 5.4 Laboratory milling procedure for oats. (a) Oat dehuller; (b) milling fractions of oats (1, oats; 2, hulls; 3, groats; 4, cut groats; 5, rolled groats; 6, flaked groats).

6. Place groats in a steamer for heat treatment for 30 minutes. This thermal treatment is aimed toward the inactivation of endogenous lipases and to prepare kernels for rolling. Calculate the yield of steam-treated groats and reserve a sample for moisture content determination.

7. If rolled oats are desired, first allow groats to equilibrate at room temperature and then flake them through the set of flaking rolls. Using a caliper, measure the average thickness and dimensions (length and width) of at least 10 randomly selected flakes.

8. If groats or oatmeal/flour is desired, skip step 7 and place steamed groats on perforated pan for 30 minutes toasting in a convection oven set at 140°C to 150°C. During the dry heat treatment, make sure to stir contents at least three times (every 10 minutes).

9. Calculate the yield of heat-treated groats and reserve a sample for moisture content determination.

10. Alternatively, the groats can be roller-milled into a whole or refined meal or flour. For refined groat flour production, remove bran using a 35-mesh sieve. Calculate the yield of bran (overs of the 35 mesh sieve) and meal or flour.

11. Reserve samples for chemical, color, particle size distribution, shelf life, and sensory analyses.

5.2.5 DRY-MILLING OF SORGHUM AND MILLETS—PRODUCTION OF DECORTICATED KERNELS, GRITS, AND FLOURS

Although sorghum and millets are rarely used for the production of human foods in America and Europe, these grains are of upmost importance in some parts of Asia and most African countries. Similar to rice, these grains are, in most instances, first decorticated and then milled into grits or flours to produce the wide array of traditional foods produced daily in Africa and Asia. Basically, these kernels can be traditional or mechanically decorticated and milled. Most dehulling equipment consist of abrasive disks that gradually remove the fiber-rich outer layers by friction. Most sorghums are usually decorticated to remove 15% to 30% of the grain weight, yielding endosperm-rich pearled kernels practically free of pericarp and germ. Thus, decorticated kernels are low in pigments (phenolic compounds), fiber, fat, and minerals and rich in starch (Munck 1995; Rooney and Serna-Saldivar 2000). Similar to rice, the hard endosperm genotypes yield higher amounts of unbroken pearled kernels but need more manual or mechanical work. The size and form of grains also affect the behavior during decortication. Decorticated and partially degerminated kernels are further milled into a wide array of refined or semirefined fractions. These are used for the preparation of most traditional foods.

Traditionally, sorghum and millet meals are produced by hand-pounding using a wooden pestle and mortar. The smallest seeded millets, such as teff and fonio, are practically impossible to decorticate for the production of refined fractions. Therefore, they are ground whole for the production of full-fat meals and flours. This process is still practiced in rural households but is declining. Indian villages still use stone mills to produce a coarse meal that is used for *roti* and other traditional foods. In recent years, mechanized milling processes have been developed especially for grain sorghum. The most common is by abrasive decortication followed by the reduction of particle size via hammer or roller milling. Most commercial operations use batch type, semicontinuous, or continuous mills equipped with abrasive disks or carborundum stones to progressively remove the sorghum outer layers rich in pericarp, germ, testa, and aleurone tissues.

Sorghum is usually decorticated to remove the pericarp and part of the germ tissues and then subjected to milling. The International Development Research Center (IDRC) and tangential abrasive dehulling device (TADD) mills are good examples of laboratory equipments. The IDRC mill is equipped with a set of abrasive disks that gradually abrade the pericarp and outer layers, including the germ (Reichert 1982; Oomah and Reichert 1981).

5.2.5.1 Production of Decorticated Kernels and Refined Flours from Sorghum or Millets

A. *Samples, Ingredients, and Reagents*
- Sorghum grain samples

B. *Materials and Equipment*
- Digital scale
- Dockage test meter
- Clipper with sieves for sorghum or millet
- Laboratory air aspirator
- Boerner divider
- Mechanical dehuller

C. *Procedure*
1. Clean the lot of sorghum or millet grain, preferably using a dockage meter. Weigh the removed extraneous materials and express the quantity based on the original weight.
2. Determine the grain moisture content and physical properties (test weight, 1000 kernel weight, density, hardness, etc.).
3. Weigh a predetermined amount of grain to be decorticated. Most pilot plant dehullers (Figure 5.5) are batch and optimally decorticated 3 kg to 5 kg.
4. Place the predetermined amount of cleaned kernels in the decorticator. Start the milling operation, making sure to remove the partially decorticated sample at 1-minute intervals.
5. After each minute of decortication, remove the sample from the dehuller and clean it with the air aspirator, dockage test meter, or clipper. Obtain the different milled fractions and weigh them with a precision of 1 g. Separate the milled sample into at least three fractions: decorticated kernels, broken kernels, and bran.
6. Return all milled fractions to the dehuller and proceed to decorticate for an additional minute and repeat step 5.
7. Calculate the matter loss (removed bran and outer layers) for each minute until achieving at least 40% loss.
8. Graph percentage of decortication (y axis) vs. accumulated milling time (x axis). 100 − (decorticated kernel weight/original grain weight × 100).
9. Calculate the correlation, slope (m), Y value (b) at intersection and the regression equation ($Y = mx + b$).
10. Analyze the decorticated kernels, bran, and other milled fractions in terms of fiber, fat, starch, and ash. In addition, determine the 1000

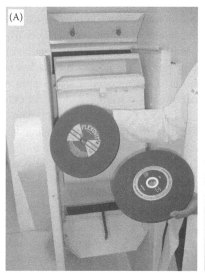
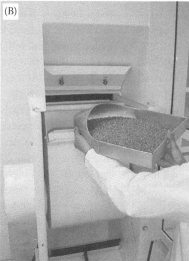
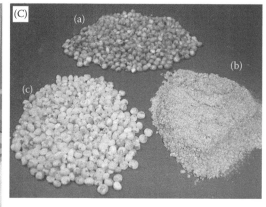

FIGURE 5.5 IDRC decorticator used for the production of pearled sorghum. (A) Decorticator showing abrasive disks; (B) sorghum decortication; (C) sorghum dry-milled fractions (a, whole sorghum; b, abraded sorghum bran; c, decorticated sorghum).

weight of decorticated kernels, color difference between whole and decorticated grains, and the May–Gruenwald dye test in the set of decorticated kernels with different extents of decortications (refer to procedure in Section 5.3.2.1).

5.2.5.2 Production of Refined Grits and Flours from Decorticated Sorghum or Millets

1. Obtain a representative sample of decorticated kernels from the procedure described above. Make sure to select kernels with the desired degree of decortication.
2. Weigh the decorticated grain sample with an accuracy of 0.1 g.
3. Mill kernels using hammer or roller mills. If a hammer mill is chosen, make sure to select the most appropriate screen because it will affect granulation. Likewise, if roller mills are selected, make sure to select the type of roller mill and properly adjust the gap between rollers.
4. Construct a set of sieves with 20 (coarse grits), 35 (medium grits), 60 (fine grits), 100 (meal), and collector pan (flour) and classify the ground sample. Make sure to weigh the original sample and the fractions. Express yields of each fraction based on the original weight. If finer granulation is desired, regrind coarser samples until the desired particle size is achieved.
5. Analyze the different milled fractions or product in terms of fiber, fat, starch, ash, and color scores.

5.2.6 Research Suggestions

1. Using the degerming-tempering (D-T) procedure, mill three different and contrasting types of maize (white regular with intermediate to hard endosperm texture, quality protein maize with soft endosperm texture, and soft-textured blue maize) and determine the yields of flaking grits, coarse grits, regular grits, fine grits, meal, and flour. Determine and compare the quality of the resulting dry-milled fractions.
2. Using the D-T procedure, mill samples of maize that have been attacked by insects, molds, or a have been sprouted (refer to procedure in Section 4.2.1.2). Determine the physical properties of the sound and damaged kernels and the yields of flaking grits, coarse grits, regular grits, fine grits, meal, and flour. Determine and compare the quality of the resulting dry-milled fractions, especially in terms of color, starch damage, insect fragments, mycotoxins, and fat oxidation (procedures in Sections 3.2.1, 4.3.2.2, 4.3.3.2, 6.4.3.1, and 2.6.2.1).
3. Using any of the roller mill laboratory or pilot plant procedures, mill three different types of wheats differing in grain size or 1000 kernel weight (i.e., 22, 28, and >32 g/1000 kernels). Determine flour extraction rate and compare the quality of the resulting flours in terms of color and dough rheological properties (procedures in Section 5.3.4).
4. Using any of the roller mill laboratory or pilot plant procedures, mill samples of the same soft wheat to produce a refined flour and a whole wheat flour supplemented with 15% bran. Determine and compare the chemical composition of the flours and color. In addition, process the wheat into cookies and compare the properties of these finished products (refer to procedure in Section 10.3).
5. Design a laboratory milling procedure to optimize the yields of refined semolina. Make sure to select the proper durum wheat and design cleaning, tempering, roller milling, and classification processes. Determine the yield and quality of the resulting semolina in terms of color, starch damage, and pasta properties (refer to procedures in Sections 11.2.1.1 or 11.2.2.2).
6. Using the laboratory rice milling procedure, mill three different and contrasting types of rough rices (long, short, and a rice with a high incidence of stress cracks). Determine the yields of head, second head, and grits. Determine and compare the quality of the head white rice in terms of color, starch composition (percentage of amylose), elongation, and cooking properties.
7. Select a sample of rough rice with a high incidence of stress cracks or fissures. Parboil half of the sample. After parboiling and drying, and using the laboratory rice milling procedure, mill the regular and parboiled rough rice into white rice. Determine the yields of head white rice, second head, and grits. Then, determine and compare the quality of the regular and parboiled white rice in terms of color, comparative chemical composition (ash, starch, protein, fat, fiber, B vitamins, and enzyme susceptible starch), viscoamylograph properties, and texture after cooking.
8. Design a laboratory procedure to obtain stabilized groats and meal or flour. Process samples at varying steaming times. Determine the yields of hulls and groats and compare the quality of the groats and ground meal in terms of color, starch, and dietary fiber contents, peroxide value, and cooking properties.
9. Using the IDRC or abrasive decorticator, mill three different and contrasting types of sorghums (hard-textured, soft-textured, and a high-tannin sorghum). Determine the optimum decortication time to remove 20% of the sorghum weight and the yield of decorticated and broken kernels. Then, determine and compare the quality of the decorticated kernels in terms of color and comparative chemical composition (ash, starch, protein, fat, fiber, phenolics, and tannins). Reserve a sample of decorticated kernels and mill it into a flour. Determine and compare the particle size distribution of resulting flours and their

quality in terms of color and comparative chemical composition (ash, starch, protein, fat, fiber, total phenolics, and tannins).

10. Select a soft sorghum or pearl millet and parboil half of the sample using the technique suggested by Young et al. (1990). After parboiling and drying, and using the IDRC or abrasive decorticator, mill the different regular and parboiled kernels. Determine the optimum decortication time to remove 20% of the kernel weight and the yield of decorticated kernels. Then, determine and compare the quality of the decorticated kernels in terms of color and comparative chemical composition (ash, starch, protein, fat, fiber, total phenolics, and enzyme-susceptible starch). Reserve a sample of decorticated kernels and mill it into a flour. Determine and compare the particle size distribution of resulting flours and their quality in terms of color and comparative chemical composition (ash, starch, protein, fat, fiber, total phenolics, and enzyme susceptible starch).

5.2.7 RESEARCH QUESTIONS

1. Define the following terms widely used in dry-milling operations:
   A. Tempering
   B. Classification
   C. Extraction rate
   D. Bran
   E. Patent flour
   F. Middlings
   G. Roller mill
   H. Gravity table
   I. Aspirator
   J. Purifier
   K. Plansifter
   L. Scalper
   M. Specks
   N. Reel
   O. Second-head rice

2. Compare maize, rice, and wheat dry-milling processes and products.

3. Why are grain-cleaning operations critical for any milling process? List at least five reasons why it is critically important to thoroughly clean grains before milling.

4. What are the physical maize grain properties that favor yield and quality of flaking grits? Why is it recommended to temper the cleaned maize kernels before degermination?

5. During maize dry-milling, an array of refined fractions are obtained. What are their particle sizes and main uses? Which of the refined dry-milled products is the most expensive? Why?

6. What is considered the most critical or important operation in rough rice dry-milling? Why?

7. In a flowchart, describe the milling steps commonly used to produce white-polished rice. How do the different rice classes and parboiling affect rice milling?

8. What is parboiling? Why is parboiling still widely practiced around the world? Why is parboiled rice considered to have more nutritional attributes compared with normal rice?

9. Why is it necessary to temper or condition wheat before dry-milling? What are the tempering and conditioning time requirements of the three major classes of wheat?

10. If you want to temper 80 tons of cleaned hard wheat with an original moisture content of 14.2% to 16.5% moisture, how much tempering water would you add?

11. What are the main differences between break and reduction roller mills in terms of equipment design and operation?

12. What are the differences between plansifters and purifiers in terms of equipment design and sorting particles with different sizes?

13. What are differences among straight grade, patent, and clear flours? How are they commercially produced?

14. What are differences between whole wheat and whole grain flours?

15. How is a chlorinated soft wheat flour (cake flour) industrially produced? What are the major effects of chlorination?

16. Why is it necessary to heat-treat oats before milling? Why do dry-millers consider oats as the most difficult cereal to process? Draw a flowchart of the oat-milling process.

17. What are the differences in chemical composition between oats and groats? Why are rolled groats considered hypocholesterolemic?

18. What kind of nutritional, nutraceutical, and chemical changes occur when whole sorghum is decorticated? What are the main traditional food uses of decorticated sorghum and flour in Africa and Asia?

19. What would happen to the tannin content of a high-tannin or type III sorghum subjected to abrasive decortication to remove 25% of its weight?

5.3 ASSESSMENT OF QUALITY OF DRY-MILLED FRACTIONS

The efficiency of the various dry-milling processes described previously is associated with the chemical, physical, and functionality changes of the dry-milled fractions. These products are chemically and physically analyzed to predict its functionality as raw materials for the production of a wide array of cereal-based end products. The quality control measurements of incoming grains or raw materials are detailed in Chapters 1 and 2, in which physical grain properties and chemical compositions are thoroughly discussed. The most common way to determine milling efficiency is by the quantification of ash (AACC 2000, Methods 08-03 and 08-12) because the degree of refining is inversely related to the mineral content. Other less important tests are the determination of fat (AACC 2000, Method 30-10) and fiber (AACC 2000, Method 32-10). This is because bran contains higher amounts of minerals, fat, and fiber compared with the starchy endosperm.

All milling processes aimed toward the production or refined flours concentrate the starch because of the selective removal of hulls, bran, germ, and aleurone layer. Thus, many different assays are commonly used to determine the chemical, physical, and functional properties of the starch fraction. There are various methods used to quantify the total starch content in foods. In most of these assays, the starch is first gelatinized and then enzymatically hydrolyzed into glucose that is colorimetrically assayed after reaction with glucose oxidase, peroxidase, and dihydrochloride o-dianasidine (refer to Chapter 2). Starch can also be quantified by the polarimetric method (AACC 2000, Method 76-20). Basically, the starch is first solubilized in an alkaline solution (mercury chloride and ethanol) that is treated with calcium chloride acidified with acetic acid and further treated with stanium chloride. The filtrated sample is polarimetrically analyzed with a sodium light beam. The ratio between amylose and amylopectin is critically important because it greatly affects starch functionality. Amylose is usually quantified by a colorimetric assay in which iodine binds with amylose to produce a blue complex that is read in a spectrophotometer, whereas amylopectin is calculated by difference. Native starch is usually quantified by birefringence; observing the amount of starch granules showing the typical Maltese cross under a microscope equipped with polarized filters (refer to procedure in Section 6.3.1.3). The analysis of mechanically or enzymatically damaged starch is based on the susceptibility of the granule to α- or β-amylases and amyloglucosidases. One accepted and quick way to determine starch damage, mainly associated with wheat flour, is the falling number assay (AACC 2000, Method 56-81B).

Starch functionality is usually assessed by the Brabender or rapid viscoamylographs, which measure the viscosity changes of starch slurries with a certain amount of solids that are subjected to a standardized and programmed temperature regime (Thomas and Atwell 1999). The amylograph curve is considered as the fingerprint of starches because it determines the initial change in viscosity related to gelatinization temperature, peak viscosity during heating, the viscosity fall after the peak (shear thinning), and viscosity changes through the cooling cycles related to retrogradation (refer to procedure in Section 6.4.1.1). Other important starch functionality tests are performed using differential scanning calorimetry. This instrument is used for the quantitative determination of starch gelatinization as an enthalpy (ΔHg) of gelatinization. The temperature at which gelatinization is initiated generally agrees with values reported from loss of birefringence measurements. In addition, the temperature needed to provide maximum starch disruption and high viscosity are in accordance with the maximum or peak viscosity development in the Brabender viscoamylograph (Zobel 1984).

Protein is one of the chemical compounds that affect functionality the most, especially in wheat products. The amount of protein is closely related to gluten, which affects optimum water absorption, dough mixing time, and dough stability. Protein is analyzed by the traditional wet-chemical Kjeldahl method (AACC 2000, Method 46-10) or the quick near-infrared analyzer (NIRA) instrument (AACC 2000, Method 39-10; see Chapter 3). The NIRA is equipped with electronic detectors that measure the amount of electromagnetic radiation that is reflected or transmitted through the sample. The sample is irradiated with light at several wavelengths, usually ranging from 400 nm to 2500 nm. The principle is that practically all organic constituents have molecular bonds that absorb certain wavelengths of infrared radiation. It is capable of scanning in the infrared spectra whole grains, whole milled or refined milling samples, and processed products. The value and reliability of the assay greatly depends on the standard curve.

The evaluation of the color of flour and other dry-milled products is important because this is related to milling efficiency and extraction rate and influences the quality of the finished products. The whiteness of wheat flours is affected by type of wheat, milling extraction rate, flour aging, and extent of oxidation of carotenoid pigments by bleaching compounds. Color is usually measured by light reflectance within the blue range of the light spectrum. The Kent Jones and Agtron color meters are the most common instruments used by the wheat industry. Hunter Lab colorimeters and NIRA analyzers have also been used for this determination. The advantage of the Hunter Lab is that it determines L, a, b, hue, and chroma parameters (Rasper and Walker 2000). The color of refined wheat flour (AACC 2000, Method 14-30) or semolina is generally performed in an Agtron colorimeter operating in the green mode (546 nm). Similar assays (AACC 2000, Methods 14-21 and 14-22) are also used to measure pasta and noodle color. For durum wheats, the rapid quantitation of carotenes is performed using a spectrophotometer or colorimeter (AACC 2000, Method 14-50).

There are many functionality tests especially devised for the various types of dry-milled fractions obtained from maize, wheat, rice, and other cereals. The rice industry commonly determines the cooking quality parameters of rice that is affected by endosperm texture, kernel size, amount and type of starch, and parboiling. There are a wide array of functionality tests used to analyze soft and hard wheat flours and semolinas obtained from the wheat milling industries. The tests are broadly subdivided into simple and dough rheological properties. The simple tests are quick assays devised to predict wheat functionality or used as screening tools especially for new hard wheat genotypes developed by plant breeding programs. The results of these assays are highly related to the gluten content and strength. The most common are the Glutomatic, Pelshenke, and sedimentation tests. The most important wheat flour functionality tests are the one that determine dough rheological properties. These assays study the rheological properties of optimally hydrated and mixed dough. They are of upmost importance because they are strongly associated with processing (optimum water absorption and mixing time) and quality of bakery products. Among the various instruments used to test dough rheological properties, most measure directly or indirectly the force or gluten strength and

the dough extensibility or elasticity. The results obtained after analyzing the graphs are used by all segments of the wheat industry. In the milling industries, these rheological tests are used to make important decisions related to blending different types of wheats for the production of certain types of flours. In addition, the instruments are used to determine the amount of dough strengtheners and other additives needed to standardize formulations (Mailhot and Patton 1988).

TABLE 5.1

Quality Control Parameters Most Commonly Used to Assess Quality of Dry-Milled Maize Products

Quality Control	Equipment, Instrument/Method	Importance
Moisture	NIRA, electric conductivity moisture meters and balances, air oven method (AACC 2000, 44-15A)	Moisture is one of the most important parameters because it affects stability during storage and affects water required for optimum conditioning.
Particle size	Rotap equipped with different sieves	The particle size determination of dry milled fractions greatly affects extrusion processes and quality of end products.
Specks	Visual determination	The amount of specks (i.e., black specks in maize grits, bran specks in flours) can negatively affect the appearance of processed products. Specks are present in dry-milled fractions due to broken sieves or the improper calibration of purifiers.
Extraneous material, filth, insect fragments, rodent hairs, and rodent excreta	(AACC 2000, Methods 28-00, 28-19, 28-40, 28-41-A, 28-50, and 28-51)	Dry milled samples are digested with diverse chemical reagents and resulting hydrolysate treated with mineral oil and other chemical compounds to separate extraneous material, insect fragments, etc. The number and types of extraneous material are viewed in a wide-field microscope.
Rodent feces	Microscope technique (AACC 2000, Method 28-50)	Dry milled samples are treated with trichloromethane and carbon tetrachloride to separate feces. Excreta fragments are viewed in a microscope.
Mycotoxins	Aflatest, fumonitest, ochratest, and other related analyses	The use of ELISA columns to selectively isolate mycotoxins followed by their quantification via fluorescence allows a quick and reliable determination of these important metabolites regulated by most regulatory agencies.
Color score	Color meters	Color of dry-milled fractions affects color of end products.
Ash content	Muffle furnace (AACC 2000, Method 08-01)	This is one of the most important parameters associated with milling efficiency. Most dry-milled products should contain less than 1% ash.
Fat content	NIRA, Goldfisch, or Soxhlet apparatus (AACC 2000, Method 30-25)	This is one of the most important parameters associated with milling efficiency. Most dry-milled products should contain less than 1% fat. The lower the fat content, the better the expansion rate in direct extrusion processes.
Starch content	NIRA, analytical determination of total starch (AACC 2000, Method 76-11)	Is the most important single component of dry milled fractions and greatly affects functionality.
Starch gelatinization	Birefringence with microscope equipped with polarized filters	Microscopic technique used to determine the relative amount of gelatinized vs. native starch granules (starch granules show a Maltese cross).
Starch damage	AACC 2000, Method 76-11 or viscoamylograph	Starch damage due to faulty storage or sprouting can be determined via hydrolysis with alpha amylase or indirectly determined by a measurement of the viscosity of slurry prepared from the ground grits or flour. The lower the viscosity, the greater the starch damage.
Starch properties	Viscoamylograph (Shuey and Tipples 1982)	One of the most important functional tests because after analyzing the viscoamylograph curve it could be determined temperature at start of gelatinization, peak viscosity, shear thinning, and set back viscosity (retrogradation). These properties greatly influence processing characteristics and quality of end-products.
Protein content	NIRA (AACC 2000, Method 39-10)	The amount of protein can be rapidly determined using an infrared analyzer that was previously calibrated with a set of standards.
	Kjeldahl methods (AACC 2000, Methods 46-10, 46-12, or 46-13)	These are the most widely analytical procedures to determine nitrogen and protein. The main disadvantage is that they take a long analysis time.
	Udy dye method (AACC 2000, Method 46-14A)	

Source: AACC (2000); Serna-Saldivar (2008); Shuey and Tipples (1982).

5.3.1 Quality of Dry-Milled Maize Fractions

Maize is milled into an assortment of dry-milled products ranging from large flaking grits (U.S. no. 3.5–6 mesh sieves) to fine flour (U.S. –100 mesh sieve). The flaking grits are pieces of endosperm almost exclusively traditionally used to manufacture cornflakes. These grits are low in fiber and contain less than 1.2% oil. Coarse and fine grits are used for the production of extruded puffs, breakfast cereals, and as a brewing adjunct for the production of European beers. These grits contain less than 1% oil. Refined maize meals and flours are used for the production of corn bread and as a key ingredient for the production of batters and breadings. The chemical composition of meals and flours are similar to grits.

Table 5.1 depicts the most common procedures to evaluate the quality of refined maize dry-milled fractions. The most relevant tests are particle size distribution, color, presence of specks, ash, fat, protein, total starch, and starch damage.

5.3.1.1 Determination of Particle Size Distribution of Dry-Milled Maize Fractions

A. Samples, Ingredients, and Reagents
- Dry-milled fractions

B. Materials and Equipment
- Digital scale
- Brush
- Rotap (sieves nos. 6, 20, 35, 60, 80, and 100)
- Rotap collection pan
- Sifting balls and triangle sieve cleaners
- Spatula

C. Procedure
1. Weigh 200 g of the dry-milled product to evaluate.
2. Prepare the nest of sieves including the bottom collection pan for rotaping. The selection of the proper sizes is critical for this test. For instance, for refined maize grits, prepare a set of sieves (U.S. nos. 6, 20, 40, 60, 80, and 100).
3. Make sure to place the lid on the first sieve and the collection pan at the bottom of the set and to include sifting balls, sifting aids, and plastic triangle cleaners on each sieve to improve particle separation (Figure 5.6).
4. Place dry-milled product on the first sieve.
5. Turn on rotap for 5 to 10 minutes. The optimum rotaping time should be determined beforehand when the separated fractions achieve constant weight (Figure 5.6).
6. Collect and weigh each fraction, including the bottom collecting pan.
7. Calculate yield of each fraction based on the original sample weight or the total weight of the collected fractions.
8. Tabulate the particle size or granulation distribution of the sample.
9. Analyze the chemical composition, starch content, and damage and color of each fraction.

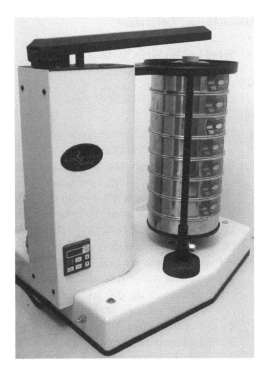

FIGURE 5.6 Rotap apparatus for determination of particle size distribution of dry-milled fractions.

5.3.2 Quality of White Rice

The aim of the rough rice milling procedure is to obtain the maximum yield of white polished rice which is used in many industrial processes. The white polished rice free of husks and pericarp is very low in fiber and, because of the removal of the germ and aleurone, contains less than 0.6% oil. The broken rice is in demand in the brewing industry and is also used for the production of extruded puffs and breakfast cereals.

The most relevant tests for rice are its cooking properties, color, total starch, and percentage of amylose. The texture and cooking properties of the different classes of rice differ because of the different ratios of amylase/amylopectin. Short rices are usually waxy (>95% amylopectin) and sticky or glutinous.

5.3.2.1 May–Gruenwald Dyeing Procedure

The efficiency of brown rice decortication or extent of pericarp removal can be determined using the May–Gruenwald dye test which dyes the pericarp green or blue when reacting with methylene blue, and the exposed endosperm pink when reacting with eosine Y. This simple test was developed by Barber and Benedicto de Barber (1976) to objectively evaluate the efficiency of the rice milling procedure.

A. Samples, Ingredients, and Reagents
- Distilled water
- Methylene blue
- Methanol
- Eosine Y

B. *Materials and Equipment*
- Scale
- Set of five beakers (500 mL)
- Plastic or wire perforated basket for rice kernels
- Dark glass bottle
- Laboratory clock

C. *Procedure*

1. Obtain a representative sample of the milled white rice (10–20 kernels).
2. Beforehand, prepare the May–Gruenwald dye solution as follows: weigh 1 g of eosine Y and 1 g of methylene blue and dilute them in 200 mL of methanol (stock solution). The May–Gruenwald stock solution should be kept in a dark glass bottle under refrigeration (5°C).
3. Prepare the work solution by mixing one part stock solution with three parts methanol.
4. Place approximately 300 mL of the work solution in a 500-mL beaker. Label this beaker as the dye beaker. Place 300 mL of pure methanol in three other beakers (label these beakers as 1, 2, 3 wash solutions). Place one empty beaker at the end of the row to serve as the drain beaker (Figure 5.7).
5. Place the representative white rice sample in the perforated wire basket for dyeing.
6. Submerge the grains in the basket in the dye beaker for 15 seconds.
7. Remove the basket from the dye solution and allow excess dye to drain. Then, place the basket in each of the methanol wash beakers in sequence for 10 seconds. Finally, place the basket in the empty beaker to allow drainage of excess methanol.
8. Place the colored sample on a light-colored surface for the subjective rating of pericarp removal and exposed starchy endosperm. The fiber-rich material associated with the pericarp and aleurone will stain blue-green, whereas the starchy endosperm will stain light pink.

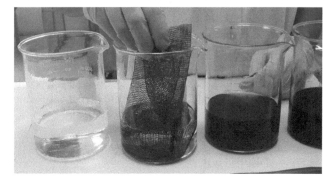

FIGURE 5.7 May–Gruenwald dyeing procedure to estimate extent of decortication or bran removal.

5.3.2.2 Analysis of Amylose in White Polished Rice

The ratio of linear amylose/branched amylopectin in rice greatly affects the cooking and organoleptic properties, especially in terms of water absorption and cooked rice texture. Basically, rice is divided into regular endosperm (25% amylose and 75% amylopectin), heterowaxy (10–20% amylose and the rest amylopectin), and waxy or glutinous (containing less than 5% amylose). The waxy rices are preferred for the production of sushi. Most large and short rices are classified as regular and waxy endosperm, respectively. Needless to say, rice breeders rely on quick measurements of amylose as one of the most important and relevant criteria for selection (Juliano 1971).

A. *Samples, Ingredients, and Reagents*
- Different white rice samples
- Amylose (potato)
- Distilled water
- Ethanol
- Sodium hydroxide (NaOH)
- Acetic acid
- Iodine solution

B. *Materials and Equipment*
- Analytical scale
- Laboratory Udy mill
- Beaker (100 mL)
- Volumetric flasks (100 mL)
- Water bath shaker
- Pipettes 1, 5, and 10 mL
- Spectrophotometer (vis)

C. *Procedure*

1. Add exactly 40 mg of potato amylose (NBC, Sigma Chemical, Co.) in a 100-mL volumetric flask. Dilute the amylose with 1 mL ethanol and 9 mL 1 N NaOH. Heat the resulting solution in a water batch set at 100°C for 10 minutes. Remove flask from the water bath and allow contents to cool down and then bring to the 100 mL mark with distilled water. Pipette 1, 2, 3, 4, and 5 mL in 100 mL volumetric flasks and add 0.2, 0.4, 0.6, 0.8, and 1.0 mL of 1 N acetic acid to each respective aliquot. Then, bring to the 100 mL volume mark with distilled water. Shake contents and then read color at 620 nm. Graph absorbance values vs. amylose concentration (dry matter). Use a dilution factor of 20. Calculate the slope of the resulting graph and its correlation factor.
2. Using the laboratory Udy mill, grind at least 25 g of polished white rice. If another mill is used, make sure to grind rice to pass the 80-mesh sieve.
3. Scale with an accuracy of 0.0001 g 60 mg of ground rice and carefully transfer to a 100-mL beaker.
4. Add 1 mL of ethanol and then 6 mL of 1 N NaOH and allow the reaction at room temperature for 12 hours.

5. Stir the sample before pippeting exactly 5 mL of the solution and transfer to another 100 mL volumetric flask. Then, add 1 mL of 1 N acetic acid and 2 mL of the iodine solution and bring to the 100 mL mark with distilled water.

6. Prepare a blank solution following the above procedure except for the addition of the rice sample.

7. After exactly 20 minutes, obtain an aliquot of the solution and determine the color (percentage of transmittance) with a spectrophotometer. The equipment should be calibrated with the blank solution to have 100% transmittance.

8. Calculate the percentage of amylose by using the standard curve of step 1.

5.3.2.3 Elongation Factor of Cooked Rice

A. Samples, Ingredients, and Reagents
- Different samples of white rice

B. Materials and Equipment
- Distilled water
- Thermometer
- Wire basket
- Beakers (500 mL)
- Hot plate or stove
- Graduated cylinders (200 mL or 500 mL)
- Ruler with millimeter scale

C. Procedure
1. Longitudinally place 10 representative milled rice kernels for the estimation of the average kernel length. Divide the number by 10 to calculate average length.

2. Place approximately 20 to 100 polished rice kernels in a wire basket for cooking.

3. In a beaker containing 300 mL of distilled water tempered at room temperature, soak the kernels contained in the wire basket for exactly 30 minutes.

4. Then, transfer the basket with the soaked kernels to a beaker containing 300 mL of boiling distilled water for exactly 10 minutes of cooking.

5. Remove basket from the boiling water and immediately quench or cool down cooked kernels by immersing the basket in a beaker containing 300 mL of distilled water at room temperature.

6. Randomly remove 10 cooked kernels and place them longitudinally for determination of the average length described in step 1.

7. Calculate cooked rice elongation by dividing the average cooked rice length by the average rice kernel length.

5.3.3 Simple Tests for Quality of Wheat Flour and Dough Properties

The relationship between milling yield and color or flour ash content is a good indicator of grain quality and the efficiency of the experimental mill. The quality of refined dry-milled fractions are usually assessed by determining particle size distribution, color, presence of specks, ash, fat, protein, and starch damage (Halverson and Zeleny 1988).

There are many simple and complex functional tests to assess the quality and characteristics of wheat flours and doughs. The range of assays includes easy and quick tests that can be performed with common laboratory glassware and detailed, complex, and time-consuming assays which require sophisticated and expensive instruments. These are mainly devised to determine the type of wheat flour (soft, hard, all purpose) and gluten quality.

These quick assays were devised to predict or screen wheat functionality, especially in new potential hard wheat genotypes being developed by plant breeders. The results of these assays differ according to the amount of gluten and gluten strength.

5.3.3.1 Pelshenke Test

The Pelshenke assay (AACC 2000, Method 56-50) is based on the formation of a dough ball with active yeast. After mixing and yeast activation, the resulting dough ball is placed in a graduated cylinder with water and a fermentation cabinet adjusted to 30°C. The time that the dough ball requires to be disrupted is related to gluten quality. High-protein and strong gluten doughs take longer to disintegrate. For instance, soft wheats usually take approximately 20 to 30 up to 100 to 175 minutes whereas hard wheats up to 400 minutes to disintegrate. The Pelshenke index is calculated by dividing the disintegration time by the protein content and is widely used in plant breeding programs to screen bread wheats.

A. Samples, Ingredients, and Reagents
- Wheat flour
- Compressed or dry yeast
- Distilled water

B. Materials and Equipment
- Digital scale
- Agitator
- Beakers (25 mL and 200 mL)
- Graduated cylinder (100 mL)
- Pipette (5 mL)
- Fermentation cabinet
- Thermometer
- Chronometer
- Hot plate

C. Procedure
1. Determine the flour moisture content (refer to procedure in Section 2.2.1.1).

2. Mix 10 g of fresh compressed yeast or 3.33 g of dry yeast in 100 mL of distilled water tempered to 30°C.

3. Prepare four separate runs of the same flour. In a 25-mL beaker, place 4 g of 14% mb flour with 2.25 mL of the yeast suspension and mix it with an agitator (Figure 5.8).

4. Continue mixing the dough ball by hand and then place the dough ball in a 100-mL graduated

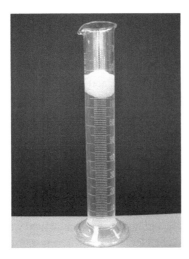

FIGURE 5.8 Determination of wheat flour quality with the Pelshenke test.

cylinder containing 80 mL of water tempered to 30°C (Figure 5.8).

5. Register the time when the dough ball was placed in the graduated cylinder and the time when the dough ball disintegrated (in some instances, when the disintegration is not evident, mark the time the dough ball causes turbidity or produces dispersed particles). If three of the samples disintegrate with more than 5% of the average value, the test should be repeated.

6. Classify the strength of the wheat flour according to Table 5.2.

5.3.3.2 Sedimentation or Zeleny Test

The Zeleny (Zeleny 1947), sedimentation, and microsedimentation (AACC 2000, Methods 56-60, 56-61A, and 56-63) tests are used to estimate the bread-baking and gluten qualities of wheat flours. They are simple, rapid, practical, and reliable tests that are valuable for use in grading different types of wheats. Samples with high gluten content have higher sedimentation values because of the higher gluten water absorption and swelling capacity. The Zeleny test is based on the swelling reaction of wheat flour proteins on treatment with lactic acid. Likewise, the sedimentation test is based on the 5-minute sedimentation volume of a fixed flour–water slurry stained with bromophenol and a weak

acidic acetic–isopropanol solution. The sedimentation values are commonly adjusted according to protein content.

A. *Samples, Ingredients, and Reagents*
  - Wheat flours
  - Isopropyl alcohol
  - Lactic acid
  - Methylene blue
  - Bromophenol blue

B. *Materials and Equipment*
  - Sieve (U.S. no. 70) with collection pan
  - Stoppered graduated cylinder (100 mL)
  - Chronometer

C. *Procedure (Sedimentation Test Method 56-60)*
  This method was previously described in AACC (2000).

1. Determine the flour moisture content (refer to procedure in Section 2.2.1.1).
2. Place 10 g of flour on a U.S. 70 mesh sieve with a collection pan. Sift the flour for 1.5 minutes with circular movements.
3. Collect the flour in the collection pan and weigh exactly 4 g of flour. Place flour in the 100 mL graduated cylinder.
4. Add 50 mL of distilled water and two to three drops of methylene blue or bromophenol blue indicator to the graduated cylinder. Place stopper on the graduated cylinder and mix the flour with the liquid reagents. Mix the contents by inverting and returning to the upright position 12 times. The time for moving to each direction should be for 5 seconds. After this 2-minute mixing protocol, the flour should be completely suspended in the water (Figure 5.9).
5. Mix contents for 30 seconds as follows: completely invert the graduated cylinder and return to the original position. Repeat this procedure 18 times in 30 seconds. Allow flour suspension to rest for 1.5 minutes.
6. Add 25 mL of isopropyl alcohol and lactic acid solution (12.5 mL isopropyl and 12.5 mL lactic acid) and after placing the stopper, immediately mix contents by inverting the graduated cylinder as explained in step 5. Allow flour suspension to rest for 1.75 minutes (Figure 5.9).
7. Agitate contents for 15 seconds as explained in step 6 and immediately place graduated cylinder in the original position to rest for 5 minutes.
8. At exactly the end of the fifth minute, record the volume of the sediment. The volume in milliliters is the sedimentation value of the flour.
9. Multiply the sedimentation value by the appropriate flour moisture factor detailed in Table 5.3.
10. Classify the strength of the wheat flour according to the corrected sedimentation value: 8 to 15 for soft wheat flours and 55 to 80 for hard wheat flours.

TABLE 5.2
Wheat Flour Classification According to the Pelshenske Test or Time Required for a Fermenting Dough Ball to Disintegrate

Soft Flours	Minutes	Hard Flours	Minutes
Very weak	<30	Weak	150–225
Regular	30–50	Medium–strong	225–300
Medium–strong	50–100	Strong	300–400
Strong	100–175	Very strong	>400

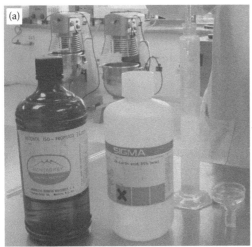 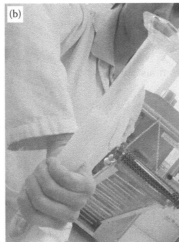 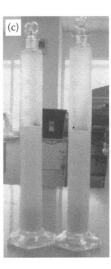

FIGURE 5.9 Procedure for the determination of wheat flour quality with the sedimentation test. (a) Addition of isopropilic alcohol and lactic acid; (b) agitation of the wheat flour slurry; (c) determination of sedimentation value.

5.3.3.3 Alkaline Water Retention Test (Method 56-10)

This method was previously described in AACC (2000).

The alkaline water retention test has been very useful in predicting the performance of soft wheat flours for cookies. The test was devised to determine the amount of alkaline water retained by a 14% mb wheat flour. The flour is hydrated with a certain amount of alkaline water and then centrifuged to calculate the weight of the pellet. This simple test is widely used to predict flour quality used in chemical leavened bakery items such as cookies.

A. *Samples, Ingredients, and Reagents*
- Soft wheat flours
- Distilled water
- Sodium bicarbonate solution (0.1 N)

B. *Materials and Equipment*
- Digital scale
- Centrifuge
- Centrifuge tubes (15 mL with plastic lids)
- Volumetric flask (1 L)
- Chronometer

- Stirring rod
- Rack for tubes
- Graduated cylinder (25 mL)
- Pipette (5 mL)

C. *Procedure*
1. Prepare a 0.1-N sodium bicarbonate by dissolving 8.4 g of sodium bicarbonate in 1 L of distilled water.
2. Determine the moisture content of the test flour (refer to procedure in Section 2.2.1.1).
3. In an analytical scale, first weigh the centrifuge tube and then weigh 0.95 g to 1.00 g of the flour. Register the exact weight of the empty tube and sample.
4. With a pipette, add 5 mL of the 0.1 N sodium bicarbonate solution.
5. Place the lid of the centrifuge tube in preparation for agitation. Manually agitate contents every 5 minutes for 20 minutes. During the first agitation, make sure to dissolve the flour.
6. Place centrifuge tubes in the centrifuge making sure to properly distribute weights. If the centrifuge is not properly balanced, fill one centrifuge tube with 6 mL of water to counteract the weight of the tube containing the sample. Set the speed of the centrifuge rotor to $1000 \times g$ for 15 minutes.
7. Decant the supernatant and position tubes in a 45-degree angle for 45 minutes to enhance water draining. Clean the top part of the tubes with tissue paper and then place tubes in the rack at a 90-degree angle. Allow water to drain for an additional 5 minutes.
8. Weigh the centrifuge tube with the wet flour pellet. Determine the percentage of alkaline water absorption using the following equation:

TABLE 5.3
Sedimentation Value Correction Factor According to Original Flour Moisture Content

Flour Moisture (%)	Factor	Flour Moisture (%)	Factor
8.0	0.93	12.5	0.98
8.5	0.93	13.0	0.98
9.0	0.95	13.5	0.99
9.5	0.95	14.0	1.00
10.0	0.96	14.5	1.02
10.5	0.96	15.0	1.04
11.0	0.97	15.5	1.07
11.5	0.97	16.0	1.10

alkaline water absorption % = [(weight of centrifuge tube with wet flour pellet – weight of empty tube)/ flour weight] * 100

Adjust value according to moisture content

$$AWRC_{14\%mb} = AWRC * (86/100 - flour\ moisture) * 100.$$

5.3.3.4 Gluten Content

Gluten is the functional component of the protein and determines many dough and processing characteristics of wheat flour. The wheat gluten consists of the two proteins: glutenin and gliadin. It is not until a dough has been hydrated and mechanically mixed that it actually forms gluten. This is why it is not possible to determine gluten in wheat without actually making a dough. During dough mixing, disulfide bonding is created between the glutelin and the gliadin. These flour proteins absorb two to three times their weight in water.

There are several assays aimed toward the determination of gluten content (AACC 2000, Methods 38-10 and 38-11). The simplest consists of using water to wash a developed dough ball to gradually remove starch and soluble proteins. The resulting wet residue, with elastic and cohesive properties or gluten, is mainly composed of glutelins and prolamins or gliadins. The wet or dried gluten weight is expressed based on the original flour weight. The gluten yield is strongly related to protein content and flour functionality. Traditionally, a flour yielding 12% to 15% dry gluten and 35% to 45% wet gluten has been considered satisfactory for bread making.

A. Samples, Ingredients, and Reagents
  - Different types of flours
  - Distilled water

B. Materials and Equipment
  - Scale
  - Porcelain cup
  - Spatula
  - Desiccator
  - U.S. no. 80 sieve
  - Petri dishes
  - Convection oven
  - Tongs
  - Laboratory clock or chronometer

C. Procedure (Gluten Method 38-10)

This method was previously described in AACC (2000).

1. Determine the flour moisture content (refer to procedure in Section 2.2.1.1).
2. Weigh 25 g of flour and place it in a porcelain cup. Add 15 mL of distilled water and mix contents to form a dough ball. Using a spatula, make sure to remove the dough which adheres to the mortar sides (Figure 5.10).
3. Place dough ball in a beaker half-filled with 26.7°C tap water for 1 hour.
4. Remove dough ball from the water and place it on a U.S. no. 80 sieve. While massaging the dough, open the water faucet and allow running water to gradually remove all the soluble material (starch, soluble proteins, and sugars).

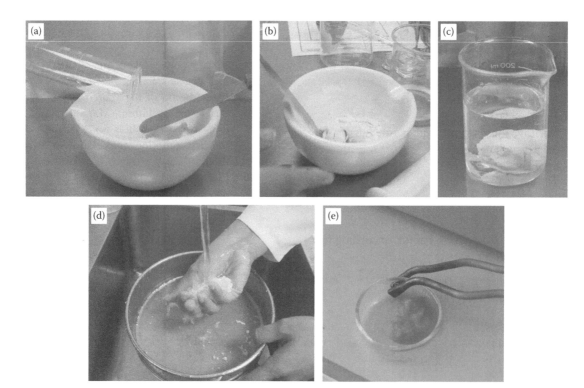

FIGURE 5.10 Procedure for the determination of hand-washed gluten content. (a) The addition of water; (b) dough mixing; (c) hydration of dough ball; (d) hand-washing of dough ball; (e) wet gluten.

5. The washing process should be stopped when the squeezed water contained by the insoluble gluten mass is crystal-clear. The gluten mass requires more washing if the water is turbid or has a milky appearance.

6. Allow wet gluten mass to rest for 1 hour. Manually compress the wet gluten to remove excess water.

7. Place wet gluten in a glass Petri dish for weighing and drying. Record the exact weight of the wet gluten mass (Figure 5.10).

8. Dehydrate the gluten at 60°C for 24 hours or until a constant weight is achieved.

9. Allow dry gluten to cool down for 20 minutes in desiccators. Register the exact weight of the dry gluten (Figure 5.10).

10. Calculate the wet and dry gluten yield using the following equation:

dry flour weight = sample weight × [(100 − percentage moisture content)/100]

percentage of wet gluten = wet gluten weight/dry flour sample weight

percentage of dry gluten = dry gluten weight/dry flour sample weight

5.3.3.5 Glutomatic Assay

The Glutomatic is an automatic apparatus developed based on the principle described above. The Glutomatic system is used worldwide by thousands of grain traders, flour millers, breeders, and pasta/noodle manufacturers. The quality of dough-based products, such as breads, pasta, or noodles, is highly dependent on the gluten quantity and quality of the flour. This means that everyone in the wheat chain, from breeder to baker, benefit from analyzing and controlling gluten properties. The instrument is widely used by quality control personnel because of its short assay time. The Glutomatic consists of a scale, dosifier of a 2% salt solution, dough mixer, the system to automatically wash the dough, a centrifuge, and a dryer. The instrument determines the yield of centrifuged wet gluten and dehydrated gluten (dried for only 4 minutes in between a couple of hot plates). Values are corrected according to protein content and widely used to select and classify wheats. The Glutomatic system is designed to measure protein quality based on wet gluten content, dry gluten content, water binding of gluten, and gluten strength determined as gluten index.

A. *Samples, Ingredients, and Reagents*
- Test wheat flour or ground wheat
- Distilled water
- Sodium chloride

B. *Materials and Equipment*
- Digital scale
- Air-convection dryer
- Aluminum dishes
- Tweezers
- Desiccator
- Spatula
- Dispenser
- Volumetric flask (1 L)
- Laboratory mill
- Glutomatic apparatus
- Gluten index centrifuge
- Glutork for gluten drying

C. *Procedure (Method 38-12)*
This method was previously described in AACC (2000).

1. Determine the flour or whole meal moisture content. If whole wheat is tested make sure to grind it with a laboratory mill. Prepare the sodium chloride solution by mixing 20 g reagent grade sodium chloride with distilled water in a 1-L volumetric flask. After dissolving the salt make sure to add distilled water to the 1-L volumetric mark.

2. Weigh 10.0 g ± 0.01 g of whole meal or flour and place it into the Glutomatic wash chamber with an 88 micron polyester sieve (Figure 5.11).

3. Dispense 4.8 mL of 2% sodium chloride or salt solution to the flour samples.

4. Mix flour and the salt solution to form a dough for 20 seconds. Place the washing chamber in the Glutomatic and press the start button.

5. The instrument will mix the dough for 20 seconds and then automatically wash the resulting dough for five minutes with 2% salt solution.

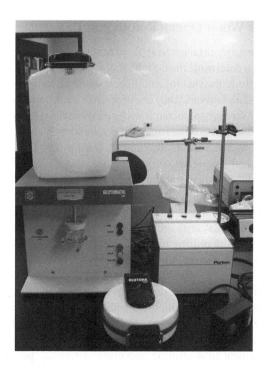

FIGURE 5.11 Glutomatic apparatus used to determine wet and dry gluten associated with wheat flour.

For wheat meal the sample is transferred to a chamber equipped with a coarse 840 micron sieve allowing bran particles to be washed out.

6. Remove wet gluten from the washing chamber and place it in the centrifuge holder for centrifugation.

7. Centrifuge the undivided wet gluten piece for exactly 30 seconds after washing. Using the Then, transfer to a special sieve cassette and centrifuge one minute at 6000 ± 5 rpm.

8. Scrape off with a spatula the fraction that passed through the sieves and collect the wet gluten fraction remaining on the inside of the sieve. Weigh the total wet gluten weight.

9. Dehydrate the wet gluten piece for 4 minutes at 150°C in the Glutork. After drying, weigh the dry gluten (Figure 5.11).

10. Calculate the gluten index by weighing the amount of gluten remaining on the centrifuge sieve in relation to the total wet gluten weight. A high gluten index indicates strong gluten.

11. Classify the flour according to wet gluten content and gluten indexes:
    a. Wet gluten
       1. 35% wet gluten for high-protein or strong gluten wheat
       2. 23% wet gluten for low-protein or weak gluten wheat
    b. Gluten index
       1. >85% strong gluten flour
       2. 70% to 85% intermediate gluten flour
       3. <70% weak gluten flour

5.3.4 Wheat Dough Rheological Properties

The most important wheat flour functionality tests are the ones that determine the dough's rheological properties. These assays study the rheological properties of a dough optimally hydrated and mixed. They are of upmost importance because they are strongly associated with processing (optimum water absorption and mixing time) and end-product quality.

Among the various instruments used to test the dough's rheological properties, most measure directly or indirectly the force or gluten strength and the dough extensibility or elasticity. The results obtained after analyzing the graphs are used by all segments of the wheat industry. In grain elevators, rheological tests are used to classify incoming wheats, whereas in the milling industry, these tests are used to make important decisions related to blending different types of wheats for the production of certain types of flours. In addition, the instruments are used to determine the amount of dough strengtheners and other additives needed to standardize the flour. In the baking, cookie, cracker, and even in the pasta industries, these rheological tests are considered the most critical to determine important processing parameters (water absorption, mixing time, and dough stability) and predict product quality.

5.3.4.1 Determination of Dough Properties with the Farinograph (Method 54-21)

This method was previously described in AACC (2000).

The farinograph has been the method most commonly used to evaluate rheological properties of dough. The popularity of the instrument resides in its ease of operation and in the fact that measurements are empirical and thus do not require the user to have an in-depth knowledge of rheological mathematics to interpret results (D'Appolonia and Kunerth 1984). The apparatus is a dynamic, physical dough testing instrument that records the torque applied during dough mixing. The resistance the dough offers to the mixing blades during mixing is transmitted to a dynamometer hooked to a recording device (D'Appolonia and Kunerth 1984). The instrument has eight basic parts: mixing bowl, dynamometer, level system, scale system, recording mechanism, dashpot, thermostat, and a buret. There are instruments that process either 50 g or 300 g of flour. The assay is based first on the determination of the optimum amount of water to achieve a maximum consistency of 500 farinograph units (FU). Several prefarinograms are run to center the curve on the 500 FU. The amount of water required to produce this consistency is the flour–water absorption. Then, the flour with its optimum water absorption is run again for up to 20 minutes to determine optimum mixing time and the behavior of the flour before and after attaining maximum consistency. The analysis of the typical farinograph curve yields important parameters such as arrival time to first achieve 500 FU, optimum mix time also called dough development time (time required to achieve maximum consistency), departure time or last time in which the dough had a 500 FU consistency and dough stability (calculated by time difference between departure and arrival times). Another important parameter is the mixing tolerance index calculated as the drop in consistency, 5 minutes after achieving dough development time. Both dough stability and mixing tolerance index are important factors, especially for bakers, because they are closely related to gluten strength and the dough tolerance to overmixning (AACC 2000; Bloksma and Bushuk 1988; D'Appolonia and Kunerth 1984). The preferred flours for yeast-leavened products have high water absorption (62–64%), 4 to 6 minutes dough development time, 8 to 12 minutes dough stability and a mixing tolerance index of approximately 40 FU.

A. Samples, Ingredients, and Reagents
- Test wheat flour
- Distilled water
- Ink

B. Materials and Equipment
- Farinograph with all accessories including graph paper
- Farinograph buret
- Digital scale
- Plastic scraper
- Desiccator
- Aluminum dishes
- Tweezers

C. *Procedure (Constant Flour Weight)*

1. Turn on the thermostat and circulating pump at least 1 hour before analysis. Make sure the temperature of the mixing bowl is 30°C ± 0.2°C, the chart paper runs properly, and put a few drops of ink in the recording pen.

2. Determine flour moisture content and adjust flour weight according to the original moisture content. Allow flour to equilibrate at room temperature especially if it was frozen or refrigerated.

3. Place 300 g ± 0.1 g or 50 g ± 0.1 g flour (14% mb) for the large or small farinograph bowls, respectively. Make sure to adjust weight according to the moisture content according to the following equations: for the 300 g farinograph accurately weigh [258 g/(100 − % flour moisture)] × 100 and for the 50 g farinograph weigh [43 g/(100 − % flour moisture)] × 100 (Figure 5.12).

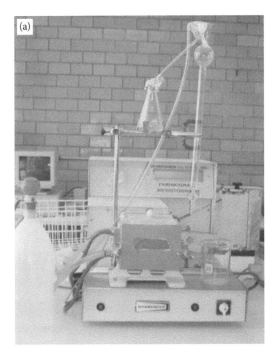

4. Fill buret with water at room temperature. Make sure that the tip is full and the automatic zero adjustment is working properly.

5. Put a few drops of ink in a pen and place in contact at the 9-minute position on the chart.

6. Turn on the machine to high speed and run for 1 minute until the zero minute line is reached. At this instant start adding water to the right front corner of bowl to the exact predetermined absorption volume value.

7. When the dough begins to form scrape down sides of bowl with plastic scraper, starting on the right side, front, left side and back. Cover immediately with the glass plate to prevent water losses.

8. If the farinograph curve levels off at a value higher than 500 FU cautiously add more water. For every 20 FU add 0.6% to 0.8% more water. Make sure to cover bowl with glass plate to prevent water evaporation.

9. If the farinograph curve levels off at a value lower than 500 FU register the maximum consistency and stop the instrument.

10. After cleaning the equipment, repeat the procedure adjusting the water absorption until the 500 FU consistency varies less than 20 FU. Make sure to deliver corrected water absorption within 25 seconds after opening the buret. Remember that when the correct absorption is achieved, the curve at maximum dough development is centered on the 500 FU line.

11. Allow the machine to run until an adequate curve is obtained (generally 20 minutes after water addition).

12. Report absorption values to nearest 0.1%. Adjust water absorption on 14% mb using the following equations: Absorption % for 300 g farinograph = $(x + y − 300)/3$, where x = mL water to produce curve with optimum consistency (500 FU) and y = g flour used. Absorption % for 50 g farinograph = $(x + y − 50)*2$ where x = mL water to produce curve with optimum consistency (500 FU) and y = g flour used.

13. Determine the following properties of the optimized farinograph curve (Figure 5.12):

    a. Arrival time: time is required for the top of the curve to first reach the 500 FU line after the mixer has been started and the water introduced.

    b. Dough development time. The time to the nearest half minute between the first addition of water and the dough's maximum consistency. This value is also referred as "peak time." If two peaks are observed the second should be considered as the development time.

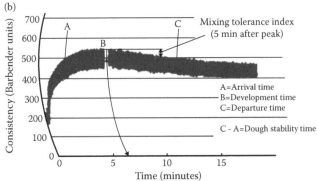

FIGURE 5.12 Farinograph used to determine the rheological properties of wheat dough with its characteristic curve. (a) Farinograph; (b) farinograph curve.

c. Departure time. The time to the nearest half minute from the first addition of the water until the top of the curve leaves the 500 FU line.

d. Stability. Defined as the difference in time to the nearest half minute between arrival and departure times.

e. Mixing tolerance index (MTI). The MTI is the difference in farinograph units between the top of the curve at peak (development time) and the top of the curve measured exactly 5 minutes afterwards.

14. Classify the tested flour according to either of the following values:

a. Very strong flour for baking or suited to blend with weaker flours. Water absorption >63%, dough development time >10 minutes, and MTI < 10 FU.

b. Strong flour. Water absorption >58%, dough development times between 4 and 8 minutes, and MTI between 15 and 50 FU.

c. Medium strength flour. Water absorption 54% to 60%, dough development times between 2.5 and 4 minutes, and MTI between 60 and 100 FU.

d. Weak flour. Water absorption <55%, dough development time <2.5 minutes and MTI >100 FU.

5.3.4.2 Determination of Dough Properties with the Extensograph (Method 54-10)

This method was previously described in AACC (2000).

The extensograph is an instrument that measures rheological properties of optimally mixed and formed dough (optimum water absorption and mixing time) obtained with the farinograph. The dough is prepared from flour, 2% salt, and the optimum water based on the farinograph. Pieces of dough (150 g) are formed into a cylinder that is proofed under controlled temperatures (30°C ± 2°C) and relative humidity. The dough cylinder is then cramped to the extensograph arms and then subjected to a constant

(a)

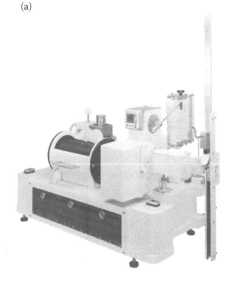

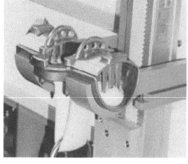

(b)

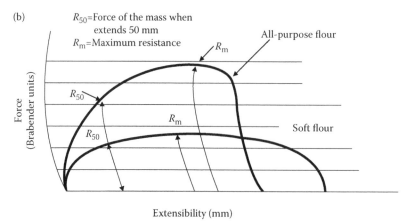

R_{50}=Force of the mass when extends 50 mm
R_m=Maximum resistance

FIGURE 5.13 Extensigraph used to determine the rheological properties of wheat dough with its characteristic curve. (a) Extensigraph; (b) extensigraph curve.

displacement until rupture (AACC 2000, Method 54-10; Rasper and Preston 1991; Bloksma and Bushuk 1988.). The dough resistance to stretching is graphed in the typical extensograph curve shown in Figure 5.13. The instrument records the resistance R on the y axis (R50 mm when the dough was stretched 50 mm and R_{max} when reaches the maximum height) and the extensibility (E) in the x axis. The ratio R/E is an important parameter because it relates gluten strength and dough extensibility and therefore flour functionality. The integration of the area under the curve is proportional to the energy (W) that is required to bring about rupture of the test piece and is also highly related to gluten strength. The assay is usually repeated after fixed amounts of times (45, 90, and 135 minutes) so the dough behavior throughout different proofing times can be determined.

A. Samples, Ingredients, and Reagents
- Test wheat flours
- Salt
- Distilled water
- Cooking oil

B. Materials and Equipment
- Extensograph with all accessories including graph paper
- Digital scale
- Planimeter
- Ink
- Convection oven
- Desiccator
- Aluminum dishes
- Tweezers
- Brush

C. Procedure

Dough Preparation

1. Prepare a dough following the 300-g farinograph procedure described before. The differences are that the flour is supplemented with 6 g salt, the addition of 2% less water due to salt addition, and that the farinograph mixes the dough for 1 minute and stops for 5-minute intervals until maximum consistency or dough development time is achieved.
2. Before dough resting, make sure to fill the humidified chamber containers with distilled water and to slightly grease the metal forms where the center of the dough cylinders will rest.
3. After dough mixing, cut and weigh 150 g ± 0.1 g of dough and place it in the special device that mechanically rounds the dough. Shape the dough ball into a cylinder using the special forming device. Then, place clamps at the ends of the cylinder and store the dough in the extensograph chamber with strict temperature (30°C) and relative humidity controls.

Dough Testing

1. Dough can be tested at 30, 60, and 90 minutes or after 45, 90, and 135 minutes. Remove dough cylinder with clamps from the humidified chamber and place it under the stretching hook arm. Adjust recording pen to zero in the extensograph paper.
2. Start the dough-stretching action until the dough ruptures. The instrument should graph the typical extensogram (Figure 5.13).
3. Remove dough and repeat the dough ball forming and resting procedures after 30- or 45-minute intervals. The same reshaped dough should be tested at least three times.

Determination of Extensogram Parameters

1. Determine the following properties of the extensograms (Figure 5.13):
   a. Resistance to stretching (R_{max} and R50 mm). Obtained as the maximum curve height (EU) and after 50 mm dough stretching. Values are measured on the y axis.
   b. Extensibility (E). Obtained after measuring the length (cm) of the curve on the x axis.
   c. Work (W) or energy calculating the area under the curve. It is calculated using a planimeter and represents the work required to stretch the dough.
   d. Calculate the R_{max}/E ratio values.
2. Classify the tested flour according to either of the R_{max}/E values:
   a. Very strong flour for baking or suited to blend with other flours

$$R_{max}/E\ 0.5\text{--}1$$

   b. Strong flour

$$R_{max}/E > 0.35$$

   c. Intermediate flour

$$R_{max}/E > 0.10$$

   d. Weak flour

$$R_{max}/E < 0.1$$

5.3.4.3 Determination of Dough Properties with the Mixograph (Method 54-40)

This method was previously described in AACC (2000).

The mixograph is an instrument that works with the same principles as the farinograph. The interpretation of the characteristic mixograph curve yields important parameters such as optimum dough mixing or peak time, stability, the height of the curve, the angle and curve thickness especially before and after the optimum dough development time, and the area under the curve. However, the analysis of the curve is not as extensive as the farinograph curve but is the preferred method by plant breeders because it only requires a 10- or 35-g sample and the assays only lasts 7 to 8 minutes (AACC 2000, Method 54-40; Finney and Shogren 1972; Rath et al. 1990; Walker et al. 1997). The wheat quality laboratories use the mixograph extensively to evaluate thousands of early generation wheat lines. Mixogram curves will be evaluated for peak times and tolerance scores. Wheat breeders can then make decisions about discarding lines with no end-use quality potential. The amount of water and sample weight varies according to protein and moisture, respectively. The instrument graphs a curve that shows a time point of maximum consistency (dough development time).

A. *Samples, Ingredients, and Reagents*
- Test wheat flour
- Distilled water

B. *Materials*
- Mixograph with all accessories including graph paper
- Scale
- Buret (10 mL or 25 mL)
- Ink
- Convection drying oven
- Desiccator
- Aluminum dishes
- Tweezers
- Thermometer
- Laboratory clock

C. *Procedure*
1. Check the speed of the mixing head (85–90 rpm) and the arm (AACC 2000, Method 54-40).
2. Adjust the range and sensibility of the instrument according to the official method (AACC 2000, Method 54-40).
3. Place ink in the pen and adjust mixograph paper so the test starts at zero.
4. Determine beforehand the flour moisture and protein content. The first parameter value will affect sample weight and the second will affect water absorption. After analysis, keep samples in sealed containers to avoid moisture gain or loss.
5. Before the test, temper the test flour, water, and mixing bowl to 25°C.
6. Calculate the sample weight according to the following equations. For the 35 g mixograph, accurately weigh [30.1 g/(100 − % flour moisture)] × 100, and for the 10 g mixograph, weigh [8.6 g/(100 − % flour moisture)] × 100. Accurately weigh the predetermined sample (±0.05 g).
7. Carefully place flour in the tempered mixing bowl (Figure 5.14).

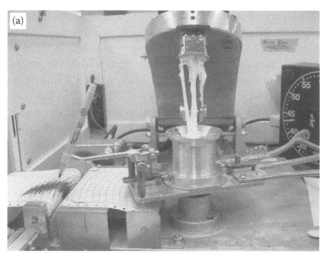

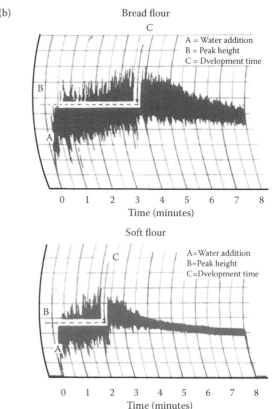

FIGURE 5.14 Mixograph used to determine the rheological properties of wheat dough with its characteristic curve. (a) Mixograph; (b) mixograph curve.

8. Calculate the desired water absorption which usually relates to the protein content. Add 50% to the flour protein to estimate percentage of water absorption. For instance, for 9%, 10.5%, 12%, and 14% protein flours add 59%, 60.5%, 62%, and 64% distilled water, respectively. Convert the percentage of water absorption for the 35 g or 10 g mixograph using the following equations:

Water (mL) for 35 g mixograph = (% water absorption/100 × 35) + (35 − sample weight)

Water (mL) for 10 g mixograph = (% water absorption/100 × 10) + (10 − sample weight)

9. Fill burette with water tempered to 25°C. With a 25- or 10-mL buret, carefully deliver the predetermined amount of water to the mixing bowl.

10. Place mixing bowl with flour sample and water, making sure to secure bowl with the two pegs. Then, lower the mixing head.

11. Make sure the graph paper and pen are properly set and placed.

12. When the marking pen reaches the vertical line, turn on the mixing head and allow dough to mix for 8 minutes (Figure 5.14). If a laboratory clock is used, the 8-minute mixing can be automatically controlled.

13. Turn off mixing head. Immediately check and register the dough temperature.

14. Determine the following properties of the mixograph curve: the height of the curve, the angle and curve thickness especially before and after the optimum dough development time, and the area under the curve:

   a. Area under the curve. Calculate the area under the 8-minute curve considering the center of the curve width.

   b. Time to reach maximum curve height (peak time). Calculate the time (nearest half minute) and height (cm) of the mixogram. These parameters are related to optimum dough development time and flour strength.

   c. Ascending and descending angle rays from the peak point. The center of the peak curve point is taken as the vertex of the angle whereas the ascending and descending rays should be drawn before the estimation of the angle.

   d. Mixing tolerance index. The width of the mixogram curve and the angle of descent indicate the tolerance of the dough to overmixing. Well-defined curves with wide bands and low angles of descent indicate strong tolerance to overmixing and superior protein quality.

5.3.4.4 Determination of Dough Properties with the Alveograph (Method 54-30)

According to Faridi et al. (1987), in the 1920s, Marcel Chopin devised several prototypes to test the physical condition of developed dough and related the tests to the breadbaking process. The key and most noteworthy design was the injection of air to a developed round disc of dough to form a bubble until it burst. During its inflation, the dough piece is extended in two directions: along a parallel and along a meridian of the bubble. This mode of deformation is called biaxial extension. The final design was named the alveograph. This apparatus differs from other dough rheological instruments because it is the only one that measures biaxial extension. This simulates gas retention during fermentation. The characteristic alveograph curve yields important dough rheological parameters that are closely related to wheat quality and type. The main evaluated parameters are maximum overpressure (P), index of swelling, average abscissa at rupture (L), deformation energy (W), and the P/L ratio. The P/L ratio is an excellent indicator of flour functionality. Strong gluten flours usually yield curves with high P and W values. The assay consists of mixing 250 g of flour for 8 minutes with a 2.5% salt solution (AACC 2000, Method 54-30; Dubois et al. 2008; Rasper and Walker 2000). The amount of water is adjusted according to the flour moisture content. The resulting dough is divided into four equal parts that are rolled on a sheet to obtain a fixed thickness (12 mm). The dough sheets are cut into discs with a given diameter and then rested in an isothermic box. The alveograph curves are generally obtained 20 minutes after dough cutting. The disc of dough is placed in the equipment in preparation for air injection. The air is injected at a constant pressure until the dough bubble bursts. Strong gluten flours usually have high P and W values.

A. *Samples, Ingredients, and Reagents*
- Test wheat flour
- Distilled water
- Sodium chloride (reagent grade) solution (2.5%)
- Paraffin or vegetable oil

B. *Materials and Equipment*
- Alveograph with all accessories
- Digital scale
- Graduated cylinder (100 mL)
- Plastic spatula
- Convection drying oven
- Volumetric flask (1 L)
- Desiccator
- Aluminum dishes
- Tweezers
- Brush
- Laboratory clock or chronometer
- Eye dropper

C. *Procedure*
1. Prepare the following reagent:
   a. Sodium chloride solution. Dissolve 25 g of sodium chloride in distilled water and make up to the 1000 mL mark.
2. Determine beforehand the flour moisture content because this value will affect sample weight. After analysis, keep samples in sealed containers to avoid moisture gain or loss.
3. Turn on alveograph and verify that the temperature of the mixer and proof chamber is 24°C and 25°C, respectively. The optimum temperature

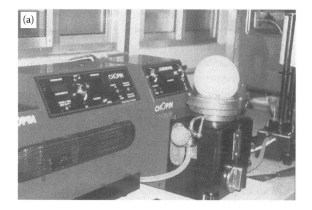

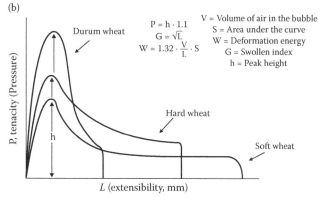

FIGURE 5.15 Alveograph used to determine the rheological properties of wheat dough with its characteristic curve. (a) Alveograph; (b) alveograph curve.

and relative humidity ranges of the laboratory should be between 18°C and 22°C and 55% and 70% relative humidity.

4. Temper the test flour and salt water solution to 18°C to 25°C.

5. Place 250 g ± 0.5 g of oil in the alveograph mixer (Figure 5.15). Make sure the extrusion gate is closed. Secure the lid by tightening the two screws. Start the motor and the timer. With the mixer running, add the required quantity of sodium chloride solution through the hole in the lid. The amount of solution will vary according to the flour moisture content. The saline solution should be delivered within 20 seconds, preferably by using the graduated burette of the equipment. The alveograph burette is graduated for moisture contents ranging from 11.6% to 17.8%.

6. After 1 minute of mixing, stop the motor, remove the lid, and use a plastic spatula to scrape down the dough adhered to walls of the lid and combine with the rest of the dough. The operation should not take more than 45 seconds.

7. Restart the motor and allow dough mixing to continue for an additional 6 minutes.

8. While the dough is being mixed, use an eye dropper to place 4 drops of paraffin or vegetable

oil on the plate attached to the extrusion gate, 16 drops on each glass plate of the sheeting plates, 5 drops on the roller, and 5 drops on each resting plate. Spread the oil drops uniformly across all surfaces with a brush.

9. After completing the mixing schedule, stop the motor and open the extrusion gate by raising the slide of the shutter and securing it in its right position with the knurled knob. Reverse the direction of the kneader and turn on the motor to obtain the strip of extruded dough.

10. Cut off and discard the first 2 cm of the strip with the metal spatula supplied with the instrument. Cut the extruded dough with the spatula when the strip reaches the two small indented notches on the receiving plate. Pull out the extrusion plate and slide the dough onto the previously oiled glass plate of the sheeting plate.

11. Extrude and cut five pieces of dough (Figure 5.15). Place two pieces on each of the two sheeting plates and leave the fifth on the receiving plate of the mixer.

12. Sheet the dough pieces on the glass plates by rolling them with the oiled roller. The sheeting operation consists of three rapid back-and-forth movements followed by three slow ones (12 passes).

13. Using the alveograph circular cutting device, cut the dough on the glass plate in a single movement. Lift away the surplus dough before carefully lifting the cutter containing the dough piece. Transfer the round dough piece to the resting plate.

14. Immediately place the resting plate with the dough piece in the resting compartment of the alveograph. Repeat the procedure for the other three or four dough pieces. Make sure to sequentially arrange dough pieces in the resting compartments.

15. During dough resting, prepare the recorder by placing a sheet of alveograph chart on the recording drum. Fill the pen with ink, trace the zero pressure line, and return the drum to its original position.

16. Let the dough pieces rest in the resting compartment until 28 minutes have elapsed from the beginning of the dough mixing operation.

17. Prepare the alveograph for the stretching operation. Make sure that the operating lever is at position 1. Raise the upper plate by rotating it counterclockwise for two revolutions. Spread four drops of oil on the fixed brass plate and two drops of oil on the brass stopper.

18. Take the resting plate with the circular dough ball from the resting compartment exactly 28 minutes after the start of dough mixing. Slide the dough to the center of the fixed plate

with the aid of a plastic spatula. Carefully position the dough onto the center. Replace the stopper and secure it with the brass collar. Flatten the dough piece by slowly lowering the upper plate, rotating it clockwise (two turns in 20 seconds). Wait 5 seconds, then remove the collar and the stopper.

19. Turn the operating lever to position. Then, turn the air valve handle to the horizontal position and press the rubber bulb with the thumb and forefinger until the two fingers touch. While the rubber bulb is still compressed, close the air valve by turning its handle to the vertical position. Switch the operating level to position 3 quickly. This will cause the dough piece to start inflating and the recording drum to revolve.
20. Turn the operating level to position 4 as soon as the dough bubble ruptures (Figure 5.15).
21. Repeat the procedure with the four remaining dough pieces. Make sure to add two drops of oil on the fixed plate and one drop on the brass stopper after each test.
22. Evaluate the following parameters of the alveogram curves (Figure 5.15). If one of the curves deviates greatly from the other four, it can be discarded.
    a. Maximum overpressure (P). Using the special alveograph chart, measure in millimeters the maximum heights of the curves. The arithmetic mean of these values is multiplied by 1.1 to obtain the P value.
    b. Index of swelling (G). This index is read on the XX′ scale of the conversion chart at the point corresponding vertically with the abrupt drop in pressure caused by the rupture of the bubble.
    c. Average abscissa at rupture (L). This value is measured in millimeters on the baseline from the origin of the curve to the point of rupture.
    d. P/L ratio. This dimensionless value is calculated by dividing the maximum overpressure or P by the average abscissa at rupture or L.
    e. Deformation energy (W). The deformation energy value is calculated by determining the area under the alveograph curve. The most rapid and efficient way to measure the area is with the planimeter scale provided with the equipment. The deformation energy W is calculated with the following formula: $W = (1.32)(V/L)(S)$, where V is the volume of air displaced (mL) and is equal to the square of the swelling index G, L is the average abscissa at rupture, and S is the area under the alveograph curve in square centimeters.

23. Classify the tested flour according to the alveogram parameters:
    a. Strong wheat flour

    $$P/L > 0.7$$

    $$W > 230$$

    b. Intermediate wheat flour

    $$P/L > 0.3 \text{ to } <0.7$$

    $$W > 140 \text{ to } <230$$

    c. Weak flour

    $$P/L < 0.3$$

    $$W < 120$$

5.3.4.5 Determination of Dough Properties with Mixolab (Method 54-60.01)

The mixolab is a relatively new device that enables users to measure the consistency of dough over time with a gradual increase in the applied temperature. The instrument was introduced in 2004 by Chopin Technologies. It is designed to test both protein and starch characteristics of the flour and also provide information about the rheological properties of dough (Dubat 2010). The apparatus is used to characterize the rheological behavior of flour subjected to a dual mixing and temperature constraint. The analysis protocol of this device is completely customizable (i.e., mixing speed, temperature, water absorption) and permits to analyze, with only one test, both protein and starch functionality. The computerized analysis of the curve also yields the Mixolab Profiler. The flour profile facilitates the selection and improvement of flours based on functionality and terminal use (AACC 2000).

The instrument is designed to test ground wheat or refined flours and is based on the principles of the farinograph and amylograph because it first determines the dough mixing characteristics and gluten strength and then the pasting, viscosity, and retrogradation properties of the same dough system. Therefore, it is the only instrument enabling the complete characterization of a gluten protein and starch functionality in a single assay. The instrument has a 50-g flour capacity and it is fitted with two blades which turn in opposite directions. The resistant torque exerted on the blades during mixing is measured by a sensor located on the axis of one of the blades. The computerized test is conducted under a strict temperature program and water addition.

The flour is first mixed with the optimum amount of water and viscosity tested similarly as in the farinograph. Then, the temperature of the dough is gradually increased to test changes in viscosity through heating and cooling cycles.

Integrated to the instrument is a simulator that automatically calculates water absorption, dough development time, and stability and viscosities mainly dependent of starch characteristics. The instrument is also suited to test starch damage, amylase activity, and ingredient functionality.

To provide comparable results between samples, the instrument works on a constant dough basis (75 g total mass). The instrument automatically calculates the quantity of flour to be weighed according to its original moisture content and the water absorption at which the test will be conducted. Recently, Codină et al. (2010) evaluated the relationship between the alveograph, falling number, and mixolab values of 60 flours. The authors found significant correlations between most of the alveograph parameters: maximum pressure (*P*), deformation energy (*W*), extensibility (*L*), alveograph ratio (*P/L*), and simulator mixolab stability. Using the mixolab standard option "Chopin+" protocol, a close association was found between some mixolab parameters: stability and protein weakening (C2, difference of the points C1 − C2) and the alveograph values (*P, W*). From the point of view of the correlations established with the falling number index, very good results were obtained with the parameters obtained using mixolab which measures starch gelatinization (C3, difference of the points C3 − C2), amylolitic activity (C4, difference of the points C3 − C4), and starch gelling (C5, difference of the points C5 − C4).

A. *Samples, Ingredients, and Reagents*
- Test wheat flours
- Distilled water
- Sodium chloride reagent grade or salt solution (2.5%)
- Paraffin or vegetable oil

B. *Materials and Equipment*
- Mixolab apparatus with all accessories
- Digital scale
- Laboratory mill fitted with 0.8 mm screen (Perten LM 120 or LM 3100)
- Convection drying oven
- Desiccator
- Aluminum dishes
- Tweezers

C. *Procedure*
1. If the sample is whole wheat, grind it using a laboratory mill fitted with a 0.8-mm screen.
2. Determine flour moisture content because the instrument will automatically adjust flour weight according to the moisture value. Input the test conditions (flour moisture content and desired water absorption, 60%).
3. Accurately weigh 45 g ± 0.05 g of the test flour and place it into the mixolab mixer (Figure 5.16). Then position the water injector.
4. Conduct a preliminary test to determine if the selected water absorption is adequate for the run. Start the assay and verify that during the

(a)

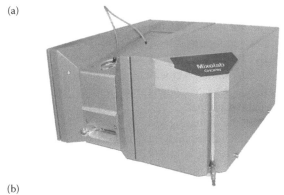

(b)

CHOPIN curve of Mixolab

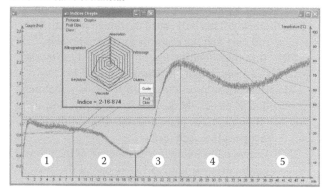

(c)

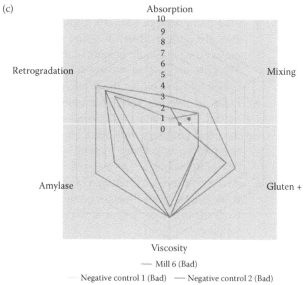

FIGURE 5.16 Mixolab used to determine the rheological and viscosity properties of wheat dough with its characteristic curve and the flour profiler graph. (a) Mixolab; (b) mixolab curve; (c) flour profiler graph.

first 5 minutes, the torque is within 1.10 nm ± 0.07 nm. If in range, allow test to continue. If not, stop the test and repeat procedure with the new water absorption.
5. Allow instrument to complete the test.
6. Evaluate the five different phases of the mixolab curve (Figure 5.16).

a. Phase I (hold at 30°C for 8 minutes). Evaluation of dough formation and weakening. The most important parameters are maximum consistency, time to maximum consistency, and dough stability (measured as the time in minutes in which torque is higher than maximum consistency, 11%).

b. Phase II (30–60°C). Evaluation of weakening proteins in function of the reduction of torque. The two most relevant parameters are minimum consistency and dough temperature at minimum consistency.

c. Phase III (60–90°C). Evaluation of starch gelatinization properties. The two most relevant parameters are minimum consistency and dough temperature at minimum consistency. These values are related to starch characteristics and amylase activity.

d. Phase IV (hold at 90°C). Evaluation of stability during baking. The most important parameters are gel stability (difference between minimum consistency of phase III and IV phases) minimum consistency during baking and dough temperature at minimum consistency.

e. Phase V (90–60°C). Evaluation of starch retrogradation. The most important parameter is the increase in torque between minimum consistency of phase IV and maximum consistency of phase V. Retrogradation is correlated to bread staling (Dubat 2010).

7. Obtain the mixolab flour profiler graph (Figure 5.16) and relate the six factors (mixing, absorption, retrogradation, viscosity, amylase, and gluten) to a reference or control flour.

5.3.5 Quality of Groats

The aim of the oat-milling procedure is to obtain the maximum yield of stabilized groats free of hulls. The groats rich in both soluble and insoluble dietary fiber should have an adequate stability throughout storage. Groats are further processed into regular and instant flaked oats or milled into meals or flours for the production of bakery products. The most relevant tests for oats are cooking properties, color, protein, dietary fiber, total starch, and fat stability or rancidity.

5.3.6 Quality of Decorticated Sorghum and Refined Meals and Flours

The aim of the sorghum-milling procedure is to obtain the maximum yield of decorticated kernels free of pericarp and germ. The pearled kernels can be transformed into grits, meals, or flours for the production of many traditional foods. Thus, the decorticated kernels or refined dry-milling fractions are low in fiber and preferably contain less than 1% oil.

The extent of pericarp removal is usually evaluated with the May–Gruenwald dyeing technique (Scheuring and Rooney 1979) previously detailed in procedure in Section 5.3.2.1. The most common quality control procedures to evaluate the quality of refined sorghum fractions are color, particle size distribution, ash, fat, total starch, and amylose/amylopectin ratio.

5.3.7 Research Suggestions

1. Compare the chemical properties, color, and damaged starch of white and yellow refined maize grits.

2. Compare the cooking properties, elongation factor, and amylose content of a short waxy rice, a long regular rice, and a long parboiled rice.

3. Compare Pelshenke, sedimentation, and gluten content values of two contrasting wheat flours (i.e., soft and hard wheat) and then relate these simple test parameters with farinograph and alveograph data.

4. For a given sample of refined wheat flour, determine and compare gluten assayed by the hand-wash procedure and the automatic Glutomatic.

5. Compare color, ash, damaged starch, and rheological dough properties of straight grade and patented flours obtained from the same wheat.

6. Evaluate the effects of the addition of potassium bromate and ascorbates (20 ppm and 100 ppm, respectively) or sodium bisulfite (20 ppm) to refined wheat flour. How do these additions affect the dough rheological properties evaluated with the farinograph, extensigraph, and alveograph.

7. Evaluate the effects of soft wheat flour chlorination on the dough rheological properties evaluated with the farinograph, extensigraph, alveograph, and mixolab.

8. Compare extensograph parameters obtained after analyzing the same sample with the Brabender extensograph and the Kieffer dough and gluten extensibility rig of the TAXT2 texture analyzer.

9. Obtain mixolab curves and the flour profiler graph (mixing, absorption, gluten, viscosity, amylase, and retrogradation) of hard, soft, and all-purpose flours with different falling number values.

10. Compare the chemical properties, color, particle size distribution, gelatinized starch, and susceptibility to rancidity of oat flour obtained after milling with and without steaming.

11. Compare the chemical properties, color, particle size distribution, and damaged starch of refined sorghum meals obtained after 20% decortication and milling of hard white and soft red sorghums.

5.3.8 Research Questions

1. Define the following terms widely used in quality control of dry-milling operations:
   a. Slick test
   b. Pelshenke test

    c. Zeleny test
    d. Glutomatic
    e. Mixolab
    f. Water absorption
    g. Mixing tolerance
    h. Oxidizing agents
    i. Matured flour
    j. Granulation
    k. Dough development time
    l. Mixolab profiler graph

2. What are the main color meters used by millers? Describe the principles of at least three different color meters?

3. During maize dry-milling, an array of refined fractions are obtained, what are their particle sizes and main uses? Which of the refined dry-milled products is the most expensive? Why?

4. What kind of considerations, in terms of raw materials and changes in the corn dry-milling process, would you make to optimize yields of flaking grits (U.S. no. 6)? What is the typical chemical composition of flaking grits?

5. Compare the chemical composition and typical extraction rate of brewing maize and rice grits. Which grits are preferred for the production of light-colored beers? What is the typical particle size and fat content of these brewing grits?

6. What is the assay or factor most related to the cooking characteristics of rice? List three other methods related to rice cooking?

7. What is the principle and use of the May–Gruenwald test?

8. What is parboiling? Why is parboiling still widely practiced? Why is parboiled rice considered to have more nutritional attributes compared with regular rice?

9. Compare the properties and cooking characteristics of a regular white vs. a parboiled white rice.

10. Why is the alkaline water absorption test widely used for cookie flours made with alkaline solution?

11. What are the principles of the Pelshenke and sedimentation tests?

12. What kind of compounds are removed during the hand or machine gluten washing process? What is the typical chemical composition of vital gluten?

13. Draw the typical farinograph curve and name the four major parameters that are obtained after analyzing the curve.

14. Draw the typical extensogram curve and name the three major parameters that are obtained after analyzing the curve.

15. Draw and compare typical mixograph curves for soft and hard wheat flours and name the three major parameters that are obtained after analyzing the curve.

16. What are the differences and similarities between the farinograph and mixograph?

17. Draw the typical alveogram curve and name the three major parameters that are obtained after analyzing the curve.

18. What are the reasons for why saline solutions are used to produce doughs for the alveograph and extensograph tests?

19. What would happen to the farinograph, mixograph, and alveograph parameters if the test flour is supplemented with 20 ppm of sodium bisulfite?

20. What is the main advantage of the mixolab compared with other rheological instruments? Investigate how a flour profiler graph is obtained after obtaining the various mixolab parameters.

21. List at least three quality control measurements closely related to the quality of refined oatmeal.

22. List at least three quality control measurements closely related to the quality of decorticated sorghum.

23. What is the general effect of the different dry-milling processes on the nutraceutical properties of cereals? Which important phytochemicals or nutraceutical compounds are partially lost during milling?

REFERENCES

American Association of Cereal Chemists (AACC). 2000. *AACC Approved Methods of Analysis.* 10th ed. St. Paul, MN: AACC.

Amato, G. W., and S. Silveira. 1991. *Parbolizacao do Arroz no Brasil.* Porto Alegre, Brasil: Fundacao de Ciencia e Tecnologia. Governo do Estado do Rio Gande do Sul.

Barber, S., and C. Benedicto de Barber. 1976. "An Approach to the Objective Measurement of the Degree of Milling." *Rice Process Engineering Center Report* 2(2):1.

Battacharya, K. R. 1985. "Parboiling of Rice." In *Rice: Chemistry and Technology*, edited by B. O. Juliano. St. Paul, MN: American Association of Cereal Chemists.

Bloksma, A. H., and W. Bushuk. 1988. "Rheology and Chemistry of Dough." In *Wheat Chemistry and Technology*, vol. 2, edited by Y. Pomeranz. St. Paul, MN: American Association of Cereal Chemists.

Codină G. G., S. Mironeasa, D. Bordei, and A. Leahu. 2010. "Mixolab versus Alveograph and Falling Number." *Czech Journal of Food Sciences* 28(3):185–191.

D'Appolonia, B. L., and W. H. Kunerth. 1984. *The Farinograph Handbook.* 3rd ed. St. Paul, MN: American Association of Cereal Chemists.

Doehlert, D. C., and W. R. Moore. 1997. "Composition of Oat Bran and Flour Prepared by Three Different Mechanisms of Dry-Milling." *Cereal Chemistry* 74:403–406.

Doehlert, D., and M. S. McMullen. 2000. "Genotypic and Environmental Effects on Oat Milling Characteristics and Groat Hardness." *Cereal Chemistry* 77(2):148–154.

Doehlert, D. C., M. S. McMullen, and R. R. Baumann. 1999. "Factors Affecting Groat Percentage in Oat." *Crop Science* 39:1858–1865.

Dubat, A. 2010. "The New AACC International Approved Method to Measure Rheological Properties of a Dough Sample." *Cereal Foods World* 55(3):150–153.

Dubois, M., A. Dubat, and B. Launay. 2008. *The Alveo Consistograph Handbook.* 2nd ed. AACC International, St. Paul, MN.

Duensing, W. J., A. B. Roskens, and R. J. Alexander. 2003. "Corn Dry-Milling: Processes, Products, and Applications." In *Corn Chemistry and Technology*, 2nd ed., edited by P. J. White and L. A. Johnson. St. Paul, MN: American Association of Cereal Chemists.

Faridi, H., V. F. Rasper, and B. Launay. 1987. *The Alveograph Handbook*. St. Paul, MN: American Association of Cereal Chemists.

Finney, K. F., and M. D. Shogren. 1972. "A Ten Gram Mixograph for Determining and Predicting Functional Properties of Wheat Flours." *Bakers Digest* 46(2):32–35,38–42,77.

Halverson, J., and L. Zeleny. 1988. "Criteria of Wheat Quality." In *Wheat Chemistry and Technology*, vol. 1, edited by Y. Pomeranz. St. Paul, MN: American Association of Cereal Chemists.

Juliano, B. O. 1971. "A Simplified Assay for Milled Rice Amylose." *Cereal Science Today* 16:34.

Juliano, B. O. 1985. *Rice: Chemistry and Technology*. American Association of Cereal Chemists: St. Paul, MN.

Mailhot, W. C., and J. C. Patton. 1988. "Criteria of Flour Quality." In *Wheat Chemistry and Technology*. vol. 2, edited by Y. Pomeranz. St. Paul, MN: American Association of Cereal Chemists.

Munck, L. 1995. "New Milling Technologies and Products: Whole Plant Utilization by Milling and Separation of the Botanical and Chemical Components." In *Sorghum and Millets: Chemistry and Technology*, edited by D. A. V. Dendy. St. Paul, MN: American Association of Cereal Chemists.

Oomah, B. D., and R. D. Reichert. 1981. "A Novel, Multisample, Tangential Abrasive Dehulling Device (TADD)." *Cereal Chemistry* 58:392.

Peplinski, A. J., R. A. Anderson, and S. R. Eckhoff. 1984. "A Dry-Milling Evaluation of Trickle Sulfur Dioxide Treated Corn." *Cereal Chemistry* 61:289.

Posner, E. S., and A. N. Hibbs. 1997. *Wheat Flour Milling*. St. Paul, MN: American Association of Cereal Chemists.

Rasper, V. F., and K. R. Preston. 1991. *The Extensigraph Handbook*. St. Paul, MN: American Association of Cereal Chemists.

Rasper, V. F., and C. E. Walker. 2000. "Quality Evaluation of Cereals and Cereal Products." In *Handbook of Cereal Science and Technology*, edited by K. Kulp and J. G. Ponte. New York: Marcel Dekker, Inc.

Rath, C. R., P. W. Gras, C. W. Wrigley, and C. E. Walker. 1990. "Evaluation of Dough Properties from Two Grams of Flour Using the Mixograph Principle. *Cereal Foods World* 35(6):572–574.

Reichert, R. D. 1982. "Dry-Milling." In *Sorghum in the Eighties. Proceedings of the International Symposium on Sorghum*, 547–563. Pachanteru, India: ICISAT.

Rooney, L. W., and S. O. Serna-Saldivar. 2000. "Sorghum." In *Handbook of Cereal Science and Technology*, 2nd ed., edited by K. Kulp and J. G. Ponte. New York: Marcel Dekker, Inc.

Scheuring, J. F., and L. W. Rooney. 1979. "A Staining Procedure to Determine the Extent of Bran Removal in Pearled Sorghum." *Cereal Chemistry* 56:545.

Serna-Saldivar, S. O., H. D. Almeida Dominguez, M. H. Gomez, A. J. Gomez, A. J. Bockholt, and L. W. Rooney. 1991. "Method to Evaluate Ease of Pericarp Removal on Lime-Cooked Corn Kernels." *Crop Science* 31:842–844.

Shuey, W. C., and K. H. Tipples. 1982. *The Amylograph Handbook*. St. Paul, MN: American Association of Cereal Chemists.

Thomas, D. J., and W. A. Atwell. 1999. *Straches*. St. Paul, MN: Eagan Press.

Walker, C. E., J. L. Hazelton, and M. D. Shogren. 1997. *The Mixograph Handbook*. Lincoln, NE: National Manufacturing Division, TMCO.

Young, R., M. Haidara, L. W. Rooney, and R. D. Waniska. 1990. "Parboiled Sorghum: Development of a Novel Decorticated Product." *Journal of Cereal Science* 11:227–289.

Zeleny, L. 1947. "A Simple Sedimentation Test for Estimating the Bread-Baking and Gluten Qualitites of Wheat Flour." *Cereal Chemistry* 24:465.

Zobel, H. F. 1984. Gelatinization of starch and mechanical properties of starch pastes. In *Starch Chemistry and Technology*, 2nd ed., edited by R. L. Whisler, J. N. Bemiller, and E. F. Paschall. San Diego, CA: Academic Press.

6 Wet-Milling Processes and Starch Properties and Characteristics

6.1 INTRODUCTION

One of the most significant uses of cereals is as a raw material for the production of refined starches. The various types of wet-milling industries aim toward the extraction of the maximum possible amount of native or undamaged starch granules. By far, maize is the main source of all the refined starch in the world because of its availability, relatively low cost, high starch content, and the value of its by-products such as gluten, germ, bran, and steep solids. It is estimated that more than 80% of the world's starch comes from maize and most of this output is bioconverted into an array of sweeteners, biofuels, and potable alcohol (which is covered in Chapter 14 of the textbook). The aim of the various starch milling industries is to obtain the highest possible yield of native starch that meets specifications for color, functional properties, and maximum amount of protein. The starch is further modified to obtain starches with different functionalities or bioconverted into an array of syrups or, in some instances, fermented into bioethanol. In the particular case of wheat, the goal of the wet-milling industry is the production of both vital gluten and refined starch. The first is in high demand by the baking industry to upgrade bread quality especially when processing whole wheat products. Starches from regular and waxy maize and wheat are the preferred and most frequently industrially used. These starches have different amylograph properties, pasting behaviors, and functionalities; therefore, they are frequently used to impart different characteristics to cereal-based foods.

6.2 WET-MILLING PROCESSES

6.2.1 WET-MILLING OF MAIZE

Most of the industrially produced starch is obtained from yellow dent maize. The optimum grain physical properties for wet-milling are soft textured dent kernels with test weights of 67.5 kg/hL and thousand kernel weights greater than 300 g. These kernels contain higher amounts of starch and their starch granules are easier to extract. In addition, the soft endosperm structure kernels hydrate faster during the critical step of steeping, which is considered as the bottleneck of the process. The industry also selects those lots of sound grains with high thousand kernel weight because they favor the ratio of endosperm to germ and pericarp (Johnson and May 2003; May 1987; Serna-Saldivar 2008; Watson 1984). Yellow-colored grains are preferred because they generally cost less and favor the production of highly pigmented gluten demanded by the poultry and feed industries.

After cleaning the grain with air aspirators to remove dust, chaff, and other light particles and screening to remove pieces of cob, sand, stones, and other undesirable extraneous material, kernels are steeped in a warm solution (48–50°C) containing 0.1% to 0.2% sulfur dioxide. This reducing agent softens the endosperm structure, avoids germination, and promotes the development and growth of the *Lactobacillus* bacteria. The synergistic effects of the sulfur dioxide treatment and the proteolytic action of the bacteria break disulfide bonds, weakening the protein matrix that engulfs the starch granules. The sulfur dioxide steeping operation is carried countercurrently so that the oldest sulfur dioxide solution rich in *Lactobacillus* treats the new incoming kernels whereas the new and stronger solution is used to treat the exiting kernels. Steeping usually lasts from 30 to 48 hours. During this time, the grain with original moisture of 12% to 14% gradually absorbs the sodium bisulfite solution increasing the moisture to 48% to 50%. Most of the sulfur dioxide solution is absorbed during the first 15 hours of steeping. During steeping, approximately 5% to 7% of kernel solids are solubilized. These solids, rich in albumins and globulins, lactic acid, minerals, phytic acid, and B vitamin kernels, are concentrated and used in the pharmaceutical industries. Industrially, the steeped kernels are wet-ground in plate or disc attrition mills equipped with pins that counterrotate at speeds of up to 1800 rpm. During this first milling step, the kernel is coarsely ground to release the germ. The ground particles diluted in water are transported into a series of hydrocyclones to separate the less dense rubbery germ from the rest of the kernel components (Johnson and May 2003; May 1987; Serna-Saldivar 2008; Watson 1984; Eckhoff et al. 1993, 1996).

The denser endosperm chunks still associated with pericarp tissue are milled in an entoleter or impact mill to release the pericarp in flakes. These fiber-rich pieces are separated in a metal sieve. The endosperm particles that passed the sieve are milled into a fine slurry with plate or attrition disc mills equipped with more pins and operated in such a way so as to release the starch granules from the protein matrix with minimal mechanical damage. The next steps are aimed at separating the less dense gluten from the denser starch granules. This is accomplished by first passing the starch–gluten slurry in a series of continuous centrifuges followed by a secondary purification using a series of hydrocyclones. Most of the protein or gluten is removed in the centrifuges but these yield starch with 2.5% to 5% residual protein. The rest of the protein or gluten is removed in hydrocyclones so that, at the end of the process, the starch contains less than 0.35% protein. The resulting refined starch is continuously dehydrated in drying tunnels to decrease its moisture to approximately 6%. The gluten stream is first dewatered in basket centrifuges, concentrated with a vacuum filter, and dehydrated to 12% moisture in rotary or drum driers (Watson 1984). The yields of prime starch and gluten meal from unclean maize are approximately 61% and 12%, respectively.

The wet-milling of maize yields solids that are rich in nutrients which are generally used by pharmaceutical industries as growth media for molds and other microorganisms in the production of antibiotics and related products. Other coproducts are the germ, which is generally used by the oil industry to obtain crude and refined oil, the protein meal (the pericarp), which is commonly used by the feed industry, and the gluten rich in yellow carotenoids, which is highly demanded by the poultry industry.

6.2.1.1 Laboratory Wet-Milling Process of Maize

Many laboratory procedures for simulating wet-milled maize have been developed during the past decades (Johnson and May 2003; Eckhoff et al. 1993). Most of these procedures are based on the classic sodium bisulfite laboratory wet-milling procedure developed by Watson et al. (1951). The basic steps of the various laboratory and pilot plant milling assays are steeping in sodium bisulfite and lactic acid solution, milling of the steeped kernels, and then, separation and drying of the milled fractions. The procedures are useful because they are relatively fast, require small amounts of grain, and the recovery of the starch is very reproducible. Nowadays, the Eckhoff et al. (1996) wet-milling procedure is recognized as the standard method. Continuous countercurrent steeping systems have been developed for use in the laboratory (Steinke et al. 1991; Johnson and May 2003) to emulate commercial operations. These methods allow the recovery of prime and tail starches and coproducts (fiber, germ, and gluten) that are further characterized (i.e., color, residual protein content, viscoamylograph properties).

A. Samples, Ingredients, and Reagents
- Yellow dent maize
- Sodium bisulfite
- Lactic acid
- Distilled water

B. Materials and Equipment
- Air aspirator
- Clipper with maize-cleaning sieves
- Digital scale
- Level
- Ruler with millimeter markings
- Peristaltic pump
- Stirrer
- Thermometer
- Glass containers (1-L capacity) with lids
- Laboratory blender
- Sieves (nos. 40, 60, and 80 and collection pan)
- Stainless steel sedimentation table (3 m long)
- Volumetric flasks (1 L)
- Beakers (400 mL)
- Graduated cylinder (1 L)
- Incubator (50°C)
- Buchner flask
- Buchner funnel
- Filter paper for Buchner funnel
- Plastic buckets
- Aluminum dishes for moisture determination
- Drying containers or sheets
- Convection oven

C. Procedure
1. Place the 3-m-long stainless steel sedimentation table on a surface and position the table with an angle of exactly 0.7 degrees. Check that the table is leveled.
2. Clean the lot of grain, preferably with an air aspirator and clipper furnished with maize cleaning sieves. Alternatively, manually clean the lot of maize.
3. Determine the cleaned maize's physical (test weight, thousand kernel weight, and density) and chemical composition (moisture, proximate composition, and starch content).
4. Prepare the steeping solution by mixing 1.48 g of sodium bisulfite and 4.7 mL of 85% lactic acid per liter of distilled water.
5. Weigh 500 g of maize (dry weight) and place kernels in a glass container. Add 1 L of the steeping solution and place the container's lid.
6. Steep kernels for 48 hours at 50°C in an incubator. The steeping time can vary according to grain properties. If you want to create a water uptake curve, sample the steeped kernels for moisture determination after 0.5, 1, 2, 4, 8, 16, 24, 32, and 48 hours.
7. After steeping, recuperate the steeping solution and measure its exact volume and the amount of suspended solids.
8. Weigh the steeped maize kernels and sample kernels for moisture determination.
9. Place steeped kernels in a laboratory blender with blunt blades and add an equal weight of distilled water. Mill kernels for 2 minutes at low speed (Figure 6.1).
10. Place ground contents on a U.S. no. 40 mesh sieve. The overs are returned to the blender and mixed with 500 mL of distilled water for 1 minute of additional grinding at medium speed. Repeat the procedure and collect the overs, which are considered the fiber-bran and germ fraction. Place this fraction in a convection oven set at 60°C for drying. Collect all the throughs for further processing.
11. Place the throughs in the blender for 2 minutes of grinding at high speed.
12. Separate the fine bran by sieving through a U.S. no. 80 sieve or alternatively through a U.S. no.

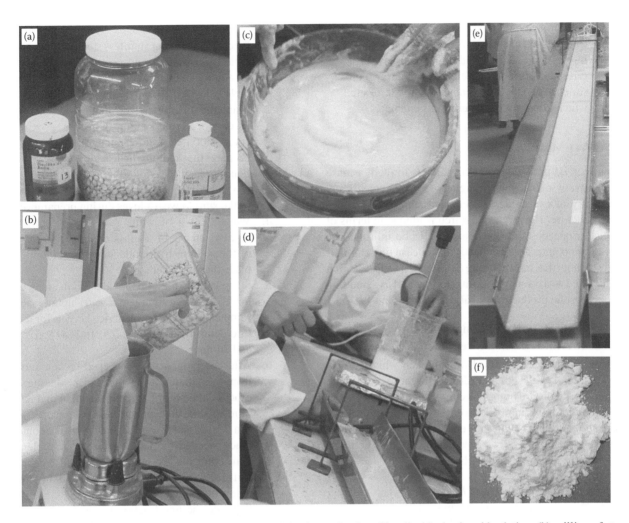

FIGURE 6.1 Laboratory maize wet-milling procedure. (a) Steeping maize in sulfur dioxide–lactic acid solution; (b) milling of steeped maize kernels; (c) sieve separation of fiber from gluten-starch suspension; (d) pumping starch-gluten suspension onto the separation table; (e) separation of starch from gluten in the sloping table; (f) dried and ground starch.

100 mesh sieve. The throughs are considered the starch/gluten suspension.

13. Allow gluten and starch solids to decant for 30 minutes. Carefully remove approximately half of the volume and save the other half for washing.

14. Place the gluten starch suspension in a container for tabling (Figure 6.1). Keep solids suspended with a stirrer and then adjust peristaltic pump to deliver 100 mL/min through the sedimentation table. Place a bucket at the end of the table to recuperate the gluten suspension. During the first stages of pumping, make sure to distribute the suspension in a crisscross pattern along the front of the sedimentation table to facilitate the sedimentation of the starch. Pump all the suspension and then add the rest of the water volume from step 13 for the first step of starch washing. Pump all the wash water first and then again pump 250 mL of distilled water (second washing step).

15. Allow sedimented solids to partially dehydrate at room temperature for 2 to 12 hours. Collect all the sedimented starch of the first 270 cm of the table and label as prime starch. Then, collect the remaining 30 cm and label as tailings or low-grade starch.

16. Filter the contents of the bucket to recuperate the gluten solids with a Buchner flask, funnel, and filter paper operating under vacuum.

17. Dehydrate the prime starch, starch tailings, and gluten for 8 hours in a convection oven set at 50°C.

18. Remove the samples from the oven and allow to cool down and equilibrate for 30 minutes at room temperature. Then, weigh the partially dehydrated samples and determine residual moisture.

19. Calculate yields of prime starch, starch tailings, gluten, fiber-germ, and steep solids.

20. Grind samples to determine chemical composition. For the specific case of prime starch,

determine color (Chapter 3), residual protein (procedure in Section 2.2.3.1), ash (procedure in Section 2.2.2.1), and functional properties (viscoamylograph, differential scanning calorimetry or DSC, percentage of amylase, etc.), which are described later in this chapter.

6.2.2 WET-MILLING OF RICE

The commercial production of rice starch is limited because of the relatively high cost of rice relative to other cereals and the difficulty of extracting the starch because of the endosperm's structure. However, rice starch is unique in terms of functional properties and functionalities. Upon milling, rice produces compound starch granules that release tiny angular-shaped subunits that only measure 3 μm to 10 μm. Rice starch is mainly used as a cosmetic dusting powder and as a pudding especially for the production of baby foods (Juliano 1984).

6.2.2.1 Laboratory Wet-Milling Procedure of White Polished Rice

Most rice starches are obtained from broken white kernels which are treated with sodium hydroxide because most of the endosperm proteins are high-molecular weight glutelins. The alkali enhances the solubilization of the endosperm proteins and the softening of the vitreous endosperm (Juliano 1984). The broken rice is generally steeped at 50°C for 24 hours in a weak alkali solution (0.3–0.5% NaOH).

A. *Samples, Ingredients, and Reagents*
- White rice (whole or broken kernels)
- Sodium hydroxide (NaOH)
- Distilled water

B. *Materials and Equipment*
- Scale
- Level
- Ruler with millimeter markings
- Peristaltic pump
- Stirrer
- Thermometer
- Glass containers (1 L capacity) with lids
- Laboratory blender
- Set of sieves (U.S. no. 80)
- Stainless steel sedimentation table (3 m long)
- Volumetric flasks (1 L)
- Colander
- Graduated cylinder (1 L)
- Incubator (50°C)
- Buchner flask
- Buchner funnel
- Filter paper for Buchner funnel
- Plastic buckets
- Aluminum dishes for moisture determination
- Drying containers or sheets
- Convection oven
- Plastic laboratory gloves

C. *Procedure*
1. Place the 3-m-long stainless steel sedimentation table on a surface and position the table with an angle of exactly 0.7 degrees. Check that the table is leveled.
2. Manually clean the rice sample and determine its chemical composition (moisture, proximate composition, and starch content).
3. Prepare the sodium hydroxide steeping solution by placing 4 g of sodium hydroxide in a 1 L volumetric flask containing distilled water. Make sure to wear gloves during preparation.
4. Weigh 500 g of white rice (dry weight) and place contents in a glass container. Add 1 L of the sodium hydroxide steeping solution and place the container's lid.
5. Steep kernels for 24 hours at 50°C in an incubator. If you want to create a water uptake curve, sample the steeped broken rice kernels for moisture determination after 0.5, 1, 2, 4, 8, 12, 16, and 24 hours.
6. After steeping, separate steeped broken kernels from the solution using a colander. Measure the exact volume of the steeping solution and determine its solid content and weigh the steeped broken kernels and determine their moisture content.
7. Place steeped kernels in a laboratory blender with blunt blades and add an equal weight of distilled water. Mill kernels for 2 and 3 minutes at low and high speed, respectively.
8. Separate the fine fraction by sieving through a U.S. no. 80 sieve or, alternatively, through a U.S. no. 100 mesh sieve. The overs can be ground with distilled water for 2 more minutes in the blender and resifted. Collect the overs, place them in a container for dehydration at 50°C for 8 hours. The throughs are considered the starch/protein suspension.
9. In a bucket, collect and place the throughs or starch/protein suspension and allow to decant for 30 minutes. Carefully remove approximately half of the volume. Save the other half for washing.
10. Place the starch-protein suspension in a container for tabling. Keep solids suspended with a stirrer and then adjust peristaltic pump to deliver 100 mL/min through the sedimentation table. Place a bucket at the end of the table to recuperate the protein suspension. During the first stages of pumping, make sure to distribute the suspension in a crisscross pattern along the front of the sedimentation table to facilitate the sedimentation of the starch. Pump all the suspension and then add the rest of the water volume from step 11 for the first step of washing. Pump all the wash water first and then again pump 250 mL of distilled water (second washing step).

11. Allow sedimented solids to partially dehydrate at room temperature for 2 to 12 hours. Collect all the sedimented starch of the first 270 cm of the table and label as prime starch. Then, collect the remaining 30 cm and label as tailings or low-grade starch.

12. Filter the contents of the bucket to recuperate the protein solids with a Buchner flask, funnel, and filter paper operating under vacuum.

13. Dehydrate the prime starch, starch tailings, and protein for 8 hours in a convection oven set at 50°C.

14. Remove samples from the oven and allow samples to cool down and equilibrate for 30 minutes at room temperature. Then, weigh the partially dehydrated samples and determine residual moisture.

15. Calculate yields of prime starch, starch tailings, protein, and steep solids.

16. Grind samples to determine chemical composition. For the specific case of prime starch, determine color (Chapter 3), residual protein (procedure in Section 2.2.3.1), ash (procedure in Section 2.2.2.1), and functional properties (viscoamylograph, DSC, percentage of amylase, etc.) described later in this chapter.

6.2.3 WET-MILLING OF WHEAT AND VITAL GLUTEN PRODUCTION

Wheat wet-milling is usually performed with two main goals: the production of prime starch and vital gluten. Wheat starch has analogous uses as maize starch whereas vital gluten is a food additive widely used in the baking and meat processing industries. There are several industrial processes to obtain wheat starch. The most important is the denominated Martin process, which is aimed toward the production of vital gluten and starch (Knight and Olson 1984). Other less relevant processes are the Halle, Fesca, and acid methods (Cornell and Hoveling 1998; Knight and Olson 1984).

The Martin process is the most practiced method of obtaining wheat starch. This method uses wheat flour as a raw material and starts when the flour is mixed with water to form a dough which is further washed with water to obtain starch and vital gluten. The resulting prime starch and wet gluten are dewatered and dehydrated to decrease its moisture content to approximately 10%. The Martin, or dough ball, process yields approximately 65% starch and 14% vital gluten (Knight and Olson 1984).

A similar process is the Alfa Laval/Raiso method, in which wheat flour is blended with water and the resulting dough screened and passed through a splitter decanter that separates the starch from the gluten. The advantage of this system is the savings in the consumption of water (Cornell and Hoveling 1998).

6.2.3.1 Wet-Milling Laboratory Procedure for Wheat Flour

The Martin process is the most practiced way of obtaining wheat starch. This method uses wheat flour as a raw material and starts when the flour is mixed with water in a 2:1 ratio to form a dough. Hard wheat flours require more water compared with lower protein flours. The flour and water are mixed and kneaded until a uniform, consistent, properly developed, and smooth dough is attained. The starch is extracted by simply washing the dough with water. The washing step gradually releases the starch granules without breaking the gluten into small particles. The industry uses several washing devices, such as a rotary drum, mixers with twin screws, and mixers equipped with a couple of sigma blades that counterrotate at different speeds. Regardless of the equipment, the water extracts most of the starch granules and some soluble proteins (albumins and globulins). The insoluble part stays on the screens and consists mainly of wet gluten (prolamins or gliadins and glutelins). Excess gluten water is removed by compression through a pair of rolls and the resulting gluten dehydrated to 8% to 10% moisture in vacuum or drum driers. The starch suspension with approximately 10% solids is first passed through a set of vibrating screens to remove small pieces of gluten and other contaminants. The denser starch is easily separated from contaminants such as soluble proteins with continuous centrifuges or hydrocyclones. The resulting starch is dewatered and dried to decrease its moisture content to approximately 10%. The industrial specification for prime wheat starch does not allow more than 0.3% protein (Knight and Olson 1984).

A. *Samples, Ingredients, and Reagents*
  - Refined wheat flour
  - Distilled water

B. *Materials and Equipment*
  - Digital scale
  - Level
  - Ruler with millimeter markings
  - Peristaltic pump
  - Stirrer
  - Squeeze bottle (1 L)
  - Dough mixer with hook attachment
  - Mixing bowl
  - Set of sieves (U.S. nos. 80 and 100)
  - Stainless steel sedimentation table (3 m long)
  - Volumetric flasks (1 L)
  - Graduated cylinder (1 L)
  - Plastic buckets
  - Aluminum dishes for moisture determination
  - Drying containers or sheets
  - Convection oven

C. *Procedure*
  1. Place the 3-m-long stainless steel sedimentation table on a surface and position the table with

an angle of exactly 0.7 degrees. Check that the table is leveled.

2. Determine the chemical composition of the refined wheat flour (moisture, proximate composition, and starch content).

3. Weigh 500 g of wheat flour (dry weight) and place it in a mixing bowl. Add 250 mL of water and start blending at low speed for 1 minute. Then, change speed to medium and mix contents until dough development is attained. The dough should be cohesive and taut. Record the weight of the resulting dough.

4. Place dough in a wide container with 3 L of water and allow dough to rest for 30 minutes.

5. After dough soaking, massage the dough ball for 5 minutes (while avoiding the loss of solids). Allow gluten to soak for an additional 10 minutes and repeat the massaging procedure. Reserve the suspension for further processing.

6. Place the remaining gluten on a U.S. no. 60 mesh sieve positioned on top of a bucket. Wash gluten with 1 L of water placed in a squeeze bottle. Keep rubbing the wet gluten on the sieve while delivering the water. If the wash water still has a white-milky appearance, repeat the procedure.

7. Mix the wash water with the starch suspension of step 5. Pass the suspension through a U.S. no. 80 sieve and collect and mix the overs with the gluten mass.

8. Weigh and place gluten in a drying container. Disrupt the gluten mass for better dehydration at 50°C for 8 hours.

9. Place the starch-rich suspension in a container for tabling. Keep solids suspended with a stirrer and then adjust peristaltic pump to deliver 100 mL/min through the sedimentation table. Place a bucket at the end of the table to recuperate soluble protein and sugars. During the first stages of pumping, make sure to distribute the suspension in a crisscross pattern along the front of the sedimentation table to facilitate the sedimentation of the starch. Pump all the suspension and then wash sedimented starch with 0.5 L of distilled water.

10. Allow sedimented starch solids to partially dehydrate at room temperature for 2 to 12 hours. Collect the starch of the first 270 cm of the table and label as prime wheat starch. Then, collect the remaining 30 cm and label as tailings or low-grade starch.

11. Filter the contents of the bucket to recuperate the protein solids with a Buchner flask, funnel, and filter paper operating under vacuum.

12. Dehydrate the prime starch, starch tailings, and soluble solids for 8 hours in a convection oven set at 50°C.

13. Remove samples from the oven and allow samples to cool down and equilibrate for 30 minutes at room temperature. Then, weigh the partially dehydrated samples and determine residual moisture.

14. Calculate yields of vital gluten, prime starch, starch tailings, and soluble solids.

15. Grind samples to determine chemical composition and functional properties. For the specific case of vital gluten, determine residual moisture, protein content, and chemical composition. For the prime starch, determine color (Chapter 3), residual protein (procedure in Section 2.2.3.1), ash (procedure in Section 2.2.2.1), and functional properties (viscoamylograph, DSC, percentage of amylase, etc.) described later in this chapter.

6.2.4 RESEARCH SUGGESTIONS

1. Using the conventional wet-milling procedure, mill three different and contrasting types of maize (white regular with intermediate to hard endosperm texture, yellow maize with soft endosperm texture, and a waxy yellow maize). Determine the moisture content of the steeped kernels after 48 hours, yields of prime starch and protein content of the starch. In addition, compare the viscoamylograph properties of the different starches (procedures in Sections 6.4.1.1 or 6.4.1.2) and the chemical and color properties of the gluten meal.

2. Compare wet-milling processes of preground maize steeped with sulfur dioxide, sulfur dioxide supplemented with cell wall–degrading enzymes, and sulfur dioxide supplemented with a protease after 24 and 48 hours of steeping at 50°C. Determine prime starch and protein contents of the starch. In addition, compare the viscoamylograph properties of the different starches (procedures in Sections 6.4.1.1 or 6.4.1.2).

3. Compare wet-milling yields of two contrasting refined wheat flours; one from a soft wheat (7–8.5% protein) and the other from a hard wheat (10.5–13% protein) following the Martin process. Determine yields of prime starch and vital gluten and the protein contents of these products. Then, compare the viscoamylograph properties of the two starches (procedures in Sections 6.4.1.1 or 6.4.1.2).

4. Using the laboratory rice wet-milling procedure, compare starch yields of a regular endosperm white rice (25% amylose and 75% amylopectin) and a waxy rice (>95% amylopectin). Determine protein contents and amylose of the starches and compare their viscoamylograph properties (procedures in Sections 6.4.1.1 or 6.4.1.2).

5. Using the International Development Research Center or abrasive decorticator, mill three different and contrasting types of sorghums (white hard-textured, white soft-textured, and a white waxy sorghum). Determine

the grain physical properties and the optimum decortication time to remove 20% of the sorghum weight and the yield of decorticated kernels. Then, process the whole and decorticated sorghums following the laboratory maize wet-milling procedure. Determine the moisture content of the steeped kernels after 48 hours, yields of prime starch, and protein content of the starch. In addition, compare the viscoamylograph properties of the different sorghum starches with that of maize (procedures in Section 6.4.1.1 or 6.4.1.2).

6.2.5 RESEARCH QUESTIONS

1. Define the following terms used in wet-milling operations:
   a. Sulfur dioxide
   b. Hydrocyclon
   c. Prime starch
   d. Waxy starch
   e. Native starch
   f. Gluten feed
   g. Vital gluten
   h. Martin process
   i. Steep liquor
2. Compare maize, rice, and wheat wet-milling processes and products.
3. What are the main grain physical factors that affect sodium bisulfite steeping requirements?
4. What are the effects of sulfur dioxide on maize milling operations? Why does the lactic acid generated by *Lactobacillus* act synergistically with the sulfur dioxide?
5. How much dry matter is commonly lost during conventional sulfur dioxide steeping? What kind of chemical compounds are mainly lost? What is the industrial use for these solids?
6. What is the typical oil content of maize germ obtained in wet-milling operations? Why does this germ contain more oil compared with germ obtained from dry-milling operations?
7. What are the physical properties of maize grain that favor starch yield and quality of by-products? Why is most of the world's starch obtained from maize?
8. During maize wet-milling, an array of products and by-products are obtained. What are their main uses?
9. What is considered the most critical or important operation in maize wet-milling operations? Why?
10. In a flowchart, describe the milling steps commonly used to produce wheat starch and vital gluten.
11. Why is it necessary to temper or condition rice with a weak sodium hydroxide solution before wet-milling? What are the main and industrial uses of rice starch?
12. Describe how continuous centrifuges and hydroclones work in milling operations.
13. What are viscoamylograph differences among maize, wheat, and rice starches?

6.3 MORPHOLOGHY AND DYEING OF STARCHES

Starch granules contain linear and branched molecules called amylose and amylopectin, respectively. Amylose is essentially a linear polymer composed of glucose units linked with α1-4 glycosidic bonds whereas amylopectin also has several α1-6 glycosidic bonds. In amylopectin, only 4% to 5% of the total glycosidic bonds are α1-6. Amylose is usually composed of approximately 1500 glucose units, whereas amylopectin is a larger molecule containing up to 600,000 glucose units. The ratio of amylose/amylopectin in regular starches is generally 25:75, whereas in waxy starches, it is more than 95% amylopectin. Although amylose is called a linear starch, the molecule forms helixes. The helicoidal conformation allows amylose to complex with iodine, free fatty acids, alcohols, and emulsifiers. One important characteristic of amylose is that it stains purple with iodine and is the most important molecule related to retrogradation and the formation of cohesive gels (Serna-Saldivar 2008).

Native starch granules are water-insoluble and swell reversibly when placed in water. The most important feature of native starches is that they show birefringence when exposed to the polarized light plane. This phenomenon occurs because of the high organization within starch granules that make these structures behave like pseudocrystals. As indicated previously, amylopectin is the predominant starch molecule and is much larger than amylose. Because of its larger size and more complex structure, amylopectin stains brownish red with iodine. Amylopectin has a low retrogradation and forms weak and sticky gels (Martinez and Prodoliet 1996; Shelton and Lee 2000; Shuey and Tipples 1982; Snyder 1984; Zobel 1984).

There are various methods used to quantify the total starch content in foods. In most of these assays, the starch is first gelatinized and then enzymatically hydrolyzed into glucose that is colorimetrically assayed after reaction with glucose oxidase, peroxidase, and dihydrochloride *o*-dianasidine (refer to Chapter 2).

The ratio between amylose and amylopectin is critically important because it greatly affects the functionality of starch. Amylose is usually quantified by iodine colorimetric assays in which iodine binds with amylose to produce a blue-colored complex that is read in a spectrophotometer, whereas amylopectins are calculated by difference. Native starch is usually quantified by birefringence by observing the amount of starch granules showing the typical Maltese cross under a microscope equipped with a polarized filter. Starch damage is based on the susceptibility of the starch to α-amylase and β-amylase (or both) and amyloglucosidases. Undamaged starch granules are resistant to β-amylase whereas damaged counterparts are attacked at a measurable rate. One accepted and quick method to determine starch damage, mainly associated with wheat flour, is the falling number assay [American Association of Cereal Chemists (AACC) 2000; Method 56-81B]. The test is based on the principle that heat-damaged or enzymatically damaged (sprouted) wheat flours that are hydrated and thermally treated generate lower viscosities compared with undamaged flours. The instrument is named falling number because it measures the time it takes for a plunger to move through the viscous gelatinized slurry. The longer it takes, the more viscous the slurry is, and the less damaged the starch is in the originally presented sample.

6.3.1 Starch Granule Morphology and Dyeing Techniques

The starch associated with cereal grains is tightly packed within a granular structure that, in its native form, presents quasicrystalline, water-insoluble, and dense properties. Starch granules range in size and shape from nearly perfect spheres typical of small wheat granules, disc-shaped granules of wheat and rye, to polyhedral forms in rice and maize. The morphology of starch granules is dictated by the particular structure and biochemistry of the starch-synthesizing organelle known as chloroplast or amyloplast. Most mature starch granules show concentric "growth rings" which are shells of alternating high and low refractive index. At the center of the granule is the original growing point botanically known as the *hilum*. The starch granules from oats and rice are compound because they contain many subgranules which appear to have developed simultaneously within a single amyloplast (Bechtel 1983; Bewley and Black 1978; French 1984).

The different types of cereal grains contain different starch compositions and functionalities. The waxy genotypes contain more than 95% amylopectin, and consequently, different functional properties such as gelatinization, gellation, retrogradation, and synerisis. There are many quick dyeing tests used to differentiate waxy from regular starch, identify pregelatinized starches, and if a processed product such as beer wort still has some nonhydrolyzed starch. The most common dye is iodine. This halogen compound has the property of binding to the inside of the starch helix, forming a hydrophobic clathrate. Structurally speaking, the linear starch or amylose reacts more readily with iodine compared with branched amylopectin. The amylose forms a purple-colored compound whereas amylopectin forms a red-brownish compound. The action of α-amylases on starch produces a very rapid decrease in iodine color, thus, the iodine test is widely used to determine the degree of starch hydrolysis during mashing in the brewing industry.

As mentioned previously, the internal structure or architecture of native starch granules is very well organized. It is characterized by the presence of amorphous and crystalline zones. Because of this internal organization, all native starch granules show birefringence when viewed under polarized light. The starch granules lose birefringence or the Maltese cross when chemically, physically, or enzymatically damaged. These starch granules stain red when treated with Congo red dye, whereas the native counterparts remain colorless (Khurana et al. 2001; Lamb and Loy 2005).

One of the most important characteristics of the various types of starch is the gelatinization temperature. The birefringence end-point temperature (BEPT) is a polarizing microscopy test in which hydrated starch granules are gradually heated to estimate the temperatures at which granules start to lose birefringence and the end-point temperature at which 95% of the granules lose the Maltese cross.

6.3.1.1 Iodine Dye Test

When starch is mixed with iodine in solution, an intensely dark blue color develops because of the formation of starch-iodine complex. The Lugol solution is a solution of elemental iodine and potassium iodide in water. This iodine-based reagent is widely used in cereal chemistry for the detection of starch. This solution is used as an indicator test for the presence of starches in organic compounds. A blue-black color results if starch is present. If amylose is not present, then the color will stay orange or yellow. Starch amylopectin does not produce the color, nor does cellulose or disaccharides such as sucrose. Elemental iodine will stain starches because of iodine's interaction with the internal helicoidal structure of amylose. Because of the structural differences between amylose and amylopectin, the iodine will stain linear starch blue or purple whereas the branched starch or amylopectin stains purple or red.

> A. *Samples, Ingredients, and Reagents*
>   - Different types of starches
>   - Different types of bisected cereal grains
>   - Elemental iodine
>   - Potassium iodide
>   - Distilled water
> B. *Materials and Equipment*
>   - Digital scale
>   - Laboratory clock or chronometer
>   - Dark bottles
>   - Drop dispenser bottle
>   - Beaker (200 mL)
>   - Volumetric flask (500 mL)
>   - Spatula
> C. *Procedure*
>   1. Prepare the iodine stain solution by mixing 1 g of elemental iodine and 10 g of potassium iodide. Place both reagents in a 500 mL volumetric flask and add distilled water to approximately three-fourths of the volume. Shake contents until the reagents completely dissolve and then add water to the 500 mL mark. Transfer dye solution to a dark bottle.
>   2. Place iodine solution in a drop dispenser bottle and add a few drops onto regular, waxy, and high-amylose starches or directly onto the exposed endosperm of different types of bisected cereal grains.
>   3. Observe the color 5 minutes after adding the dye solution.
>   4. Classify starches according to the color (purple or red).

6.3.1.2 Congo Red Dye Test

Congo red is the sodium salt of benzidinediazo-bis-1-naphthylamine-4-sulfonic acid (formula, $C_{32}H_{22}N_6Na_2O_6S_2$; molecular weight, 696.66 g/mol) classified as a secondary diazo dye. It is soluble in water and organic solvents, such as ethanol, yielding a red colloidal solution. When added to gelatinized or cooked starch, it stains because of a reaction with the amylose.

A. *Samples, Ingredients, and Reagents*
- Different types of starches
- Congo red
- Distilled water

B. *Materials and Equipment*
- Digital scale
- Chronometer
- Hot plate with agitation
- Thermometer
- Dark bottles
- Drop dispenser bottle
- Beaker (400 mL)
- Volumetric flask (100 mL)
- Spatula
- Plastic gloves
- Eye goggles

C. *Procedure*
1. Prepare a 10% starch (native or ungelatinized) solution by mixing 10 g of starch and 90 mL of distilled water. Place starch solution in a beaker.
2. Gradually heat the starch solution while agitating to 85°C. Immediately suspend heat and allow starch slurry to cool down.
3. Wearing eye goggles and plastic gloves, prepare the Congo red solution by dissolving 100 mg of the powder into 100 mL of distilled water.
4. Place Congo red solution in a drop dispenser bottle and add a few drops onto the starch slurry before (native starch) and after heat treatment (gelatinized starch).
5. Observe the color and determine whether or not the starch is gelatinized.

6.3.1.3 Starch Microscopy

Considerable information on starch granule structure may be gathered from microscopy (Bechtel 1983; Cortella and Pochettino 1994). These microscopic examinations have been extensively used by various segments of the cereal industries. The techniques used include light microscopy, scanning electron microscopy (SEM), and transmission electron microscopy. In light microscopy, oil immersion is a technique used to increase the resolution of a microscope. This is achieved by immersing both the objective lens and the specimen in a transparent oil of high refractive index, thereby increasing the numerical aperture of the objective lens. In light microscopy, stains may be used. The advent of SEM in the 1960s facilitated the analysis of starches because the images were more easily interpreted and sample preparation was not difficult compared with electron microscopy. Specimens for the transmission electron microscope must be sufficiently thin for the electron beam to pass through them. Each species of plant has a unique size, shape, and crystallization pattern of starch granules. Under the microscope, native starch grains stained with iodine and illuminated from behind with polarized light show a distinctive Maltese cross. Each cereal has a unique starch granular size and form: rice starch is relatively small (~2 μm) whereas maize or sorghum starches are larger granules.

Upon gelatinization, starch becomes water-soluble. The starch granules swell and eventually burst and the internal crystalline structure is disrupted and lost. The smaller amylose molecules leach out of the granules, forming a viscous network or paste that holds water. During cooling or prolonged storage of the previously gelatinized starch, the amylose molecules start to reassociate or retrogradate. This phenomenon causes more viscosity and the expelling of water that was present in the interphase between amylose molecules. This last phenomenon is known as syneresis. Retrogradation is responsible for bread and tortilla staling and for the release of water on top of starch gels (syneresis).

A. *Samples, Ingredients, and Reagents*
- Starches
- Immersion oil
- Distilled water

B. *Materials and Equipment*
- Light microscope
- Two polarizing lenses or filters
- Heating mounting stage
- Microscope slides
- Cover glass
- Spatula
- Drop dispenser bottle

C. *Procedure*

Observation under Light

1. Place a small amount of the starch on a clean microscope slide and then add one or two drops of water. Mix the starch with the water to disrupt lumps and distribute starch granules.
2. Place the cover glass on top of the starch solution. Make sure to avoid the formation of air bubbles.
3. Under the microscope, using different magnifying lenses or objectives, observe the form (round, oval, angular, polyhedral, lenticular, etc.), dimensions, presence of concentric rings, and hilum of the starch granules. Draw the observed starch granules. For compound starch granules (rice or oats) observe if the granules are intact or in subunits.

Observation of Starch under Polarized Light

1. Prepare samples as explained for regular light microscopy.

2. Equip the microscope with two polarizing light lenses or filters and the special heated mounting stage or slide heater. One polarizing filter is placed on the illuminator located at the base of the microscope whereas the other is placed above the objective lenses.

3. Place a small amount of the starch on a clean microscope slide and then add one or two drops of water. Mix the starch with the water to disrupt lumps and distribute starch granules.

4. Place the cover glass on top of the starch solution. Make sure to avoid the formation of air bubbles.

5. After adjusting the coarse and fine focus, observe the starch granules under the microscope with different magnifying lenses or objectives. Then, gradually rotate the bottom polarizing lens placed on the illuminator until the observation of the Maltese crosses (Figure 6.2).

6. By counting the number of total starch granules on the microscopic field, determine the percentage of granules showing birefringence or Maltese crosses.

6.3.1.4 Birefringence End-Point Temperature

The BEPT test is measured using the same basic principle but the microscope is equipped with a starch slurry heating device that heats at a controlled rate. BEPT is considered the temperature at which 95% of the granules lose birefringence.

A. *Samples, Ingredients, and Reagents*
- Starches
- Immersion oil
- Distilled water

B. *Materials and Equipment*
- Light microscope
- Two polarizing lenses or filters
- Heated mounting stage
- Microscope slides
- Cover glass

- Spatula
- Drop dispenser bottle

C. *Procedure*
1. Prepare samples and furnish the microscope as explained for polarized microscopy (procedure in Section 6.3.1.3).

2. Observe starch granules under polarized light to observe birefringence. Count the total number of starch granules on the field and those having Maltese crosses.

3. Turn on heat of the special mounting or slide heater. Continuously observe starch granules in the range of temperature from 50°C to 85°C. Register the exact temperature when 50% and 98% of the starch granules lose birefringence. The BEPT is considered the temperature when 98% of the granules lose birefringence.

6.3.1.5 Scanning Electron Microscopy

The SEM is a type of electron microscope that images a sample by scanning it with a high-energy beam of electrons in a scan pattern. The electrons interact with the atoms that make up the sample, producing signals that contain information about the specimen surface topography, texture, and composition. Conventional SEM requires samples to be imaged under vacuum because a gas atmosphere rapidly spreads and attenuates electron beams. Areas ranging from approximately 1 cm to 5 μm in width can be imaged in a scanning mode using conventional techniques. The microscope is capable of magnifying from 20× to approximately 30,000× at a spatial resolution of 50 nm to 100 nm. A typical SEM instrument is furnished with an electron column, sample chamber, energy dispersive X-ray spectroscopy detector, electronics console, and visual display monitors. The fundamental principle of SEM is that the accelerated electrons carry significant amounts of energy which is dissipated as a variety of signals produced by electron–sample interactions when the incident electrons are decelerated in the solid sample. SEM analysis is considered to be "nondestructive" because the X-rays generated by electron interactions do not lead to loss of the sample. Sample preparation can be

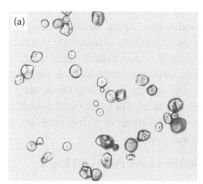
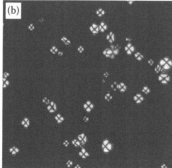
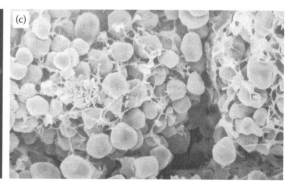

FIGURE 6.2 Native maize starch viewed under normal light (a) polarized light (b) and SEMs (c). (Courtesy of C. McDonough and Dr. L. Rooney, Texas A&M University).

minimal for SEM analysis, providing that the sample fits into the SEM chamber and after some accommodations to prevent charge buildup on electrically insulated samples. Most electrically insulated samples are coated with a thin layer of conducting material, commonly carbon, gold, or some other metal or alloy. Metal coatings are most effective for high-resolution electron imaging applications. Alternatively, an electrically insulated sample can be examined without a conductive coating in an instrument capable of "low vacuum" operation. Consequently, samples that produce a significant amount of vapor, such as wet biological samples, need to be dried.

SEM techniques have been used for the examination of the structure of bisected cereal grains, native and enzyme-damaged starches, flour samples, freeze-dried dough structures, and many cereal-based products (Fannon et al. 1992; Sargent 1988; Cortella and Pochettino 1994).

A. *Samples, Ingredients, and Reagents*
- Starches or ground meals from cereals
- Cereal-based products
- Gold palladium alloy

B. *Materials and Equipment*
- SEM
- Freeze-drier or vacuum-drier
- Glue tabs
- Aluminum tabs
- Sputter coater

C. *Procedure*
1. If the cereal-based product (bread, tortilla, or starch slurry) has a moisture content higher than 10%, it is necessary to dehydrate the product, preferably using a freeze-drier or a vacuum-drier.
2. Mount the dry sample specimen on a glue tab attached to an aluminum tab. Alternatively, coat specimen with a sputter coater, applying a gold palladium coat of 300 A in preparation for examining at 10 kV.
3. Observe the three-dimensional topographic characteristics of the sample in a water vapor environment of 2 to 10 torr at an accelerating voltage of 20 kV (Figure 6.2).

6.3.2 Research Suggestions

1. Compare the morphology of refined potato, cassava, rice, wheat, regular maize, waxy maize, and sorghum using light microscopy under regular and polarized light and SEM. Measure the average size and morphological features of each type of starch.
2. Determine and compare the iodine test and BEPT results of native regular and waxy starches.
3. Compare the birefringence and size of starch granules associated with raw maize transformed into a tortilla (refer to procedure in Section 7.2.3.1). The

samples should be carefully dehydrated before conducting the comparative tests.

4. Determine the Congo red test of a native maize starch that is subjected to heat treatment in a jet cooker used for ethanol production.
5. Using the SEM, compare the morphology and topography of native maize starch granules after hydrolysis with α-amylase.

6.3.3 Research Questions

1. Define the following terms:
   a. Birefringence
   b. BEPT
   c. Iodine test
   d. Congo red test
   e. Maltese cross
2. Describe the internal morphology of a native starch granule. What is the difference between a simple and compound starch granule? Which cereals produce compound starch granules?
3. Compare the microscope techniques of light, SEM, and transmission electron microscopies. What are their advantages, disadvantages, and main uses.
4. Investigate the way starch granules are synthesized during grain maturation on the field?
5. What are the structural differences between starch granules from the soft or chalky endosperm and the horny or hard endosperm?
6. Explain the principle of the iodine dye test.
7. Explain the principle and usefulness of the Congo red dye test.
8. Mention at least two ways to mechanically, chemically, and enzymatically damage starch granules.
9. Explain the procedure and principle of the BEPT microscopy test. What is considered the final BEPT temperature?

6.4 EVALUATION OF THE FUNCTIONAL PROPERTIES OF STARCHES

6.4.1 Viscoamylography

The viscoamylograph is the most widely used instrument to measure the functional properties of starch and starch-rich flours or processed products because it is capable of measuring viscosity changes of starch slurries when heated above the gelatinization temperature and during cooling. The assay is conducted with a certain amount of solids that are subjected to a standardized and programmed temperature regime. The classic instrument is the Brabender viscoamylograph. The instrument consists of a pin style stirrer/sensor that is inserted in a bowl that contains the starch suspension. The temperature is regulated by a thermoregulator that may be set at a constant temperature or may be raised or lowered at a rate of 1.5°C/min. During the assay, the bowl rotates at a constant speed (75 rpm) and the stirrer registers the viscosity.

The complete viscoamylograph curve is obtained after four distinctive and sequential stages: temperature increase, hot temperature hold, temperature decrease or cooling, and cold temperature hold. The instrument records the viscosity of the starch slurry expressed on viscoamylograph units. Generally, the assay starts at 50°C with a temperature increase of 1.5°C/min until the maximum temperature of 95°C is achieved. Next, the temperature is held for 15 to 30 minutes followed by gradual cooling (−1.5°C/min) until reaching 50°C. The final stage is the temperature hold at 50°C (Figure 15.3). The entire test or run can last 120 minutes (Thomas and Atwell 1999).

6.4.1.1 Amylograph Properties of Starches and Starch-Rich Products

A. *Samples, Ingredients, and Reagents*
- Test starches or flours or processed products
- Distilled water
- Hydrochloric acid (0.1 N)
- Sodium hydroxide (0.1 N)
- Dessicant (activated alumina)

B. *Materials and Equipment*
- Amylograph
- Laboratory mill
- Digital scale
- Convection oven
- Airtight dessicator
- Tweezers
- Aluminum dishes
- Spatula
- Beakers (600 mL)
- Volumetric flask (500 mL)

C. *Procedure*
1. Determine the moisture content of the test sample (starch, flour, and processed product). If the sample is a cereal-based food product, make sure to first dehydrate the sample at low temperature (<50°C) or in a freeze-drier and then grind it using a laboratory mill. Determine the residual moisture content of the sample.
2. Weigh the predetermined sample (the sample size will vary according to starch content). Most starches are tested based on 10% solids and diluted with water tempered to 25°C to produce a 500 mL dispersion. It is advisable to determine the optimum solid concentration based on a preliminary assay aimed toward the amount needed to produce 500 BU peak viscosity.
3. If the assay is run with a fixed pH, then adjust the desired pH with 0.1 N HCl or sodium hydroxide solutions.
4. Transfer the 500 mL suspension to the amylograph stirring bowl. Lower amylograph head with the agitator making sure that the thermoregulator transport switch is in the neutral position, with the heat off and the cup or bowl rotating at 75 rpm (Figure 6.3).

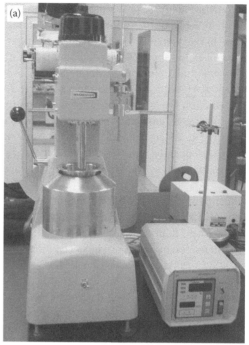

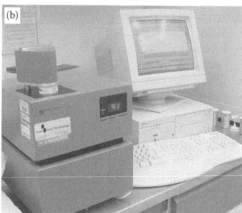

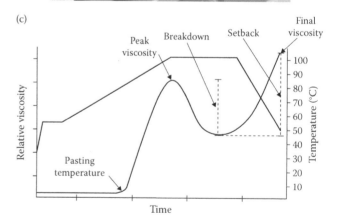

FIGURE 6.3 Viscoanalyzers commonly used to test amylograph properties of starches. (a) Brabender viscoamylograph; (b) rapid viscoamylograph; (c) typical viscoamylograph curve with its main parameters.

5. Adjust the recording pen to zero viscosity and then turn on cooling water with cooling switch in controlled position and adjust regulating thermocouple to 50°C.

6. Turn on heat switch and allow sample to equilibrate at 50°C. This is indicated by alternate cyclings of the heater lamp and the cooling water.

7. Place transport switch in the up position and heat at 1.5°C/min until the sample reaches 95°C (30 minutes). This step is called the "heating cycle."

8. Move transport switch to neutral and hold the 95°C temperature for 30 minutes. This cycle is known as "hot temperature hold."

9. Move transport switch to the down position and gradually cool the slurry at 1.5°C/min for 30 minutes (from 95°C to 50°C). This is known as the "cooling cycle."

10. Move transport switch to neutral and hold the 50°C temperature for 30 minutes. This cycle is known as "cold temperature hold."

11. If the viscosity exceeds the 1000 BU line, place extra weights to lower the viscosity to 500 BU. This will allow recording viscosity especially during the cold temperature hold stage.

12. Determine the viscoamylograph properties of the sample (Figure 6.3). The most relevant parameters are
    a. Temperature at start of gelatinization
    b. Peak viscosity
    c. Viscosity at 95°C
    d. Viscosity at end of hot temperature hold (first holding period)
    e. Drop in viscosity between "d" and "c" known as shear-thinning
    f. Viscosity of cooked paste after cooling to 50°C
    g. Viscosity at end of cold temperature hold

6.4.1.2 Rapid Viscoamylograph Properties of Flour and Starches

The rapid viscoanalyzer or RVA is an instrument that is operated based on the same principles of the Brabender amylograph. The advantage of the RVA is that it significantly shortens the run time while maintaining a high correlation with the Brabender viscoamylograph (Crosbie and Ross 2007; Deffenbaugh and Walker 1989; Thiewes and Steeneken 1997; Walker and Hazelton 1996). In addition, it requires lower sample size. Regardless of the type of instrument, the amylograph curve is considered as the fingerprint of starches because it determines the initial change in viscosity related to gelatinization temperature, peak viscosity during heating, the viscosity fall after the peak (shear-thinning), and viscosity changes through the cooling cycles related to retrogradation. These instruments are the most frequently used to determine native and modified starch properties related to gelatinization, viscosity, and retrogradation.

A. *Samples, Ingredients, and Reagents*
- Test starches, flours, or processed products
- Distilled water
- Hydrochloric acid (0.1 N)
- Sodium hydroxide (0.1 N)
- Dessicant (activated alumina)

B. *Materials and Equipment*
- Rapid viscoamylograph
- Digital scale
- Canisters
- RVA paddle
- Airtight dessicator
- Tweezers
- Aluminum dishes
- Spatula
- Beakers (250 mL)
- Volumetric flask (100 mL)

C. *Procedure (Variable Temperature Profile, Method 76-21)*
1. Determine the moisture content of the test sample (starch, flour, or processed product). If the sample is a cereal-based food product, make sure to first dehydrate the sample at low temperature (<50°C) or in a freeze-drier and then grind it using a laboratory mill (AACC 2000). Determine the residual moisture content of the sample.

2. Weigh 3.5 g ± 0.02 g of flour or 3 g ± 0.02 g of starch (14% mb) and place it in test canister. Add 25 mL ± 0.05 mL of distilled water and manually stir contents with the paddle.

3. Place the canister into the instrument and initiate heating profile cycle by depressing the motor tower (Figure 6.3). The instrument will automatically start the test at 50°C (1 minute holding), then it will heat contents to 95°C over a specified period (3.8 minutes), hold at 95°C for a specific time (2.4 minutes) and cool back to 50°C over a specified period (3.8 minutes).

4. Determine the rapid viscoamylograph properties of the test sample. The most relevant parameters are:
    a. Temperature at start of gelatinization
    b. Peak viscosity
    c. Viscosity at 95°C
    d. Viscosity at end of hot temperature hold (first holding period)
    e. Drop in viscosity between "d" and "c" known as shear-thinning
    f. Viscosity of cooked paste after cooling to 50°C

6.4.2 DIFFERENTIAL SCANNING CALORIMETRY (THERMAL PROPERTIES)

The DSC is a thermoanalytical assay in which the difference in the amount of heat required to increase the temperature of a sample is measured as a function of temperature (temperature increases linearly as a function of time). The instrument measures the specific heat capacity, heat of transition, and the temperature of phase changes and melting points. These differences determine variations in material composition, crystallinity, and oxidation. In cereals, DSC analysis of starch-rich and starch–water slurries have been used to quantitatively determine starch gelatinization as an enthalpy ($-\Delta$Hg) of gelatinization. Enthalpy measurements can also be used to measure the return to crystallinity in aged starch gels. The endotherm excursions show a broad temperature range over which crystal structure is being melted. The temperature at which gelatinization is initiated generally agrees with values reported from loss of birefringence measurements. In addition, the temperature needed to provide maximum starch disruption and high viscosity are in accordance with the maximum or peak viscosity development in the Brabender viscoamylograph (Zobel 1984). The instrument is used to determine the degree of gelatinization in bakery products and measure their rate of retrogradation. The parameters usually evaluated are enthalpy of crystal fusion, onset temperature, and transition temperature. The T_g glass transition is the temperature at which amorphous polymers or an amorphous part of a crystalline polymer goes from a hard brittle state to a soft rubbery state. The T_m melting point is the temperature at which a crystalline polymer melts and the ΔH is the energy absorbed when melting.

A. Samples, Ingredients, and Reagents
- Starch or starch-rich products
- Indium
- Calibration sample kit

B. Materials and Equipment
- DSC
- Stainless steel sample pans

C. Procedure
1. Turn on equipment 20 minutes before testing. Calibrate the DSC (Figure 6.4) with a calibration sample kit provided by the manufacturer. Once the calibration is performed, the DSC is calibrated automatically and continually. Occasionally, reference material (indium) should be tested to assure that the DSC is well-calibrated.
2. Weigh approximately 23 mg of sample and mix it with double-distilled water.
3. Place sample in the center of a stainless steel sample pan and then encapsulate the pan.
4. Keep one empty pan for reference.
5. Place the reference pans, followed by the test pans, in the center of the DSC sample holder.
6. Program the DSC to hold at 40°C for 2 minutes and then increase the heat from 40°C to 90°C at 10°C/min.
7. Obtain the ΔH, onset, end, and peak of gelatinization provided by the DSC software. The degree of gelatinization is determined by

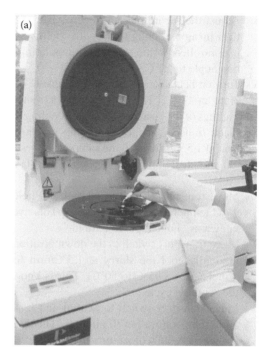

(a)

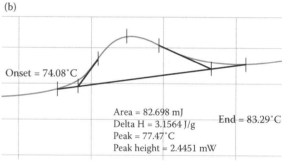

(b)

Onset = 74.08°C

Area = 82.698 mJ
Delta H = 3.1564 J/g
Peak = 77.47°C
Peak height = 2.4451 mW

End = 83.29°C

FIGURE 6.4 DSC (a) used for the evaluation of starch properties with its typical curve (b).

comparing ΔH of a sample and a reference or control sample, the higher the ΔH, the lower the degree of gelatinization (Figure 6.4).

6.4.3 DETERMINATION OF STARCH DAMAGE AND DIASTATIC ACTIVITY

The Brabender and RVA have successfully been used to indirectly measure starch damage and diastatic activity, mainly of wheat or rye flours because sprouted kernels with high starch damage or diastatic activity yield less viscous slurries compared with sound or undamaged counterparts. Sprouting in wheat and other cereals, as indicated by high enzyme activity, produces sticky doughs that could cause problems during processing and result in products with poor color and weak texture. Additionally, the viscoanalyzers can be used as an effective tool to determine the optimum amount of diastatic malt to supplement wheat flour for bread production.

6.4.3.1 Determination of Diastatic Activity of Wheat Flour with the Amylograph (Method 22-10)

This method was previously discussed in AACC (2000).

A. Samples, Ingredients, and Reagents
- Wheat flours with different diastatic activities or sprout damage
- Monohydrated citric acid
- Anhydrous disodium phosphate
- Dessicant (activated alumina)

B. Materials and Equipment
- Amylograph
- Laboratory mill
- Digital scale
- Convection oven
- Airtight dessicator
- Tweezers
- Aluminum dishes
- Spatula
- Graduated cylinder (50 mL)
- pH meter
- Beakers (600 mL)
- Volumetric flask (1 L)
- Agitator

C. Procedure
1. Prepare a concentrated buffer solution dissolving 14.8 g of anhydrous disodium phosphate (Na_2HPO_4) and 10.3 g of citric acid in 1 L of distilled water. Dilute 46 mL of the concentrated buffer in 460 mL of water. Verify that the resulting solution has a pH between 5.3 and 5.35. The stock buffer solution should be stored in a refrigerator.
2. Place 100 g of flour (14% mb) in a 1-L beaker. For instance, if the flour contains 15% moisture content, weigh 101.17 g of flour [(100 − 14% moisture)/(100 − 15% moisture) × 100 g] in the beaker and decrease the total buffer content addition by 1.17 mL. Add 360 mL of the diluted buffer solution.
3. Place the dissolved sample in the amylograph bowl. Rinse the beaker with 100 − 1.17 mL diluted buffer and add it to the bowl. Lower the amylograph head with the stirrer making sure that the thermoregulator transport switch is in the neutral position, the slurry is tempered to 30°C, and the cup or bowl speed set at 75 rpm.
4. Adjust recording pen to zero viscosity and then turn on heat switch and allow sample to heat at 1.5°C/min until the sample reaches 95°C (43.3 minutes).
5. After completing the heating cycle, turn off the instrument and clean the stirring bowl. Record the maximum viscosity (BU), which is known as the malt index. If a duplicate sample was run, the standard deviation should be less than 10 BU.

6.4.3.2 Determination of Diastatic Activity with the Rapid Viscoamylograph (Stirring Number, Method 22-08)

1. Determine the moisture content of the wheat flour sample (AACC 2000).
2. Weigh 3.5 g ± 0.02 g of flour or 3 g ± 0.02 g of starch (14% mb) and place it in a test canister. Add 25 mL ± 0.05 mL of distilled water and manually stir contents with the paddle using 10 up-and-down strokes.
3. Load the canister into the instrument and initiate the heating profile cycle by depressing the motor tower. The instrument temperature and time will be set at 95°C and 3 minutes, respectively.
4. Determine the rapid viscoamylograph properties of the flour sample. The peak viscosity values are closely correlated to the falling number. Flours with low stirring numbers have low falling numbers.

6.4.3.3 Determination of Diastatic Activity with the Pressurometer (Method 22-11)

This method was previously discussed in AACC (2000).

A. Samples, Ingredients, and Reagents
- Test flours
- Fresh compressed yeast
- Distilled water

B. Materials and Equipment
- Digital scale
- Fermentation or proof box (30°C, 85% relative humidity)
- Pressurometers with wrench
- Graduated pipette (10 mL)
- Spatula
- Laboratory clock
- Thermometer
- Relative humidity recorder or gauge

C. Procedure
1. Adjust the fermentation or bioclimatic chamber to 30°C and 85% relative humidity.
2. Weigh 10 g of flour, 7 mL of distilled water, and 0.3 g of fresh compressed yeast or its dry yeast equivalent (~0.1 g).
3. Place ingredients in the pressurometer and then mix contents with the spatula (Figure 6.5).
4. Screw lid on the pressurometer and tighten with the special wrench. Make sure the pressurometer is properly sealed.
5. Place pressurometer in the fermentation box and allow contents to ferment for 5 minutes. Release the pressure by pressing the poppet valve stem until the internal pressure drops to zero. Mark this time as zero.

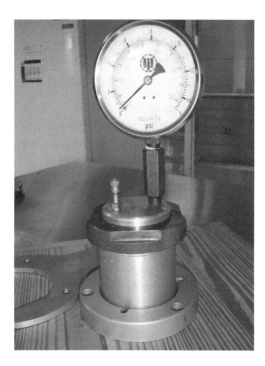

FIGURE 6.5 Pressurometer used to test gas-releasing properties of yeast and flour damage.

6. Record the pressure during 5 hours of fermentation. Take at least 10 readings, with more frequency at the beginning of the test.

7. Graph results of pressure (mm Hg) in the y axis vs. time (minutes) in the x axis. Calculate the slope of the curve which is related to the carbon dioxide production throughout the assay time. The higher the slope value, the higher the diastatic activity of the flour.

6.4.3.4 Falling Number Method (Method 56-81B)

One of the most accepted and rapid procedures to determine starch damage, mainly associated with wheat flour, is the falling number assay (AACC 2000, Method 56-81B). The instrument analyzes viscosity by measuring the resistance of a flour-and-water paste to a falling stirrer. The test is based on the principle that heat or enzymatically damaged (sprouted) wheat flours that are hydrated and thermally treated generate lower viscosities compared with undamaged flours. Falling number results are recorded as an index of enzyme activity in a wheat or flour sample, and the results are expressed in time as seconds. A high falling number (e.g., >300 seconds) indicates minimal enzyme activity and sound quality wheat or flour. A low falling number (e.g., <250 seconds) indicates substantial enzyme activity and sprout-damaged wheat or flour. When grinding a wheat sample to perform a falling number test, it should be at least 300 g to assure a representative sample. The level of enzyme activity measured by the falling number test affects product quality. Yeast in bread dough, for example, requires sugars to develop properly and therefore needs some level of enzyme activity in the dough.

Too much enzyme activity, however, means that too much sugar and too little starch are present. Because starch provides the supporting structure of bread, too much activity results in sticky dough during processing and poor texture in the finished product. If the falling number is too high, enzymes can be added to the flour in various ways to compensate. If the falling number is too low, enzymes cannot be removed from the flour or wheat, which results in a serious problem that makes the flour unusable (www.wheatflourbook.org).

A. *Samples, Ingredients, and Reagents*
- Wheat flours with different sprout damage or diastatic activities
- Glycerol, ethylene glycol, or isopropyl alcohol
- Distilled water

B. *Materials and Equipment*
- Falling number apparatus
- Thermometer (0.1°C scale)
- Laboratory mill
- Automatic pipette that dispenses 25 mL ± 0.3 mL
- Brush
- Air-forced convection oven

C. *Procedure*
1. When grinding a wheat sample to perform a falling number test, it should be at least 300 g to assure a representative sample. The whole wheat sample needs to be ground in a laboratory mill to obtain the following particle size distribution: more than 500 μm, 0% to 10%; 210 μm to 500 μm, 25% to 40%; and less than 210 μm, 50% to 75%.

2. The flour or whole wheat moisture should be in the range of 8% to 16%. If the sample contains less moisture, water should be added to increase the moisture content to 12%. If the sample moisture is too high, allow sample to dehydrate at low temperature (<50°C) in a regular or vacuum-drier. Make sure to remove sample from the oven when moisture decreases to 10% to 12% and allow sample to equilibrate at room temperature.

3. Determine the exact moisture content (refer to procedure in Section 2.2.1.1) of the flour. Adjust sample weight according to moisture content (Table 6.1).

4. Fill the water bath of the apparatus to approximately 1 in. (2.54 cm) below the top.

5. Place the thermometer in the interior part of the test tube until a constant temperature is achieved. If the temperature is between 98.0°C and 99.8°C, adjust to 100°C by adding ethylene glycol or glycerol. The amounts needed are summarized in Table 6.2.

   a. If the temperature of the water bath is lower than 98°C, the falling number cannot be performed at 100°C because of the danger of spilling the tube's contents. Instead, the falling number should be determined at the

TABLE 6.1

Falling Number Sample Weight According to Original Flour Moisture Content

Sample Moisture Content (%)	Sample Weight (14% mb, g)	Sample Moisture Content (%)	Sample Weight (14% mb, g)	Sample Moisture Content (%)	Sample Weight (14% mb, g)
8.0	6.54	10.8	6.75	13.6	6.97
8.2	6.56	11.0	6.76	13.8	6.98
8.4	6.57	11.2	6.78	14.0	7.00
8.6	6.59	11.4	6.80	14.2	7.02
8.8	6.60	11.6	6.81	14.4	7.03
9.0	6.62	11.8	6.83	14.6	7.04
9.2	6.63	12.0	6.84	14.8	7.07
9.4	6.64	12.2	6.86	15.0	7.08
9.6	6.66	12.4	6.87	15.2	7.10
9.8	6.67	12.6	6.89	15.4	7.12
10.0	6.69	12.8	6.90	15.6	7.13
10.2	6.70	13.0	6.92	15.8	7.15
10.4	6.72	13.2	6.94	16.0	7.17
10.6	6.73	13.4	6.95	16.2	7.18

temperature at which boiling occurs. After adjusting the temperature to 97.5°C, add 13.6% ethylene glycol and again determine the falling number. Graph both values against temperature and prolong the slope of the line to reach the 100°C value. Determine the falling number at this temperature or point.

b. If the water bath temperature exceeds 100°C, add 0.1% isopropyl alcohol for every 0.1°C to the water. The isopropyl alcohol will reduce the boiling temperature to 100°C. This step is not necessary unless the water temperature is higher than 100.2°C.

6. Mix the 7 g (14% mb) sample of ground wheat or flour with 25 mL of distilled water in a glass tube. Place cork and manually shake contents to form a slurry. Before running the test, make sure to remove flour adhered to the test tube with the falling number agitator-plunger.

7. Place the tube in the water bath and immediately turn on the instrument that will automatically heat and stir the sample (Figure 6.6). During this operation, the starch will gelatinize and form a thick paste.

8. After approximately 1 minute, the instrument will automatically measure the time it takes the stirrer to drop through the paste. This is the falling number value. Adjust the falling number according to 14% mb using the following equation: Falling number × (100 − 14)/(100 − % sample moisture).

TABLE 6.2

Recommended Amounts of Ethylene Glycol or Glycerol Needed to Bring the Water Bath Temperature to 100°C

	Amount to Add	
Temperature Increase (°C)	Ethylene Glycol (% v/v)	Glycerol (% v/v)
0.2	1.9	2.5
0.4	3.9	4.9
0.6	5.8	7.4
0.8	7.8	9.8
1.0	9.7	12.3
1.2	11.3	14.2
1.4	12.9	16.1
1.6	14.4	18.1
1.8	16.0	20.0
2.0	17.6	21.9

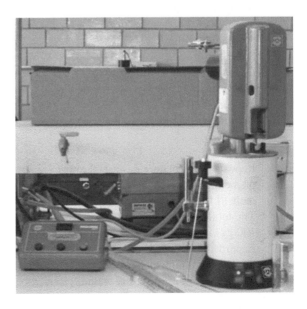

FIGURE 6.6 Falling number instrument widely used to assess diastatic properties of wheat flours.

9. Classify the wheat sample according to the falling number value. If the value was less than 150, it contains high diastatic or amylolytic activity, meaning that that sample was field-, sprout-, or storage-damaged. If the value is between 200 and 250, the flour is considered normal, and if the value is higher than 300, the sample is sound but it will need diastatic malt for bread making.

10. Immediately after concluding the test, make sure to remove the tube with the stirrer from the water bath. Clean the tube and stirrer-plunger with running water.

6.4.3.5 Determination of Optimum Malt Supplemented to Wheat Flour for Baking Purposes with the Amylograph

The diastatic activity of most baking flours is adjusted by adding different amounts of diastatic barley malt. The α-amylase and β-amylase of the barley malt will hydrolyze part of the starch to yield fermentable sugars that are used by the fermenting yeast. The supplementation of barley malt is especially important in those breads that do not contain added sugars (i.e., French bread).

A. *Samples, Ingredients, and Reagents*
- Wheat flours
- Diastatic malt
- Monohydrated citric acid
- Anhydrous disodium phosphate
- Dessicant (activated alumina)

B. *Materials and Equipment*
- Amylograph
- Laboratory mill
- Digital scale
- Convection oven
- Airtight dessicator
- Tweezers
- Aluminum dishes
- Spatula
- Graduated cylinder (50 mL)
- pH meter
- Beakers (600 mL)
- Volumetric flask (1 L)
- Agitator

C. *Procedure*
1. Repeat the procedure described above by supplementing different concentrations of diastatic malt (0.1–1 g/100 g flour) to the wheat flour. The total sample weight in all assays should be 100 g (14% mb).
2. Record the malt index for each run and determine the optimum malt concentration to achieve the desired peak viscosity value.* Remember

that increasing malt concentrations significantly lowers peak viscosity.

6.4.4 Research Suggestions

1. Determine and compare the viscoamylograph properties of the following starches: acid, acetylated, cross-linked, and pregelatinized.
2. Compare complete viscoamylograph curves of regular starch and refined wheat flour obtained from the Brabender and RVAs.
3. Determine and compare the viscoamylograph and DSC properties of raw maize and its processed dry *masa* flour (refer to procedure in Section 7.2.4.1).
4. Determine and compare iodine and Congo red dye tests and viscoamylograph and DSC properties of the following white polished rices: short waxy, regular long, and parboiled–regular.
5. Determine and compare the endotherm curves (specific heat capacity, heat of transition, temperatures of phase changes, and melting points) of the following maize starches: regular, waxy, acid, acetylated, cross-linked, and pregelatinized.
6. Compare falling numbers and pressurometer values of flours obtained from the same hard wheat that was purposely stored at high moisture for 2 weeks (refer to procedure in Section 4.2.1.2).

6.4.5 Research Questions

1. Define the following terms:
   a. Gelatinization
   b. Peak viscosity
   c. Shear-thinning
   d. Retrogradation
   e. Synerisis
   f. Endotherm curve
   g. Enthalpy
   h. Clathrate
   i. Diastatic activity
2. What is the principle of the viscoamylograph? What are the four consecutive stages of the complete viscoamylograph curve? In which stage is peak viscosity and retrogradation obtained?
3. Compare the viscoamylograph properties of regular maize starch, waxy maize starch, wheat starch, and rice starch. Why are waxy starches in high demand by the food industry?
4. Using the same solids, compare the viscoamylographic properties of potato starch, regular maize, cross-linked maize starch, and acetylated maize starch. Which starch produces the highest peak viscosity? Which starch is more stable during heating? Why?
5. What is the principle of the DSC? What are the values generally obtained from the endotherm curves?
6. What is the principle of the falling number test? Why is this test widely used by wheat millers?

---

* The same assay can be used to compare different sources of malt at a fixed diastatic malt concentration (i.e., 0.2% malt).

7. Why does damaged starch produce less viscous slurries compared with undamaged starch? What are the main types of starch damage?

8. Why should pressurometer tests be performed under strict temperature controls?

9. Why does a sprouted-damaged wheat flour produce lower viscosity as measured with the viscoamylograph or falling number apparatus?

10. Why does a high diastatic wheat flour contain more fermentable sugars and promote higher yeast activation?

11. What is the significance of the following wheat flour falling numbers: lower than 150, 200 to 250, and higher than 300. Which of these flours needs more malt supplementation for baking purposes? Why?

REFERENCES

American Association of Cereal Chemists (AACC). 2000. *AACC Approved Methods of Analysis.* 10th ed. St. Paul, MN: American Association of Cereal Chemists.

Bechtel, D. B. 1983. *New Frontiers in Food Microstructure.* St. Paul, MN: American Association of Cereal Chemists.

Bewley, J. D., and M. Black. 1978. *Physiology and Biochemistry of Seeds. Vol. 1: Development, Germination and Growth.* Berlin: Springer Verlag.

Cornell, H. J., and A. W. Hoveling. 1998. *Wheat Chemistry and Utilization.* Lancaster, PA: Technomic Publishing Co.

Cortella, A. R., and M. L. Pochettino. 1994. "Starch Grain Analysis as a Microscopic Diagnostic Feature in the Identification of Plant Material." *Economic Botany* 48(2):171–181.

Crosbie, G. B., and A. S. Ross. 2007. *The RVA Handbook.* St. Paul, MN: American Association of Cereal Chemists.

Deffenbaugh, L. B., and C. E. Walker. 1989. "Comparison of Starch Pasting Properties in the Brabender Viscoamylograph and the Rapid Visco-Analyzer." *Cereal Chemistry* 66:493–499.

Eckhoff, S. R., K. D. Rausch, E. J. Fox, C. C. Tso, X. Wu, Z. Pan, and P. Buriak. 1993. "A Laboratory Wet-Milling Procedure to Increase Reproducibility and Accuracy of Products Yields." *Cereal Chemistry* 70:723.

Eckhoff, S. R., S. K. Singh, B. E. Zher, K. D. Rausch, E. J. Fox, A. K. Mistry, A. E. Haken, Y. X. Niu, P. Buriak, M. E. Tumbelson, and P. L. Keeling, 1996. "A Laboratory Wet Corn-Milling Procedure." *Cereal Chemistry* 73:54–57.

Fannon, J. E., R. J. Hauber, and J. N. Bemiller. 1992. "Surface Pores of Starch Granules." *Cereal Chemistry* 69(3):284–288.

French, D. 1984. "Organization of Starch Granules." In *Starch Chemistry and Technology*, edited by R. L. Whistler, J. N. Bemiller, and E. F. Paschall. San Diego, CA: Academic Press, Inc.

Johnson, L. A., and J. B. May. 2003. "Wet Milling: The Basis for Corn Biorefineries." In *Corn Chemistry and Technology*, 2nd ed., edited by P. J. White and L. A. Johnson. St. Paul, MN: American Association of Cereal Chemists.

Juliano, B. O. 1984. Rice strach: Production properties and uses. In *Starch Chemistry and Technology*, 2nd ed., R. L. Whistler, J. N. BeMiller and E. F. Paschall. Orlando, FL: Academic Press.

Khurana, R.,V. N. Uversky, L. Nielson, and A. L. Fink. 2001. "Is Congo Red an Amyloid-Specific Dye?" *Journal of Biological Chemistry* 276(25):22715–22721.

Knight, J. W. and R. M. Olson. 1984. "Wheat Starch: Production, Modification and Uses." In *Starch: Chemistry and Technology*, 2nd ed., edited by R. L. Whistler, J. N. Bemiller, and E. F. Paschall, Orlando, FL: Academic Press.

Lamb, J. and T. H. Loy. 2005. "Seeing Red: The Use of Congo Red Dye to Identify Cooked and Damaged Starch Grains in Archaeological Residues." *Journal of Archaeological Science* 32:1433–1440.

Martinez, C., and J. Prodoliet. 1996. "Determination of Amylose in Cereal and Non-Cereal Starches by a Colorimetric Assay: Collaborative Study." *Starch* 48(3):81–85.

May, J. B. 1987. "Wet Milling: Process and Products." In *Corn Chemistry and Technology*, edited by S. A. Watson and P. E. Ramstad. St. Paul, MN: American Association of Cereal Chemists.

Sargent, J. A. 1988. "The Application of Cold Stage Electron Microscopy to Food Research." *Food Microstructure* 7:123–135.

Serna-Saldivar, S. O. 2008. "Manufacturing of Cereal Based Dry-Milled Fractions, Potato Flour, Dry *Masa* Flour and Starches." In *Industrial Manufacture of Snack Foods.* London, UK: Kennedys Publications Ltd.

Shelton, D. R., and W. J. Lee. 2000. "Cereal Carbohydrates." In *Handbook of Cereal Science and Technology*, 2nd ed., edited by K. Kulp and J. G. Ponte. New York, NY: Marcel Dekker, Inc.

Shuey, W. C., and K. H. Tipples. 1982. *The Amylograph Handbook.* St. Paul, MN: American Association of Cereal Chemists.

Snyder, E. M. 1984. "Industrial Microscopy of Starches." In *Starch: Chemistry and Technology*, edited by R. L. Whistler, J. N. Bemiller, and E. F. Paschall, 2nd ed. Orlando, FL: Academic Press.

Steinke, J. D., L. A. Johnson, and C. Wang. 1991. Steeping maize in presence of multiple enzymes. II. Continuous countercurrent steeping. *Cereal Chemistry* 68:12–17.

Thiewes, H. J., and P. A. M. Steeneken. 1997. "Comparison of the Brabender Viscograph and the Rapid Visco Analyser." *Starch* 49(3):85–92.

Thomas, D. J., and W. A. Atwell. 1999. "Starch Analysis Methods." In *Starches.* St. Paul, MN: Eagan Press.

Walker, C. E., and J. L. Hazelton. 1996. *Application of the Rapid Visco Analyser.* Warriewood, NSW, Australia: New Port Scientific.

Watson, S. A. 1984. Corn and sorghum starches: Production. In *Starch: Chemistry and Technology*, 2nd ed., edited by R. L. Whistler, J. N. BeMiller and E. F. Paschall. Orlando, FL: Academic Press.

Watson, S. A., C. B. Williams, and R. D. Wakely. 1951. "Laboratory Steeping Procedure Used in a Wet-Milling Research Program." *Cereal Chemistry* 28:105.

Zobel, H. F., 1984. "Gelatinization of Starch and Mechanical Properties of Starch Pastes." In *Starch Chemistry and Technology,* 2nd ed., edited by R. L. Whisler, J. N. Bemiller, and E. F. Paschall. San Diego, CA: Academic Press.

7 Production of Maize Tortillas and Quality of Lime-Cooked Products

7.1 INTRODUCTION

Lime-cooking or nixtamalization consists of cooking maize kernels in a calcium hydroxide solution followed by stone-grinding to produce *masa*, which is considered the backbone for the production of many industrial and traditional foods. For table tortillas, the *masa* is sheeted and formed into thin discs and then baked. Soft tortillas are still the main staple for Mexicans and Central Americans. An average Mexican consumes more than 80 kg of maize tortillas annually. For corn chips (refer to Chapter 12), the *masa* is formed into different configurations and the resulting pieces directly deep fat–fried, whereas tortilla chips are manufactured from pieces of baked tortillas that are fried. Taco shells are the American version of tostadas, with the only difference that they are usually fried bent. Latin Americans living in the southwestern states first introduced tortilla products into the United States in the middle of the 20th century. The rapid and exponential growth of the production and sales of lime-cooked snacks took place mainly during the last two decades of the 20th century. Tortillas represent 30% of all baked product sales in the United States and continue being the most popular food in Mexico. Approximately 120 million tortillas are consumed yearly in the United States, making this the second most popular baked product, after white bread.

There are basically two ways to produce table tortillas and related snacks: fresh *masa* or dry *masa* flour. In Mexico, more than 4.8 million tons of dry *masa* flour is produced annually. Dry *masa* flour provides approximately 40% of the total tortilla market. In the United States and in other parts of the world, dry *masa* flour is the preferred way of producing nixtamalized foods. Dry flours are convenient because they have a shelf life of up to 1 year in dry storage and require only water to reform or reconstitute the *masa*. The major advantage of using dry flour is product flexibility (Rooney and Serna-Saldivar 2003; Serna-Saldivar et al. 1990). *Masa* flours for the production of white and yellow table tortillas, restaurant-style chips, tortilla chips, corn chips, and tamales are available. Additionally, these can be easily blended with other dry ingredients (i.e., preservatives, gums, and enrichment mixes) before processing.

7.2 QUALITY TESTS FOR NIXTAMALIZED PRODUCTS

The three major operations for soft tortilla production are lime-cooking, stone-grinding, and tortilla baking. Lime-cooking is considered the most important part of the process because it affects the functionality and characteristics of the product. Stone-grinding also plays a key role because it disrupts swollen pregelatinized starch granules and distributes the hydrated starch and protein around the ungelatinized portions of the endosperm, forming *masa* with a given granulation. Cooking and degree of grinding dictates the type of *masa* produced. Fine-grinding produces *masa* suitable for table tortillas whereas coarse *masa* is for fried snacks (Serna-Saldivar 2008a,b; McDonough et al. 2001). *Masa* is transformed into tortillas after a baking step that forms the typical tortilla structure. In addition, baking inactivates all microorganisms and affects the color and sensory properties of tortillas. Generally, approximately 146 kg of table tortillas with 44% to 46% moisture can be obtained from 100 kg of cleaned maize.

Maize is generally cooked with 2.5 to 3 parts water and 1% food-grade lime based on grain weight. Cooking time varies greatly from a few minutes to an hour, with 15 to 45 minutes as the range of time most often cited. In general, temperatures higher than 68°C are thought to be required for cooking to occur. Cooking depends on the characteristics of the maize and the interaction of temperature, time, lime concentration, size of cooking vessel, and frequency of agitation. Optimum cooking and steeping are determined subjectively by evaluating the extent of pericarp removal (Serna-Saldivar et al. 1991), kernel softening, and overall appearance of the *nixtamal*. For table tortillas, longer cooking times are required and *nixtamal* is steeped without quenching. *Nixtamal* for corn and tortilla chips is cooked to a lesser extent, either by decreasing the cooking time or by quenching the steeping liquor to approximately 68°C by the addition of water (Serna-Saldivar et al. 1990, 1993). After steeping, the lime-cooked maize or *nixtamal* and steeping liquor are pumped or dropped by gravity to mechanical washers to remove the *nejayote* (cook and wash water solution containing pericarp, soluble, and excess lime). The clean and wet *nixtamal* is ground using a system of two matching, carved volcanic or synthetic (aluminum oxide) stones. The milling face of the stones is typically radially carved. The grooves become progressively shallower as they approach the perimeter of the stone. The number, design, and depth of the grooves vary with the intended product. For example, stones carved for table tortillas contain more shallow grooves, and thus a finer dough is produced. Stones for corn and tortilla chips contain fewer and deeper grooves (Serna-Saldivar et al. 1990; McDonough et al. 2001).

Masa is commercially formed into tortillas using different forming equipment such as two rotating, smooth Teflon-coated rolls that automatically press the *masa* into a thin sheet of approximately 2 mm, or equipment consisting of a mixer, extruder, and former. In the latter equipment, the extrusion system forces the *masa* through a slot at the bottom of the unit and a gate cutter controls the discharge and regulates the shape and size of the *masa* product (Serna-Saldivar et al. 1990). Regardless of the type of forming device, the formed *masa* pieces are almost always baked into tortillas on a triple-pass, gas-fired oven at temperatures ranging from 280°C to 302°C for 30 to 60 seconds. These ovens are built with atmospheric gas combustion or proportional mix burners. The baking belts are either slat-type or woven wire. One side of the tortilla bakes twice as long as the other side. During baking, approximately 10% to 12% moisture is lost from the *masa*. Baking causes starch gelatinization, protein denaturation, color, and flavor development due to Maillard or browning reactions, and the inactivation of microorganisms. The baked tortillas are cooled for up to 30 minutes through a series of open tiers that discharge into the packaging area. Tortilla shelf life greatly depends on the effectiveness of cooling (Serna-Saldivar et al. 1990).

A useful quality control guide for the production of nixtamalized foods is included in the *Corn Quality Assurance Manual* of the Snack Food Association (Rooney 2007). The fresh and dry *masa* flour industries have developed numerous measurements to control the quality of raw materials and the intermediate and finished products. The quality of raw kernels is tested similar to other milling industries (refer to Chapter 1). The main quality control parameters for fresh *masa* and dry flours are particle size distribution, degree of starch gelatinization, water absorption, color, and pH (Almeida Dominguez et al. 1996). The extent of pericarp removal and the evaluation of optimum cooking and incurred dry matter losses are very useful to standardize processing conditions and quality. Pericarp removal can be effectively determined after lime-cooking maize and dyeing the resulting kernels with the May–Gruenwald solution (Serna-Saldivar et al. 1991) and lime-cooking properties in the method devised by Serna-Saldivar et al. (1993; Table 7.1). The industry prefers kernels that easily lose their pericarp because pericarp-free cooked kernels yield flours with better color scores and functionality. The most important factor to control during alkaline cooking is the extent of cooking. Most processors evaluate cooking by observing the condition of the *nixtamal*. Analytical approaches that have been applied include tests for enzyme-susceptible starch, loss of birefringence, viscosity with consistometers, amylograph peak viscosity, mixograph tests (Lobeira et al. 1998), and Instron shear force (Bedolla and Rooney 1984). The viscoamylograph (Shuey and Tipples 1982) and rapid viscoanalyzer are effective and fast ways to determine the extent of *nixtamal* cooking (Almeida Dominguez et al. 1997). One of the simplest tests to indirectly determine gelatinization is the water absorption and solubility indexes proposed by Anderson et al. (1969). The industry also relies on viscosity tests in which a certain amount of flour is mixed with water to produce a slurry. More viscous slurries are obtained from flours with higher cooking or starch gelatinization and these tend to flow less (Lobeira et al. 1998) when placed on an inclined ramp

or a table marked with concentric circles. The determination of peak viscosity with the regular or rapid viscoamylograph correlates well with the extent of cooking, although values change when hydrocolloids are added beforehand to *masa* flours. Lobeira et al. (1998) developed rapid viscoanalyzer, consistometer, and mixograph methods to evaluate the pasting, hydration, and mixing properties of dry *masa* flours.

The quality control parameters summarized in Table 7.1 are the most frequently used tests to assess the quality of *nixtamal, masa,* and tortillas.

7.2.1 NIXTAMAL COOKING AND QUALITY

Lime-cooking for the production of *nixtamal* is considered the most important step of the tortilla-making process. The maize kernels are usually cooked with 2.5 to 3 parts water and 1% food-grade lime based on grain weight. Cooking time varies from a few minutes to an hour according to the physical properties of the grain, the desired type of *masa,* and the cooking conditions especially in terms of temperature. For table tortillas, longer cooking times are required and *nixtamal* is steeped without quenching. *Nixtamal* for corn and tortilla chips is cooked to a lesser extent, either by decreasing the cooking time or by quenching the steeping liquor to approximately 68°C by the addition of water (refer to Chapter 12; Serna-Saldivar et al. 1990, 1993; McDonough et al. 2001). Optimum cooking and steeping are determined subjectively by evaluating the extent of pericarp removal (Serna-Saldivar et al. 1991), kernel softening, and overall appearance of the *nixtamal.*

7.2.1.1 Ease of Pericarp Removal Test

Lime-cooking of maize causes hydrolysis of fiber components associated with cell walls mainly located in the pericarp tissue. Therefore, the amount of pericarp removed during lime cooking, steeping, and *nixtamal* washing affects the product's color, *masa* texture and machinability, and tortilla and chips quality. The ease of pericarp removal during lime cooking is an inherited trait and therefore is closely linked to genotype. The extent of pericarp removal is affected by type and strength of the alkali, cooking time and temperature, and type of maize kernels. Serna-Saldivar et al. (1991) devised a method to efficiently determine the extent of pericarp removal during nixtamalization using the May–Gruenwald dye, which is commonly used to determine the dry-milling efficiency of rice and sorghum.

A. *Samples, Ingredients, and Reagents*
- Maize
- Food-grade reactive lime (CaO)
- Eosine-Y
- Methylene blue
- Methanol

B. *Materials and Equipment*
- Digital scale
- Graduated cylinders
- Cooking vessel

TABLE 7.1
Quality Control Parameters Most Commonly Used to Assess Quality of *Nixtamal*, *Masa*, and Tortillas

Quality Control Test	Equipment Instrument	Importance
	Nixtamal	
Moisture	NIRA, microwave, moisture meters/balances, air-oven method (AACC 2000, 44-15A)	The moisture content of the cooked-steeped *nixtamal* is correlated to the extent of cooking and degree of starch gelatinization.
pH	Potentiometer calibrated with buffers	The pH of the *nixtamal* correlates to the lime absorbed during cooking and steeping and the amount of washing. The pH affects flavor, texture, and color of tortillas and related products.
Pericarp removal test	Use of May–Gruenwald dye (Serna-Saldivar et al. 1991)	Maize kernels are placed inside nylon bags for lime-cooking for a given amount of time (20 minutes) and then stained with a May–Gruenwald dye containing methylene blue and eosine-Y. After washing excess dye, kernels are evaluated by determining the blue-greenish stained pericarp (Serna-Saldivar et al. 1991). Insufficient removal of the pericarp causes darker colorations in tortillas and off-colors in snacks.
Optimum lime-cooking time and dry matter loss	Mini-cooking trial (Serna-Saldivar et al. 1993)	A known amount of maize kernels are placed inside nylon bags and lime-cooked for three different times and then steeped in the cooking solution overnight. Optimum cooking time is calculated using regression equations solving the time required to achieve a certain *nixtamal* moisture level (50% for table tortillas and 48% for tortilla chips) and dry matter loss is calculated by estimating the loss incurred during the cooking process. Both parameters are of utmost importance for the production of fresh *masa* and tortillas.
	Masa	
Moisture	NIRA, microwave, moisture meters/balances, air-oven method (AACC 2000, 44-15A	The moisture content of *masa* greatly affects texture, rheological properties and machinability.
Particle size distribution	Use of sieves to fractionate wet *masa* (Pflugfelder et al. 1988)	A *masa* sample is fractionated in a set of sieves (U.S. nos. 35, 60, and 100 mesh sieves and filter paper) with the aid of water sprayed with a squeeze bottle. The amount of sample recovered from each sieve is weighed and dried. The particle size distribution can be expressed on wet or dry matter basis. The method is fast and ideally suited to adjust grinders in processing plants.
Color value	Color meters (Hunter Lab and others)	The color of the *masa* is greatly affected by the color of the raw grain, the amount of lime used during cooking/steeping and the amount of lime removed during *nixtamal* washing. The color of the *masa* correlates with the color of table tortillas and fried tortilla chips.
Starch gelatinization	Birefringence with microscope equipped with polarized filters	Microscopic technique used to determine the relative amount of gelatinized vs. native starch granules (starch granules show Maltese cross).
	Glucoamylase method with subsequent measurement of glucose (AACC 2000, Method 76-16)	Chemical analysis in which the *masa* is subjected to amyloglucosidase hydrolysis followed by the determination of glucose with glucose oxidase. The ESS assay correlates with degree of cooking and starch gelatinization.
Starch properties	Viscoamylograph (Shuey and Tipples 1982)	One of the most important functional tests because, after analyzing the viscoamylograph curve, temperature at the start of gelatinization, peak viscosity, shear thinning, and set back viscosity (retrogradation) could be determined. These properties greatly influence the processing characteristics and quality of end products. Peak viscosity is closely related to the amount of starch gelatinized during the lime-cooking and grinding processes.
WAI and WSI	Centrifugation of slurry (Anderson et al. 1969)	These parameters are greatly affected by the degree of starch gelatinization or extent of cooking.
Masa hardness	Instron or TAXT2. texture analyzer, compression test	A given piece of *masa* is compressed at a constant rate to obtain a force–deformation curve.
Masa texture	Penetrometer	The force required to deform *masa* obtained after hydration with a given amount of water gives an indication of the amount of cooking or starch gelatinization.
	Adhesiveness test (Ramirez Wong et al. 1993)	The adhesiveness of *masa* can be rapidly evaluated with a mechanical stickiness device consisting of two rectangular bars in a parallel arrangement. A block of *masa* is formed between the bars and partially split with a cutter and the adhesiveness measured by raising the movable bar until the *masa* detaches from it. The degree of adhesion of *masa* to the upper bar gives an adhesiveness index.

(continued)

TABLE 7.1 (Continued)

Quality Control Parameters Most Commonly Used to Assess Quality of *Nixtamal, Masa,* and Tortillas

Quality Control Test	Equipment Instrument	Importance
	Texture analyzer or Instron. TPA (Bosiger 1997)	The TPA consists of a two-bite compression assay developed to determine adhesivity, cohesiveness, firmness, springiness, and other rheological parameters of *masa* using a texture analyzer. The technique was developed for quality control purposes and is sensitive to different degrees of lime-cooking, *masa* particle size, other processing conditions, and the addition of gums and other additives.
		Tortillas
Moisture	NIRA, microwave, moisture meters/balances, air-oven method (AACC 2000, 44-15A)	The moisture content of baked or equilibrated tortilla affects oil absorption during frying.
Pilot plant alkaline cooking	Tortilla pilot plant	Procedure to evaluate alkaline cooking properties of 3 to k kg lots of maize. Kernels are placed in a perforated nylon bag, lime-cooked, steeped, washed, and stone-ground into *masa*. The *masa* is sheeted, formed into tortillas or tortilla pieces in a small-scale three-tier baking oven. Yields of tortillas are calculated by obtaining the original moisture content of the grain and the amount of tortillas obtained. Resulting tortillas can be used for texture, color, organoleptic, and shelf life stability tests.
Texture tests	Texture analyzer or Instron equipped with Kramer shear tests	The texture of tortillas could be determined using the bending test described by Suhendro et al. (1998b). The bending technique is sensitive to changes in tortilla texture throughout storage or equilibration.
	Rollability test (Suhendro et al. 1998a,b)	The objective rollability test uses a custom-designed rollability fixture consisting of an acrylic cylindrical dowel and a metal chain that connects the cylinder dowel to the texture analyzer arm. The force and work required to pull the axle is determined. The technique is fast, simple, and sensitive to changes in tortilla texture.
Color value	Color meters (Hunter Lab and others)	The color of the tortilla correlates with the color of the fried product.
Blistering or pillowing	Visual observation	The number and frequency of blisters or pillows in table tortillas and raw tortilla chips greatly affects the texture of the finished products. For chips, it is considered as the most important defect because pillowing will exacerbate during frying. Blistering is controlled by the particle size of the *masa*, percentage of moisture in the *masa* and by the temperature profile during baking.

Source: AACC 2000; Almeida Dominguez et al., *Cereal Foods World* 41:624–630, 1996; Anderson et al., *Cereal Sci. Today* 14:1, 1969; Bosiger, 1997; Lobeira et al., *Cereal Chem.* 75(4):417-420, 1998; Pflugfelder et al., *Cereal Chem.* 65:127–132, 1988; Ramirez Wong et al., *Cereal Chem.* 70(3):286–290, 1993; Rooney and Suhendro, *Snack Foods Processing*, Technomic Publishing Co., Inc. Lancaster, PA, 2001; Serna-Saldivar et al., *Advances in Cereal Science and Technology*, American Association of Cereal Chemists, St. Paul, MN, 1990; *Crop Sci.* 31:842–844, 1991; *Cereal Chem.* 70:762–764, 1993; Serna-Saldivar 2003; Shuey and Tipples 1982, and Suhendro et al., *Cereal Chem.* 75(3):320–324, 1998a; *Cereal Chem.* 75:854–858, 1998b.

- Agitator
- Perforated nylon bags
- Thermometer
- Laboratory clock or chronometer
- Beakers (500 mL capacity)
- Wire or plastic basket that fits inside the beakers

C. *Procedure*

This procedure was previously discussed in Serna-Saldivar et al. (1991).

1. Place 15 g to 20 g of the different maize samples in perforated nylon bags. Make sure to identify nylon bags containing the different kernel

samples and tie the nylon bag to resist the cooking procedure (Figure 7.1).

2. Heat 25 L or 50 L of water to a gentle boiling (98–100°C) in a covered cooking vessel such as a jacketed steam cooker. A 25-L cooking vessel can test 75 different maize samples placed in nylon bags.

3. Add 83.3 g or 166.6 g of food-grade reactive lime to 25 L or 50 L of boiling water. Mix the lime thoroughly with the hot water.

4. Add all the perforated nylon bags (36 perforations/cm^2) to the hot lime solution and start the

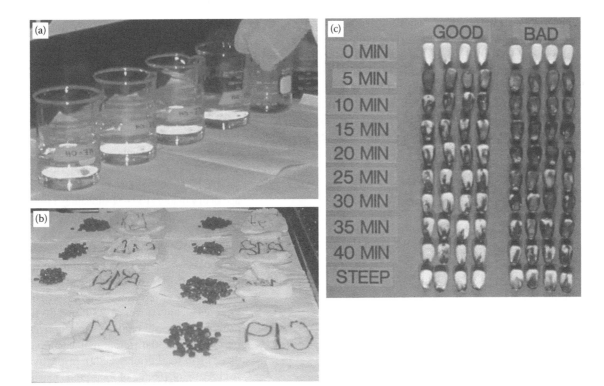

FIGURE 7.1 Steps for determining ease of pericarp removal of *nixtamal* using the May–Gruenwald dye. (a) Immersion of *nixtamal* into May–Gruenwald solution; (b) subjective evaluation of pericarp removal; (c) progressive removal of pericarp as affected by lime-cooking time and steeping.

laboratory clock for exactly 20 minutes of cooking. The solution should reboil 2 to 3 minutes after adding the samples.

5. Make sure to agitate contents every 3 minutes and maintain all nylon bags submerged in the cooking solution.

6. After exactly 20 minutes of cooking, turn off the heating source and remove nylon bags from the cooker. The nylon bags should be quenched in a bucket containing running tap water.

7. After quenching and washing, open the nylon bag and obtain a random sample of 10 to 20 kernels. Place kernels in a perforated wire basket in preparation for staining.

8. Prepare, beforehand, a May–Gruenwald stock solution by dissolving 1 g of eosine-Y and 1 g of methylene blue in 200 mL of methanol. The stock solution should be stored in a dark bottle under refrigeration. The working solution is prepared a few minutes before starting the procedure by diluting one part of the stock May–Gruenwald solution with three parts of methanol.

9. Submerge the wire basket containing the lime-cooked maize sample for 15 to 20 seconds in the working dye solution (Figure 7.1).

10. Rinse excess dye by submerging the wire basket in three consecutive beakers containing 250 mL to 300 mL of methanol. Each rinsing step should last from 5 to 10 seconds. Replace the methanol rinsing solution after 50 samples.

11. Determine subjectively the amount of pericarp removal by observing the blue-green stained pericarp remaining on the kernel. A scale of 1 to 5 is recommended, in which 1, pericarp totally removed; 2.5, 50% of the pericarp was removed; and 5, all pericarp is still attached to the kernel. Make sure to evaluate all kernels and obtain an average pericarp removal value.

7.2.1.2 Mini Lime-Cooking Trial: Optimum Cooking and Dry Matter Loss

The extent of cooking and dry matter losses can be determined by the mini-cooking trial (Serna-Saldivar et al. 1993). Fixed amounts of maize kernels with known initial moisture contents are placed in perforated nylon bags for different lime-cooking times (i.e., 0, 20, and 40 minutes) and then steeped overnight. Resulting *nixtamals* are washed, blotted on paper towels to remove excess water, and immediately tested for moisture and dry matter. For each maize type, regression equations can be calculated to predict optimum cooking times and percentage of dry matter loss. Generally, as cooking time increases, water absorption increases due to higher starch gelatinization. *Nixtamal* for table tortillas and chips is usually cooked to increase the moisture content to 50% and 48% moisture, respectively. This method is aimed toward the prediction of the optimum lime-cooking time because it greatly affects *masa* machinability, tortilla properties, and yield of product. In addition, the method calculates dry matter losses incurred during lime cooking, steeping, and washing.

A. *Samples, Ingredients, and Reagents*
- Maize
- Food-grade reactive lime (CaO)

B. *Materials and Equipment*
- Digital scale
- Air-forced oven
- Graduated cylinders
- Cooking vessel with lid
- Agitator
- Perforated nylon bags
- Colander
- Thermometer
- Laboratory clock or chronometer

C. *Procedure*
This procedure was previously discussed in Serna-Saldivar et al. (1993).

1. Clean the different maize samples by discarding foreign material and broken kernels. Determine moisture content of all maize samples.
2. Weigh quadruplicate maize samples of 100 g and place them in perforated nylon bags (17 cm × 12.5 cm). Register the weight with an accuracy of 0.1 g and then calculate the dry matter of the 100-g sample by multiplying sample weight by percentage of dry matter (100 – % moisture). For instance, a 100-g sample with 14% moisture contains 86 g of solids or dry matter. Make sure to identify nylon bags and tie it to avoid sample loss during the cooking-steeping procedure (Figure 7.2).
3. Heat 25 L or 50 L of water to a gentle boil (98–100°C) in a covered cooking vessel such as a jacketed steam cooker. A 25 L and 50 L capacity cooking vessel can test quadruplicate samples of 15 and 30 different maize samples (6 kg or 12 kg of total grain weight), respectively.
4. Add 83.3 g or 166.6 g of food-grade reactive lime to the 25 L or 50 L of boiling water. Thoroughly mix the lime with the hot water.

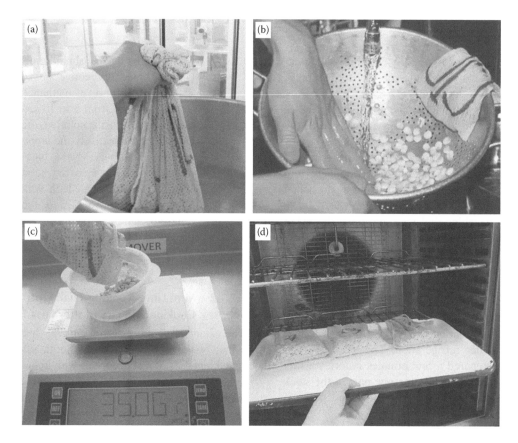

FIGURE 7.2 Sequential steps for determining the lime-cooking properties and *nixtamal* dry matter losses using the nylon bag mini-cooking trial. (a) Lime-cooking of maize samples placed in nylon bags; (b) washing of *nixtamal*; (c) weighing of cleaned *nixtamal* sample; (d) drying of *nixtamal* placed in nylon bags.

5. Assign quadruplicate samples to 0, 15, 30, and 45 minutes cooking time. Add first all the perforated nylon bags assigned to the 45-minute cooking schedule. After exactly 15 and 30 minutes, add the second and third lots of samples to the hot lime solution. Finally, after exactly 45 minutes, add the last set of samples and immediately shut off the heat source or discontinue heat. Make sure to agitate contents every 3 minutes during the whole cooking procedure and maintain all nylon bags submerged in the cooking solution. Place the lid of the cooker to achieve a uniform heat decrease during steeping.

6. Allow maize samples to steep for 14 to 16 hours in the cooking vessel equipped with the lid.

7. Drain steep water or *nejayote* and place all nylon bags with the maize samples in a bucket containing tap water. Then, open each bag and wash the sample by first placing the *nixtamal* in a colander in preparation for cleaning with running tap water for 40 seconds. Then, blot the cleaned *nixtamal* in a paper towel to remove excess water.

8. Weigh and register the cleaned *nixtamal* with an accuracy of 0.1 g. Then, return the cleaned *nixtamal* to its corresponding nylon bag for drying (Figure 7.2).

9. Dry the nylon bag containing the *nixtamal* sample for 24 hours in an air-forced oven set at 100°C.

10. After drying, place nylon bags in a desiccator for 30 minutes of cooling. Then, open the bag and weigh its contents with an accuracy of 0.1 g. Register the dry *nixtamal* weight (Figure 7.2).

11. Calculate the dry matter loss and *nixtamal* moisture for each cooking time using the following equations:

Nixtamal moisture = [(wet *nixtamal* weight – dry *nixtamal* weight)/dry grain weight] × 100.

Dry matter loss = [(dry grain weight – dry *nixtamal* weight)/dry grain weight] × 100.

12. Calculate the optimum cooking time for each sample using linear regression. Relate the *nixtamal* moisture (*y* axis) with the different cooking times (*x* axis; 0, 15, 30, and 45 minutes). For the preparation of corn tortillas and tortilla chips, the optimum cooking is considered the time needed to increase the *nixtamal* moisture to 48% to 50% and 46% to 48% moisture, respectively.

13. Calculate the dry matter loss for each sample using linear regression. Relate the solid losses (*y* axis) with the different cooking times (*x* axis). Then, calculate the dry matter loss at an optimum cooking time.

7.2.2 MASA QUALITY

Masa is produced after stone-grinding of the clean and hydrated *nixtamal* by a system of two matching carved volcanic or synthetic stones. The milling faces of the stones are radially carved. The grooves become progressively shallower as they approach the perimeter of the stone. The number, design, and depth of the grooves vary with the intended product. For example, stones carved for table tortillas contain more shallow grooves, and thus a finer dough is produced. Stones for corn and tortilla chips contain fewer and deeper grooves. The grinding operation consists of forcing the *nixtamal* through a center opening of one of the stones that conducts it into the gap between the stones. Water is added during the grinding operation to cool the stones, prevent excessive wear, reduce *masa* temperature, and increase the moisture content in the *masa*. *Masa* particle size is the result of several interacting factors, (1) degree of *nixtamal* cooking, (2) carving design of the grinding stones, (3) pressure between stones, (4) amount of water added during milling, and (5) type of maize (Serna-Saldivar et al. 1990).

Stone-grinding for the production of *masa* is considered critically important for both the tortilla and snack industries. The moisture content, pH, color, particle size distribution, degree of starch gelatinization, and rheological properties are usually assessed (Table 7.1).

Pflugfelder et al. (1988) developed a simple method to determine the particle size distribution of wet *masa* consisting of wet-sieving of the particles through a set or nest of sieves. Likewise, the granulation of dry *masa* flours plays an important role in functionality and product quality. It is generally determined with the Rotap furnished with coarse (U.S. no. 20–35 mesh), medium (U.S. no. 60–80 mesh), and fine (U.S. no. 100 mesh) sieves and a collection pan (refer to procedure in Section 5.3.1.1).

Plasticity, cohesiveness, and stickiness are some of the subjective rheological properties of *masa* that are used to judge optimum cooking conditions. The stickiness of *masa* can be rapidly evaluated with a mechanical stickiness device consisting of two rectangular bars in a parallel arrangement. A block of *masa* is formed between the bars and partially split with a cutter and the stickiness measured by raising the movable bar until the *masa* detaches from it. The degree of adhesion of *masa* to the upper bar gives an adhesiveness index (Ramirez Wong et al. 1993).

A texture profile analysis (TPA) of *masa*, consisting of a two-bite compression test, was developed to determine adhesivity, cohesiveness, firmness, springiness, and other important rheological parameters. The texture analyzer technique was developed for quality control purposes and is sensitive to different degrees of lime-cooking, *masa* particle size, and the addition of gums and other additives (Bosiger 1997).

7.2.2.1 Color

The color of the *masa* is greatly affected by the color of the raw grain, the amount of lime used during cooking/steeping, and the amount of lime removed during *nixtamal* washing. The color of the *masa* correlates with the color of the raw and fried tortilla chips. For objective color determinations, refer to procedures detailed in Chapter 3.

7.2.2.2 Determination of pH

Masa pH is highly related to the lime absorbed during *nixtamal* cooking and steeping and the extent of washing. pH affects the flavor, texture, and color of tortillas and related products.

A. Samples, Ingredients, and Reagents
- Different *masas*
- Standard buffer solutions (pH 4, 7, and 9)

B. Materials and Equipment
- Hot plate
- Laboratory blender
- pH meter
- Beakers (250 mL and 500 mL)
- Graduated cylinders (100 mL and 200 mL)
- Laboratory clock

C. Procedure
1. Bring to a boil distilled and deionized water, suspend heat and allow water to equilibrate to room temperature.
2. Scale 20 g of dry *masa* flour or 40 g of fresh *masa* with an accuracy of 0.1 g. Place the sample in the bowl of the laboratory blender.
3. For dry *masa* flour and fresh *masa*, add 180 mL and 160 mL of the boiled distilled and deionized water, respectively.
4. Blend the mix at low speed for 1 minute.
5. Allow resulting suspension to rest for exactly 20 minutes.
6. Determine pH with a pH meter that was previously calibrated with at least two standard buffer solutions of pH 4, 7, or 9. Make sure to adjust the pH meter to the temperature of the laboratory.

7.2.2.3 Particle Size Distribution of Hydrated *Masa*

The particle size distribution of *masa* is greatly affected by the physical properties of the grain, extent of lime-cooking–steeping, and the settings of the stone grinder. The granulation of the *masa* is carefully controlled in both table tortilla and chips operations because this factor greatly affects quality. In general, *masa* for table tortillas is ground finer compared with *masa* for corn chips and tortilla chips (refer to Chapter 12). Pflugfelder et al. (1988) developed a quick and simple method to determine the granulation of hydrated *masa* consisting of wet-sieving the particles through a set of sieves and weighing the resulting fractions. This assay can be effectively used in processing plants to control the setting of the grinder.

A. Samples, Ingredients, and Reagents
- *Masa* samples
- Distilled water
- Dessicant (activated alumina)

B. Materials and Equipment
- Scale
- Air-forced oven
- Airtight desiccator
- Tongs
- Moisture dishes
- Laboratory tweezers
- Set of 7.5 cm diameter sieves (U.S. nos. 20, 35, 60, and 100 mesh)
- Buckner filter
- Whatman paper filter
- Kitasato flask for vacuum filtering
- Squeeze bottle
- Laboratory brush

C. Procedure
This procedure was previously discussed by Pflugfelder et al. (1988).
1. Obtain a representative *masa* sample.
2. Weigh exactly 10 g of wet *masa* (Figure 7.3).
3. Construct a set of sieves (U.S. nos. 20, 35, 60, and 100 mesh) on top of a Buckner filter furnished with Whatman filter paper (Figure 7.3).
4. Place the *masa* on top of the U.S. no. 20 mesh sieve. With the squeeze bottle spray water and carefully distribute the *masa* with the brush. Carefully recover and weigh the overs of the U.S. no. 20 mesh sieve. Repeat the procedure with each of the following sieves. After recovering the overs of the U.S. no. 100 mesh sieve, place the Buckner filter on a Kitasato flask for vacuum filtering.

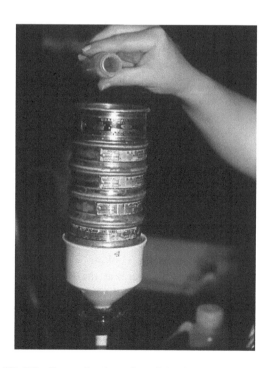

FIGURE 7.3 Determination of particle size distribution of wet *masa*.

5. Spray water on top of the filter paper and vacuum filter. The filter paper will retain the starch-rich material. Recover and weigh the starch-rich material from the filter paper by carefully scraping.

6. Register the wet weight of each fraction and then place fractions in an air-forced oven for drying at 100°C for 8 hours.

7. Remove samples from the air-forced oven and immediately transfer them to a desiccator for 30 minutes of equilibration. Weigh dry sample weights with an accuracy of 0.01 g.

8. Express particle size distributions based on the total wet and dry matter weights.

7.2.2.4 Determination of *Masa* Stickiness

Ramirez Wong et al. (1993) developed an instrumental assay to objectively evaluate *masa* stickiness. The assay consists of two rectangular bars fastened at one end in a parallel arrangement with a 12-mm gap between them. A block of *masa* is formed between the bars and partially split with a special cutter. Then, one end of the movable upper bar is raised until the *masa* detaches. The test measures the degree of *masa* adhesion to the upper bar, yielding an adhesiveness index.

A. *Samples, Ingredients, and Reagents*
- Different lots of *masas*

B. *Materials and Equipment*
- Digital scale
- Plastic film
- Ruler
- Knife
- Mechanical stickiness device consisting of two smooth, flat-surfaced rectangular bars made of aluminum (25 × 1.6 × 1.5 cm in length, width, and height, respectively). A screw in the bottom stationary bar allows the upper bar to move upwards. When paralel, the bars had a 1.2-cm gap between them (Ramirez Wong et al. 1993).
- V-shaped *masa* cutter consisting of two guitar strings in a rectangular frame with no bottom and one end made of 3-mm Plexiglas (dimensions, 30 × 1.5 × 1.6 cm in length, width, and height, respectively). The guitar strings (no. 4) are attached to the side walls at the other end of the device so that both wires are horizontally and V-shaped in position (Ramirez Wong et al. 1993).

C. *Procedure*

This procedure was previously discussed by Ramirez Wong et al. (1993).

1. Clean the interior surfaces of the aluminum bars of the mechanical stickiness device.

2. Position bars in parallel with the aid of the screw.

3. Weigh 175 g of *masa* and roll it by hand on a surface covered with a plastic sheet. The resulting cylinder should be 15 cm in length and 3 cm in diameter.

4. Lift the upper bar to allow the *masa* cylinder to be placed at the bottom stationary bar. Then, compress the *masa* between the two bars. With a sharp knife, remove the masa flowing outside the bars. The block of *masa* remaining in between the bars should weigh approximately 42 g ± 2 g.

5. Longitudinally split the *masa* with the cutting device.

6. Slowly raise the upper bar until the *masa* detaches from the bar.

7. Measure the length of the *masa* still adhering to the upper bar.

8. Calculate the percentage of adhesiveness using the following equation:

$$\% \text{ adhesiveness} = (\text{cm of } masa \text{ adhering to the} \\ \text{upper bar}/15 \text{ cm}) \times 100.$$

A noncohesive *masa* gives values lower than 12%, an optimum cooked *masa* 10% to 35%, and sticky *masa* values are higher than 73%.

7.2.2.5 Determination of *Masa* Consistency with the Penetrometer

Masa texture is critical for tortilla- and related snack-making processes. *Masa* should be adhesive enough to slightly stick to the sheeting rollers and to separate properly. When *masa* is overcooked, it becomes sticky, and when undercooked, it is noncohesive and generally yields a less desirable *masa* especially in terms of machinability.

A. *Samples, Ingredients, and Reagents*
- Different lots of *masas*

B. *Materials and Equipment*
- Digital scale
- Penetrometer (precision penetrometer)
- Aluminum cone (35 g)
- 50 g or 100 g weights
- 1.5 kg or 2 kg weight
- Wire cutter
- Graduated cylinder (100 mL)
- Beaker (250 mL)
- Mixer
- Chronometer
- Mold (7.5 cm diameter × 3.75 cm deep)

C. *Procedure*

1. Determine the wet *masa* moisture content and particle size distribution (refer to procedures in Sections 2.2.1.1 and 7.2.2.3). For dry *masa* flour testing, mix 500 g of dry flour with 550 mL of water for 4 minutes at low speed. Place resulting wet *masa* inside a plastic bag for 10 to 15 minutes before testing. The amount of water can be modified to produce *masa* for table tortillas or snacks. For table tortillas, a ratio

of 1.2 to 1.3 water/kg *masa* flour is generally used. For snacks, the ratio generally used and recommended is 1 to 1.1 water/kg *masa* flour. Determine the moisture content and particle size distribution of the reconstituted *masa* flour.

2. Form a *masa* cylinder using the 7.5 cm (3 in.) diameter × 3.75 cm (1.5 in.)–deep mold. Make sure to overfill the mold. Place a 1.5 kg to 2 kg weight on top and allow to compress for 1 minute. Remove weight and cut excess *masa* using the wire cutter.

3. Carefully remove the preformed *masa* cylinder and place it on the penetrometer's base.

4. Set up the penetrometer with a 100 g weight. Set to zero and move cone until it is barely touching the sample.

5. Release the rod and hold for 15 seconds.

6. Read penetration in millimeters.

7.2.2.6 *Masa* Texture with the Instron Compression Tension Test

Ramirez Wong et al. (1993) developed an assay to objectively evaluate *masa* texture with the Instron. The compression tension test compresses a preformed *masa* disk between two flat plates to a thickness of 2 mm, and then the sample is put under tension. This test is capable of obtaining important factors such as adhesiveness, hardness, and the compression tension factor. This assay proved to be reproducible and capable of discriminating *masas* with different moistures, cooking schedules, and degrees of gelatinization.

A. *Samples, Ingredients, and Reagents*
- Different types of *masas*

B. *Materials and Equipment*
- Instron universal testing machine
- Cylindrical plastic container (31 mm in diameter and 6 mm in height)
- Two smooth, flat, stainless steel plates of 6.9 cm diameter. The stationary top plate is attached to the compression tension load cell (1000 lb) of the Instron texture analyzer. The bottom plate is attached to the crosshead that moves up or down at a constant speed of 0.5 cm/min.

C. *Procedure*
This procedure was previously discussed by Ramirez Wong et al. (1993).

1. Equip the Instron universal testing machine with a 1.000-lb load cell and calibrate the crosshead speed to 0.5 cm/min and the chart speed to 10 cm/min. Calibrate the recorder to zero at the center of the chart.

2. Weigh 5 g ± 0.05 g of *masa* and shape it into a sphere. Then, flatten the piece of masa into a cylindrical plastic container 31 mm in diameter and 6 mm in height.

3. Place the resulting *masa* disk between the stainless steel plates.

4. Start the previously calibrated and programmed Instron machine by first compressing the sample and then moving the lower plates apart to apply tension loading. The compression loading proceeds until the plates are 2 mm apart. Then, the crosshead movement stops and automatically moves in the opposite direction.

5. Register the compressive and tensile forces with a chart speed of 10 cm/min.

6. Interpret the force–distance curve. Hardness (Pa) is defined as the maximum compression force, adhesiveness or stickiness (N/m area under the negative curve) as the maximum tensile force or tensile work, and the compressive to tensile force or work as the ratio of maximum compression to tensile force or work.

7.2.2.7 TPA of *Masa*

The TPA of *masa* consists of a two-bite compression test that measures hardness/firmness, adhesiveness, cohesiveness, chewiness, gumminess, springiness, and resilience. The texture analyzer technique was developed for quality control purposes and is sensitive to different degrees of lime-cooking, *masa* particle size, other processing conditions, and the addition of gums and other additives (Bosiger 1997). Sample preparation procedure is critical to assure acceptable sensitivity to test the *masa* texture characteristics. Freshness and geometry of *masa* samples are critical control parameters.

A. *Samples, Ingredients, and Reagents*
- Different types of *masas*
- Plastic shortening

B. *Materials and Equipment*
- Digital scale
- Texture analyzer TAXT2 (Texture Tech.)
- Cylindrical probe (6 cm diameter)
- Graduated cylinder (1 L)
- Chronometer
- Dough mixer with paddle
- Polyethylene bag
- Acrylic mold (1.5 in. diameter 1.5 in. deep)
- Acrylic plunger to fit 1.5 in. mold
- Wire cutter
- 4 lb weight

C. *Procedure*
1. Collect a representative sample of fresh-milled *masa* and place it immediately in a plastic bag. If dry *masa* flour is to be analyzed, determine beforehand its moisture content and particle size distribution. Decide the amount of water to add to produce the targeted moisture content in the rehydrated *masa* flour. *Masa* for table tortillas usually contains 56% to 58% moisture, whereas tortilla chips usually have 54% moisture (Bosiger 1997). Calculate the amount of water required to reach the desired *masa*

moisture content. For instance, if 500 g of dry *masa* flour containing 10% moisture will be hydrated to 58%, add 571 mL of water.

Water to add = (100 − % moisture of *masa* flour)/(100 − desired *masa* moisture content) − 1] × amount of dry *masa* flour = [(90/42) − 1] × 500 = 571.4 mL water.

2. Place the dry *masa* flour in a mixing bowl and add the predetermined amount of water and blend at low speed for 5 minutes. Make sure to scrape flour that adheres to the sides of the bowl. Place *masa* in a polyethylene bag and rest for 15 minutes before testing (resting allows uniform distribution of water and full hydration of particles).

3. Lightly grease the center of the mold with shortening. Weigh approximately 80 g of *masa* and manually roll it into a cylinder less than 1.5 in. thick. Push *masa* into the center of the mold and apply just enough pressure with your thumb to fill the gaps of air.

4. Place the 4-lb weight on top of the *masa* and mold for 1 minute to standardize the packing of the *masa* into the mold. Scrape the excess *masa* off the top of the mold with the wire slicer.

5. Place *masa* cylinder on the analyzer platform and run test using the TPA setup (test speed 5 mm/sec, contact force 0.048 N). Test the cylinder surface that was in contact with the polyethylene film. Clean probe after each test.

6. Record the TPA parameters for springiness, cohesiveness, chewiness, gumminess, adhesiveness, hardness, and resilience.

7.2.3 Tortilla Production and Quality

There are basically two ways to produce table tortillas and related snacks: fresh *masa* or dry *masa* flour. The quality of the *nixtamal* and *masa* greatly affects tortilla quality. The tortilla is produced by first shaping or molding the *masa* into tortilla disks and then baking on a hot surface. Most commercial tortillas are baked on a three-tier gas-fired oven at temperatures ranging from 280°C to 302°C for 45 to 60 seconds. Thus, one side of the tortilla bakes twice as long as the other side. During the baking process, the starch and protein further gelatinizes and denatures, respectively, the plastic *masa* sets its structure into a tortilla and the product develops color and flavor due to Maillard reactions. Furthermore, the tortilla exits the oven without any microbial count. The baked tortillas are cooled and then packaged to prevent moisture and texture loss. Tortilla shelf life greatly depends on the effectiveness of the cooling operation. Improper cooling before packaging causes microbial problems, sticking of stacked and packaged tortillas, and moisture condensation inside the package (Serna-Saldivar et al. 1990).

As with most bakery products, the quality of fresh and stored tortillas is assessed in terms of texture (folding or bending capacity and firmness), color, and flavor. Another critical factor is shelf life. Texture is greatly affected by starch gelatinization and retrogradation and the softness and reheating capacity is improved when antistaling agents such as hydrocolloids or gums and emulsifiers are included in the formulation. Color is affected by the type of maize used (i.e., white, yellow, or blue), amount of lime used during cooking, extent of *nixtamal* washing, and pH, which is affected by the supplemented acidulants or lime added to the *masa* before baking. Flavor is greatly affected by pH, amount of lime that remained in the tortilla, and some additives used to prolong microbial shelf life (i.e., acidulants and preservatives).

7.2.3.1 Production of Tortillas

A. *Samples, Ingredients, and Reagents*
- Maize
- Food-grade lime
- Distilled water

B. *Materials and Equipment*
- Digital scale
- Graduated cylinders (100 mL, 200 mL, or 1 L)
- Dough mixer (hook or paddle attachments)
- Cooker (steam or conventional)
- Stone grinder
- Tortilla-forming equipment with cutters
- Three-tiered, gas-fired baking oven
- Cooling rack
- Infrared or spot thermometer (300°C)
- Chronometer

C. *Procedure*
1. Weigh a fixed amount of cleaned maize kernels and add three times as much water and 1% food-grade lime based on grain weight to the cooking vessel. Keep the maize kernels separated from the lime solution.

2. Adjust the temperature of the cooking solution (most processes cook at near-boiling or between 85°C and 100°C). When the cooking solution reaches the proper temperature, add the grain and register temperatures throughout cooking. Make sure to stir contents frequently (i.e., every 5 minutes). Cook the maize kernels for the predetermined cooking time (refer to mini lime-cooking trial), suspend heat and leave kernels to steep for at least 8 hours (optimally, 12–14 hours). Register temperatures during steeping (Figure 7.4).

3. Drain the cooking liquor or *nejayote* and wash the *nixtamal* with water. Make sure to remove excess lime and adhered pericarp tissue. Collect the *nejayote* and wash waters and measure the volume and solids. Obtain a sample of the cleaned *nixtamal* for moisture analysis.

4. Weigh the cleaned *nixtamal* and place it in the hopper of the stone mill. The stone mill should

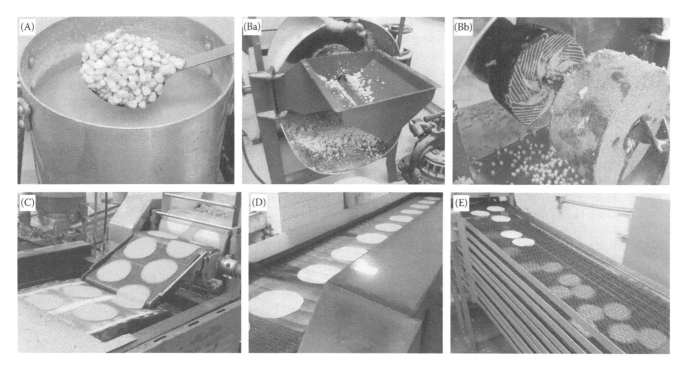

FIGURE 7.4 Sequential steps for producing table tortillas. (A) Lime-cooking; (Ba) stone-grinding of *nixtamal* into *masa*; (Bb) photograph depicting the interior face of the volcanic grinding stones; (C) sheeting and forming of dough into tortilla rounds; (D) tortilla baking; (E) tortilla cooling.

be calibrated beforehand. Calculate the amount of water to add during the milling procedure. The amount of water to grind 1 kg of *nixtamal* for table tortillas and chips is approximately 160 mL/kg and 150 mL/kg, respectively.

5. Start the stone grinder and adjust the pressure between the grinding stones to obtain the proper *masa* texture (refer to particle size distribution of fresh *masa* procedure in Section 7.2.2.3). Grind all the *nixtamal*, making sure to gradually add the water. Measure the temperature of the *masa*, collect it and place it in a plastic bag to prevent dehydration. Disassemble the stone grinder and collect and weigh all the unground *nixtamal* and *masa* particles (Figure 7.4).

6. Place *masa* in the hopper of the sheeter/former device with cutting dies to form the tortilla rounds. Adjust the thickness and weight of the *masa* pieces. For instance, *masa* pieces of table tortillas generally weigh 35 g (Figure 7.4).

7. After attaining the optimum weight of the *masa* pieces, bake them in a triple-pass, gas-fired oven set at temperatures of 240°C to 290°C for approximately 45 to 65 seconds. Adjust the temperature of each tier of the baking oven and the dwell time. It is recommended to use an infrared or spot thermometer. Generally, for table tortillas, the last tier of the oven is adjusted to a high temperature setting to enhance pillowing (Figure 7.4). Register the existing tortilla temperature and the 10-count weight.

8. Allow baked tortilla pieces to cool down. This operation is optimally performed in a continuous cooling rack (Figure 7.4). Register the tortilla temperature and 10-count weight every 5 minutes for 30 minutes.

9. After cooling, place table tortillas in plastic bags and sample for moisture and other analyses.

7.2.3.2 Tortilla Texture

The textural shelf-stability of table tortillas is of upmost importance for the industry. The quality depends on the ability of the product to retain its original texture and sensory characteristics. Staling is the main characteristic responsible for the progressive loss of tortilla texture or increase in firmness. Aged tortillas are firmer, more rigid, less rollable, and tend to crack when folded compared with fresh counterparts. Tortilla texture can be subjectively and objectively tested. The subjective assessment of tortillas is generally done by first rolling a tortilla around a dowel, followed by the evaluation of the extent of cracking by a trained human judge. As expected, the dowel test scores vary from person to person and the method is not sensitive to changes in fresh tortilla texture (Suhendro et al. 1998a,b). Thus, objective bending, rollability, and extensibility techniques were developed to assess tortilla texture with the texture analyzer (Suhendro et al. 1998a,b). The bending technique detects changes in tortilla texture throughout storage and correlates with subjective rollability and flexibility test scores. Likewise, the rollability technique, measured as the force and work required to pull an axle that causes a tortilla to roll around a dowel, was more sensitive to changes in texture and tortilla thickness compared with subjective evaluations. These techniques can be used to evaluate the effect of formulation and processing changes on fresh and stored tortillas.

7.2.3.2.1 Subjective Dowel Test

The Dowel test simply consists of rolling a tortilla around a dowel with the subsequent evaluation of the degree of tortilla cracking.

A. Samples, Ingredients, and Reagents
- Different types of tortillas

B. Materials and Equipment
- Dowel (1 cm diameter by at least 20 cm long)

C. Procedure
1. Equilibrate tortillas to room temperature.
2. Wrap and roll at least five different tortillas belonging to the same treatment around a 1-cm diameter dowel.
3. Subjectively score tortilla texture using a scale of 1 to 5, in which 1, tortilla is firm, rigid, and cracks; and 5, tortilla is soft, flexible, and does not crack. Register the subjective evaluations of the five repetitions.

7.2.3.2.2 Objective Tortilla Rollability Test

Suhendro et al. (1998a) devised a texture analyzer method to objectively test the rollability of tortillas. The assay imitates the dowel test but is more reliable because it is more sensitive and less variable. The objective method registers the force and work required to pull an axle that causes a tortilla to roll around a dowel. The method proved to be fast, simple, and sensitive to changes in the tortillas and worked effectively on commercial samples. The main advantage of this technique is that it was able to detect texture differences during the first 24 hours after baking or tortilla preparation and effectively evaluated the effects of additives such as texture improvers.

A. Samples, Ingredients, and Reagents
- Different types of tortillas

B. Materials and Equipment
- Scale
- Caliper
- Ruler
- Texture analyzer such as TAXT2
- Rollability fixture consisting of a 1.9-cm diameter acrylic cylindrical dowel and a metal chain that connects the cylinder dowel to the texture analyzer arm

C. Procedure
1. Allow packaged tortillas to equilibrate at room temperature.
2. Record the weight and average diameter and thickness of each of the tortillas to be analyzed.
3. Calibrate the probe to a distance of 160 mm from the analyzer arm to the platform with a metal wire that holds the tortilla on top of the

dowel. Then, fix the tortilla to the dowel by firmly clasping to the metal wire. Make sure to position tortillas with the double-baked side down.
4. Start the test and register the force required to pull the axle and roll the tortilla. The test should be conducted using the "force tension mode" and the "return to start" option with pre- and postspeed set at 10 mm/sec. The trigger force setting is 0.05 N and the probe moves a 50-mm distance at 3 mm/sec during the assay. The force required to roll the tortilla on the dowel by one revolution is the first peak of the rollability curve, whereas the total work required to drag and roll the tortilla around the dowel is the area under the curve.
5. Repeat the procedure with at least three different tortillas belonging to the same treatment.
6. Relate force and work results to tortilla thickness, weight, and diameter.

7.2.3.2.3 Objective Tortilla Bending Method

A. Samples, Ingredients, and Reagents
- Tortillas

B. Materials and Equipment
- Scale
- Caliper
- Ruler
- Texture analyzer (TAXT2)
- Bending attachment consisting of two clamps; one attached to the texture analyzer to hold a vertical aluminum guillotine (1.7 mm thick) and the other to the texture analyzer platform that holds the tortilla specimen horizontally (Suhendro et al. 1998b)
- Template (30 mm × 35 mm)

C. Procedure
1. Allow tortillas to equilibrate at room temperature.
2. Cut a strip from the center of the tortilla using a 30 mm × 35 mm template.
3. Calibrate the probe to a distance of 50 mm from the platform to the guillotine. The horizontal separation between sample clamp and guillotine should de adjusted to 6.45 mm. Set the probe to travel a distance of 5 mm at a speed of 1 mm/sec in such a way that the tortilla strip bends to a controlled 40 degree angle.
4. Clamp the tortilla strip with the double-baked side down in a horizontal position.
5. Start the bending test with the "return to start option" with the compression mode and trigger force of 0.05 N, and register the force required to pull the axle and roll the tortilla. The test should be conducted using the "force tension mode" and the "return to start" option with pre- and postspeed set at 10 mm/sec. The trigger force setting is adjusted to 0.05 N.

6. Register the bending modulus of deformation as determined by the slope (N/m) of the deformation curve in the linear region, force at 1 mm distance, peak force/apparent force (N), and bending work (area under the curve).

7. Repeat the procedure with at least three different tortilla strips belonging to the same treatment.

7.2.4 Dry Masa Flour Production

The use of dry *masa* flour is rapidly growing because of its convenience. Dry *masa* flour use eliminates the tedious, labor-intensive cooking, washing, and grinding of lime-cooked maize or *nixtamal* and eliminates steep water and waste disposal problems related to cooking. In addition, processors do not have to manage the selection of suitable maize and invest in cooking equipment. However, dry *masa* flour costs more and does not have the flavor of freshly cooked *masa* products.

Industrial production of pregelatinized dry *masa* flour is accomplished by lime-cooking, washing, and grinding the *nixtamal* to produce *masa,* followed by drying, sieving, regrinding coarse particles, resieving, classifying, and blending to meet certain requirements (Gomez et al. 1987; Almeida Dominguez et al. 1996). The dried *masa* is formulated into flours with carefully controlled particle size distribution, water absorption and other characteristics such as pH and supplementation of different additives.

Masa flours designed especially for the production of white and yellow table tortillas, restaurant-style tortilla chips, corn chips, and tortilla chips (refer to Chapter 12) are commercially produced. Some companies offer more than 25 different *masa* flours formulated to meet certain color, pH, particle size distribution, water absorption, and viscosity requirements. In terms of particle size distribution, three major classes of dry *masa* flours are recognized: for table tortillas, for corn chips, and for tortilla chips. Table tortillas are usually manufactured from fine flours whereas corn and tortilla chips from medium and coarse flours, respectively. In general, the particle size distribution is coarser for snacks, taco shells, and tostadas because pores are needed to vent steam generated during the critical operations of baking and frying.

Dry *masa* flours for table tortilla are usually treated with acidulants, bleaching agents, preservatives, emulsifiers, gums, and enrichment premixes. Comparatively with fresh *masa* tortillas, these additives can be easily incorporated into the flours to enhance tortilla color, texture, reheating capacity, and shelf life.

7.2.4.1 Production of Dry Masa Flours

A. Samples, Ingredients, and Reagents
- Maize
- Food-grade lime
- Distilled water

B. Materials and Equipment
- Graduated cylinder (100 mL, 200 mL, or 1 L)
- Digital scale
- Cooker (steam or conventional)
- Perforated drying sheets
- Rotap (U.S. nos. 35, 60, and 100 sieves)
- Rotap collection pan
- Stone grinder
- Air convection dryer
- Air aspirator
- Hammer or roller mill
- Dough mixer with hook or paddle attachments
- Thermometer (300°C)
- Tortilla-forming equipment with table tortilla cutters
- Three-tier baking oven
- Cooling rack
- Deep-fat fryer
- Chronometer

C. Procedure
1. Weigh a fixed amount of cleaned maize kernels and add two or three times as much water and 1% food-grade lime based on grain weight to the cooking vessel. Keep the kernels separated from the lime solution.

2. Adjust the temperature of the cooking solution (most processes cook at near-boiling or between 85°C and 100°C). When the cooking solution reaches the proper temperature, add the grain and register temperatures throughout cooking. Make sure to stir contents frequently (i.e., every 5 minutes). Cook the maize kernels for the predetermined cooking time (generally 20 to 35 minutes, depending on the physical properties of the grain) and suspend heat.

3. Drain the cooking liquor or *nejayote* and wash the *nixtamal* with water. Make sure to remove excess lime and adhered pericarp tissue. Collect the *nejayote* and wash waters and measure the volume and solids. Obtain a sample of the cleaned *nixtamal* for moisture analysis.

4. Weigh the cleaned *nixtamal* and place it in the hopper of the stone, attrition, or special hammer mill. Mill the *nixtamal* into coarse particles in preparation for drying.

5. Dehydrate the ground particles at a relatively low temperature (60°C). Register the drying curve throughout this time. The particles should be dried to a moisture content of approximately 10%.

6. Pass the dried particles first through an air-aspirator to remove light pericarp particles. Register the weight of the air-aspirated particles. Then, classify particles in plansifters or a set of sieves ranging from U.S. no. 20 to 100 mesh. Register the yield of each fraction.

7. Select the large particles that need regrinding. For dry *masa* flours for table tortillas, practically all particles should pass the U.S. no. 60 mesh sieve, whereas for tortilla chips, having

approximately 20% of coarse particles is preferable (mesh sizes >60 and <40).

8. Reground coarse particles in a hammer or roll mill. Reclassify the ground material into streams with different particle sizes.

9. Select and blend milled fractions with optimum particle size distribution for different applications.

10. Calculate yield of dry *masa* flour and by-products including solids lost in the *nejayote*.

11. Alternatively, supplement resulting dry *masa* flours with fixed amounts of hydrocolloids, acidulants, preservatives, bleaching agents, and selected vitamins and minerals before packaging. These additives are added to enhance microbial and textural shelf life, optimize color, and improve the levels of micronutrients checked by regulatory agencies.

12. Analyze the resulting flour in terms of moisture, water activity, particle size distribution, pH, *masa* texture, color, and functionality (refer to table tortilla procedure).

7.2.4.2 Production of Tortillas from Dry *Masa* Flour

A. Samples, Ingredients, and Reagents
- Dry *masa* flours
- Distilled water

B. Materials and Equipment
- Digital scale
- Graduated cylinder (100 mL, 200 mL, or 1 L)
- Cooker (steam or conventional vessel)
- Dough mixer with hook attachment
- Tortilla-forming equipment with cutters for table tortillas
- Three-tier baking oven
- Cooling rack
- Deep-fat fryer
- Chronometer
- Thermometer (300°C)

C. Procedure
1. Weigh a fixed amount of dry *masa* flour and place it in a mixing bowl.

2. Calculate the amount of water needed to yield *masa* using the following equation: [(100 − % moisture of dry *masa* flour)/(100 − desired *masa* moisture content)] − 1] × amount of dry *masa* flour. For instance, 1 kg of 10% moisture flour needs 1.14 L of water to yield a *masa* with 58% moisture.

3. Add the water to the mixing bowl and mix until a proper *masa* texture is attained. It usually requires only 3 to 5 minutes to achieve proper texture. Overmixing can cause stickiness.

4. After mixing, place the resulting *masa* in a plastic bag for 5 minutes resting.

5. Place *masa* in the hopper of the sheeter/former device with cutting dies to form the tortilla rounds. Adjust the thickness and weight of the *masa* pieces. For instance, the *masa* pieces of table tortillas commonly weigh 35 g.

6. After attaining the optimum weight of the *masa* pieces, bake them in a triple-pass gas-fired oven set at temperatures of 240°C to 290°C for approximately 45 to 65 seconds. Adjust the temperature of each tier of the baking oven and the dwell time. It is recommended to use an infrared or spot thermometer. Generally, the last tier of the oven is adjusted to a high temperature for table or soft tortillas. Register the existing tortilla temperature and the 10-count weight.

7. Allow baked tortilla pieces to cool down. This operation is optimally performed in a continuous cooling rack. Register the tortilla temperature and 10-count weight every 5 minutes for 30 minutes.

8. After cooling, place table tortillas in plastic bags and sample for moisture and other analyses.

7.2.4.3 Determination of Water Absorption and Solubility Indexes

The water absorption index (WAI) and the water solubility index (WSI), first developed by Anderson et al. (1969), can be effectively used to estimate these parameters in dry *masa* flour. The WAI and WSI quantify the content of water-soluble solids and the ability of particles to absorb water, respectively (Rooney 2007). A ground sample is incubated in water at room temperature (25°C), promoting the dispersion of particles and allowing the solubilization of soluble solids and absorption of water by particles. Soluble solids are separated with the supernatant, dried, and weighed. The gel-like material produced after particles absorb water is separated by centrifugation from the solution phase, weighed and then used to calculate the WAI (Rooney 2007). Both indexes are affected by starch content and gelatinization.

A. Samples, Ingredients, and Reagents
- Dry *masa* flour
- Distilled water
- Fresh *masa*
- Dessicant (activated alumina)

B. Materials and Equipment
- Centrifuge test tubes
- Centrifuge
- Analytical balance
- Reciprocating tube shaker
- Pipette (10 mL)
- Spatula
- Convection or air-forced oven
- Airtight dessicator
- Aluminum tins
- Tweezers
- Laboratory clock or chronometer

C. *Procedure*

Water Absorption Index

1. Determine moisture content of the samples to be analyzed (Anderson et al. 1969; Rooney 2007).
2. Weigh the equivalent of 1 g of dry sample with an accuracy of 0.001 g and place it in a test tube. For instance, if dry *masa* flour with 10% moisture or fresh *masa* with 56% moisture are assayed, weigh approximately 1.1 g or 2.25 g, respectively. Add 15 mL of distilled water to each test tube.
3. Shake contents and incubate for 30 minutes at room temperature (25°C) with horizontal shaking in a reciprocating shaker set at low speed (184 cycles/min).
4. Place test tubes in the centrifuge, making sure to distribute tubes to balance the weight of the rotor. If the number of samples is odd, then place 16 mL water in one tube to equilibrate the weight of the rotor. Centrifuge for 20 minutes at 5000 rpm (768 × *g*).
5. Carefully decant excess water into tared aluminum tins and weigh the pellet. Keep decanted water for solids determination needed to calculate WSI.
6. Calculate the WAI using the following equation:

WAI = wet pellet weight/dry sample weight.

Water Solubility Index

1. Place the decanted water from step 5 of the previous list into tared aluminum tins.
2. Place aluminum tin with the sample in a convection oven set at 100°C for 3 hours or until a constant weight is achieved.
3. With the tweezers, take aluminum dishes out of the air-forced oven and immediately place them in a dessicator. Allow for 30 minutes of equilibration at room temperature and weigh using an analytical balance. Calculate the difference between the empty aluminum dish (tare weight) and the aluminum dish with the solids of the suspension.
4. Calculate the WSI using the following equation:

WSI = (weight of soluble solids/dry sample weight) × 100.

7.2.4.4 Consistency of Dry *Masa* Flour Slurries

The consistency of slurries produced from dry *masa* flour is a simple and easy to perform assay to determine quality. The principle of the test is that flours with a high degree of starch gelatinization produce more consistent or viscous slurries and, therefore, run less when they are allowed to free flow.

This test is commonly used to adjust cooking times in dry *masa* flour operations (Lobeira et al. 1998).

A. *Samples, Ingredients, and Reagents*
- Different types of dry *masa* flours
- Distilled water

B. *Materials and Equipment*
- Digital scale
- Consistometer or consistency flow meter
- Beaker
- Graduated cylinders (50 mL or 100 mL)
- Spatula
- Chronometer
- Thermometer
- Ruler

C. *Procedure*
1. Determine moisture content of the dry *masa* flour to be analyzed.
2. Weigh 25 g of dry *masa* flour with an accuracy of 0.01 g and place it in a beaker. Calculate the water required to produce a 22% solid slurry using the following equation: [(100 – dry masa flour moisture/100 – 78) – 1] × amount of dry *masa* flour to test. For instance, the amount of water to add to 25 g of dry *masa* flour with 10% moisture is 77.27 mL.
3. Add the predetermined amount of water (22–25°C) to the beaker and mix thoroughly for exactly 1 minute with the spatula.
4. Pour the slurry into the testing compartment and immediately release the slurry. Allow the slurry to run through the ramp for exactly 2 minutes.
5. Measure the distance (cm) traveled by the slurry or consistometer reading.

7.2.4.5 Determination of Dry *Masa* Flour Consistency

The ability of dry *masa* flour to flow freely when mixed with excess water is widely used by the industry because the consistency is affected by the degree of starch gelatinization, which is affected by cooking time. A diluted slurry is placed on a Bostwick consistometer and allowed to flow for a controlled time. The traveled distance can be used as an index for consistency. Flours for table tortillas with higher water absorption capacity and cohesiveness will flow shortened distances compared with counterparts tailored for snacks.

A. *Samples, Ingredients, and Reagents*
- Different lots of dry *masa* flours
- Water

B. *Materials and Equipment*
- Digital scale
- Bostwick consistometer
- Spatula
- Beaker (250 mL)
- Graduated cylinder (100 mL)
- Chronometer

C. *Procedure*

1. Determine the dry *masa* flour moisture content and particle size distribution (refer to procedures in Sections 2.2.1.1 and 5.3.1.1).

2. Calculate the amount of flour needed for 15 g of solids using the following equation: dry *masa* flour weight = 15/(100 − % moisture/100). Weigh the sample within an accuracy of two digits and place it in a 100 mL beaker.

3. Calculate the amount of distilled water needed to produce a slurry containing 78% moisture. First, calculate the amount of water contained in the sample = dry *masa* flour weight − 15 g. Then, calculate the amount of water needed to produce a slurry with exactly 78% moisture = 15/(100 − 78/100). Subtract the water contained in the sample from the water needed to produce the slurry. For instance, for a flour with 10% moisture content, 16.666 g of flour needs to be weighed. This quantity of flour will contain 1.666 g water. Thus, the amount of distilled water needed to add to the sample is 68.182 − 1.666 = 66.516 mL water.

4. Weigh the dry *masa* flour and place it in a 250 mL beaker. Measure the amount of water required to produce the 78% moisture slurry in a graduated cylinder and add it to the beaker which contains the *masa* flour.

5. Mix water with dry *masa* flour for 45 seconds using the spatula. Make sure to completely disperse solids.

6. Pour slurry into testing compartment of Bostwick consistometer. Then, scrape out adhered particles using a spatula.

7. Immediately release sample by pressing the lever that opens the gate. Allow slurry to travel on the platform and read distance after exactly 120 seconds.

8. Register the distance traveled in centimeters.

7.2.5 RESEARCH SUGGESTIONS

1. Determine and compare pericarp removal, optimum lime cooking time, and dry matter losses of three contrasting maizes (i.e., white with intermediate endosperm texture, yellow with soft texture, and soft blue maize).

2. Determine and compare the soft tortilla-making properties of three contrasting maizes (i.e., white with intermediate endosperm texture, yellow with soft texture, and soft blue maize). Compare yields, *masa* texture, tortilla-bending capacities throughout 5 days of storage at room temperature, and design a sensory evaluation test (refer to Chapter 3) aimed toward color, texture, flavor, and overall acceptability.

3. Determine and compare the soft tortilla-making properties of a white dent maize processed into tortillas via traditional fresh *masa* process or via further processing of dry *masa* flour. Compare *masa* textures, tortilla-bending capacities throughout 5 days of storage at room temperature, and design a triangular evaluation test (refer to Chapter 3) aimed toward determining color, texture, flavor, and overall preference.

4. Prepare a dry *masa* flour from a given lot of white maize and then supplement three lots of flour with (1) 0.2% fumaric acid and 0.2% potassium sorbate; (2) 0.2% lecithin, 0.1% sodium stearoyl 2-lactylate, and 0.2% carboxymethylcellulose; (3) 0.2% fumaric acid, 0.2% potassium sorbate, 0.2% lecithin, 0.1% sodium stearoyl 2-lactylate, and 0.2% carboxymethylcellulose. Determine the dry *masa* flour consistency, color, and pH. Process the control and supplemented flours into tortilla packages and then determine differences in terms of pH, microbial stability throughout 10 days at room temperature, *masa* texture, tortilla-bending or folding capacity, and preference with a sensory evaluation panel. The objective is to determine which tortilla system is the best in terms of overall acceptability and shelf life.

5. Prepare dry *masa* flours from a given lot of white maize via traditional nixtamalization and thermoplastic extrusion. The idea is to emulate as much as possible the properties of the extruded dry *masa* flour so that various lime concentrations, extrusion temperatures, and tempering water should be tested. Compare the control dry *masa* flour with the extruded flours in terms of pH, *masa* texture, viscoamylograph properties, particle size distribution, flour and tortilla color, tortilla-bending or folding capacity, and preference with a sensory evaluation panel.

6. Determine and compare the soft tortilla-making properties of a white dent maize and a white food-grade sorghum used as whole and decorticated to remove 20% of the external layers. First, determine the optimum cooking times using the nylon bag laboratory technique, and then process the maize, whole sorghum, and decorticated sorghum into table tortillas. Compare *masa* textures, tortilla color, tortilla-bending capacities throughout 5 days of storage at room temperature and design a sensory evaluation test (refer to Chapter 3) aimed toward determining differences among the three different tortillas.

7.2.6 RESEARCH QUESTIONS

1. Define the following terms which are widely used in *masa* operations:
   a. *Nixtamal*
   b. *Nejayote*
   c. *Masa*
   d. Food-grade lime
   e. Dowel test
   f. TPA

2. What are the principles of the May–Gruenwald pericarp removal test which is used to screen *nixtamal* samples? What are the main kernel properties related to the extent of pericarp removal during nixtamalization?
3. What are the effects of residual lime on color, texture, flavor, and microbial shelf life of soft tortillas? How are high-alkaline or limed tortillas produced in Mexico?
4. Draw a general scheme describing the processes for the production of *nixtamal, masa,* dry *masa* flour, table tortillas, corn chips, and tortilla chips.
5. How are grain properties related to dry matter losses incurred during lime-cooking and steeping? What is the best test to estimate dry matter losses incurred during lime-cooking and steeping?
6. Why is the *nejayote* considered as one of the worst industrial effluents? What kinds of maize solids are lost in the *nejayote*?
7. Why is white dent maize generally preferred for the production of *masa* and dry *masa* flour?
8. What are the major differences in lime-cooking of *nixtamal* suited for table tortillas and tortilla chips? Which tests can you apply to determine the differences between the two sorts of cooked *nixtamals*?
9. How is the *nixtamal* transformed into *masa* during stone-grinding operations? Why is it difficult to substitute volcanic stones to perform this operation? What happens to the starch during stone-grinding?
10. What are the major differences in grinding of *nixtamal* to produce *masa* suited for table tortillas and tortilla chips? Which tests can you apply to determine the differences between the two *masas*?
11. What are the principles of the WAI and WSI? Why are these assays very useful in the tortilla industry?
12. What are the major chemical changes that occur during lime-cooking and tortilla baking?
13. If you want to produce sorghum tortillas similar to maize counterparts, what kind of sorghum will you select? What changes in the processing will you make? What kinds of quality control tests will you run?
14. Investigate at least two novel technologies to produce *masa* or dry *masa* flour suited for tortillas or chips.
15. What are the major differences in baking of preformed pieces of *masa* suited for soft tortillas and tortilla chips?
16. Define two strategies to produce a long shelf-life tortilla. Which microorganisms are mainly responsible for tortilla spoilage?
17. Define two strategies to enhance tortilla texture (better folding or bending and decreased cracking) and enhanced reheatability. Which texture studies will effectively detect differences between tortillas stored for different periods of time at different temperatures and supplemented with different amounts of antistaling agents?
18. How does lime-cooking affect the nutritional value of maize? Investigate why pellagra (vitamin B_3 or niacin deficiency) is virtually unknown in Mexico and other tortilla-consuming countries.
19. What are the major differences between dry *masa* flour for table tortillas and tortilla chips, in terms of degree of starch gelatinization, particle size distribution, and supplemented additives?
20. Investigate the nutritional and nutraceutical properties of blue maize and quality protein maize tortillas.
21. What is the effect of pH on the appearance and coloration of blue corn tortillas (i.e., tortillas with a pH of 5.8, 7, and 9)? Which kind of pigments are the major responsible for the blue coloration?
22. What is the bioavailability of the calcium present in nixtamalized products?

REFERENCES

Almeida Dominguez, H. D., M. Cepeda, and L. W. Rooney. 1996. "Properties of Commercial Nixtamalized Corn Flours." *Cereal Foods World* 41:624–630.
Almeida Dominguez, H. D., E. L. Suhendro, and L. W. Rooney. 1997. "Corn Alkaline Cooking Properties Related to Grain Characteristics and Viscosity (RVA)." *Journal of Food Science* 62:516–519, 523.
American Association of Cereal Chemists (AACC). 2000. AACC, *Approved Methods of Analysis*, 10th ed. St. Paul, MN: American Association of Cereal Chemists.
Anderson, R. A., H. F. Conway, V. F. Pfeifer, and E. L. Griffin. 1969. "Gelatinization of Corn Grits by Roll and Extrusion Cooking." *Cereal Science Today* 14:1.
Bedolla, S., and L. W. Rooney. 1984. "Characteristics of US and Mexican instant maize flours for tortilla and snack preparation." *Cereal Foods World* 29:732–735.
Bosiger, I. 1997. Evaluation of Masa Texture. MSC Thesis. College Station, TX: Texas A&M University.
Gomez, M. H., L. W. Rooney, R. D. Waniska, and R. L. Pflugfelder. 1987. "Dry Corn Masa Flours for Tortilla and Snack Food Production." *Cereal Foods World* 32:372–377.
Lobeira, R., H. D. Almeida Dominguez, and L. W. Rooney. 1998. "Methods to Evaluate Hydration and Mixing Properties of Nixtamalized Corn Flours." *Cereal Chemistry* 75(4):417–420.
McDonough, C. M., M. H. Gomez, L. W. Rooney, and S. O. Serna-Saldivar. 2001. "Alkaline Cooked Corn Products." In *Snack Foods Processing*, 1st ed., edited by E. Lusas and L. W. Rooney. 73–114. Lancaster, PA: Technomic Publishing Co., Inc.
Pflugfelder, R. L., L. W. Rooney, and R. D. Waniska. 1988. "Dry Matter Losses In Commercial Corn Masa Production." *Cereal Chemistry* 65:127–132.
Ramirez Wong, B., V. E. Sweat, P. I. Torres, and L. W. Rooney. 1993. "Development of Two Instrumental Methods for Corn Masa Texture Evaluation." *Cereal Chemistry* 70(3):286–290.
Rooney, L. W. 2007. *Corn Quality Assurance Manual.* 2nd ed. Arlington, VA: Snack Food Association.
Rooney, L. W., and S. O. Serna-Saldivar. 2003. "Food Uses of Whole Corn and Dry Milled Fractions." In *Corn Chemistry and Technology*, 2nd ed., edited by P. White and L. Johnson, 495–535. St. Paul, MN: American Association of Cereal Chemists.

Rooney, L. W., and E. L. Suhendro. 2001. "Food Quality of Corn." In: *Snack Foods Processing*, 1st ed., edited by E. Lusas and L. W. Rooney, 37–72. Lancaster, PA: Technomic Publishing Co., Inc.

Rooney, L. W., H. D. Almeida Dominguez, E. L. Suhendro, and A. J. Bockholt. 1995. "Critical Factors Affecting the Food Quality of Corn." In *49th Annual Corn and Sorghum Research Conference of the American Seed Trade Association*, 80–96. Washington, DC.

Serna-Saldivar, S. O. 2003. *Manufactura y Control de Calidad de Productos Basados en Cereales*. Mexico DF: AGT Editor.

Serna-Saldivar, S. O. 2004. "Foods from Maize." In *Encyclopedia of Grain Science*. 1st ed., edited by C. Wrigley, C. Walker, and H. Corke, 242–253 Oxford, UK: Elsevier.

Serna-Saldivar, S. O. 2008a. "Manufacturing of Cereal-Based Dry Milled Fractions, Potato Flour, Dry Masa Flour and Starches." In *Industrial Manufacture of Snack Foods*. London, UK: Kennedys Publications Ltd.

Serna-Saldivar, S.O. 2008b. "Snacks from Alkaline Cooked Maize Products." In *Industrial Manufacture of Snack Foods*. London, UK: Kennedys Publications Ltd.

Serna-Saldivar, S. O., M. H. Gomez, and L. W. Rooney. 1990. "Technology, Chemistry, and Nutritional Value of Alkaline-Cooked Corn Products." In *Advances in Cereal Science and Technology*. Vol. 10, edited by Y. Pomeranz. St. Paul, MN: American Association of Cereal Chemists.

Serna-Saldivar, S. O., H. D. Almeida Dominguez, L. W. Rooney, M. H. Gómez, and A. J. Bockholt. 1991. "Method to Evaluate Ease of Pericarp Removal on Lime-Cooked Corn Kernels." *Crop Science* 31:842–844.

Serna-Saldivar, S. O., M. H. Gomez, A. R. Islas-Rubio, A. J. Bockholt, and L. W. Rooney. 1992. "The Alkaline Processing Properties of Quality Protein Maize." In *Quality Protein Maize*, edited by E. T. Mertz. St. Paul, MN: American Association of Cereal Chemists.

Serna-Saldivar, S. O., M. H. Gomez, H. D. Almeida Dominguez, A. Islas Rubio, and L. W. Rooney. 1993. "A Method to Evaluate the Lime Cooking Properties of Corn (*Zea mays*)." *Cereal Chemistry* 70:762–764.

Serna-Saldivar, S. O., M. H. Gomez, and L. W. Rooney. 2000. "Food Uses of Regular and Speciality Corns and Their Dry Milled Fractions." In *Speciality Corns*, 2nd ed., edited by A. R. Hallauer. Boca Raton, FL: CRC Press, Inc.

Shuey, W, C., and K. H. Tipples. 1982. *The Amylograph Handbook*. St. Paul, MN: American Association of Cereal Chemists.

Suhendro, E. L., H. D. Almeida Dominguez, L. W. Rooney, and R. D. Waniska. 1998a. "Objective Rollability Method of Corn Tortilla Texture Measurement." *Cereal Chemistry* 75(3):320–324.

Suhendro, E. L., H. Almeida Dominguez, L. W. Rooney, R. D. Waniska, and R. G. Moreira. 1998b. "Tortilla Bending Technique: An Objective Method for Corn Tortilla Texture Measurement." *Cereal Chemistry* 75:854–858.

8 Functionality Tests for Yeast and Chemical Leavening Agents

8.1 INTRODUCTION

There are two main ways to generate gas for the production of leavened wheat-based products. One is with the utilization of yeast or other biological agents, whereas the other is with the use of chemical leavening agents. The trapped gas causes the dough or batter to spring, imparting porous open texture, or crumb to the finished products. Yeast (*Saccharomyces cerevisceae*) is almost always used as biological fermenting agent to produce the wide array of yeast-leavened bakery products, whereas chemical leavening agents are commonly used for the production of cookies, cakes and pancakes, wheat flour tortillas, muffins, and biscuits.

Chemical-leavened products are manufactured from an array of chemical agents that can release gas during the mixing of the dough or batter or during the baking stage under the influence of the heat of the oven. Carbon dioxide is produced faster by chemical reaction than by yeast fermentation. Therefore, chemical-leavened products are produced in significantly lower processing times.

8.2 FUNCTIONALITY TESTS FOR YEAST ACTIVITY

Bakers and cereal scientists and technologists have long recognized the close relationship between sugar metabolized, total gas production and product quality. In addition, yeast metabolizes sugar in wheat doughs into an array of organic acids and many other flavorful and aromatic metabolites.

Yeast is a chemosynthetic, unicellular, nucleated, and immobile microorganism that reproduces asexually by budding. The size of the yeast cell varies from 4 μm to 8 μm wide and from 5 μm to 16 μm long. Yeast ferments simple sugars (i.e., glucose, fructose, mannose, galactose, sucrose, maltose, and maltotriose) into ethanol, carbon dioxide, and energy. The by-products of its metabolism or alcoholic fermentation are key compounds that impart the typical bread flavor and aroma. The chemical composition of fresh compressed yeast is 70% water, 13.5% protein, 12% soluble carbohydrates, 2% ash, 1.1% crude fat, and 1.5% cellulose. There are various types of commercial yeast: fresh, compressed-fresh, and dehydrated. Industrially, yeast cells are cultivated in large reactors containing a medium of molasses, minerals, sulfur compounds, vitamins, including biotin, and small amount of nitrogenous salts (i.e., ammonium salts). Yeast is cultivated with strict controls of temperature, aeration, and agitation and reproduces by budding in a period of several days. The

yeast cells are harvested, concentrated by centrifugation, washed, and then press-filtered to obtain compressed cells with approximately 70% moisture. For the production of dry yeast (92% solids), the compressed yeast is mixed with phospholipids and other protecting agents and cold-extruded and shaped to form thin strips in preparation for dehydration. Drying is performed in continuous dryers in which air flows countercurrently to the yeast or alternatively by bed drying at low temperature (30°C–60°C). The objective is to minimize damage to cell membranes. In practical terms, 1 kg of fresh compressed yeast is equivalent to approximately 0.45 kg dry yeast. The advantage of dry yeast is that it has a prolonged shelf-life especially when it is vacuum packaged. The disadvantage is that it takes longer to reactivate and start hydrolyzing the dough substrate.

Yeast breaks down monosaccharide, disaccharide, and trisaccharides, yielding organic acids (i.e., acetic, butyric, lactic, succinic) responsible for lowering the dough pH, besides other chemical compounds such as aldehydes and ketones, which affects flavor and aroma (i.e., acetaldehyde, formaldehyde, propionaldehyde, isobutylaldehyde, methyl-ethyl ketone, isovaleraldehyde, 2-methyl butanol, etc.) and carbon dioxide (Poitrenaud 2006; Maloney and Foy 2003; Reed and Peppler 1973). The carbon dioxide is the main factor responsible of the leavening effect because it is trapped by the elastic gluten network. Yeast fermentation or proofing is generally performed at temperatures ranging from 26°C to 30°C in proof cabinets normally containing a relative humidity of 85%. The amount of dry yeast generally used in bread formulations varies from 1% to 2%, which is equivalent to 3% to 6% of fresh compressed yeast. There are various instruments especially designed to measure yeast activity. The principle in all is to measure gas or CO_2 production under standardized conditions. The Brabender fermentograph, maturograph, and rheofermentometer measure yeast activity in doughs, whereas others in solutions rich in fermentable sugars.

8.2.1 FERMENTOGRAPH

The fermentograph is designed to test yeast activity by measuring production of carbon dioxide under controlled fermentation conditions (Figure 8.1). The equipment is especially useful in the baking and yeast-manufacturing industries. For bakers, the fermentograph allows the determination of the optimum yeast concentration. The fermentograph operating principle is based on measuring the rise of a piece of dough during yeast fermentation due to the formation of carbon

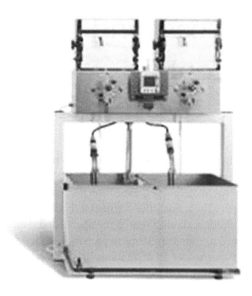

FIGURE 8.1 Fermentograph used to test yeast activity.

dioxide. Briefly, a weighed amount of yeasted dough of a well-defined weight is placed into a rubber balloon, which is then suspended from a pivoted counter poised arm and immersed into a temperature-controlled water tank. As gas is produced in the dough, the balloon becomes more buoyant and gradually raises, moving the supporting arm. A pen draws a line on a moving sheet of recording paper. The gas generated by the fermenting yeast is measured through pressure changes generally at different time intervals (90, 60, and 60 minutes). In each interval, the dough is degassed or punched to release the pressure. The fermentograph emulates fermentation times usually applied in the industry.

8.2.1.1 Determination of Yeast Activity with the Fermentograph

A. *Samples, Ingredients, and Reagents*
- Test fresh bakers or dry yeasts
- Sucrose
- Salt
- Wheat flour
- Shortening
- Distilled water

B. *Materials and Equipments*
- Digital scale
- Thermometer
- Chronometer or laboratory clock
- Fermentograph
- Recording pen

C. *Procedure*
1. Turn on the fermentograph and adjust the temperature of the water tank. Generally, the temperature is set at 30°C or 35°C.
2. Test different types of yeasts or concentrations on a typical bread formulation. Prepare doughs preferably using the 300 g farinograph (refer to procedure in Section 5.3.4.1). Mix the dough until

attaining optimum properties (optimum dough mixing time). The dough can be produced with different types of yeast and formulations depending on the purpose of the fermentograph study. Try to produce the testing dough using the same flour, amount of water, and other ingredients (i.e., sugar, salt, shortening, malt, etc.). In addition, follow the same mixing protocol for all doughs and try to minimize experimental error.

3. Weigh exactly 250 g of prepared dough and after 5 minutes place dough in the fermentograph plastic balloon.
4. Suspend the sealed plastic balloon from the pivoted counterpoised fermentograph arm and immerse the balloon into the temperature-controlled water tank. Make sure that the temperature of the water tank is well adjusted.
5. Place the recording pen on time zero of the moving sheet of recording paper and allow doughs to ferment for 90 minutes at the predetermined temperature.
6. After the first fermentation period, remove the plastic balloon, open it, and manually expel or punch all the gas trapped by the fermenting dough.
7. Repeat step 5 and allow dough to ferment for 60 minutes (second fermentation).
8. Repeat steps 6 and 7 and ferment the dough for 60 more minutes (third fermentation).
9. Obtain the pressure vs. fermentation time graphs of the first, second, and third fermentation periods and calculate the maximum gas pressure at the end of each fermentation time and the slope of the lines.

8.2.2 Maturograph and Oven Rise Recorder

The Brabender maturograph and oven rise recorder instruments are used by the milling and baking industries and manufacturers of baking additives (Figure 8.2). The maturograph records gas production and loss by measuring the changes in height of a fermenting dough subjected to periodic punching at 2 minute intervals in a conditioned compartment. After the analysis of the maturograph curve, optimum proofing conditions and fermentation tolerance can be established. The difference between top and bottom values of the curve band reflects changes in the height of the dough due to punching and recovery related to elasticity (Seibel 1968; Rasper and Walker 2000). On the other hand, the oven rise recorder measures the change in volume of a dough-bread during the entire baking process. The fermented dough is heated inside a temperature-conditioned oil bath. The oven rise recorder measures and records the rise of the dough due to the increase in volume (both dough and bread volume) and the oven rise. Both instruments are effectively used to test functionality of improving baking additives and flour ingredients. For these tests, a dough with all common ingredients (flour, salt, sugar,

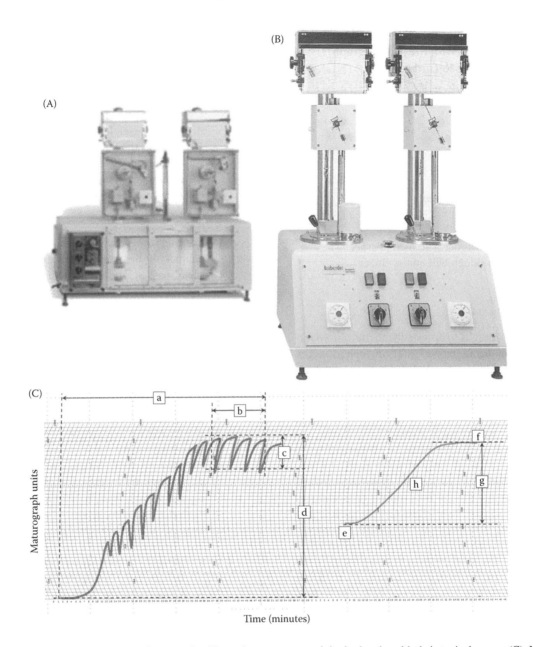

FIGURE 8.2 Maturograph (A) and oven rise recorder (B) used to test yeast activity in doughs with their typical curves (C). Maturograph: a = final proving time (maximum or optimum fermentation maturity); b = proving stability (time at maximum fermentation); c = elasticity (bandwidth); d = dough level (maximum dough volume). Oven-rise recorder: e = dough volume (dough height at the start of the baking period); f = baking volume (the height of the curve at the end of a test); g = oven rise (the oven rise is the difference between final volume (f) and dough volume (e)); h = final rise (measured from the middle of the curve after 11 minutes).

yeast, fat) is prepared varying only the test ingredient (i.e., yeast, sugar, oxidizing agents, etc.).

Optimally, both the maturograph and oven rise apparatus are used together. In the maturograph, one dough is used to register proof time and other identical piece of dough is proofed in the fermentation cabinet of the apparatus for use in the oven rise instrument. The oven rise dough suffers the same fermentation time as the other piece without receiving the periodical loading being applied. At the point of maximum maturity the second dough is placed in a metal basket of the oven rise recorder. Then, the metal basket containing the dough is immersed in the oil bath and its suspension hook connected to the scale head,

which in turn is linked to the strip chart recorder. The oven rise recorder records the change in volume of a dough during the whole baking process. Due to the transfer of contact heat at exact temperature control, the temperature can be determined at any point of the curve. The oil temperature is controlled by the thermoregulator and increased from 30°C to 100°C within 22–28 minutes. This corresponds to the typical temperature curve in the interior of the bread. While baking, the volume of the dough augments and the bread increases depending on the flour quality, yeast activity, and addition of functional ingredients. These changes are registered by the scale system and recorded in oven rise units.

8.2.2.1 Determination of Dough Properties and Bread Volume with the Maturograph and Oven Rise Recorder

A. *Samples, Ingredients, and Reagents*
- Test fresh bakers or dry yeasts
- Test wheat flours
- Sucrose
- Shortening
- Salt
- Distilled water

B. *Materials and Equipments*
- Digital scale
- Maturograph
- Oven rise recorder with metal basket
- Brabender dough ball homogenizer

C. *Procedure*

Maturograph

1. Prepare doughs to be tested with the desired formulation using the 300 g farinograph as mixer. It is highly recommended to mix contents at 30°C, add the optimum water absorption and stop the farinograph at optimum development time.

2. Set the maturograph fermentation chamber at 30°C ± 1°C. Place two pieces of dough (150 g) in the fermentation compartments of the maturograph for fixed periods of time (i.e., emulate fermentation times used during conventional baking of pan bread). Between proofs, it is recommended to punch and round the fermenting dough in the molding box of the ball homogenizer. When the instrument is switched on, the round base plate rotates eccentrically rounding the dough to a homogeneous ball. The recommended rounding time is 10 to 20 sec.

3. Record the maturograph fermentation behavior of a dough during the proofing times by means of a sensing probe that touches the dough. The most important measurement is during final proofing (temperature 30°C ± 1°C and relative humidity 80%–85%).

4. Determine the four maturogram parameters from the curve:
   a. Final proving time. This is the time in minutes from the start of the final proof to the first drop of the curve after the maximum. This specific parameter relates to the time needed to obtain optimum fermenting maturity and is sensible to supplemented baking improvers.
   b. Proving stability. The proving stability can be evaluated with a provided gauge in the range of the curve's maximum. This parameter relates to the time tolerance during which the loaf has to be placed into the oven

and when an optimum bread volume can be obtained.
   c. Elasticity. Calculated as the band width in the range of the maximum peak. It is a very important criterion of flour quality and can be influenced by various flour improvers.
   d. Dough level. It is calculated during the final proof as the maximum fermentation volume of the dough. This value is expressed in maturograph units from the zero line to the maximum peak of the curve.

Oven rise recorder

1. Transfer the separate piece fermented in the cabinet of the maturograph to the oven rise metal basket. The oven rise dough should have had the same fermentation time as the maturograph piece without receiving the periodical loading applied during the maturograph test.

2. Immerse the metal basket containing the dough in the oil bath after attaching the suspension hook to the scale head, which in turn is linked to the strip chart recorder. The oil temperature is regulated to increase from 30°C to 100°C within 22 minutes. A circulation pump guarantees that the temperature is kept uniform all over the oil bath.

3. Register the change in dough-bread volume versus heating time. This action is automatically measured by the scale system and recorded in oven rise units on a chart.

4. Determine the following parameters from the oven rise curve:
   a. Dough volume. Measured as the height of the curve at the beginning of a test.
   b. Baking volume. Measured as the height of the curve at the end of a test (after 22 minutes baking).
   c. Oven rise. The oven rise is the difference between final bread volume and initial dough volume. This parameter is also known as oven spring.
   d. Final rise. The final rise is measured from the middle of the curve after 11 minutes and represents the curve of the bread in the range of higher temperatures. The suppression and shrinkage of the baked goods is recorded numerically.

8.2.3 Rheofermentometer

The Chopin rheofermentometer measures fermentation with a weight placed on the developed dough (Figure 8.3). The instrument registers the dough height with a sensor and gas developed by a pressure sensor. It is an instrument especially devised to measure gas production and gas retention in doughs placed inside a sealed chamber with controlled

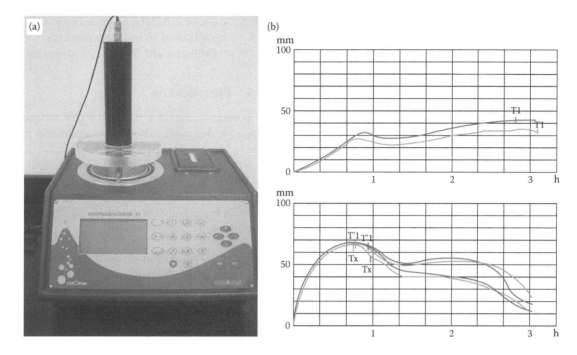

FIGURE 8.3 Rheofermentometer (a) used to test yeast activity in doughs with its characteristic curve (b).

temperature. The advantage of this apparatus is that measures total gas volume related to yeast activity and dough gas retention related to gluten strength (Rasper and Walker 2000). It is designed to evaluate the fermentative capacity of flours and yeast activity. It is especially useful to measure the development of dough during fermentation. The instrument records dough development, the speed of carbon dioxide release and the quantity produced, and the volume of the carbon dioxide retained in the dough.

The main parameters determined include maximum dough height (Hm), maximum height of gas release (Hm0) and carbon dioxide production (Czuchajowska and Pomeranz 1993).

8.2.3.1 Determination of Fermenting Dough Gas Production and Retention with the Rheofermentometer

A. Samples, Ingredients, and Reagents
- Test bakers fresh or dry yeasts
- Wheat flour
- Sucrose
- Shortening
- Salt
- Distilled water

B. Materials and Equipments
- Digital scale
- Rheofermentometer

C. Procedure
1. Prepare a dough was with 100 units of flour, fresh compressed or dry yeast (4.5% or 1.5% fresh or dry yeast, respectively), sugar (20% flour weight basis), water (optimum amount determined with the farinograph), 1.5% salt, 3.5% shortening using a Hobart mixer equipped with a hook attachment. The dough should be mixed until the gluten network is optimally developed.
2. Place dough in the rheofermentometer F3 (Chopin, Villeneuve-La-Garenne Cedex, France) movable basket of the gas meter with a 2000-g cylindrical weight and the cover of the vat was fitted with an optical sensor. Make sure the graph paper and pen are properly working.
3. Conduct the test for 3 hours at 30°C.
4. Obtain the rheofermentometer graph.

8.2.4 GASOGRAPH

The gasograph is an instrument intended to measure gas produced by different concentrations of yeast mixed with 10 g flour (Rubenthaler et al. 1980). The gasograph consists of stoppered reaction bottles that are placed in a water bath for strict temperature control. The reaction bottles contain tubing connected to water reservoirs and aluminum rods that contain plastic pens that mark on a continuously moving chart (100 gasograph units). The temperature is controlled within less than 0.05°C by a combination of a thermostat, heater, and circulating pump. Values are recorded as gasograph units (GU), which can be readily expressed as millimeters of mercury or cubic centimeters of gas. Gasograph channel to channel reproducibility is at least equal to that of different manometric-type and gauge-type nonrecording instruments. The instrument has the capacity to run 12 different samples per test so it is ideally suited to determine the optimum amount of yeast for bakery formulations. The test consists of mixing different amounts of yeast (3.5 up to 7.5) to batters made with 6% sugar, 1.5% salt, and 150% water based on the original flour weight (10 g). Samples are placed in closed flasks inside a water bath with strict temperature controls. Each flask is provided with a perforated plastic lid connected to a system that measures pressure throughout time.

According to Rubenthaler et al. (1980), the average of the coefficients of variability of treatments within laboratories was 0.55% and within channels between laboratories was 0.75%. Typical gasograms demonstrate the high reproducibility of the actions of formula ingredients, yeast, sugar, and diastatic malt because the coefficient of variability was only 0.69%. The gasograph can be used to indicate the presence or absence of inhibitors or stimulators of yeast respiration and to investigate the interaction of formula ingredients and fermentation rates during various stages of the fermentation and proofing of dough. Traces of α-amylase in wheat and flour can be easily detected with this instrument.

8.2.4.1 Determination of Yeast Activity with the Gasograph

A. *Samples, Ingredients, and Reagents*
- Different types of flours
- Sodium chloride (NaCl)
- Sucrose
- Fresh and/or dry yeast
- Distilled water

B. *Materials and Equipments*
- Gasograph
- Half-pint reaction bottles
- Rubber stoppers
- Glass stirrer
- Chart paper

C. *Procedure (Rubenthaler et al. 1980)*
1. Place distilled water in the gasograph and adjust to the desired temperature (30°C).
2. In the reaction bottles weigh 10 g flour, 0.15 g NaCl, 0.6 g sugar, and different amounts of fresh bakers yeast (0.2, 0.3, 0.5, or 0.75 g) or the equivalent of dry yeast (0.066, 0.1, 0.166, or 0.25). Add 15 mL distilled water and mix contents until attaining a paste. Alternatively, malt, yeast food, sugars, and other additives can be tested at different concentrations.
3. Place gasograph reaction bottles in the water bath, and after 2 minutes, place stopper.
4. Make sure the marking pens are working in each of the gasograph channels.
5. Allow doughs to ferment for 2 hours.
6. Obtain the gas production vs. fermentation time plot. Register the maximum value and the slope in the linear part of the curve using the following equation $(y2 − y1)/(x2 − x1)$. Express results in gasograph units, millimeters mercury, and

cubic centimeters. The conversion factor of gasograph units to millimeters mercury and cubic centimeters are 7.3 and 2.38, respectively.

8.2.5 PRESSUROMETER

The pressurometer is a special metal airtight container equipped with a gauge designed to measure gas pressure produced by a yeasted suspension of flour (Figure 8.4). The test is usually carried for 5 hours under strict temperature conditions (30°C) in a proof cabinet or in a water bath (AACC 2000, Method 22-11). The instrument is used to determine yeast activity although it could be also used to indirectly determine malt diastatic activity.

8.2.5.1 Determination of Yeast Activity with the Pressurometer

A. *Samples, Ingredients, and Reagents*
- Wheat flour
- Different types of yeast
- Sugar
- Distilled water

B. *Materials and Equipments*
- Digital scale
- Pressurometers
- Fermentation cabinet
- Stirring glass rod
- pH meter
- Spatula
- Pipette (10 mL)
- Volumetric flask (1 L)
- Chronometer

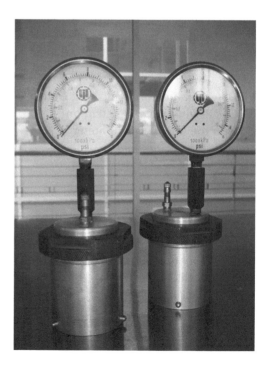

FIGURE 8.4 Pressurometer used to test yeast activity.

C. *Procedure (AACC 2000, Method 22-11)*

1. Prepare a 5% sugar solution (50 g in a 1-L volumetric flask).
2. Weigh 2 g fresh baker's yeast or its equivalent of dry yeast (0.66 g) and place it in the pressurometer container. Add exactly 10 mL of the 5% sugar solution and with the stirring glass rod blend contents. Measure the initial pH of the mix. Close the pressurometer with the pressurometer wrench.
3. Place the pressurometer in the fermentation cabinet set at a predetermined temperature (30°C). After 5 minutes, release the internal pressure by punching the pressure air valve until the gauge marks zero.
4. Thereafter, register the pressure every 10 minutes during 90 minutes of fermentation.
5. After 90 minutes release the pressure by punching the pressure air valve until the gauge marks zero. Open the pressurometer and register the pH of the fermented broth. If needed, close the pressurometer and repeat the procedure for 60 more minutes.
6. Plot the first and second fermentation tests (pressure vs. fermentation time). Calculate the slope of the curves.

8.2.6 RESEARCH SUGGESTIONS

1. Compare the performance of dry yeast vs. compressed fresh yeast of and standard bread dough. The dry yeast will be added one third of the quantity recommended for fresh compressed yeast. Test and graph yeast activity vs. fermentation time of the doughs using the fermentograph, gasograph, and/or pressurometer procedures.
2. Prepare four different types of standard bread doughs only differing in the type of antimold agent. One control and the others supplemented with 0.2% calcium propionate, 0.2% potassium sorbate, or 0.2% parabens. Test and graph yeast activity vs. fermentation time of the doughs using the fermentograph, gasograph, and/or pressurometer procedures.
3. Prepare two different types of standard French bread doughs (the standard formulation does not contain sugar) only differing in the supplementation of diastatic malt. Test and graph yeast activity versus fermentation time of the doughs using the fermentograph, maturograph, and rheofermentometer.
4. Prepare five different types of standard bread doughs containing the same type and concentration of yeast only differing in the supplemented additives. One control and the others supplemented with 0.2% SSL, 20 ppb and 100 ppb of potassium bromate and sodium ascorbate, respectively, 0.5% of a commercial yeast food preparation, and 0.2% diastatic malt. Test the resulting doughs with the fermentograph, rheofermentometer, maturograph, and oven rise recorder assays.
5. Compare the rheofermentometer or maturograph properties of two different types of standard bread doughs only differing in the supplementation of 2% vital gluten. The gluten supplemented dough should be mixed with 3% more water compared to the standard dough.
6. Study the inhibition of conventional yeast used for the production of bioethanol as affected by type of grain. Compare yellow maize, white sorghum, and high-tannin sorghums hydrolyzates obtained after liquefaction with α-amylase and saccharification with amyloglucosidase. At the end of the test determine the pH and ethanol content of the fermented broth.

8.2.7 RESEARCH QUESTIONS

1. What are the principles of the following apparatus used to test yeast activity?
   a. Fermentograph
   b. Gasograph
   c. Pressurometer
2. What are principles of the rheofermentometer and maturograph? What are the main advantages of these apparatus?
3. Investigate at what temperature and processing conditions (pH, A_w) yeast inactivates.
4. What are the main functionalities of yeast in bread making processes? Why is compressed fresh yeast still widely used by the industry despite its lower shelf life?
5. What are the major factors that affect the carbon dioxide retention capacity of a fermenting dough? Explain how these properties affect bread quality.
6. Draw a flowchart of the biotechnological processes to industrially produce fresh compressed and dry yeasts. In general terms, what is the conversion factor of dry to fresh compressed yeast? Why do most bakers still prefer to use fresh compressed yeast?
7. What are the main chemical components generated during a typical wheat dough fermentation procedure? Which of these metabolites are lost during the baking process?

8.3 FUNCTIONALITY TESTS FOR CHEMICAL LEAVENING AGENTS

There is a wide array of baking goods produced from soft wheat flour and baking powder or chemical leavening agents. These raw materials are common in cookies, cake mixes, hot cakes, muffins, wafers, crackers, and wheat flour tortillas. The leavening effect is due to the carbon dioxide generated by chemical leavening agents, to the incorporation of air bubbles during mixing and the water vapor produced during baking (Faridi 1994; Faridi et al. 2000; Manley 1996; Matz 1992).

A chemical leavening system contains two functional components: a leavening base and a food grade acid-reacting chemical. The sodium bicarbonate containing 52% by weight of carbon dioxide by weight will react with the acid salt in a moist dough or batter environment to yield the leavening. During this reaction, these agents generate gas at a rate that is greatly affected by the pH. If strong acids are used the reaction takes place very fast and therefore most of the gas is lost during dough or batter preparation. Thus, most processors use weak acids. The most common leavening agents are nonocalcium phosphate, dicalcium phosphate, sodium acid pyrophospate, and sodium aluminum sulfate. Chemical leavening agents are classified into three categories: fast, slow, and double acting. Fast-acting releases most of the gas in a relatively short time during mixing or while the dough or batter is on the bench (room temperature). Therefore, fast-acting powders act during mixing and proofing. Examples are tartrate and orthophosphate baking powders. On the other hand, slow-acting powders release most of the gas during baking. The sodium aluminum sulfate (SAS) and sodium aluminum phosphate (SAP) are considered slow acting, whereas the pyrophosphates as moderately slow acting. Double-acting baking powders contain both fast- and slow-acting ingredients so they release carbon dioxide at both ambient, and baking temperatures.

Monocalcium phosphate (MCP) in double-acting baking powders is mainly used for angel cake, pancake, and cookie mixes. It is the natural replacement of cream of tartar. The main use of sodium acid pyrophosphate (SAPP) is for doughnut mixes, regular biscuits and muffins, and refrigerated canned biscuits. The major problem of SAPP is the aftertaste. Sodium aluminum phosphate (SALP) is used in pancakes biscuits and muffins, whereas the dicalcium phosphate is used for the production of cake mixes.

Most commercial baking powders are manufactured from a blend of selected chemical leavening agents, acidulants, and an inert compound (generally starch). Both the acid and acid salts are the key elements to control the release of the carbon dioxide. An important property of chemical leavening agents is the neutralization value that is defined as the parts of sodium bicarbonate that neutralizes 100 parts of the chemical leavening agent under controlled baking conditions. For example, MCP has a neutralization value of 80 whereas dicalcium phosphate of only 33. The sodium aluminum salts (phosphate and sulfate) have values of 100. The salts should not have any toxic effects on humans, affect gluten formation nor negatively affect the organoleptic properties of finished products. In addition, they should be cost-effective and easy to handle. The use of acids is important especially in regular or nonchlorinated flours or in those products where the pH is neutral. The most used acids are tartaric with a neutralization value of 116, derived from the wine industry, and glucodelta-lactone with a neutralization value of 45. The inert or carrier agent is necessary to minimize loss of leavening power because it significantly lowers the interaction between salts and the acidulant. Examples of fast-acting baking powders are tartaric acid 6%, cream of tartar 44.9%, sodium

bicarbonate 26.7% and starch 22.4%, or MCP 33.4%, sodium bicarbonate 26.7%, and starch 39.8%. A typical slow-acting formulation contains 40.4% sodium acid pyrophosphate, 30.6% sodium bicarbonate, and 29% starch (Faridi 1994; Faridi et al. 2000). There are many examples of double-acting baking powders. One typical formulation consists of MCP (6.7%–13.2%), sodium aluminum sulfate (19%–21%), sodium bicarbonate (26.7%), and starch (40%–45%).

8.3.1 NEUTRALIZATION VALUE

The most important functional test for chemical leavening agents is the neutralization value. These tests are based on the acid required to neutralize chemical leavening agents. The neutralization value is usually expressed as parts of sodium bicarbonate equivalent to 100 parts by weight of acid-reacting material.

8.3.1.1 Determination of Neutralization Values of Monocalcium Phosphate, Monohydrate or Anhydrous

A. *Samples, Ingredients, and Reagents*
  - MCP, monohydrate or anhydrous leavening agents
  - Sodium hydroxide (0.1 N NaOH)
  - Hydrochloric acid (0.2 N HCl)
  - Phenolphthalein (1 in 95% ethanol)
  - Sodium chloride (NaCl)
  - Sodium citrate (10% solution)
  - Standard pH solutions

B. *Materials and Equipments*
  - Digital scale
  - White porcelain casserole No. 4
  - Glass stirring rod
  - Hop plate or Meker burner
  - Burettes (50 mL and 100 mL)
  - Beakers (250 mL)
  - pH meter

C. *Procedure*
  1. Weigh exactly 0.84 g sample of MCP, monohydrate or anhydrous, and transfer to No. 4 casserole.
  2. For monocalcium monohydrate or anhydrous first add 25 mL water and stir, then add 90 mL or 120 mL of 0.1 N NaOH, respectively.
  3. Stir intermittently during 5 minutes, then bring suspension to boil for 2 minutes and boil for 1 minute.
  4. While solution is boiling, add 0.15 mL phenolphtalein indicator and titrate with 0.2 N HCL until pink color disappears.
  5. Record the exact amount of HCl used during the titration procedure.
  6. Calculate the neutralization value using the following equation:

Neutralization value = 100 − (2 * mL 0.2 N HCl used).

8.3.1.2 Determination of Neutralization Values of Sodium Acid Pyrophosphate

A. *Samples, Ingredients, and Reagents*
- Sodium acid pyrophosphate
- Distilled water
- Sodium hydroxide (0.1 N NaOH)
- Hydrochloric acid (0.2 N HCl)
- Sodium chloride (NaCl)
- Phenolphthalein (1 in 95% ethanol)
- Standard pH solutions

B. *Materials and Equipments*
- Digital scale
- White porcelain casserole No. 4
- Glass stirring rod
- Hot plate or Meker burner
- Burettes (50 and 100 mL)
- Graduated cylinder (100 mL)
- Beakers (250 mL)
- pH meter
- Dropper bottle

C. *Procedure*
1. Weigh exactly 0.84 g of sodium acid pyrophosphate and transfer to No. 4 casserole.
2. Add 20 g NaCl and 25 mL water. Stir intermittently during 3–5 minutes with a stirring rod.
3. Add 90 mL 0.1 N NaOH and a drop of phenolphthalein indicator.
4. Titrate with 0.2 N HCl until pink color disappears.
5. Record the exact amount of HCl used during the titration procedure.
6. Calculate the neutralization value using the following equation:

Neutralization value = 90 – (2 * mL 0.2 N HCl used).

8.3.1.3 Determination of Neutralization Values of Sodium Aluminum Phosphate

A. *Samples, Ingredients, and Reagents*
- Sodium aluminum phosphate samples
- Distilled water
- Sodium hydroxide (NaOH 0.1 N)
- Sodium chloride (NaCl)
- Hydrochloric acid (HCl 0.2 N)
- Phenolphthalein (1 in 95% ethanol)

B. *Materials and Equipments*
- Digital scale
- White porcelain casserole No. 4
- Glass stirring rod
- Hop plate or Meker burner
- Burettes (50 mL and 100 mL)
- Beakers (250 mL)
- pH meter
- Graduated cylinders (25 mL and 100 mL)

C. *Procedure*
1. Weigh exactly 0.84 g of sodium aluminum phosphate and transfer into a 250-mL capacity beaker.

2. Add 20 g NaCl and 5 mL of 10% sodium citrate solution and 25 mL water.
3. Add 120 mL 0.1 N NaOH from a burette swirling during addition.
4. Place suspension on a hot plate and stir contents with a magnetic stirrer. Bring to boil in 3 to 5 minutes and then boil for exactly 5 minutes.
5. Remove form hot plate and allow the solution to cool down to 25°C.
6. Titrate with 0.2 N HCL until achieving a pH 8.5. The pH meter should be previously standardized with pH 7 buffer solution.
7. Continue stirring for 5 more minutes then add more 0.2 N HCl to a final pH of 8.5.
8. Record the exact amount of HCL used during titration.
9. Calculate the neutralization value using the following equation:

Neutralization value = 120 – (2 * mL 0.2 N HCl used).

8.3.2 RESEARCH SUGGESTIONS

1. Compare the performance of slow- and fast-acting baking powders with and without the addition of tartaric acid of and standard high-ratio cake formulation (refer to procedure in Section 10.4.4.2). Determine the neutralization value of the chemical leavening agents, batter pH, cake volume, and symmetry and crumb texture.
2. Compare the appearance, thickness, dough pH, and overall sensory properties of wheat flour tortillas prepared with the following ingredients (refer to procedure in Section 10.5.1.1): control prepared with 1.0% double-acting baking powder; 2% double-acting baking powder; 2% double-acting baking powder and 0.2% fumaric acid; 1.5% slow-acting baking powder and 0.2% fumaric acid; 1.5% fast-acting baking powder, and 0.2% fumaric acid.
3. Compare the appearance, average thickness, dough pH during the different parts of the process, texture, and overall sensory properties (i.e., flavor and aroma mainly) of crackers (refer to procedure in Section 10.2.1) prepared with 0.2% and 0.4% ammonium sulfate. The ammonium sulfate, sodium bicarbonate, and other chemical leavening agents should be added during the second stage of dough preparation.

8.3.3 RESEARCH QUESTIONS

1. Define the following terms:
   a. Baking powder
   b. Neutralization value
   c. Slow-acting baking powder

d. Double-acting baking powder
e. SAPP
f. SALP
g. Gluco-delta-lactone

2. What are the four types of leavening? What are the functionalities of chemical leavening agents in bakery products?

3. What kinds of leavening gases are produced by the reaction of ammonium bicarbonate?

4. List three ions from residual chemical leavening agents that impact quality of bakery products?

5. List three ingredients that are often increased or decreased to compensate with high-altitude baking.

6. What is the main difference between a chemical leavening agent and a baking powder? Give at least two examples of fast- and slow-acting chemical leavening agents.

7. Explain differences in the activity of chemical leavening agents in a soft wheat product elaborated with regular (pH 6.9) or chlorinated (pH 5.6) flours.

8. How much sodium bicarbonate is required to neutralize 7.5 kg of SAPP (neutralization value of 72)?

9. How much monocalcium phosphate (MCP) with a neutralization value of 80 is necessary to neutralize 2.4 kg of sodium bicarbonate?

10. Why is ammonium bicarbonate not used in most chemically leavened products?

REFERENCES

American Association of Cereal Chemists. 2000. *Approved Methods of the AACC*. St. Paul, MN: AACC.

Czuchajowska, Z., and Y. Pomeranz. 1993. "Gas Formation and Gas Retention I. The System and Methodology." *Cereal Foods World* 38:499–503.

Faridi, H. 1994. *The Science of Cookie and Cracker Production*. New York: Chapman & Hall.

Faridi, H., C. S. Gaines, and B. L. Strouts. 2000. "Soft Wheat Products." In *Handbook of Cereal Science and Technology*, edited by K. J. Lorenz and J. G. Ponte, chapter 18. 2nd ed. New York: Marcel Dekker.

Maloney, D. H., and J. J. Foy. 2003. "Yeast Fermentation." In *Handbook of Dough Fermentations*, edited by K. Kulp and K. Lorenz, chapter 3. New York: Marcel Dekker.

Manley, D. 1996. *Technology of Biscuits, Crackers and Cookies*. 2nd ed. Cambridge, UK: Woodhead Publishing.

Matz, S. A. 1992. *Cookie and Cracker Technology*. 3rd ed. Westport, CT: AVI Publishing.

Poitrenaud, B. 2006. "Yeast Chapter." In *Handbook of Food Science, Technology and Engineering*, Vol. II, edited by Y. H. Hui, chapter 69. Boca Raton, FL: CRC Press.

Rasper, V. F. 1991. "Quality Evaluation of Cereal and Cereal Products." In *Handbook of Cereal Science and Technology*, edited by K. J. Lorenz and K. Kulp, Chapter 15. New York: Marcel Dekker.

Reed, G., and H. J. Peppler. 1973. *Yeast Technology*. Westport, CT: AVI Publishing.

Rubenthaler, G. L., P. L. Finney, D. E. Demaray, and K. F. Finney. 1980. "Gasograph: Design, Construction and Reproducibility of a Sensitive 12-Channel Gas Recording Instrument." *Cereal Chemistry* 57:212–216.

9 Production of Yeast-Leavened Bakery Products

9.1 INTRODUCTION

Bread is considered the most common food for mankind since men became sedentary and practiced farming. The manufacturing of primitive types of flat breads is well documented. Different types of breads originated since prehistoric times. Bread is a sacred symbol for Christians, Jews, Greeks, and Egyptians. There are clear indications of the production of bread by the Egyptian culture in times of Ramses III 1,200 years B.C. Bread is manufactured using common ingredients (flour, water, salt, sugar) and simple utensils, and it is staple for most cultures around the globe due to its high nutritional value and highly digestible caloric value.

Modern industrial baking processes are highly mechanized and require the best quality flours because their properties affect process variables, machinability, and quality of end products. The general sequential steps for the production of bread are blending of dry ingredients, dough mixing, fermentation, punching/molding, and baking. Most yeast-leavened breads are preferably made from refined hard wheat flours. Flour quality mainly affects dough water absorption, optimum mixing time, and the final bread characteristics.

The basic ingredients needed for the production of yeast-leavened bread are flour, water, and yeast. Most formulas also contain salt, sugar, and shortening or lard. To fulfill shelf-life expectations and produce high-quality products, ingredients such as malt, preservatives, oxidizing agents, emulsifiers, yeast food, nonfat dry milk, and vital gluten are used (Matz 1972, 1987; Schunemann and Treu 1988; Sultan 1983; Quaglia 1991; Pyler 1988; Pomeranz and Shellenberger 1971).

Flour is the most important ingredient of bread formulations and affects functionality, manufacturing parameters, and properties of finished products. It affects the requirement of other ingredients such as water, malt, and vital gluten. Flour functionality is mainly dictated by the protein content and/or gluten properties. Both water and mechanical mixing work are required for properly dough development. The resulting dough forms a continuous elastic network that is capable of retaining the carbon dioxide produced by the fermenting yeast or by the gases generated by the chemical leavening agents. The most important flour characteristics are water absorption, mixing, or dough development time, and stability or mixing tolerance. Generally, bakeries have stringent flour quality control measurements. The most important are related to dough rheological properties measured with the mixolab, farinograph, extensigraph, and/or alveograph (refer to Chapter 5).

Yeast (*Saccharomyces cerevisiae*) is key for production of bread because it ferments simple sugars into carbon dioxide, ethanol, and many intermediate metabolites that greatly affect flavor and aroma (refer to Chapter 8). In most bakeries, yeast is used as fresh compressed or dehydrated. The fresh compressed and dried yeast contains about 70% and 10% water, respectively. In practical terms, 1 kg of fresh compressed yeast is equivalent to approximately 0.45 kg dry yeast. Most bread formulations are depicted in terms of fresh-compressed yeast. The advantage of dry yeast is that it has a prolonged shelf-life especially when it is vacuum packaged. The disadvantage is that it takes longer to reactivate and start hydrolyzing the dough substrate. In addition, yeast suffers damage to their cell walls during dehydration, releasing glutathione, which has a known gluten-weakening effect.

Sugars have three basic functionalities in bread systems: impart flavor and color, contribute to prolonged shelf life, and is the main regulator of yeast activity. The flavor profile is produced by means of sugar breakdown during fermentation and by the amount of residual or unfermented sugar. Sugars also greatly affect bread color, especially crust color, by Maillard reactions when exposed to the high baking oven temperatures. These carbohydrates also improve bread shelf life because they are transformed into organic acids that lower pH and water activity. Pan bread formulations usually contain 4% to 6.5% sugar while sweet pastries and baking goods up to 15% (Matz 1972, 1987; Schunemann and Treu 1988; Sultan 1983; Quaglia 1991; Pyler 1988; Pomeranz and Shellenberger 1971).

Salt is one of the four essential ingredients in bread formulations because it strengths the gluten via ionic protein modifications, stabilizes yeast fermentation rate, enhances the flavor of the final product, and slightly increases dough mixing time. It does not impart a salty taste but rather brings out the other flavors in the system at the level generally used (1% to 2%). It is known to increase sweetness of sugars and mask metallic and bitter off-flavors. Furthermore, salt counter rests the overly sweet flavor of sugars in pastry products and acts as stabilizer and controller of yeast fermentation. It also lowers water activity and therefore acts synergistically with preservatives to enhance shelf life.

Most bread formulations include hydrogenated vegetable shortening or lard because they act as lubricants improving dough texture and machinability. These fats significantly lower dough stickiness. Their main functionality is to improve the textural shelf life of baking goods. This is because the plastic shortening or lard forms thin films between the gluten network and other dough components retarding the loss of bread texture throughout storage. The main concern about the use of shortening nowadays is the level of *trans* fatty acids because of their proven negative effects on human health. Zero *trans* plastic shortenings with good oxidative stability are now available to produce healthier products. Shortening and lard are usually used in pan bread formulations at levels varying from 3% to 3.5% and in sweet baking goods at levels of up to 15%. Diastatic malt is used in bread formulation because it contains high levels of α- and β-amylases and proteases that mainly hydrolyze damaged starch granules and proteins, respectively. These enzymes gradually and slowly provide substrate for the fermenting yeast. The diastatic malt is especially important in those formulations where sugar is not used such as in French breads.

Pan and sweet bread formulations usually contain small quantities of nonfat dried milk (1% to 3.5% based on flour weight). The milk slightly increases water absorption, and improves crust color (golden color) and flavor. It is noteworthy to mention that yeast is not capable of breaking down lactose therefore this disaccharide remains unaltered until the baking process, where it contributes to the crumb color. Milk also improves the nutritional value because its protein complements the amino acid pattern of wheat proteins and supplies important amounts of calcium, magnesium, and other essential nutrients.

Dough conditioners are widely used in commercial bread production because they act as dough conditioners, and decrease very effectively, staling rate. The most popular emulsifiers are stearoyl-2 sodium lactylate, monoglycerides, lecithin, succinylated monoglycerides, ethoxylated monoglycerides, and diacetyl tartaric acid ester of monoglycerides (DATEM). The emulsifiers are commonly used in combination because of their synergistic positive effects and used in levels that vary from 0.01% up to 0.3% based on flour weight (Matz 1972, 1987; Schunemann and Treu 1988; Sultan 1983; Quaglia 1991; Pyler 1988; Pomeranz and Shellenberger 1971).

Oxidizing agents have little or no effect on yeast activity but affect the rheological dough properties and therefore the gluten gas retention capacity. Oxidizing agents enhance the formation of disulfide bonds and therefore gluten strength. These rheological changes also improve crumb texture because breads usually develop better-distributed gas cells or loci with lesser amounts of large air pockets or crumb defects. The most popular oxidizing agent is potassium bromate, but it is banned in several countries around the globe. Most formulations that contain oxidizing agents also include ascorbic acid because of their synergistic effect. The levels commonly used of ascorbic acid vary from 30 ppm to 100 ppm. Other important oxidizing agents used are azodicarbonamide and cupric sulfate. Azodicarbonamide is used instead of potassium bromate and supplemented to baking flours by millers.

To inhibit bread molds and enhance shelf life, the baking industry use propionate salts (mainly calcium propionate). The calcium propionate strongly inhibits molds without greatly affecting yeast activity. The organic acids generated during fermentation drops the pH and gradually transform the salt into the active propionic acid. Generally, breads with more acidic pHs have longer shelf life expectations. The most common maximum level allowed of preservatives used alone or in combination is 0.2% based on flour weight.

Yeast food consists of a blend of mineral salts and nitrogenous compounds included in a base. These nutrients are essential to enhance yeast activity. The minerals used are acidic calcium phosphate, dicalcium phosphate, sodium chloride, and ammonium sulfate. Most of these salts are usually mixed with dough improvers and oxidizing agents diluted in a starch or flour base. Most yeast food mixes are added 0.5% based on flour weight (Doerry 1995; Kulp and Ponte 2000).

Most breads are made by five sequential major operations: mixing of dry ingredients, dough mixing, fermentation, baking, and cooling. Dough mixing has two major objectives: distribute homogenously ingredients and gluten formation. Mixing is divided in several sequential stages: in the first stage known as water absorption, the flour absorbs the water yielding a noncohesive and sticky dough. This step generally lasts less than 1 minute. In most yeast-leavened bread formulations, the amount of water added varies from 58% to 66% based on flour weight. As mixing proceeds, the dough gradually develops elastic and cohesive properties because the hydrated gliadin–glutelin network or gluten starts interacting via formation of hydrophobic and disulfide bonds. The optimum mixing time is when the dough acquires the maximum force or strength, attains a smooth and shiny texture, and tends to retain the maximum amount of gas produced during fermentation. There are three major control parameters during the critical step of dough mixing: flour water absorption, dough mixing time, and dough temperature (Matz 1972, 1987; Schunemann and Treu 1988; Sultan 1983; Quaglia 1991; Pyler 1988; Pomeranz and Shellenberger 1971).

Commercial dough fermentation is performed under strict controls of temperature and air humidity. Generally, fermentation is performed in fermentation cabinets or continuous proofers at temperatures ranging from 26°C to 32°C under high air humidity (i.e., 85% relative humidity). A high relative humidity is required to prevent dough surface dehydration (crusty dough) that affects quality and even possibly yield of end products. Fermentation is generally subdivided into several stages: yeast activation, degassing-punching-forming, and proofing. The total fermentation time will depend on the formulation, baking system, fermentation temperature, and substrate. The aim of dough punching is to remove the carbon dioxide gas trapped by the gluten and create new cells or loci due to the subdivision of the large gas pockets. The punching operation reactivates yeast because the elimination of the high carbon dioxide concentration is trapped in the dough. The new air pockets or loci will become the crumb bread cells affecting texture and appearance. The fermenting dough is generally degassed by forcing it through rolls or by pressing to a rotating cone. During these mechanical operations, the trapped gas is released and new small gas bubbles form.

The properly degassed dough is formed and in some instances placed inside baking pans in preparation for proofing. The forming operation is usually performed in special equipments or in some instances by hand. Finally, the preformed piece of dough is proofed for a given amount of time before baking. The proofing time is chiefly affected by proofing temperature, type of flour, and type of bread.

The preformed, fermented, and proofed piece of dough is transformed into bread after baking at temperatures that commonly range from 200°C to 230°C for 12 to 25 minutes depending on the type and size of bread. During the initial baking stage, the dough increases its height and volume because the yeast is still alive and yields carbon dioxide. The trapped gas expands due to the higher temperature and the formation of water vapor. This phenomenon is commonly known as oven-spring. Generally, high-quality protein flours have more oven spring compared with low-protein counterparts. Yeast cells die approximately 8 minutes after baking at temperatures of about 220°C. In addition, the gluten denatures and sets giving the foundation for the piece of bread, the hydrated starch granules gelatinize and eventually acquire a strong water-holding capacity and the bread develops its characteristic crust color due to Maillard and caramelization reactions. During most baking schedules, there is sufficient time to destroy all microorganisms and spores. Thus, breads exit the oven practically sterile. This is critically important to design good sanitation and cooling procedures so to avoid cross-contamination that could compromise shelf life.

The microbial bread shelf life greatly depends on the effectiveness of the cooling operation and storage conditions. The rate of cooling depends on the bread size, the temperature in the cooling room and whether or not fans are used. Most breads are subjected to cooling schedules of at least 20 to 30 minutes. Optimally, the bread temperature should be lowered to less than 28°C. Improper cooling causes water condensation or sweating inside the package, loss of bread texture, and microbial problems.

Breads are produced by straight dough, sponge dough, or continuous procedures. The last employs a liquid sponge undergoing high fermentation. Straight dough procedures are usually practiced in small bakeries and consist of mixing all ingredients to form a dough that is further processed into bread. The sponge dough is the most common way to prepare pan bread. It is known as sponge because the flour is divided into two lots of approximately 60% and 40%. The sponge flour is mixed with almost all the water and total yeast required. After 5 to 8 hours of fermentation the fermenting sponge is mixed with the rest of the flour and other ingredients until developing the dough. The advantages of the sponge procedure are the reduced in-plant fermentation and proofing times and the properties of the finished bread. These breads have stronger flavor and possess a better crumb texture. The continuous liquid sponge procedures are highly mechanized and aimed toward a considerable reduction of processing time. Thus, these systems require less labor but require better quality flours and strict quality controls of ingredients and processing conditions (Matz 1972, 1987; Schunemann and Treu 1988; Sultan 1983; Quaglia 1991; Pyler 1988; Pomeranz and Shellenberger 1971).

9.2 PRODUCTION AND QUALITY OF YEAST FERMENTED BREADS

9.2.1 CHINESE STEAMED BREAD

The Chinese or mantou bread is highly popular in China and neighboring countries. Historically, this bread has been staple for more than 2,000 years. More than 40% of the Chinese wheat is currently used for the traditional and commercial production of steamed breads. Steamed breads and buns have evolved continuously throughout Chinese history so that today there are many types or varieties (Huang 1999). Among breads, it is unique because the formed pieces of dough are steamed instead of baked. A lean formulation consisting of refined wheat flour with intermediate protein content, water, yeast, and salt is used for its production. After dough mixing, the dough is sheeted, rolled, and hand-formed and uniformly cut into pieces ranging from 130 g to 150 g. In some instances, the pieces of dough are formed into animal configurations. The bread has a white colored crust because steaming is a mild cooking process and no sugar is used. The bread is steamed for approximately 30 minutes, the dough increases its volume and the cooked bread has a very fine and firm crumb texture and a bland flavor. However, the bread is comparatively denser (0.3 g/cm^3 to 0.55 g/cm^3) compared with other more aerated breads. The Chinese bread is widely used to accompany other foods and to prepare sandwiches. The bread is divided into two broad categories: northern and southern styles. The northern type is denser with a fine crumb, elastic, cohesive, chewy, and not sticky, whereas the southern counterparts are softer, more open, and even and fine crumb and with a slight sweet flavor.

The recommended amount of water is 76% to 80% of the farinograph water absorption.

9.2.1.1 Production of Chinese Steamed Bread

A. Samples, Ingredients, and Reagents
- Refer to Table 9.1

B. Materials and Equipments
- Digital scale
- Graduated cylinder (100 mL or 200 mL)
- Dough mixer
- Dough cutter and rounder
- Fermentation cabinet
- Plastic or stainless steel containers for proofing
- Baking sheets
- Punching or degassing roll unit
- Steamer
- Rapeseed displacement volume meter
- Bread knife
- Thermometer
- pH meter
- Chronometer
- Heat-resistant gloves

C. Procedure
1. Weigh 200 g of all-purpose or intermediate protein flour (14% mb) and divide it into two lots one containing 78% of the flour (sponge)

TABLE 9.1
Typical Formulations for Production of Chinese Steamed Breads

Ingredients	Northern Style Sponge (%)	Northern Style Dough (%)	Southern Style Sponge (%)	Southern Style Dough (%)	Sweet Southern Style Sponge (%)	Sweet Southern Style Dough (%)
Refined flour (all-purpose)	78.0	22.0	78.0	22.0	78.0	22.0
Water	36.6	10.0	34.6	9.0	36.6	10.0
Fresh compressed yeast	3.0	–	3.0	–	3.0	–
Salt	–	–	–	–	–	0.5
Sugar	–	–	–	–	–	15.0
Shortening	–	–	–	–	–	3.0
Baking powder	–	–	–	–	–	0.5
Nonfat dry milk	–	–	–	–	–	0.5
Emulsifier	–	–	–	–	–	0.1

and the other the remaining 22% of the flour (Table 9.1).

2. Mix the sponge flour, yeast, and water into a sponge dough and allow it to ferment for 90 minutes at 30°C. Register the pH at the beginning and end of fermentation (Figure 9.1).

3. Place the sponge dough, rest of the flour, water, and other ingredients and mix in a dough mixer for gluten development. After mixing, register the mix time, dough consistency and temperature, and pH.

4. Allow the dough to rest in the proofing cabinet for 10 minutes.

5. Sheet the piece of dough through a set of rolls adjusted at a gap of 0.48 cm or 3/16 inch. Manually roll the resulting dough sheet into a cylinder making sure to seal borders. Register the subjective dough consistency and pH.

6. Cut the dough cylinder into three equal parts, and register the weight of each dough piece. Alternatively, these pieces of dough can be rounded by hand (Figure 9.1).

7. Place the molded dough pieces for 20 minutes of proofing in a fermentation cabinet.

8. Place the pieces of dough into a steamer. The cooker should contain a lid and enough water to produce a gentle boiling during the cooking process. Steam the pieces of dough in the closed steamer for 15–20 minutes (Figure 9.1).

9. After steaming, allow the pieces of Chinese bread to cool down at ambient temperature.

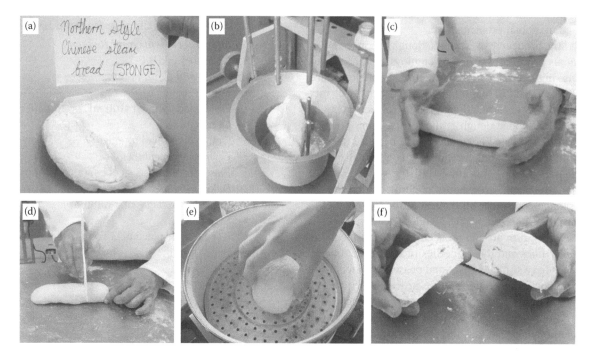

FIGURE 9.1 Steps for the production of Chinese steamed bread. (a) Sponge dough; (b) dough mixing; (c) dough forming; (d) dough cutting; (e) steaming; and (f) Chinese steamed bread.

10. Upon cooling, evaluate the properties of resulting steamed breads in terms of pH, bread height, weight, volume (rapeseed displacement), crust formation and color, crumb texture, and organoleptic properties. Calculate the bread yield based on the original formulation.

9.2.2 BAGUETTES OR FRENCH BREADS

The baguette is a descendant of bread first developed in Vienna, Austria, in the mid-19th century when deck or steam ovens were first brought into common use. Baguette, the hard crusty loaf we currently associate with France, dates only to the Industrial Revolution. A baguette is a long thin loaf of the type more commonly known as French bread. The baguette was introduced in the 1920s after a new law banned French bakers from working before 4 a.m. Bakers liked it because it was convenient to make and stayed fresh for only a few hours. Hence, customers visited bakeries two or three times a day. Consumers liked the baguette because it was whiter and sweeter compared with sourdough breads.

French bread and baguettes are commonly manufactured by the straight baking procedure and using a very simple formulation consisting of flour, water, salt, yeast, and malt. The amounts of these ingredients vary but a typical formulation contains 60% to 66% water, 2% salt, 1.5% to 2% dry yeast, and from 0.1% to 0.5% malt. The amount of water depends on the type of flour and the type of bread. Due to the lack of extrinsic fermentable carbohydrates or sugars, the yeast has little substrate to ferment. Malt plays an important role because α and β-amylases breakdown damaged starch, yielding fermentable carbohydrates. French breads are usually subclassified into hard crusted and soft crusted. Regardless of the type, the process consists of first mixing dry ingredients and then adding the predetermined amount of water in preparation for dough mixing. The dough is mixed to fully develop the gluten and then cut, fermented for a short period (i.e., 30 minutes), hand or mechanically formed, and proofed for approximately 90–120 minutes. Before baking, the preformed pieces of dough are cut on the top part so the bread breaks during baking and acquires the typical configuration. French breads are usually baked 230°C–250°C for 15–30 minutes, depending on the type and size of bread. Soft-crusted French breads are usually baked on special ovens where steam is injected. The steam will help to produce a thin and soft crust. The formulation of hard crusted French breads use less water, and breads are normally baked without steam. The textural shelf life of baguettes is limited (1–3 days) due to the lack of shortening and dough improvers. Nowadays, and due to the longer shelf life expectations, most French bread formulations include oxidizing agents, vital gluten, emulsifiers, and in some instances little amounts of shortening (Boge 1972; Calvel 1987).

9.2.2.1 Production of French Bread or Baguettes
A. *Samples, Ingredients, and Reagents*
- Refer to Table 9.2

B. *Materials and Equipments*
- Digital scale
- Graduated cylinder (100 mL or 200 mL)

TABLE 9.2
Typical Formulations for Production of Standard, Improved, and High Fiber Soft- and Hard-Crusted Baguettes

Ingredients	Soft Crust			Hard Crust (%)
	Standard (%)	Improved (%)	High Fiber (%)	
Hard refined flour	100.0	100.0	94.0	100.0
Wheat bran	–	–	8.0	
Water	63.0	67.0	64.0	58.0
Fresh compressed yeast	6.0	6.0	6.0	6.0
Salt	2.2	2.2	2.2	2.2
Vital gluten	–	1.5	1.5	–
Nonfat dry milk	–	1.0	1.0	–
Diastatic malt	0.5	0.5	0.5	0.5
Shortening	–	1.5	1.5	–
Sugar	–	0.5	0.5	–
Ascorbic acid[a]	–	20–50 ppm	20–50 ppm	–
Potassium bromate[a]	–	20 ppm	20 ppm	–

[a] The amounts of potassium bromate and ascorbic acid for 100 g flour could be included in the water and calculated as follows:

Example:

1 ppm = 1 mg/L

1 g/L = 1000 mg/L or 1000 ppm/L

50 ppm = X L

X = 0.05 L or 50 mL solution

- Dough mixer
- Dough cutter and rounder
- Fermentation cabinet
- Proof plastic or stainless steel containers
- Baking sheets for baguettes
- Punching or degassing roll unit
- Baking oven with steam injection
- Rapeseed displacement volume meter
- Bread knife
- Thermometer
- pH meter
- Chronometer
- Heat-resistant gloves

C. Procedure

1. Weigh 200 g hard flour (14% mb) and the ingredients (Table 9.2).
2. Place the flour and ingredients in the dough mixer. Add the predetermined amount of water and start the mixer until the dough is properly developed (Figure 9.2). The properly developed dough should be cohesive, smooth, and form a thin layer when stretched by hand. An overmixed dough usually develops stickiness.
3. After mixing, register the mix time, dough consistency and temperature, and pH. Then, divide the dough into two equal parts and place first the dough balls first in a greased proofing container and then in a proofing cabinet set at 28°C and 85% RH.
4. After 30 minutes of proofing, punch the dough through a set of degassing rolls adjusted at a gap of 0.48 cm or 3/16 inch. Manually roll the resulting dough sheet into a cylinder making sure to

seal borders. Register the subjective dough consistency and pH.
5. Place the molded dough pieces on baking sheets especially designed for baguettes for 60–80 minutes of proofing in a fermentation cabinet. After 2/3 proofing, cut with a knife or scalper the upper side of the fermenting dough pieces with the characteristic baguette configuration (perpendicular and inclined cuts).
6. Return the baking sheets for final proofing.
7. Place the baking sheets with the fermented dough pieces in an oven set at 220°C for 15 to 25 minutes of baking (Figure 9.2). For soft crust baguettes make sure to inject steam during baking. If the oven is not equipped with a steam injector, it is advisable to place a container with distilled water so to produce an internal environment with high moisture. For hard crust baguettes, make sure to perform baking without steam.
8. After baking, allow the pieces of bread to cool down at ambient temperature.
9. Upon cooling, evaluate the properties of resulting breads in terms of pH, proof height, weight, volume (rapeseed displacement), crust color, crumb texture, and organoleptic properties. Calculate the bread yield based on the original formulation.

9.2.3 Arabic Flat Breads

Arabic flat breads are among the most ancient breads because they did not need oven or even utensil for their baking.

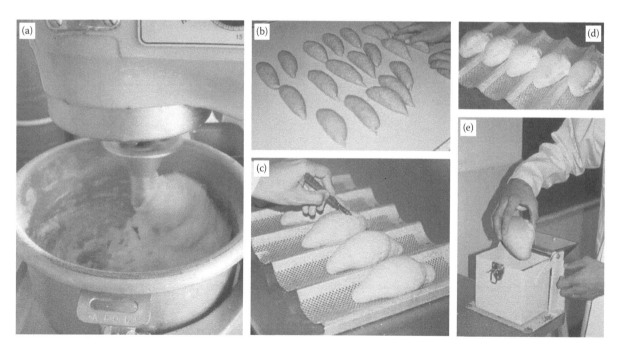

FIGURE 9.2 Steps for the production of French bread. (a) Dough mixing; (b) dough forming; (c) diagonal dough cutting; (d) baked French bread; and (e) evaluation of French bread volume.

Nowadays, the Arabic flat bread, also known as pita or pocket, is still one of the most popular breads especially in Arab countries, Israel, Greece, and the Balkans. Pita is now the western name for the Saudi Arabian bread called *khubz* (ordinary bread), other breads of Arab, Egyptian, or Syrian origin, or *kumaj* (a Turkish word meaning a bread cooked in ashes), all baked in a brick oven. Pitas are increasing in popularity in other parts of the world because it is suitable to accompany with fillings and salads and viewed by the consumer as dietetic. The typical pita formulation based on high protein bread flour is 70% water, 2% salt, 1% dry yeast or its equivalent on fresh compressed yeast, and 0.25% ascorbic acid (Quail 1996). They are defined as a slightly leavened wheat bread, flat, either round or oval with considerable variations in size. They have lower specific volumes but higher crust-to-crumb ratio compared with other breads. In addition, leavened flat breads have relatively shorter fermentation times and are normally baked at high temperature (i.e., 300°C) and short time. Some are manufactured with high fiber ingredients and other cereal grains. To produce high-quality pita breads, the flour is mixed with relatively high amounts of water (up to 68%–70% water, Table 9.3) and the resulting slack dough is folded and formed into layers so to form the characteristic internal air pocket during high temperature baking. For this reason, pitas are commonly named pocket breads. Other popular Arabic breads are *lavash*, *yufka*, and *pide* (Quail 1996).

9.2.3.1 Production of Pita Bread

A. *Samples, Ingredients, and Reagents*
- Refer to Table 9.3

B. *Materials and Equipments*
- Digital scale
- Graduated cylinder (100 mL or 200 mL)
- Dough mixer
- Dough cutter and rounder
- Fermentation cabinet
- Plastic or stainless steel containers for proofing
- Baking sheets
- Punching or degassing roll unit
- Baking oven
- Bread knife
- Thermometer
- pH meter
- Chronometer
- Heat-resistant gloves

C. *Procedure*
1. Weigh hard flour (14% mb) and dry ingredients (Table 9.3).
2. Place the flour and ingredients in the dough mixer. Add the predetermined amount of water and start the mixer until the dough is properly developed (Figure 9.3). The properly developed slack dough should be cohesive, smooth, and form a thin layer when stretched by hand. After mixing, register the mix time, dough consistency and temperature, and pH.
3. Cut and round the resulting dough into pieces. For pita bread adjusts the cutter to yield pieces of 80–90 g. Then, place the dough balls on greased proofing sheets and then in a proof box set at 28°C and 85% RH.
4. After 60 minutes of proofing, laminate dough balls into 5-mm-thick circles, then fold the sheeted dough three times to form a multilayered small piece of dough. Make sure to seal by hand the borders of the dough. This is critical important to enhance the formation of the pocket. Register the subjective dough consistency and pH.
5. Return dough balls to proof box (10 minutes).
6. Sheet dough into 20-cm-diameter and 0.5-cm-thick round pieces. Weigh pieces of dough before transferring to baking sheets. Sprinkle

TABLE 9.3
Typical Formulations for Production of Arabic Flat Breads

Ingredients	Pita Bread (%)	Lavash[a]	Yufka	Pide[b]
Hard wheat flour	100.0	100.0	100.0	100.0
Water	70.0	52.0	61.0	75.0
Vegetable oil (olive)	0	7.3	1.5	0
Egg whites	0	0	3.0	0
Sugar	0	0	0	1.5
Honey	0	11.0	0	0
Vinegar	0	0	1.5	0
Salt	2.0	1.5	1.5	1.5
Dry yeast	1.0	1.8	0	1.5
Ascorbic acid	0.25	0	0	0

[a] The *lavash* is usually sprinkled with toasted sesame seed.

[b] The *pide* dough is egg washed and sprinkled with sesame and nigella seeds before baking.

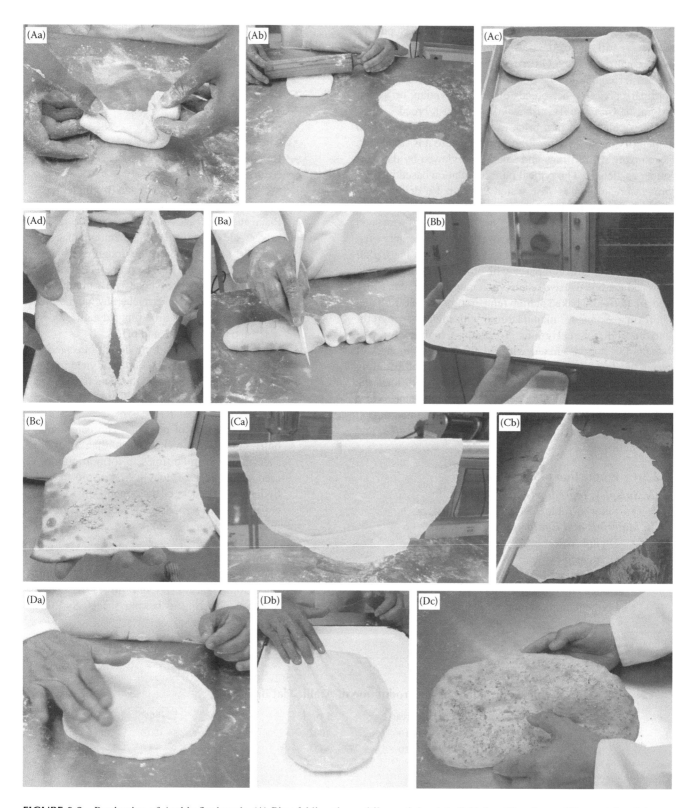

FIGURE 9.3 Production of Arabic flat breads. (A) Pita: folding the multilayered dough ball (Aa); rolling the multilayered dough into a round patty (Ab), baked pita bread (Ac), and characteristic internal pocket of pita bread (Ad); (B) *lavash*: cutting *lavash* dough (Ba), laminated *lavash* dough prior to baking (Bb), and *lavash* flat bread (Bc); (C) *yufka* lamination of *yufka* dough (Ca), baking of *yufka* sheeted dough on hot griddle (Cb); (D) pide: marking borders of the laminated dough circle (Da), finger marking of parallel horizontal rows on egg-washed dough (Db), and baked *pide* (Dc).

yellow corn meal on top of the rounded pieces of dough and ferment in the proof cabinet for 30–40 additional minutes (final proofing).

7. Place the baking sheets with the fermented dough pieces in an oven set at 250°C–280°C for 4–5 minutes of baking.

8. After baking, allow the pieces of bread to cool down at ambient temperature.

9. Upon cooling, weigh the pieces of bread and evaluate the percentage of pieces that developed an internal pocket, crust color, crumb texture, and organoleptic properties. Calculate the bread yield based on the original formulation.

9.2.3.2 Production of *Lavash*

Lavash is another popular flat cracker bread with ancient roots in Armenia. *Lavash* is a thin, soft flatbread that is served with dips and used for wraps. It is usually made with wheat flour made in a variety of shapes all over the regions of the Caucasus, Iran (where it is often so thin as to be like tissue and can be almost seen through), and Afghanistan. *Lavash* is classified as a single-layered, usually served with kebabs, and is used to scoop up food or wrap sandwiches and roll-ups (for shish kebab). *Lavash* can dry quickly and become hard and brittle. The soft form is usually preferable, due to a better taste and ease of making wrap sandwiches. The mixed dough is bulk fermented for 30–60 minutes at approximately 30°C. The dough is divided (100–300 g), rounded, allowed to ferment for approximately 15 minutes at 30°C, laminated (length 40–60 cm, width 20–40 cm, and thickness 2–3 mm) and baked in hot walls of a special *tandoor* oven and kept at oven walls for 15–40 seconds. In the *tandoor* or Middle East clay oven, the flat breads are slapped onto the vertical wall, where they bake quite quickly by a combination of radiant and convection heat (Quail 1996).

A. *Samples, Ingredients, and Reagents*
- Refer to Table 9.3

B. *Materials and Equipments*
- Digital scale
- Graduated cylinder (100 mL or 200 mL)
- Dough mixer
- Dough cutter and rounder
- Fermentation cabinet
- Plastic or stainless steel containers for proofing
- Baking sheets
- Punching or degassing roll unit
- Baking oven
- Fork
- Roller pin
- Thermometer
- Chronometer
- Heat-resistant gloves

C. *Procedure*
1. Weigh hard wheat flour (14% mb) and dry ingredients (Table 9.3).
2. Place the flour and ingredients in the dough mixer. Add the predetermined amount of warm water and start the mixer until the dough is properly developed (Figure 9.3). After mixing, register the mix time, dough consistency and temperature, and pH.

3. Once dough is kneaded, place ball of dough in oiled bowl. Roll the dough around the bowl to coat it with oil. Then shape the dough into a log and cut dough pieces of approximately 22 g to 25 g.

4. Place dough pieces in a fermentation box and allow for 60 minutes of proofing at 28°C and 85% relative humidity. After the first fermentation, lightly dust the dough balls and punch them through the degassing roll unit set at 0.48 cm or 3/16 inch.

5. Return dough pieces to proof box for 30 minutes of fermentation.

6. Roll dough pieces to thin rectangles about 20 cm × 15 cm. The sheeted dough should be paper thin. Weigh pieces of dough before transferring to greased baking sheets.

7. Puncture small holes onto the dough rectangle with a fork. Brush dough with water and sprinkle sesame seeds.

8. Place the baking sheets with the dough pieces in an oven set at 225°C for 3 minutes of baking. The crackers should be lightly browned on the top with small bubbles.

9. After baking, allow the pieces of cracked bread to cool down at ambient temperature.

10. Upon cooling, weigh the pieces of lavash and evaluate crust color, texture, and organoleptic properties. Calculate the bread yield based on the original formulation.

9.2.3.3 Production of *Yufka*

Yufka is a cream-colored and flexible Turkish flat bread. It is a thin, round, and unleavened bread about 40–50 cm in diameter similar to lavash. The flour is kneaded with water, salt, little vinegar or lemon juice, and small amounts of olive oil. Dough is divided (150–200 g), rounded and fermented for approximately 30 minutes. It is flattened into a circular sheet in homes by a rolling pin or rolled by a *yufka*-sheeting device in commercial operations. Then, dough pieces are laminated and baked for a short period of time (30 seconds to 2 minutes) depending on the temperature on a round hot griddle called a *sac* in Turkish. During baking, it is turned over once (Quail 1996). After baking, *yufka* bread has low moisture content and, depending on how low the moisture is, a long shelf life. Before consumption, dry *yufka* bread is sprayed with warm water. The moistened bread is covered with a cotton cloth and is rested for 10 to 12 minutes before consumption.

A critical step of the manufacturing it is the formation of the thin round piece of dough. It is gradually sheeted with an 80-cm long rolling pin as thin as a finger named *oklava*. Thus, it takes expertise to obtain the desired thinness. After rolling the dough with the *oklava*, the thin dough is wrapped around the *oklava*. The dough is hand-pressed to spread it toward the ends of the *oklava*. Then, the dough is unrolled and the operation repeated from another edge of the dough.

A. *Samples, Ingredients, and Reagents*
- Refer to Table 9.3

B. *Materials and Equipments*
- Digital scale
- Graduated cylinder (100 mL or 200 mL)
- Dough mixer
- Dough cutter and rounder
- Proof box
- Plastic or stainless steel containers for proofing
- Hot griddle (80 cm diameter)
- Rolling pin (80 cm long and 2 cm diameter)
- Surface thermometer
- Chronometer
- Heat-resistant gloves

C. *Procedure*
1. Weigh hard wheat flour (14% mb) and dry ingredients (Table 9.3).
2. Place the flour and ingredients in the dough mixer. Add the predetermined amount of warm water (30°C) and start the mixer until the dough is properly developed (Figure 9.3). After mixing, register the mix time, dough consistency, and dough temperature.
3. Once dough is kneaded, divide the dough into 150-g pieces and place dough balls in a proof box for 30 minutes relaxing at 28°C and 85% relative humidity.
4. Lightly dust the dough balls and punch them through the degassing roll unit set at 0.48 cm or 3/16 inch. Then roll the dough with a 80-cm long rolling pin or *oklava* into the thinnest round configuration (70 cm diameter). During the rolling operation the operator has to unroll the dough from the *oklava* and repeat the operation from another edge of the dough.
5. Bake the thin pieces of dough on a hot griddle or sac at 265–280°C for 15 seconds on each side.
6. Upon cooling, weigh the pieces of *yufka* and evaluate its moisture content, crust color, and texture. Calculate the bread yield based on the original formulation.
7. Before consumption, the dry yufka bread is wet by sprayed warm water and rested for 10 or 12 minutes.

9.2.3.4 Production of *Pide*

Pide is a kind of flat bread with round/oval shape. It is made of leavened dough of low consistency. The dough is sheeted into the typical round form of 20–30 cm diameter and 1.5 cm to 2 cm thick. Flour, salt, water, shortening, sugar, and yeast are mixed and kneaded for about 20 minutes and the resulting dough fermented for 40 minutes at 30°C. The dough is divided, rounded, and left for 30–40 minutes of proofing at 30°C. It is baked at a temperature of 300–320°C for 18 minutes (Quail 1996).

A. *Samples, Ingredients, and Reagents*
- Refer to Table 9.3

B. *Materials and Equipments*
- Digital scale
- Graduated cylinder (100 mL or 200 mL)
- Dough mixer
- Dough cutter and rounder
- Proof box
- Plastic or stainless steel containers for proofing
- Hot griddle (80 cm diameter)
- Rolling pin (80 cm long and 2 cm diameter)
- Surface thermometer
- Chronometer
- Heat-resistant gloves
- Egg yolk separator
- Brush

C. *Procedure*
1. Weigh hard wheat flour (14% mb) and dry ingredients (Table 9.3).
2. Place the flour and ingredients in the dough mixer. Add the predetermined amount of warm water (30°C) and start the mixer until the dough is properly developed (Figure 9.3). After mixing, register the mix time, dough consistency, and dough temperature.
3. Once dough is kneaded, place it in a proof box for 60 minutes of fermentation at 28°C and 85% relative humidity.
4. Divide the dough into 450-g round pieces and return them to the fermentation box for 30 minutes. Prepare the egg wash formulation by mixing 6 parts of beaten egg yolks with 3 parts olive oil.
5. Flatten each dough piece slightly or laminate it through rolls adjusted to 1.5 cm. Wet your hands, press and enlarge the dough outward into a circle. Stretch out the circle, pressing hard, particularly with the sides of your hands. When the dough is stretched to a 25-cm circle, apply onto the surface the egg wash with a brush. Using the sides of your hands, mark a border about 5-cm wide all around the edge. Dip your fingertip in egg wash; holding your hands above the circle, 4 fingertips pointing down, mark 4 horizontal rows of indentations parallel to each other with your fingertips, staying within the border. Rotate the circle halfway (180 degrees) and mark 4 rows of indentations parallel to each other and perpendicular to the previous rows. Let your fingertips go down deep, stopping short of piercing the dough.

6. Lift the *pide*, holding it at both ends, and stretch it into an oval shape of approximately 22 cm by 40 cm.
7. Apply a light egg wash with the brush and sprinkle with sesame (*Sesame indicum*) and nigella (*Nigella sativa*) seeds (2 parts sesame and 1 part nigella). Allow pide to rest for 10 minutes before baking.
8. Bake the *pide* in an oven set at 285°C for 6 to 8 minutes.

9.2.4 Bagels

Historically, bagels originated in southern Germany in the 1600s to honor the successful campaign of the Polish king Cobleskill and his Christian horsemen against the Turkish invasion of Vienna, Austria. Then, bagels followed Jewish immigration in the early 1900s from Europe to Canada and the United States. The world bagel derived from the Yiddish and German word for a round loaf of bread *bugel*. Bagels were first produced by Jewish bakers in Eastern Europe (Cross 2007) and are produced using a simple recipe that includes baking flour, sugar (3%), salt (2%), shortening (3%), and yeast (2.0 compressed or 0.8% dry yeast) (Bath and Hoseney 1994, Cross 2007, Kulp and Ponte 2000). Other formulations contain eggs, malt extract, dry milk, and hazelnuts. The dough is usually formed with only 50% water. Bagels are unique because it is the only baked product that is first cooked for about 2 minutes in simmering water (90°C–95°C) or a hot sugar solution before baking. The characteristic crust and crumb textures are due to this hydrothermal process. Toppings such as caraway, poppy, and sesame seeds, minced garlic, or onion or grated cheese are applied onto the bagel immediately before baking. Traditionally bagels are baked on redwood boards or metal plates at 200°C to 230°C for about 17 to 25 minutes. Jewish bagels do not contain added sugar or shortening. Bagels are gaining popularity because they are viewed as a low-calorie baking item.

9.2.4.1 Production of Bagels

A. *Samples, Ingredients, and Reagents*
- Refer to Table 9.4

TABLE 9.4
Typical Formulations for Production of Bagels

Ingredients (%)	Bagels	Bagels Without Sugar
Refined hard wheat flour	100.0	100.0
Water	50.0	45.0–50.0
Dry yeast	2.0	1.5
Salt	2.0	–
Shortening	3.0	1.0–2.0
Sugar	3.0	–
Nondiastatic malt	–	2.0
Emulsifier (SSL)	–	0.2
Sodium bisulfite	–	<20 ppm

B. *Materials and Equipments*
- Digital scale
- Graduated cylinder (100 mL, 200 mL, or 1 L)
- Dough mixer
- Dough cutter and rounder
- Rolling pin
- Fermentation cabinet
- Plastic or stainless steel containers
- Baking sheets
- Punching or degassing roll unit
- Baking oven
- Bread knife
- Thermometer
- pH meter
- Chronometer
- Heat-resistant gloves

C. *Procedure*
1. Weigh refined wheat flour (14% mb) and dry ingredients (Table 9.4).
2. Place the flour and ingredients in the dough mixer. Add the predetermined amount of water and start the mixer until the dough is properly developed (Figure 9.4). After mixing, register the mix time, dough consistency, and dough pH.
3. Cut and round the resulting dough into 70 g pieces. Then, manually form 20 cm by 2 cm diameter dough cylinders. Wet one end of the dough cylinder in preparation to bonding with the other end to form the typical bagel configuration.
4. Place dough pieces on a baking sheet in a refrigerator (2°C–5°C) for 18 hours. To avoid crusting and drying, lay a polyethylene film on top of the dough pieces. Register the dough pH after fermentation at refrigeration temperature.
5. Take out dough pieces from the refrigerator and allow them to equilibrate for 15 minutes at room temperature.
6. Cook dough pieces for 2 minutes on each side in simmering water (water may contain sugar). Drain excess water for 30 seconds and place cooked bagels on baking sheets in preparation for baking (Figure 9.4).
7. Bake cooked bagels in an oven set at 230°C for 13 minutes.
8. After baking, allow bagels to cool down at ambient temperature (Figure 9.4).
9. Upon cooling, weigh bagels and evaluate crust and crumb color and texture and organoleptic properties. Calculate bagel yield based on the original formulation.

9.2.5 Pretzel Bread

Soft pretzels are produced following conventional baking procedures. The main difference is that shaped (i.e., bow ties) doughs are normally dipped in a sodium bicarbonate solution. This gives the outer layer a shiny brown color.

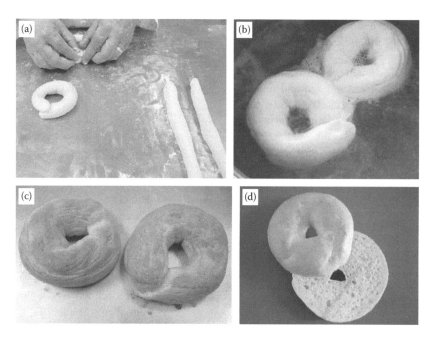

FIGURE 9.4 Production of bagels. (a) Forming dough cylinders into the bagel configuration; (b) cooking bagels in a boiling water bath; (d) baked bagels; and (d) bagel showing crumb texture.

Like other yeast-leavened breads, the best quality soft pretzels are obtained from hard wheat flours (Table 9.5). Most formulations are yeast-raised, although chemical-leavened pretzels also exist in the market. Cysteine or sodium bisulfite is often added to break down gluten and produce a softer or more relaxed dough, especially when pretzels are hand-shaped. Emulsifiers are commonly used to improve dough texture and functionality. Other ingredients including molasses and other sugars are also added to improve color and flavor. Following shaping, the dough is typically

proofed for several hours and then retarded under refrigeration until baked. Before baking, the shaped dough is dipped for about 10 seconds in a 1% sodium bicarbonate solution tempered at 90°C. Then, pretzels are sprinkled with salt and/or other toppings and baked at 240°C–260°C for 5 to 8 minutes. Resulting pretzels have a shelf life of less than 3 days (Hui et al. 2006).

9.2.5.1 Production of Soft Pretzels

A. *Samples, Ingredients, and Reagents*
   - Refer to Table 9.5

B. *Materials and Equipments*
   - Digital scale
   - Graduated cylinder (100 mL, 200 mL, or 1 L)
   - Dough mixer
   - Dough cutter and rounder
   - Rolling pin
   - Fermentation cabinet
   - Plastic or stainless steel containers
   - Baking sheets
   - Punching or degassing roll unit
   - Baking oven
   - Bread knife
   - Thermometer
   - pH meter
   - Chronometer
   - Heat-resistant gloves

C. *Procedure*

Retarded Dough

1. Weigh refined hard wheat flour (14% mb) and dry ingredients (Table 9.5).
2. Place the flour and ingredients in the dough mixer. Add the predetermined amount of water

TABLE 9.5
Recommended Formulation for the Production of Pretzel Bread

Ingredients	Soft Pretzel	
	Formulation A (Salt)	Formulation B (Sesame)
Dough Ingredients		
Hard wheat flour	100.0	–
All-purpose flour	–	100.0
Water	60.0	63.4
Shortening	2.5	–
Sugar	1.0	1.5
Dry yeast	2.4	1.5
Salt	1.5	0.5
SSL	0.2	–
Sodium bisulfite	< 20 ppm	–
Topping		
Coarse or flaked salt	7.5	–
Sesame seed (decorticated)	–	1.6

and start the mixer until the dough is properly developed. After mixing, register the mix time, dough consistency and dough pH.

3. Cut and round the resulting dough into 90 g pieces. Then, manually form 45 by 1 cm diameter dough cylinders. Wet one end of the dough cylinder in preparation to bonding with the other end. Then, manually twist the round circle into the typical pretzel configuration (Figure 9.5).

4. Place dough pieces on a baking sheet in a refrigerator (2°C–5°C) for 18 hours. To avoid crusting and drying, lay a polyethylene film on top of the dough pieces. Register the dough pH after fermentation at refrigeration temperature.

5. Take out dough pieces from the refrigerator and allow them to equilibrate for 30 minutes at room temperature.

6. Dip dough pieces for 10 to 15 seconds in a 10% sodium bicarbonate solution tempered to 90°C–100°C.

7. Then, sprinkle coarse salt or sesame on top of the pretzel form (Figure 9.5).

8. Bake bicarbonate-cooked pretzels at 220°C for 10–13 minutes.

9. After baking, allow pretzels to cool down at ambient temperature (Figure 9.5).

10. Upon cooling, weigh pretzels and evaluate crust and crumb color, texture, and organoleptic properties. Calculate pretzel yield based on the original formulation.

Without Retarding at Refrigeration

1. Weigh refined wheat flour (14% mb) and dry ingredients (Table 9.5).

2. Place the flour and ingredients in the dough mixer. Add the predetermined amount of water and start the mixer until the dough is properly developed. After mixing, register the mix time, dough consistency and dough pH.

3. Cut and round the resulting dough into 90 g pieces. Then, manually twist the round circle into the typical pretzel configuration.

4. Place dough strips on a greased container for 1 hour proofing at 28°C and 85% relative humidity.

5. After fermentation, manually form 45 by 1.25 cm long cylinders. Wet one end of the dough cylinder in preparation to bonding with the other end. Then, manually twist the round circle into the typical pretzel configuration. Return the pieces of dough to the fermentation cabinet for 20 minutes of proofing before cooking.

6. Dip pretzel configurations for 30 seconds in a 10% sodium bicarbonate solution heated to 90°C–100°C. Allow excess alkaline solution to drain and then place pretzel doughs on a greased baking sheet.

7. Alternatively, an egg wash can be applied on top of the pretzel dough. Sprinkle coarse salt or sesame on top of the pretzel form. Alternatively, an egg wash can be applied on top of the pretzel dough.

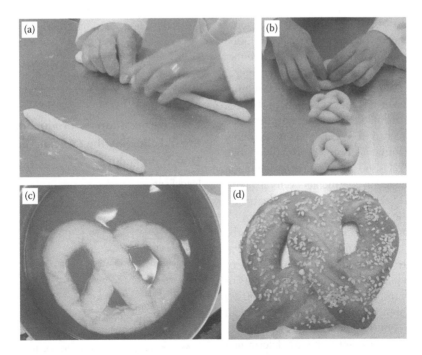

FIGURE 9.5 Production of soft pretzels. (a) Hand-rolling of pretzel dough; (b) shaping into the pretzel configuration; (c) cooking pretzel in the alkaline soda solution; and (d) baked pretzel.

8. Bake bicarbonate-cooked pretzels at 220°C for 10–13 minutes.
9. After baking, allow pretzels to cool down at ambient temperature.
10. Upon cooling, weigh pretzels and evaluate crust, crumb color and texture, and organoleptic properties. Calculate pretzel yield based on the original formulation.

9.2.6 Pan Bread

Pan bread is produced following three main baking procedures: straight dough, sponge, and liquid fermentation. Optimum flour characteristics, labor requirements, and properties of end products differ among processes. Undoubtedly, the most practiced by large bakeries is the sponge dough process that has advantages from the industrial and product quality viewpoints. The straight dough procedure is generally used by small bakeries and simply consists of mixing all ingredients for the production of the dough that is further processed into bread. The main disadvantage of the straight dough process is the high labor requirement and the long "in-plant" fermentation time. The liquid fermentation system is highly mechanized and requires liquid ingredients and less fermentation (the formulation contains more sugar and yeast and it is generally fermented at higher temperatures). It is the system that requires less labor but needs strict quality control in terms of raw materials and manufacturing steps.

The liquid fermentation system is highly mechanized and evolved from the sponge system and is therefore more efficient in terms of labor requirements, processing time, and plant space. The system is based on the elaboration of a liquid sponge commonly named brew (water, yeast, sugar, and other ingredients such as yeast food) that might contain small quantities of flour. The rest of the ingredients are delivered to the mixer in liquid form by pumping. The fermentation time is reduced because the formulations contain higher amounts of sugar and yeast. The brew and the other ingredients are generally mixed in high-speed mixers that require cool water to counteract the heat created by the high friction. The dough undergoing fermentation is cut in extruders into uniform pieces and then placed in baking pans for proofing (up to 90 minutes). The continuous proofers usually operate at higher temperatures (32°C–36°C) to reduce fermentation times. Then the dough is baked in continuous ovens at a temperature of 220°C for 20–25 minutes. The loaves of bread are cooled in cooling racks, sliced, and packaged (Kulp 1988).

The straight dough procedure consists of mixing the flour with the rest of the dry ingredients and water to form properly developed dough. The resulting dough is hand or mechanically divided and placed in fermentation cabinets or proof boxes with strict controls of temperature (25°C–30°C) and relative humidity (approximately 85%). The dough is fermented for about 2 hours, punched, formed, paned, and proofed for 50–70 minutes until the predetermined and desired proof height is achieved. The dough is baked into a loaf of bread for 20–25 minutes at temperatures of 210–230°C. The loaf of bread is cooled for about 30 minutes, sliced, and bagged preferably in moisture-proof plastic bags.

9.2.6.1 Production of Pup Loaves with the Official Microbaking Straight Dough Procedure

The method is devised for evaluating bread wheat quality and a variety of dough ingredients by a straight dough procedure in which all ingredients are incorporated in the initial mixing step (Finney 1984; AACC 2000). In the test, mixing time and water absorption are optimized and balanced. Flour and additives play a critical role in bread functionality. The microbaking test described herein is ideally suited to study flour functionality, optimum water absorption, and ingredient functionality (Finney 1984). Table 9.7 suggests possible changes in the original formulation to study flour quality and ingredient functionality.

A. Samples, Ingredients, and Reagents
- Refer to Tables 9.6 and 9.7

B. Materials and Equipments
- Digital scale
- Graduated cylinder (100 mL or 200 mL)
- Dough micromixer
- Fermentation cabinet
- Plastic or stainless steel containers
- Baking pans
- Punching or degassing roll unit
- Baking oven
- Rapeseed displacement volume meter
- Proof height ruler
- Bread knife
- Thermometer
- pH meter
- Chronometer
- Heat-resistant gloves

TABLE 9.6

Basic Formulation for Production of Pup Loaves of Bread Following the Official Microbaking Straight-Dough Procedure

Ingredients	%
Wheat flour	100.0
Water[a]	60.0–64.0
Sugar	6.0
Shortening	3.0
Compressed fresh yeast[b]	6.0
Salt	2.0
Diastatic malt[c]	0.3

[a] Water absorption should be adjusted according to type of flour.

[b] Dry yeast can be used at a suggested level of 2%.

[c] Amount varies according to the starch damage or falling number value of the flour.

TABLE 9.7

Suggested Treatments to Study the Effects of Ingredients and Additives on the Properties of Pup Loaves Following the Straight-Dough Procedure

Treatment	Composition	Objective
1	Hard wheat flour (62%–64% water absorption) plus ingredients listed in Table 9.6	Control dough and bread used for comparison purposes
2	Treatment 1 + 2% more water absorption	Study the effect of more water on dough and bread properties
3	Treatment 1 + 2% less water absorption	Study the effect of adding less water on dough and bread properties
4	Hard wheat flour (92%) + 8% wheat bran	Study the effect of adding wheat bran on dough and bread properties
5	Hard wheat flour (62%–64% water absorption) (92%) + 8% oat flour	Produce composite breads and to study the effect of adding oat flour in terms of bread volume, density, color, and flavor
6	Hard wheat flour (62%–64% water absorption) (92%) + 8% defatted soybean flour (US mesh – 100)	Produce high-quality protein breads and to study the effect of a nongluten flour in terms of bread volume, density, color, and flavor (Finney et al. 1963)
7	Treatment 6 + 0.5% SSL	Study the effect of SSL addition on the properties of a soybean supplemented bread
8	Soft wheat flour (58% water absorption)	Study the effect of a soft wheat flour on bread properties
9	Treatment 8 + 20 ppm $KBrO_3$ + 100 ppm ascorbic acid	Study the effect of adding oxidizing agents on properties of bread
10	Treatment 9 + 2% vital gluten (add 3% more water compared to treatment 8)	Study the effect of adding vital gluten on properties of bread
11	Treatment 1 + 50 ppm sodium bisulfite	Study the detrimental effect of adding reducing agents on properties of bread
12	Treatment 1 with half the recommended amount of yeast	Study the functionality of yeast on properties of dough and bread
13	Treatment 1 without sugar	Study the functionality of yeast on properties of dough and bread
14	Treatment 1 + 2% nonfat dried milk	Study the effect of adding milk solids on properties of dough and bread (color and flavor)
15	Treatment 1 + 0.2% calcium propionate	Study the functionality of calcium propionate on dough and bread microbial shelf life
16	Treatment 1 + 0.2% potassium sorbate	Study the functionality of potassium sorbate on dough and bread properties and microbial shelf life

C. *Procedure to Study Flour Quality and Ingredient Functionality (AACC 2000, Method 10-10B)*

1. Weigh 200 g wheat flour (14% mb) and the ingredients needed for this amount of flour listed in Tables 9.6 and 9.7.
2. Place the flour and ingredients in the micro dough mixer. Add the predetermined amount of water tempered to 28.8°C and start the mixer until the dough is properly developed (Figure 9.6). The properly developed dough should be cohesive, smooth, and form a thin layer when stretched by hand. An overmixed dough usually develops stickiness. It is recommended to run a series of preliminary tests to determine optimum water absorption and mix times.
3. After mixing, register the mix time, dough consistency and temperature, and pH. Then, divide the dough into two equal parts and place the dough balls first in a greased proofing container and then in a proofing cabinet set at 28.8°C and 85% RH for 52 to 105 minutes of resting. All doughs should be proofed for a fixed time.
4. Dust the dough with small amounts of flour in preparation for sheeting. Sheet or laminate the piece of dough through 0.48-cm or 3/16-in. roll spacing. The resulting dough sheet should be folded in half and in half again and returned to the fermentation cabinet. Register the subjective dough consistency and pH.
5. After 25 minutes of proofing, dust the dough in preparation for punching through a set of degassing rolls adjusted at a gap of 0.48 cm or 3/16 in. The resulting dough sheet should be folded in half and in half again and returned to the fermentation cabinet (Figure 9.6).
6. After 13 minutes additional proofing, dust and sheet the dough through a set of rolls adjusted to a gap of 0.79 cm or 5/16 in. Manually roll the resulting dough sheet into a cylinder making sure to seal bottom and side borders. Register the subjective dough consistency and pH.
7. Place the molded dough pieces on baking pans previously greased on the bottom and three of its sides. The fourth side should be only greased approximately 1/3 from the bottom to enhance bread breaking (Figure 9.6).
8. Place the panned doughs for 37 minutes of proofing at 28.8°C and 85% relative humidity.
9. Before baking measure proof height using the proof height meter (Figure 9.6). Then,

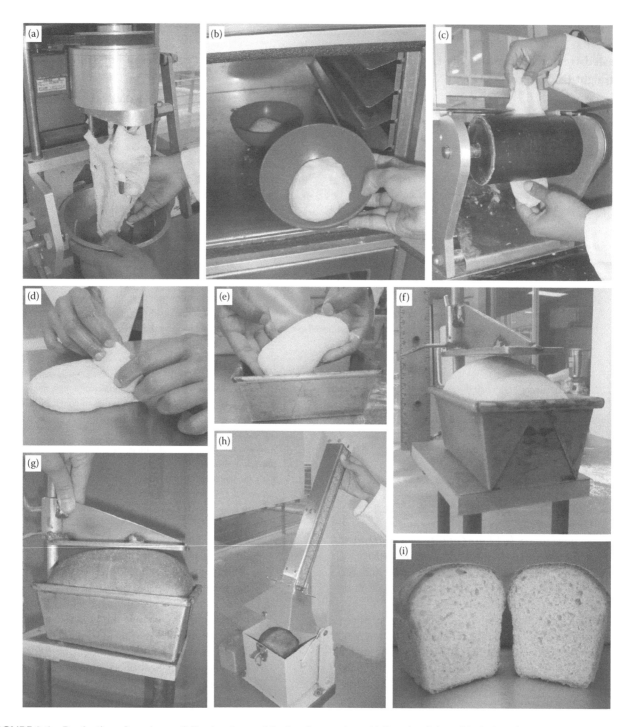

FIGURE 9.6 Production of pup loaves following the straight dough procedure. (a) Dough mixing; (b) placing dough in fermentation cabinet; (c) punching of fermented dough; (d) dough forming; (e) placing dough cylinder into baking pan; (f) measurement of proof height; (g) measurement of bread height; (h) measurement of bread volume by rapeseed displacement; and (i) evaluation of crumb texture.

bake panned doughs for 20 minutes at 220°C. While bread is still in the baking pan measure its height for calculation of oven spring (bread height–proof dough height). Then, depan loaves of bread for weight and volume measurements. Calculate bread yield based on the original formulation and determine bread volume using a previously calibrated rapeseed displacement volume meter. Calculate apparent

bread density by applying the following equation: bread weight/bread volume. Make sure to handle hot baking pans and breads with heat-resistant gloves.

10. Allow loaves of bread to cool down at ambient temperature for 30 minutes.

11. Upon cooling, evaluate the properties of resulting loaves of bread in terms of pH, crust color and color, and texture. For crumb grain texture

evaluation, carefully cut loaves in half and score texture from 1 to 7 using the following benchmark values: 1 = poor; 3 = regular; 5 = good; 7 = excellent.

9.2.6.2 Production of Pan Bread from Sponge Doughs

Most commercial pan breads are produced by the sponge procedures because this system presents advantages from the processing and quality viewpoints. The manufacturing procedure is considered semicontinuous because the sponge and dough mixing steps are batch, whereas the rest of the process is continuous. It is named sponge because part of the flour (60%–70%) is mixed with all the yeast and almost all the water required by 100 units flour (Table 9.8). The sponge is placed in troughs in large fermentation rooms and allowed to ferment for 4 to 6 hours at 28°C and 85% relative humidity. During the sponge phase, the yeast will first activate and then ferment the dough gradually decreasing the pH. The dough volume will increase due to the trapped carbon dioxide generated during fermentation. The in-plant processing starts when the sponge dough is placed in the mixer and the rest of the ingredients incorporated (salt, sugar/sweeteners, shortening, malt, additives, and preservatives). The dough is carefully kneaded until the gluten fully develops. The mix time requirement is reduced because the sponge dough is already hydrated and undergoing fermentation. The in-plant fermentation time is greatly reduced to approximately 30–40 minutes because the yeast is already active. The pieces of dough are punched, formed into cylinders, and proofed for 50–70 minutes before baking. The advantages of this process is that the in-plant processing time is reduced, lowering labor

requirements and that the bread has a stronger flavor and better crumb texture compared with the other baking procedures. Sponge doughs are used for the production of white pan bread, high fiber breads, and composite breads.

A. *Samples, Ingredients, and Reagents*
   - Refer to Table 9.8

B. *Materials and Equipments*
   - Digital scale
   - Graduated cylinder (100 mL or 200 mL)
   - Microdough mixer
   - Fermentation cabinet
   - Plastic or stainless steel containers
   - Baking pans
   - Punching or degassing roll unit
   - Baking oven
   - Rapeseed displacement volume meter
   - Proof height ruler
   - Bread knife
   - Thermometer
   - pH meter
   - Chronometer
   - Heat-resistant gloves

C. *Procedure*
   1. Weigh the ingredients listed on the sponge dough column listed in Table 9.8 (14% mb). Consider that 750 g or 600 g of dough are needed to produce large or medium loaves, respectively.
   2. Place the flour and sponge ingredients in the dough mixer. Add the suggested amount of water tempered to 28.8°C and mix ingredients for about only 1–2 minutes.

TABLE 9.8
Recommended Formulations for Production of Various Types of Pan Breads with Sponge Doughs

Ingredients	White Pan Bread		Pan Bread with Bran		Whole Wheat	
	Sponge	Dough	Sponge	Dough	Sponge	Dough
Refined hard wheat flour	65.0	35.0	65.0	23.0	–	–
Whole wheat flour	–	–	–	–	65.0	35.0
Wheat bran	–	–	–	12.0	–	–
Oat meal	–	–	–	–	–	–
Water	40.0	24.0	39.0	24.0	40.0	25.0
Sugar	–	6.0	–	6.0	–	6.0
Shortening	–	3.5	–	3.5	–	4.0
Nonfat dry milk	–	2.0	–	2.0	–	2.0
Salt	–	2.0	–	2.0	–	2.0
Dry yeast	1.5	–	1.5	–	1.5	–
Diastatic malt	–	0.2	–	0.2	–	0.2
Yeast food	0.5	–	0.5	–	0.5	–
Lecithin/SSL	–	0.5	–	0.5	–	0.5
Calcium propionate	–	0.2	–	0.2	–	0.2
Vital gluten	–	–	–	1.5	–	2.0

[a]   Water absorption should be adjusted according to type of flour.

[b]   Fresh compressed yeast can be used at a suggested level of 5%.

3. Place the resulting sponge dough in a greased container and then in a proofing cabinet set at 28.8°C and 85% RH for 4–6 hours. Register the initial pH and the evolution of pH throughout fermentation.

4. Place the fermented sponge in the mixing bowl and then add the dough stage ingredients listed in Table 9.8. Turn on the mixer until the dough is fully developed. The properly developed dough should be cohesive, smooth, and form a thin layer when stretched by hand. Register the mix time, dough consistency and temperature, and pH. Then, divide the dough into the desired weight. Baking pans for 750-, 600-, or 300-g dough pieces are commonly processed into large, medium, or small loaves of bread. If twisted loaves of bread are desired then subdivide the dough piece into two identical portions. Place the individual pieces of dough inside previously greased containers for proofing at 28.8°C and 85% RH for 30 minutes (Figure 9.7).

5. Dust dough pieces with small amounts of flour in preparation for sheeting through 0.48-cm or 3/16-in. roll spacing. The resulting dough sheet should be folded in half and in half again and returned to the fermentation cabinet for 15

minutes of proofing. Register the subjective dough consistency and pH.

6. After 15 minutes of proofing, dust dough pieces with small amounts of flour in preparation for sheeting and forming. Sheet or laminate the piece of dough through 0.79-cm or 5/16-in. roll spacing. Register the subjective dough consistency and pH. Manually roll the resulting dough sheet into a cylinder making sure to seal bottom and side borders.

7. Place the molded cylindrical dough pieces on baking pans previously greased on the bottom and all internal sides. For regular pan bread, place the cylindrical dough piece inside the baking pan. For twisted formed breads, place side by side the two cylindrical pieces of doughs and twist the two cylinders (Figure 9.7). Then place the twisted dough pieces making sure to place the two terminal parts of each of the dough ends on each corner of the baking pan.

8. Place the panned doughs for 65–70 minutes of proofing at 28.8°C and 85% relative humidity.

9. Before baking measure proof height using the proof height meter (Figure 9.7). Then, bake panned doughs for 25 minutes at 220°C. While bread is still in the baking pan measure its height

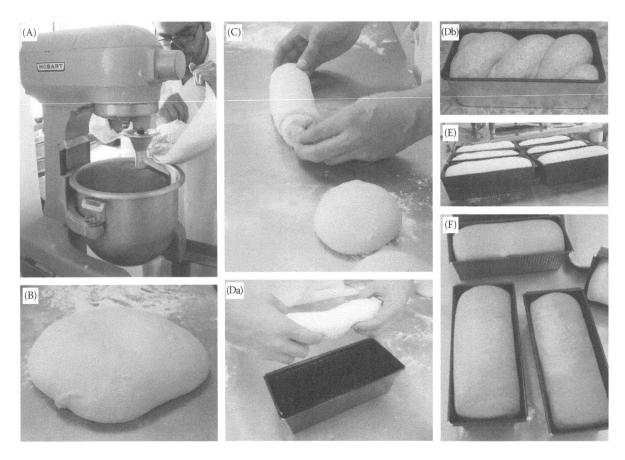

FIGURE 9.7 Production of sponge breads. (A) Mixing of fermented sponge with rest of the ingredients; (B) optimum mixed dough before cutting and scaling; (C) dough forming; (D) dough panning: cylinder (Da) and twisted dough (Db); (E) proofed doughs; and (F) bread.

for calculation of oven spring (bread height − proof dough height). Then, depan breads for weight and volume measurements. Calculate bread yield based on the original formulation and determine bread volume using a previously calibrated rapeseed displacement volume meter. Calculate apparent bread density by applying the following equation: bread weight/bread volume. Make sure to handle hot baking pans and breads with heat-resistant gloves.

10. Allow loaves of bread to cool down at ambient temperature for 30 minutes.

11. Upon cooling, evaluate the properties of resulting breads in terms of pH, crust color, and color and texture. For crumb grain texture evaluation, carefully cut loaves in half and score texture from 1 to 7 using the following benchmark values: 1 = poor; 3 = regular; 5 = good, and 7 = excellent.

9.2.7 WHOLE, VARIETY, AND MULTIGRAIN BREADS

Although breads produced from refined flours are still the most sold all over the world, variety breads are the segment that has shown the most rapid growth. Variety, whole, and multigrain breads offer consumers choices of flavors, textures, and more importantly dietary fiber and nutraceutical compounds that are present in insignificant quantities in white breads (Kulp and Ponte 2000). Whole, variety, and multigrain breads have positive health implications because they are comparatively lower in energy density and provide important amounts of known nutraceutical compounds. These healthy breads prevent constipation, hemorrhoids, and colon cancer and provide important phytochemicals that prevent oxidative stress responsible for higher incidence of cardiovascular diseases, hypercholesterolemia, diabetes, and fibrosis. However, from the processing viewpoint the addition of nonwheat flours and fiber have detrimental effects on bread quality and processing. Thus, these breads are usually supplemented with additives to counteract the negative effects in functionality and product quality. Most formulations are supplemented with vital gluten to compensate the use of fiber sources or nongluten flours. Most of these breads are also supplemented with honey and fructose syrups to improve flavor. The leading established variety breads are still wheat-based breads. The group includes whole wheat, stone-ground wheat, honey wheat, and cracked wheat. Other less popular variety breads include rye, pumpernickel (dark rye flour), oatmeal, fruit (raisin), and multigrain. The multigrain or mixed grain breads are gaining popularity because different cracked grains with different nutritional and nutraceutical properties are added to the wheat flour base. It is common to find in the market multigrain breads manufactured with six or more grains (wheat, oats, flax, sesame, rye, buckwheat, etc.). Production of these breads is generally more difficult because the fiber associated to the whole flours interferes with gluten development yielding denser loaves. Vital gluten is the key ingredient that

counteracts the deleterious effect of brans. Most commercial formulations of whole, variety, and multigrain breads contain from 1% to 3% vital gluten. Large-scale bakers usually produce variety breads by the sponge-dough process because it generally yields breads with consistently greater volume and quality. Doughs of these bread formulations are usually hydrated with less water necessary to restrict dough flow and maintain desired product symmetry. In addition, the lower water absorption avoids dough stickiness. Variety bread dough usually requires less mixing or kneading compared to white bread dough and is more prone to overmixing. In addition, these doughs are often fermented for shorter times to promote better flavor. The denser proofed doughs are generally baked for longer periods of time but at lower temperatures to ensure good loaf characteristics and maximum flavor development. After baking, the denser variety breads require longer cooling. Variety breads are playing an important role in diet and disease prevention especially due to their high dietary fiber content. The dietary fiber reduces the caloric density and aids in the prevention of obesity, colonic diseases, diabetes, cardiovascular diseases, and metabolic syndrome. Variety breads with low sodium content, high amounts of polyunsaturated omega-3 fatty acids, and lactose-free are available in the market.

9.2.7.1 Production of Whole, Variety, and Multigrain Breads

A. Samples, Ingredients, and Reagents
- Refer to Table 9.9

B. Materials and Equipments
- Digital scale
- Graduated cylinder (100 mL, 200 mL, or 1 L)
- Dough mixer with attachments
- Fermentation cabinet
- Plastic or stainless steel containers
- Baking pans
- Punching or degassing roll unit
- Baking oven
- Rapeseed displacement volume meter
- Proof height ruler
- Bread knife
- Thermometer
- pH meter
- Chronometer
- Heat-resistant gloves

C. Procedure
1. Weigh wheat and other flours and the ingredients listed in Table 9.9.
2. Place the flour and ingredients in the dough mixer. Add the predetermined amount of water tempered to 28.8°C and start the mixer until the dough is properly developed.
3. After mixing, register the mix time, dough consistency and temperature, and pH. Then, divide the dough into the desired weight pieces. Baking pans for 750, 600, or 300 g dough pieces are commonly processed into large, medium,

TABLE 9.9

Typical Formulations for the Elaboration of Whole-Wheat, Variety Pan, and Sourdough Breads Using the Straight Dough Procedure[a]

Ingredients	Whole Wheat		Variety Breads		
	Wheat (%)	Whole Wheat (%)	Oats (%)	Raisin Oatmeal (%)	Rye (%)
Refined hard wheat flour	50.0	–	60.0	50.0	60.0
Whole wheat flour	50.0	100.0	–	37.0	–
Rye flour	–	–	–	–	40.0
Oat flour	–	–	40.0	13.0	–
Water[a]	60.0–64.0	65.0–68.0	63.0–66.0	62.0–64.0	62.0–66.0
Dry yeast	1.5	1.5	2.0	1.0	2.0
Salt	2.0	2.0	2.0	2.0	2.0
Shortening	4.0	4.0	3.5	3.0	2.0
Sugar, white, or brown	6.0	6.0	7.0	6.0	5.0
Maize syrup or honey	2.2	2.2	–	–	–
Molasses	10.0	–	–	–	–
Malt-diastatic	0.2	0.1	–	–	–
Malt-nondiastatic	–	–	–	–	2.0
Vital gluten	2.0	2.0	2.0	2.5	1.5
Yeast food	0.5	0.5	0.5	0.5	0.5
Nonfat dry milk	–	2.0	–	2.0	–
Raisins	–	–	–	50.0	–
Emulsifier (SSL)	0.2	0.1	0.1	0.2	0.2
Lecithin	–	0.2	0.2	0.2	–
Calcium propionate	0.2	0.2	0.2	0.2	0.2

Source: Serna-Saldivar, S. R. O., *Manufactura y Control de Calidad de Productos Basados en Cereales*, AGT Editor, México, Mexico, 2003; Kulp, K., and Lorenz, K. J., *Handbook of Dough Fermentation*, Marcel Dekker, New York, 2003; Kulp, K., and Ponte, J. G., *CRC Crit. Rev. Food Sci. Nutr.*, 15, 1–48, 1981.

[a] Water absorption varies according to flour strength, type of flour, and fiber and vital gluten additions.

or small loaves of bread. Place the individual pieces of dough inside previously greased containers for proofing at 28.8°C and 85% RH for 90 minutes.

4. Dust the dough with small amounts of flour in preparation for sheeting. Sheet or laminate the piece of dough through 0.79-cm or 5/16-in. roll spacing. The resulting dough sheet should be folded in half and in half again and returned to the fermentation cabinet. Register the subjective dough consistency and pH.

5. After 20 minutes of proofing, dust the dough in preparation for punching and forming. Laminate the dough piece through a set of degassing rolls adjusted at a gap of 0.79 cm or 5/16 in. and then manually roll the resulting dough sheet into a cylinder making sure to seal bottom and side borders. Register the subjective dough consistency and pH.

6. Place the molded dough pieces on baking pans previously greased on the bottom and all internal sides.

7. Place the panned doughs for 60–80 minutes of proofing at 28.8°C and 85% relative humidity.

8. Before baking, measure proof height using the proof height meter. Then, bake for 25 minutes at 200°C–210°C. Wear heat-resistant gloves to remove breads from the oven. While bread is still in the baking pan, measure its height for calculation of oven spring (bread height – proof dough height). Then depan breads for weight and volume measurements. Calculate bread yield based on the original formulation and determine bread volume using a previously calibrated rapeseed displacement volume meter. Calculate apparent bread density by applying the following equation: bread weight/bread volume. Make sure to handle hot baking pans and breads with heat-resistant gloves.

9. Allow breads to cool down at ambient temperature for 30 minutes.

10. Upon cooling, evaluate the properties of resulting breads in terms of pH, crust color, and color and texture.

9.2.8 Sour Breads

The term "sourdough bread" refers to a product made with wheat and/or rye flours or other composite flours, other baking ingredients that are primarily fermented with bacteria that produce a more acidic pH compared to regular yeast breads. Cereal proteases with acidic optima pH play a central role in the rheological changes taking place during sourdough fermentation (Clarke et al. 2004; Esteve et al. 1994). Sourdoughs are inoculated with active *Lactobacillus plantarum*, *L. San francisco*, *L. fermentum*, *L. brevis*, *Leuconostoc mesenteroides*, and/or *Streptococcus thermophilus* bacteria and have been traditionally used for the production of variety breads, especially rye products (Kulp and Ponte 2000). Sours breads started by natural fermentation of doughs in which bacteria from the genus *Lactobacillus* mainly grew. Compared to regular yeast doughs, sourdoughs are easier to handle and produce breads with unique organoleptic properties and crumb texture. These breads have higher nutritional value, longer shelf life, and properties not seen in other breads.

The organic acids generated by the fermenting bacteria such as acetic, lactic, hydroxiacetic, formic, pyruvic, and others are the main flavor precursors. Acetic acid is considered the main acid. It improves dough characteristics, speeds up fermentation, and affects final bread properties. It is generated mainly from maltose and other simpler carbohydrates. Other fermenting compounds, such as free amino acids, also contribute to the typical flavor profile. These amino acids and their derivatives are generated due to proteolysis, sugar and peptide metabolism, and hydrogenation or enzymatic conversion of ketoacids. These can also come from the fermenting bacteria cells. Many other yeast species also can form part of the sourdough inoculums contributing to volatile and nonvolatile chemical species that also contribute to special characteristics of sourdough breads.

The microorganisms that ferment sourdoughs act as leavening agents, improving bread volume. An excessive inoculum concentration results in a high dough acidification and a deleterious effect on bread volume. Sourdoughs have different rheological properties and plasticity compared to regular doughs due to the low pH (5.2–5.4). As a result, sourdoughs usually have better oven-spring and yield breads with higher volumes and lower apparent densities.

Historically, the pumpernickel rye bread was produced in Germany around 1540 during a time of famine. This type of bread has a very characteristic and distinct flavor. The authentic pumpernickel bread is produced by soaking whole rye flour in hot (70°C–100°C) water with a 1:3 ratio. This soaking produces thorough hydration of the rye flour, partial starch gelatinization, and some enzyme hydrolysis that produces fermentable sugars that influence the flavor of the final product. Pumpernickel bread formulations generally consist of less than 10% of the rye flour and breads are baked in fully closed pans in special ovens where steam is introduced. The baking time is up to 24 hours depending on the baking temperature, which normally ranges from 100°C to 170°C. The characteristic taste is due to the enzymatic starch hydrolysis during sour ripening, dough preparation, proofing, and the special baking process (Kulp and Lorenz 2003).

9.2.8.1 Production of Sour Breads
A. *Samples, Ingredients, and Reagents*
- Refer to Table 9.10
B. *Materials and Equipments*
- Digital scale
- Graduated cylinder (100 mL, 200 mL, or 1 L)

TABLE 9.10

Typical Formulations for the Elaboration of Sourdough and Pumpernickel Breads Using Sponge Dough Procedures[a]

Ingredients (%)	Sourdough Bread		Pumpernickel Bread	
	Sponge	Dough	Sponge	Dough
Hard wheat flour	60.0	40.0	24.0	–
Dark rye flour	–	–	38.0	–
Medium rye flour	–	–	–	38.0
Water[a]	36.0	24.0	40.0	30.0
Dry yeast	1.5	–	1.0	–
Salt	–	2.0	–	2.5
Shortening	–	3.0	–	1.0
Sugar	–	6.0	–	–
Malt, diastatic	–	0.5	–	–
Malt, nondiastatic	–	–	–	1.0
Sourdough (initiator)[a]	10.0	10.0	10.0	–

[a] Initiator or starter dough from previous batches rich in *Lactobacillus bulgaricus*, *L. plantarum*, *L. San francisco*, *L. fermentum*, *L. brevis*, *Leuconostoc mesenteroides*, and/or *Streptococcus thermophilus*. New starter dough is produced by mixing ingredients with pure culture inoculum of pure lactic acid forming bacteria.

- Dough mixer
- Fermentation cabinet
- Plastic or stainless steel containers
- Baking pans
- Punching or degassing roll unit
- Baking oven
- Rapeseed displacement volume meter
- Proof height ruler
- Bread knife
- Thermometer
- pH meter
- Chronometer
- Heat-resistant gloves

C. *Procedure*

1. Weigh sponge dough flours, starter dough, and other ingredients listed in Table 9.10. If the starter sourdough is not available, add the pure starter culture to the sponge. Mix sponge ingredients and allow the resulting sponge to ferment at 35°C/85% HR for 24 hours or until the dough pH decreases to 4.3.

2. Place the fermented sponge in the mixing bowl and then add the dough stage ingredients listed in Table 9.10. Turn on the mixer until the dough is fully developed. Register the mix time, dough consistency and temperature, and pH.

3. Divide the dough into the desired weight. Baking pans for 750, 600, or 300 g dough pieces are commonly processed into large, medium, or small loaves of bread. Place the individual pieces of dough inside previously greased containers for proofing at 30°C–32°C and 85% RH for 30 minutes.

4. Dust the dough with small amounts of flour in preparation for sheeting. Sheet or laminate the piece of dough through 5/16 in. roll spacing. The resulting dough sheet should be folded in half and in half again and returned to the fermentation cabinet. Register the subjective dough consistency and pH.

5. After 20 minutes of additional proofing, dust the dough in preparation for punching and forming. Laminate the dough piece through a set of degassing rolls adjusted at a gap of 5/16 in. and then manually roll the resulting dough sheet into a cylinder making sure to seal bottom and side borders. Register the subjective dough consistency and pH.

6. Place the molded dough pieces on baking pans previously greased on the bottom and all internal sides.

7. Place the panned doughs for 60–80 minutes of proofing at 30°C–32°C and 85% relative humidity.

8. Before baking measure proof height using the proof height meter. Then, bake for 25 minutes at 200°C. Wear heat-resistant gloves to remove baking pans with the breads from the oven. While bread is still in the baking pan measure its height for calculation of oven spring (bread height – proof dough height). Then, depan breads for weight and volume measurements. Calculate bread yield based on the original formulation and determine bread volume using a previously calibrated rapeseed displacement volume meter. Calculate apparent bread density by applying the following equation: bread weight/bread volume. Make sure to handle hot baking pans and breads with heat-resistant gloves.

9. Allow sour breads to cool down at ambient temperature for 30 minutes.

10. Upon cooling and slicing with a bread knife, evaluate the properties of resulting breads in terms of pH, crust color, sensory properties, and crumb color and texture.

9.2.9 Hamburger and Hot Dog Buns

Hamburger and hot dog buns are manufactured following similar technologies as pan bread. However, since these breads are expected to have higher textural and microbial shelf life, the formulations contain higher quantities of shortening, emulsifiers, sugar, and other additives (Table 9.11). Most formulations also contain fresh egg or egg solids to obtain products with longer textural shelf life and better organoleptic properties. For the specific case of hot dogs, recipes normally contain egg yolks or yellow pigments (i.e., carotenoids) to yield a yellowish crumb. These buns are industrially produced using the straight or sponge dough methodologies described above. There are highly mechanized dough cutting/forming equipments integrated to continuous proof boxes ideally suited for continuous operations. Compared to pan breads, hamburger and hot dog buns are baked for shorter periods. Decorticated sesame (*Sesame indicum*) seeds are frequently used as toppings and sprinkled on top of the fermenting dough before baking for the production of hamburger buns.

9.2.9.1 Production of Hamburger and Hot Dog Buns

A. *Samples, Ingredients, and Reagents*
- Refer to Table 9.11

B. *Materials and Equipments*
- Digital scale
- Graduated cylinder (100 mL, 200 mL, or 1 L)
- Dough mixer
- Fermentation cabinet
- Plastic or stainless steel containers
- Baking pans for hot dogs or hamburger buns
- Punching or degassing roll unit
- Baking oven
- Rapeseed displacement volume meter
- Bread knife
- Thermometer
- pH meter

TABLE 9.11

Recommended Formulation for Production of Hot Dog or Hamburger Buns Using the Sponge Dough Procedure[a]

Ingredients	Sponge (%)	Dough (%)
Hard wheat flour	70.0	30.0
Water	42.0	18.5
Fresh compressed yeast	5.0	–
Salt	–	2.0
Sugar or high-fructose corn syrup	–	12.0
Nonfat dry milk	–	3.0
Whole eggs[b]	–	7.0
Shortening	–	7.5
Vital gluten	–	1.0
Yeast food	0.5	–
Diastatic malt	–	0.2
Emulsifiers (lecithin, monoglycerides, or diglycerides, DATEM, and/or SSL)	–	0.5
Calcium propionate	–	0.2
Ascorbic acid	–	0.01

[a] For hot dogs, the formulation may contain carotenoids or artificial yellow coloring agents to produce a yellowish crumb coloration.

[b] Whole fresh eggs can be substituted by dry egg solids. The whole fresh egg contains about 76% moisture and 24% solids so the equivalent egg solids with 8% moisture content are 1.8%. If egg solids are used the formulation should also be adjusted in terms of water because 7% of fresh eggs provide approximately 5.3% of water.

- Chronometer
- Heat-resistant gloves

C. Procedure

1. Weigh the ingredients listed on the sponge dough column listed in Table 9.11 (14% mb).
2. Place the flour and sponge ingredients in the dough mixer. Add the suggested amount of water tempered to 28.8°C and mix ingredients for only about 1 to 2 minutes.
3. Place the resulting sponge dough in a greased container and then in a proofing cabinet set at 28.8°C and 85% RH for 4–6 hours. Register the initial pH and the evolution of pH throughout fermentation.
4. Place the fermented sponge in the mixing bowl and then add the dough stage ingredients listed in Table 9.11. Turn on the mixer until the dough is fully developed. The properly developed dough should be cohesive, smooth, and form a thin layer when stretched by hand. Register the mix time, dough consistency and temperature, and pH. Then, divide the dough into the desired weight (50–60 g for hot dog buns and 120–140 g for hamburger buns). Place the individual rounded pieces of dough inside previously greased containers for proofing at 28.8°C and 85% RH for 30 to 40 minutes.
5. After proofing, dust rounded dough pieces with small amounts of flour in preparation for sheeting. Sheet or laminate the piece of dough through 0.48-cm or 3/16-in. roll spacing. Register the subjective dough consistency and pH.
6. After 15–20 minutes additional proofing in the fermentation cabinet, dust dough pieces with small amounts of flour in preparation for forming. For hot dogs, sheet or laminate the piece of dough through 0.79 cm or 5/16 in. roll spacing and manually roll the resulting dough sheet into a 15-cm-long cylinder. For hamburger buns, degass manually with a wood pin the round dough balls into 20–25 cm diameter round patties.
7. Place the molded cylindrical hot dog dough pieces or round shaped hamburger patties in their respective baking sheets that were previously greased.
8. Place the panned hot dog or hamburger doughs for 60 and 80 minutes of proofing at 28.8°C and 85% relative humidity.
9. Before baking measure proof height using the proof height meter. Then, bake hot dog and hamburger doughs for 12 and 15 minutes at 180°C. While bread is still in the baking pan measure its height for calculation of oven spring (bread height – proof dough height). Then depan breads for weight and volume measurements. Calculate bread yield based on the original formulation and determine bread volume using a previously calibrated rapeseed displacement volume meter.

Calculate apparent bread density by applying the following equation: bread weight/bread volume. Make sure to handle hot baking pans and breads with heat-resistant gloves.

10. Allow buns to cool down at ambient temperature for 30 minutes before slicing with a bread knife.

11. Evaluate the properties of hamburger or hot dogs buns in terms of pH, crust color, and color and texture.

9.2.10 CHEESE BREAD ROLLS

Cheese bread rolls combine the fermented bread and cheese flavors. The process to produce cheese bread rolls follows the typical dough production followed by sheeting the dough into a multilayered configuration where cheese is placed as filling. The dough is then rolled into a cylinder that is cut into 1- to 2-in. rolls that after proofing are baked. These rolls have higher caloric density, protein value, and calcium compared to regular bread because of the high fat, protein, and calcium content of cheese.

9.2.10.1 Production of Cheese Bread Rolls

A. *Samples, Ingredients, and Reagents*
- Refer to Table 9.12

B. *Materials and Equipments*
- Digital scale
- Graduated cylinder (100 mL, 200 mL, or 1 L)
- Cheese shredder
- Rolling pins
- Dough mixer
- Fermentation cabinet
- Plastic or stainless steel containers
- Baking pans
- Punching or degassing roll unit

TABLE 9.12
Recommended Formulation for the Elaboration of Cheese Bread Rolls

Ingredients	%
Refined hard wheat flour	100.0
Water[a]	44.0
Yellow cheddar cheese	31.0
Evaporated milk (26% solids)	28.0
Butter or margarine	5.6
Sugar	5.2
Salt	1.7
Dry yeast	1.5
Ascorbic acid	0.01

[a] Adjust water absorption according to the moisture content of the evaporated milk. The total water absorption (water plus water associated to evaporated milk) should be between 62% and 65% according to flour strength and quality.

- Baking oven
- Dough cutter
- Bread knife
- Thermometer
- Chronometer
- Heat-resistant gloves

C. *Procedure*

1. Weigh all ingredients listed in Table 9.12 except the cheddar cheese. The yellow cheddar cheese should be shredded beforehand. Place the flour and ingredients in the dough mixer and add the predetermined amount of water.

2. Mix ingredients until the dough is properly developed. Register optimum mix time and dough consistency.

3. Place the individual pieces of dough inside previously greased containers for proofing at 28°C–30°C and 85% RH for 45 minutes.

4. Dust doughs with small amounts of flour in preparation for sheeting. Sheet or laminate the piece of dough through 0.79-cm or 5/16-in. roll spacing. Then, with a rolling pin, thin the rectangular dough sheet to a dough of approximately 1.5 cm thick. Fold the resulting sheet in half and in half again and return the folded dough piece to the fermentation cabinet.

5. After 20 minutes of proofing, laminate the folded piece of dough first through 0.79-cm or 5/16-in. roll spacing and then with a rolling pin to a 1.5-cm-thick rectangular dough piece.

6. Spread the shredded cheese on the rectangular piece of dough, making sure to avoid about 1 in. from the periphery of the formed dough. Then, carefully roll the rectangular dough piece into a cylinder and manually seal borders. Cut the resulting cylinders into 2.5-cm-thick roll pieces.

7. Place two columns of rolls on baking pans previously greased on the bottom and all internal sides.

8. Return baking pans with cheese rolls into the fermentation cabinet and proof for 30–40 minutes.

9. Bake for 20–25 minutes at 200°C. Then depan bread rolls for calculation of yield based on the original formulation. Make sure to handle hot baking pans and breads with heat-resistant gloves.

10. Allow bread rolls to cool down at ambient temperature for 30 minutes.

11. Upon cooling, evaluate the properties of resulting breads in terms of crust color and organoleptic properties.

9.2.11 RESEARCH SUGGESTIONS

1. Prepare three different types of Chinese steamed breads varying the type of flour (i.e., soft, all-purpose, and hard wheat flour). Compare optimum water

absorptions, mix times, and the properties of the resulting steamed breads (volume, crust texture, crumb grain, and texture, apparent density) and their sensory properties.

2. Prepare soft- and hard-crusted French breads supplemented with 2% vital gluten. Indicate the proposed changes in formulation, water absorption, and baking. Determine the bread volume, crust color, apparent density, and comparative sensory properties.

3. Prepare and compare properties of pita or Arabic flat breads produced from all-purpose and hard wheat flours supplemented with 20 ppm potassium bromate and 100 ppm ascorbic acid. Compare optimum water absorptions, mix times, average bread diameter, and the properties of the resulting flat breads in terms of yield, pocket formation, crust color, and sensory properties.

4. Compare properties of pita or Arabic pocket breads produced only differing in baking temperature (i.e., compare 280°C vs. 200°C). Adjust baking times accordingly. Compare bread yield, the pocket bread formation, crust color, and sensory properties.

5. Prepare and compare properties of bagels produced from retarded or overnight refrigerated dough and a similar dough directly processed into the final product. Compare optimum proofing times and the properties of the bagels in terms of crust color, crumb texture, and sensory properties.

6. Prepare and compare properties of soft Pretzel breads dipped for 15 seconds in hot (90°C) 10% sodium bicarbonate or sodium hydroxide solutions. Compare properties of the resulting pretzels especially in terms of crust color, texture throughout storage, and flavor.

7. Compare yields, crust color and thickness, and textural shelf life of hamburger buns produced with 3% and 10% shortening that are baked in a regular baking oven and an oven that injects steam.

8. Prepare hot dog buns using fresh and dehydrated egg solids. Make sure to adjust water absorption and add the same amount of solids to the two formulations. Determine the effect of adding dehydrated solids on optimum mixing time and water absorption, dough texture and stickiness, crust color, and organoleptic properties of the two different buns.

9. Prepare white pan breads using the sponge-dough procedure. One of the bread formulations will be supplemented with 0.2% calcium propionate, the other with 0.2% potassium sorbate, and another without any antimold agents. Determine sponge pH throughout fermentation time and determine bread weight, volume, apparent density, oven spring, crumb texture, and comparative microbial shelf life.

10. Prepare whole wheat pan breads using the sponge-dough procedure. One of the bread formulations

will be supplemented with 2% vital gluten, 0.2% SSL, and 100 ppm ascorbic acid and the other without these additives will serve as control. Compare water absorptions, optimum dough mixing times and dough stickiness, and determine bread weight, volume, apparent density, crumb texture, and comparative sensory properties.

9.2.12 RESEARCH QUESTIONS

1. Define the following terms:
   a. Oven-spring
   b. Retardation
   c. Bakers formulation
   d. Proofing
   e. Crumb grain
   f. Egg wash

2. What are advantages and disadvantages of using dry or fresh compressed yeasts?

3. In a table compare culinary properties, processing, and relative caloric content of the following breads: French bread, pita, Chinese steamed bread, pan bread, bagel, and soft pretzel.

4. Mention at least two functionalities of the following bread ingredients
   a. Salt
   b. Sugar or sweeteners
   c. Shortening
   d. SSL
   e. Potassium bromate
   f. Calcium propionate
   g. Diastatic malt
   h. Nonfat dried milk

5. Why are most yeast-leavened breads made with a hard wheat flour?

6. What is gluten? What kind of proteins conform the functional wheat gluten? What are the effects of reducing or oxidizing agents on gluten strength and functionality?

7. What factors related to amino acid composition of wheat gluten are in the main responsible for producing viscoelastic gluten?

8. What are the effects of adding vital gluten to whole wheat bread formulations (water absorption, crumb texture, bread volume, overall bread quality, etc.)?

9. What are the different stages of dough mixing? Why is it critically important to determine the optimum dough development or optimum mixing time? What happens when a dough is overmixed?

10. Give at least three reasons why is it necessary to punch yeast-fermenting doughs before proofing and baking.

11. What kinds of doughs have better oven spring? Why?

12. What are the optimum flour characteristics for production of Chinese steamed bread, baguettes, and bagels?

13. What differences in formulation, water absorption, and processing are necessary for the production of a soft- and hard-crusted baguettes?

14. Explain the reason why French breads or baguettes have a limited textural shelf life?

15. What is the purpose of the alkaline water bath treatment of pretzels before baking? How does this alkali treatment differ between soft and hard pretzels?

16. What would happen to the bagel dough if it is not refrigerated before final proofing?

17. Why is it more challenging to produce whole wheat or whole grain breads compared to white counterparts?

18. Why the dough of whole wheat breads, especially those supplemented with oat flour, have more machinability problems (i.e., sticky doughs) compared to white doughs?

19. Explain how a starter is used to produce sour breads? What kinds of chemical compounds are produced by the starter during fermentation?

20. What is necessary form the formulation and processing viewpoints to produce a paper thin sheet of dough required for production of Arabic flat breads such as *lavash* and *yufka*?

21. What is staling? Investigate the effect of temperature on the rate of staling. What kind of ingredients or food additives can be used to lower the rate of bread staling?

22. Convert the following whole wheat formulation to metric system and kitchen units and express the recipe in terms of bakers formulation (based on 100 g flour).

Ingredients	English System	Metric System	Kitchen Units (Cups, Tablespoons, etc.)
Whole wheat flour	3 lb and 3 oz		
Refined hard wheat flour	3 lb and 4 oz		
Water	4 lb		
Sugar	8 oz		
Fresh compressed yeast	6 oz		
Shortening	4 oz		
Salt	2 oz		
Dry milk	4 oz		
Molasses	3 oz		

23. Why are bagels considered as a low calorie or dietetic bread? Investigate its chemical composition, and based on 100 g, calculate its total calories and calories provided by fat (remember that carbohydrates and proteins provide 4 kcal/g whereas fats provide 9 kcal/g).

24. At what temperature and relative humidity doughs are generally fermented? What kinds of chemical compounds are generated during yeast and sourdough fermentations? Give at least three reasons why doughs need to be periodically punched or degassed.

25. List at least five changes that occur during bread baking. Explain the oven-spring phenomena.

26. What are the differences, advantages, and disadvantages among the three major baking systems? Which is the most popular? Why?

27. Why are frozen doughs gaining popularity worldwide? What kind of formulation or processing changes has to be done to obtain the best-frozen doughs? What kind of commercial bakery items are mainly produced by frozen dough technology?

9.3 PRODUCTION OF SWEET PASTRIES

Sweet fermented breads are usually glazed with sugar and syrups, flavored, and in many instances filled with jellies, marmalades, fruits, cheeses, and condensed and sweetened dairy products. The fermented and sweet flavor combination is highly enjoyed and demanded by consumers. Sweet bread doughs are almost always produced from a rich formulation consisting of significant amounts of shortening, sugars, milk, and egg products. Most sweet breads formulations do not normally exceed 15% sugar to prevent yeast inhibition. After fermentation, some sugar is left over, contributing to their characteristic flavor. The crumb color of sweet breads and pastries that contain whole egg (fresh or dehydrated) normally acquires a light yellow coloration.

9.3.1 CROISSANTS

Croissants originated in Vienna, Italy in 1683 when the region suffered from a war between the Turkish and the Austrian–Hungarians. A few invading Turkish soldiers caved a tunnel to penetrate the city and surprise the enemy. The tunnel ended in a bakery. The artisan bakers heard the construction activities and immediately alerted the Austrian–Hungarians so the Turkish soldiers were surprised and defeated. The Austrian imperator conceded special privileges to the Vienna bakers, and as a gift, they manufactured bread with the emblem of the Turkish flag, a quarter crescent moon, or croissant. Years later, the princess Marie Antoinette demanded the manufacture of Vienna croissants for her wedding with King Louis XVI. Soon croissants gained popularity and disseminated throughout Europe. This tasty pastry has annual sales that exceed 100 million dollars in the United States, with an expected market annual growth of 5% to 7% (Calvel 1987; Doerry and Meloan 1986).

Croissants are manufactured from sweet or Danish pastry doughs that are laminated and folded, cut into triangles, rolled, and formed into its characteristic form. The rich formulation, yeast fermentation and folding yield a light and delightful sweet bread. Croissants are preferably elaborated from hard flours; other ingredients are added to improve organoleptic and dough handling properties. In many bakeries, the first dough fermentation is performed at refrigeration temperature for long periods (8–12 hours), although many bakers today use regular fermentation schedules. One of the most critical operations is the sheeting and folding of the dough before forming and final proofing. The croissants are formed first by sheeting into rectangular form, then a thin layer of roll consisting of whipped butter, margarine, shortening, and emulsifiers is placed onto the surface of the resulting dough, and then the dough is folded several times so to form a multilayered bread. After a brief fermentation period (i.e., 20 minutes), the operation is repeated once or twice. After these operations, the dough is sheeted to a final thickness of 2–3 mm followed by triangular cuts (11–12 cm long on the base and 17–18 cm on each of the two sides), with an average weight of each piece of 45–50 g. The triangular piece of dough is rolled starting from the base and formed into the characteristic quarter moon shape before final proofing. Then, a liquid mix of eggs and/or milk might be brushed on top of the fermented croissants before baking at 200°C–220°C for approximately 15–20 minutes. Alternatively, syrups might be applied on top of the croissants immediately after baking (Doerry and Meloan 1986).

9.3.1.1 Production of Croissants

A. Samples, Ingredients, and Reagents
- Refer to Table 9.13
- Eggs

B. Materials and Equipments
- Digital scale
- Graduated cylinder (100 mL, 200 mL, or 1 L)
- Dough mixer
- Fermentation cabinet
- Rolling pin
- Refrigerator
- Plastic or stainless steel containers
- Baking sheets
- Punching or degassing roll unit
- Baking oven
- Dough cutter
- Brush
- Thermometer
- Chronometer
- Heat-resistant gloves

C. Procedure
1. Weigh all ingredients except water and roll-in ingredients listed in Table 9.13 and place them in the dough mixer. Mix these dry ingredients for 1 to 2 minutes.
2. Add the predetermined amount of water and blend until the dough is properly developed. Register optimum mix time and dough consistency. Then, place the dough in a container for 8 to 12 hours in a refrigerator at 5°C. Alternatively, place the dough in a fermentation cabinet set at 24°C and 85% RH for 2.5 hours.
3. Dust dough with small amounts of flour in preparation for sheeting. Sheet or laminate the piece of dough through 0.79-cm or 5/16-in. roll spacing. Then with a rolling pin gradually reduce the dough sheet thickness to 0.5 cm. Place the roll-in or the combination of shortening, margarine and/or butter at a total rate of 250 g/kg dough on top of the laminated dough. The resulting dough sheet should be folded in half and in half again and returned to the fermentation cabinet for 15 additional minutes of proofing. Repeat this operation to produce a multilayered rectangular piece of dough (Figure 9.8).
4. Laminate the multilayered dough to 3- to 5-mm-thick rectangular sheets. Then, cut the dough into triangles (10–12 cm base and 18 cm sides). Make an incision of about 2 cm right in the central part of the triangle base.

    Roll the triangular pieces of dough from the base to the tip and manually fold the sides to form the typical half moon croissant configuration (Figure 9.8). Make sure to bond the tip of the triangle with the dough and place the tip contacting the surface of the baking pan.
5. Proof croissants in a fermentation cabinet for 60–70 minutes at 30°C and 85% relative humidity.
6. Egg wash the surface of the croissants with beaten eggs.
7. After proofing, bake croissants at 200°C for 20 minutes.
8. Wearing protective gloves, take the croissants out of the oven and allow croissants to cool down for 30 minutes.
9. Upon cooling, calculate yield and properties in terms of layering, crust color and texture, crumb texture, appearance, and organoleptic properties.

TABLE 9.13
Recommended Formulation for the Production of Croissants

Ingredients	%
Hard wheat flour	100.0
Water	60.0–62.5
Sugar	8.0
Yeast	3.5
Salt	2.4
Nonfat dry milk	1.5
Malt extract	1.0
Shortening	2.0
Roll-in[a]	45.0

[a] Shortening, margarine, and/or butter (250 g/kg dough) are spread on top of the sheeted dough to enhance the formation of multilayered pastries.

9.3.2 Danish Pastries

Danish bread is very similar to croissants in terms of formulation (Tables 9.13 and 9.14) and forming procedure. The main characteristic of Danish breads is that the crumb is multilayered imparting a special texture. The roll-in consisting

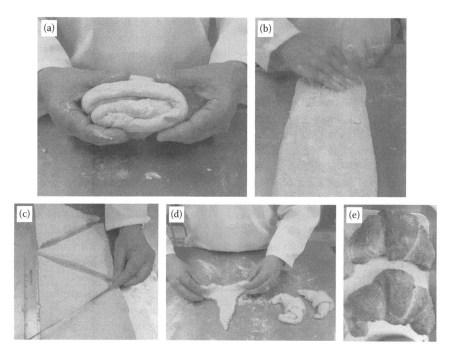

FIGURE 9.8 Production of croissants. (a) Forming a multilayered dough; (b) application of *roll-in*; (c) cutting of triangular forms; (d) rolling triangular forms into croissants; and (e) baked croissants.

of butter, margarine, and/or shortening are applied onto the surface of each layer. Traditional Danish breads were first fermented for long periods under refrigeration or low temperatures to relax the gluten and maintain the fat layers crystallized or solid. After baking, Danish pastries are usually covered with syrup or glazings.

9.3.2.1 Production of Danish Pastries

A. *Samples, Ingredients, and Reagents*
- Refer to Table 9.14

TABLE 9.14

Recommended Formulation for the Production of Danish Pastries

Ingredients	%
Hard wheat flour	100.0
Water	58.0–60.0
Sugar	10.0
Dry yeast	1.5
Salt	2.4
Nonfat dry milk	4.0
Diastatic malt	0.1
Shortening	10.0
Roll-in[a]	36.0

[a] Consists of a mixture of shortening, margarine, and/or butter. The roll-in is placed on top of the sheeted dough to enhance the formation of a multilayered pastries.

B. *Materials and Equipments*
- Digital scale
- Graduated cylinder (100 mL, 200 mL, or 1 L)
- Dough mixer
- Fermentation cabinet
- Rolling pin
- Refrigerator
- Plastic or stainless steel containers
- Baking sheets
- Punching or degassing roll unit
- Baking oven
- Dough cutter
- Brush
- Thermometer
- Chronometer
- Heat-resistant gloves

C. *Procedure*
1. Weigh all ingredients except water and roll-in ingredients listed in Table 9.14 and place them in the dough mixer. Mix these dry ingredients for 1 to 2 minutes.
2. Add the predetermined amount of water and blend until the dough is properly developed. Register optimum mix time and dough consistency. Then, place the dough in a container for 2 hour of fermentation in a refrigerator adjusted to 5°C.
3. Dust dough with small amounts of flour in preparation for sheeting. Sheet or laminate the piece of dough through 0.79-cm or 5/16-in. roll spacing. Then with a rolling pin gradually reduce the dough sheet thickness to 2 mm. Place and

spread part of the roll-in on top of the laminated dough. Then fold the dough in half and in half again and return it to the refrigerator for 30 minutes. Repeat this operation to produce a multilayered rectangular piece of dough and return the dough for 12 hours fermentation in the refrigerator (Figure 9.9).

4. Laminate the multilayered dough to 5-mm-thick rectangular sheets. Then cut the dough into 10 by 6 cm rectangles.

5. Place and spread the filling (jelly, marmalade, sweetened fruit fillings, jam) on the central part of the rectangles making sure to avoid the at least one each of the periphery. Take one side

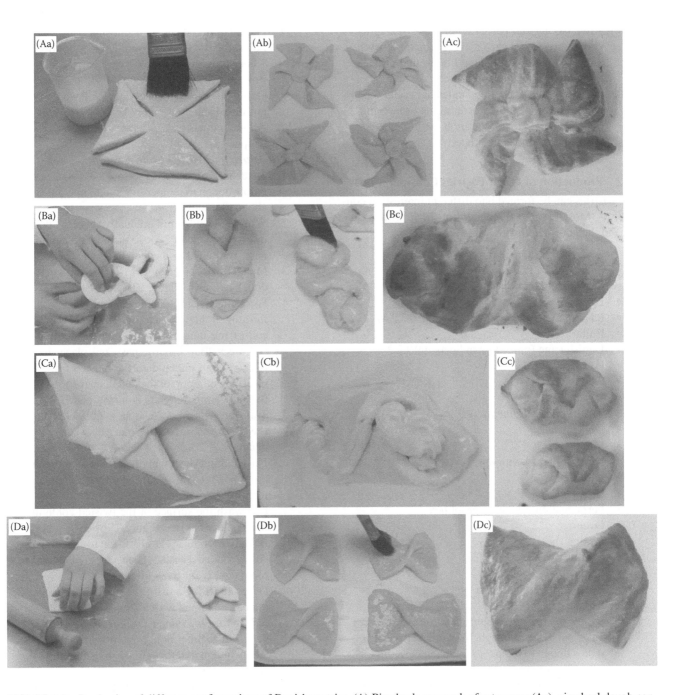

FIGURE 9.9 Production of different configurations of Danish pastries. (A) Pinwheel: egg wash of cut square (Aa), pinwheel dough configurations (Ab), and baked pinwheel (Ac); (B) twisted Danish pastry: twisting of dough cylinder (Ba), final twisted egg-washed configurations (Bb), and baked twisted Danish pastry (Bc); (C) owl face: dough configuration (Ca), application of pastry cream on owl face dough configuration (Cb), and baked owl face (Cc); (D) Bow tie: production of bow tie configurations (Da), egg wash of bow ties prior to baking (Db), and baked bow tie (Dc).

of the rectangle and fold in the middle part and then the opposite side so to form a three-layered piece of dough with the filling inside. Manually seal all edges to avoid the spill of the filling.

6. Apply with a brush an egg wash on top of the Danish pastries and place the formed dough pieces in a fermentation cabinet for 2 hours at 36°C–38°C and 85% relative humidity.

7. Wearing protective gloves, bake at 175°C for 20 minutes.

8. After baking and partial cooling (40°C), apply with a brush a sugar or syrup glazing on top of the pastry. Syrups should be heated at least three minutes before application.

9. Upon complete cooling, calculate yield and Danish pastries properties in terms of layering, crust color and texture, crumb texture, appearance, and organoleptic properties.

9.3.2.2 Production of Other Pastries Configurations

Danish pastries can be formed into different interesting configurations. Most of these products are filled with pastry cream and then decorated with Danish icing.

A. *Samples, Ingredients, and Reagents*
- Danish dough (procedure in Section 9.3.2.1)
- Eggs
- Pastry cream (procedure in Section 9.3.2.4)
- Butter
- Danish icing (procedure in Section 9.3.2.3)
- Powdered sugar
- Granulated sugar
- Powdered sugar

B. *Materials and Equipments*
- Digital scale
- Wooden pin
- Decorating bag with tips
- Knife
- Brush
- Fermentation cabinet or proof box
- Oven
- Baking sheets
- Small bowl
- Spoon
- Ruler with mm markings
- Scraper

C. *Procedure for Pinwheel Configuration*
1. Take out Danish dough from the refrigerator. Allow dough to temper to room temperature for about 30 minutes.

2. With the wooden pin gradually sheet the dough into a rectangle of 24 cm × 48 cm and 0.5 cm thickness. With the knife cut eight squares of 12 cm × 12 cm.

3. Starting from each corner of the square, make a 7-cm diagonal cut (Figure 9.9).

4. Egg wash the surface of the dough. Then, grab the tip of every other corner and fold it to the center of the square. Lightly press the tips of the dough to prevent detachment (Figure 9.9).

5. Place pastry cream in the decorating bag equipped with a 1-cm tip. Place a small amount of pastry cream in the center of the pinwheel.

6. Transfer the decorated pinwheels on a greased baking sheet. Make sure to leave space between pinwheels.

7. Place baking sheet with pinwheels in a proof box set at 30°C and 85% relative humidity for 1 hour proofing.

8. Bake pinwheels at 215°C for 10–15 minutes.

9. Optionally, hot pinwheels can be flavored with powdered sugar.

10. Allow pinwheels to cool down at room temperature.

D. *Procedure for Twisted Configuration*
1. Take our Danish dough from the refrigerator. Allow dough to temper to room temperature for about 30 minutes.

2. With the wooden pin gradually sheet the dough into a rectangle of 30 × 15 cm and 2.5 cm thickness. With the knife cut eight equal strips.

3. Manually form each strip into a 60-cm-long dough cylinder (Figure 9.9).

4. Form the twisted dough configuration by first forming a hook, then by grabbing the long end of the dough form an eight configuration (Figure 9.9Ba). Finally, pass and place the tip of the dough underneath the twisted form and insert the other tip of the dough on the top of the twisted configuration (Figure 9.9Ba and Bb).

5. Transfer twisted forms on a greased baking sheet. Make sure to leave space between twisted doughs.

6. Place baking sheet with the pieces of dough in a proof box set at 30°C and 85% relative humidity for 1 hour proofing.

7. Egg wash the surface of the twisted configurations before baking (Figure 9.9Bb).

8. Bake twisted forms at 210°C for 10–15 minutes.

9. Allow baked twisted forms to cool down at room temperature (20 minutes).

10. Decorate with Danish icing placed in a decorating bag equipped with a 2 mm to 3 mm tip.

E. *Procedure for Owl Face Configuration*
1. Take out Danish dough from the refrigerator. Allow dough to temper to room temperature for about 30 minutes.

2. With the wooden pin gradually sheet the dough into a rectangle of 24 cm × 48 cm and 0.3 cm thickness. With the knife cut eight squares of 12 cm × 12 cm.

3. Egg wash the surface of the square pieces of dough. Then, grab the tip of one corner and fold

it to the center of the square. Grab the opposite corner and fold it over to the edge of the first fold. Lightly press the tip of the dough to prevent detachment (Figure 9.9).

4. Transfer the decorated owl faces on a greased baking sheet. Make sure to leave space between dough pieces.
5. Place baking sheet with owl faces in a proof box set at 30°C and 85% relative humidity for 1 hour proofing.
6. Place pastry cream in the decorating bag equipped with a 1 cm tip. Before baking, place pastry cream on each side of the owl configuration and egg wash the surface of the decorated forms.
7. Bake decorated pieces of dough at 215°C for 10–15 minutes.
8. Allow baked owl faces to cool down at room temperature.

F. *Procedure for Bow Tie Configuration*

1. Take out Danish dough from the refrigerator. Allow dough to temper to room temperature for about 30 minutes.
2. With the wooden pin gradually sheet the dough into a rectangle of 30 cm × 32 cm and 0.5 cm thickness. With the knife cut two equal rectangles of 15 cm × 32 cm. Then cut each large rectangle into 4 pieces of 15 cm × 8 cm.
3. Twist the 15 cm × 8 cm dough piece into the typical bow tie configuration (Figure 9.9).
4. Transfer the bow ties on a greased baking sheet. Make sure to leave space between dough pieces.
5. Place baking sheet with bow ties in a proof box set at 30°C and 85% relative humidity for 1 hour proofing.
6. Bake pieces of dough at 215°C for 10–15 minutes.
7. Allow baked bow ties to cool down at room temperature. Then, with a brush apply melted butter onto the surface.
8. Immediately, place bow ties on a container with granulated sugar.

TABLE 9.15
Recommended Formulation for the Preparation of Danish Icing

Ingredients	Amount (g)
Powdered sugar	1000.0
Granulated sugar	230.0
Water	200.0
Gelatin	30.0
Shortening	20.0
Vanilla	2.0

9.3.2.3 Production of Danish Icing

A. *Samples, Ingredients, and Reagents*
- Refer to Table 9.15

B. *Materials and Equipments*
- Digital scale
- Graduated cylinder (1 L)
- Mixer with whisk attachment
- Stove or heater
- Cooking pot
- Beater with blades
- Thermometer
- Chronometer

C. *Procedure*
1. Place the granulated sugar, water, shortening, gelatin, and vanilla into the cooking pot and heat contents to boiling.
2. In a separate mixing bowl, place the powdered sugar and incorporate approximately half of the boiling mix of step one and blend at slow speed for 2 minutes. Then, gradually add the rest of the mix and keep mixing for three more minutes or until attaining a smooth consistency.

9.3.2.4 Production of Pastry Cream

A. *Samples, Ingredients, and Reagents*
- Refer to Table 9.16

B. *Materials and Equipments*
- Digital scale
- Graduated cylinder (1 L)
- Mixer with whisk attachment
- Stove or heater
- Cooking pot
- Measuring cup
- Beater with whisk attachment
- Thermometer

C. *Procedure*
1. Place the milk and half of the sugar into the cooking pot and heat contents to boiling.
2. In a separate mixing bowl, blend the corn starch, the other half of the sugar, eggs, vanilla, and coloring agent until attaining a homogenous mix.

TABLE 9.16
Recommended Formulation for the Preparation of Pastry Cream

Ingredients	Amount (g)
Regular milk	1000.0
Sugar	250.0
Eggs	150.0
Maize starch	100.0
Vanilla	2.0
FD&C yellow	0.2

3. Add one cup of the sugared boiling milk to the blend to obtain a pourable mix.

4. Gradually add contents to the rest of the boiling sugared milk and while cooking immediately blend with the whisk. The cream should thicken and form a smooth textured paste. The total cooking time should be at least 5 minutes.

5. Pour the pastry cream immediately into a bowl greased with butter.

6. Allow cream to cool down at room temperature and then keep it in close containers at refrigeration temperature.

9.3.3 Cinnamon Rolls

Cinnamon rolls are popular worldwide, especially in industrialized countries where they are generally consumed as breakfast or as a snack. Cinnamon rolls are manufactured from fermented sweet doughs rich in eggs, milk, shortening, and sugar (Table 9.17). The sheeted dough is covered with butter or margarine and sprinkled with brown sugar, raisins, pecans, and cinnamon. Then the dough is hand or machine rolled into a cylinder that is cut into many small cylindrical rolled pieces. The dough pieces are panned, fermented, and baked. Right after baking, rolls are normally glazed with sugar-based coatings.

9.3.3.1 Production of Glazed Cinnamon Rolls

A. *Samples, Ingredients, and Reagents*
- Refer to Table 9.17

B. *Materials and Equipments*
- Digital scale
- Graduated cylinder (100 mL, 200 mL, or 1 L)
- Dough mixer
- Fermentation cabinet

TABLE 9.17
Recommended Formulation for the Production of Cinnamon Rolls[a]

Ingredients	%
Hard wheat flour	100.0
Water	60.0–62.0
Whole egg solids[b]	10.0
Sugar	8.0
Shortening	6.0
Dry yeast	2.0
Nonfat dry milk	2.0
Salt	1.5

[a] *Roll-in*: 6.8 units of butter or margarine for 100 units flour. Filling: for 100 units of flour mix 3.5 units brown sugar with 0.35 units ground cinnamon. Then add 8 units of coarsely ground pecan and 8 units of raisins.

[b] If fresh eggs (36 units/100 flour units) are used instead of egg solids (10 units/100 flour units), the water absorption should be adjusted by subtracting 7.5% (52.5%–54.5%).

- Rolling pin
- Refrigerator
- Plastic or stainless steel containers
- Baking pans
- Punching or degassing roll unit
- Baking oven
- Dough cutter
- Cheese shredder
- Bread knife
- Brush
- Thermometer
- Chronometer
- Heat-resistant gloves

C. *Procedure*

1. Add all ingredients listed in Table 9.17 except the water to a mixing bowl. Mix dry ingredients for 1 to 2 minutes.

2. Add the predetermined amount of water and mix the dough until is properly developed. Register optimum mix time and dough consistency. Cut the dough into 500-g pieces.

3. Place the individual pieces of dough inside previously greased containers for proofing at 28°C–30°C and 85% RH for 60 minutes.

4. Dust doughs with small amounts of flour in preparation for sheeting. Sheet or laminate the piece of dough through 0.79-cm or 5/16-in. roll spacing. Then, with a rolling pin, thin the rectangular dough sheet to 1 cm thick. Place and spread the roll-in onto the laminated dough. Then fold the rectangular dough sheet in half and in half again and return the folded dough piece to the fermentation cabinet.

5. After 15 minutes of proofing, laminate the folded piece of dough first through 0.79-cm or 5/16-in. roll spacing and then with a rolling pin to a 1-cm-thick rectangular dough piece.

6. Spread more roll-in onto the rectangular piece of dough. Then fold the rectangular dough sheet in half and in half again and return the folded dough piece to the fermentation cabinet for 15 minutes of proofing.

7. Laminate the folded piece of dough first through 0.48-cm or 3/16-in. roll spacing and then with a rolling pin to a 1-cm thick rectangular dough piece. Spread the rest of the roll-in and then place the combination of sugar and ground cinnamon, pieces of pecan, and raisins on the rectangular piece of dough. Make sure to avoid placing pecans and raisins in close to the periphery of the rectangular piece of dough. Carefully roll the rectangular dough piece into a cylinder and manually seal borders. Cut the resulting cylinders into 3.5-cm-thick roll pieces (Figure 9.10).

8. Place two columns of rolls on baking pans previously greased leavening space between dough

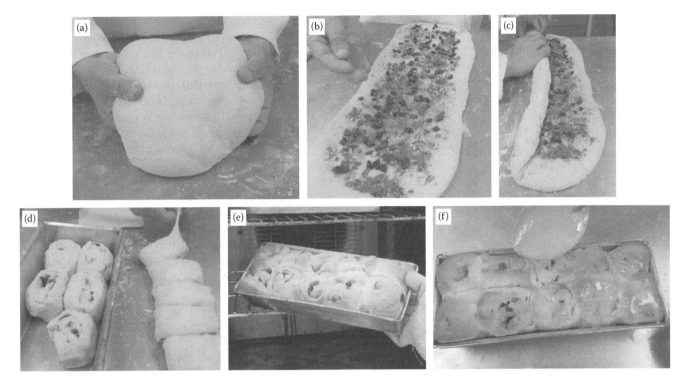

FIGURE 9.10 Production of cinnamon rolls. (a) Dough; (b) addition of flavorings to sheeted dough; (c) hand-rolling of dough; (d) cutting and panning cinnamon rolls; (e) baked cinnamon rolls; and (f) glazing of cinnamon rolls.

pieces. Then place the pans with the rolled pieces of dough in a proof box for 1.5 to 2 hours at 28°C and 85% relative humidity.

9. Wearing baking gloves, bake for 20 minutes at 175°C. Then immediately place the sugar glazing on top of the hot cinnamon rolls (Figure 9.10).

10. After cooling, depan cinnamon rolls and calculate product yield based on the original formulation and added amounts of roll-in and glazing (Table 9.18). Then, evaluate the properties of sweet cinnamon rolls in terms of layering, crust color and texture, crumb texture, appearance, and organoleptic properties.

TABLE 9.18
Recommended Formulation for Glazing Cinnamon Rolls[a]

Ingredients	%
Powdered sugar	100.0
Water	20.0
Salt	0.4

[a] Add the desired flavoring (0.6 maple flavoring or 1.25 vanilla flavoring or 0.8 cocoa). Mix the flavoring with the glazing until achieving a uniform and homogenous consistency.

9.3.4 Sweet Concha Bread

Sweet *conchas* are one of the most popular fermented sweet bread products in Latin America. The product consists of a bread manufactured from a dough rich in eggs, shortening, and sugar covered with the typical sugar-shortening covering flavored with vanilla, cocoa, and maple.

9.3.4.1 Production of Sweet Conchas

A. *Samples, Ingredients, and Reagents*
- Refer to Tables 9.19 and 9.20

B. *Materials and Equipments*
- Digital scale
- Graduated cylinder (100 mL, 200 mL, or 1 L)
- Dough mixer
- Fermentation cabinet
- Plastic or stainless steel containers
- Baking sheets
- Punching or degassing roll unit
- Baking oven
- Dough cutter and rounder
- Rolling pin
- Thermometer
- Special die for cutting the covering
- Chronometer
- Heat-resistant gloves

C. *Procedure*
1. Weigh all dough and covering ingredients listed in Tables 9.19 and 9.20. Prepare the covering by first creaming the shortening and sugar and

TABLE 9.19

Recommended Formulation for the Production of Sweet *Conchas*

Ingredients	%
Hard wheat flour	100.0
Water[a]	38.0–40.0
Whole fresh eggs[a]	30.0
Shortening	3.5
Butter	0.7
Sugar	15.0
Dry yeast	2.0
Salt	2.0
Nonfat dry milk	2.5
Emulsifier (SSL) and monoglycerides	0.2
Calcium propionate	0.2

[a] 7.6% whole egg solids are equivalent to 30% fresh eggs. If dry eggs are used adjust water absorption considering that 30% fresh eggs provide about 22.8% water.

then adding the flour until getting a smooth and homogeneous blend. Add dough ingredients, except water and eggs, to a mixing bowl and blend them for 2 minutes. Then add eggs and the predetermined amount of water.

2. Mix ingredients until the dough is properly developed. Register optimum mix time and dough consistency.

3. Place dough in a proof box for 45 minutes of fermentation at 30°C and 85% relative humidity.

4. Dust the dough with small amounts of flour in preparation for punching/sheeting. Sheet or laminate the piece of dough through 0.79-cm or 5/16-in. roll spacing and then form a large dough ball. Return the dough to the fermentation cabinet for 10 minutes.

5. Divide and round the dough into 75-g dough pieces. If a divider/rounder is not available, the

TABLE 9.20

Recommended Formulation for the Production of the Typical Sweet Covering of *Conchas*[a]

Ingredients	%
Flour	100.0
Sugar	66.6
Shortening	66.6

Note: For white vanilla covering, add 7.5 g of vanilla.
For maple flavored covering, add 10 g of maple syrup.
For chocolate dark covering add 1.4% cocoa powder.

[a] Cream the sugar and shortening and gradually add the flour. Keep blending until forming a smooth dough. Then form 30-g pieces that will cover each *concha*.

operation could be performed by hand. After getting the 75-g dough piece, press or laminate the dough ball into a 17-cm diameter and 1.5-cm thick patty (Figure 9.11).

6. Place the individual pieces of dough on a previously greased containers and then apply 30 g of covering. The covering is pressed by hand on top of the dough patty. Then, cut the covering with the special round die configuration (Figure 9.11).

7. Place baking sheets with the *conchas* for 70 to 90 minutes in a proof box adjusted to 36°C and 85% RH.

8. Bake *conchas* for 12 minutes at 180°C. Then calculate yield based on the original dough and covering formulations. Make sure to handle hot baking sheets and *conchas* with heat-resistant gloves.

9. Allow *conchas* to cool down at ambient temperature for 30 minutes (Figure 9.11).

10. Upon cooling, evaluate the properties of resulting breads in terms of volume, covering adherence, crumb texture, and organoleptic properties.

9.3.5 Yeast-Leavened Donuts

Donuts are sweet baking goods that are generally fried instead of baked. There are two broad categories: yeast and chemical leavened. The first category is the most popular because of the fermented flavor that is more appealing to the general consumer. The second category, also known as coffee donuts, is industrially produced from chemically leavened doughs that are baked and have longer shelf life expectations. Yeast-leavened donuts are usually produced from all-purpose or family flours that are processed into dough following both straight or sponge dough procedures. Straight dough is usually used to produce dough-cut donuts, whereas sponge is used to yield extruded yeast-raised donuts. The common recipe is rich in sugar, shortening, eggs, and milk solids. The properly developed dough is fermented at 28°C–30°C, sheeted, and cut or extruded into the typical donut configuration and proofed at 28°C–30°C under a low relative humidity to form a crust. The crust will decrease the amount of oil absorbed during the critical step of frying. The fermented dough pieces are generally fried at 175°C–180°C on both sides or by immersion in the hot oil for times that vary from 1 to 2 minutes. Donuts are immediately glazed with liquid sugar-based flavorings or flavored with a combination of crystallized sugar and cinnamon. Donuts generally absorb about 10% oil during frying and usually contain approximately 18%–20% fat after frying and glazing.

9.3.5.1 Production of Yeast-Leavened Fried Donuts

A. *Samples, Ingredients, and Reagents*

• Refer to Tables 9.21 and 9.22
• Frying oil

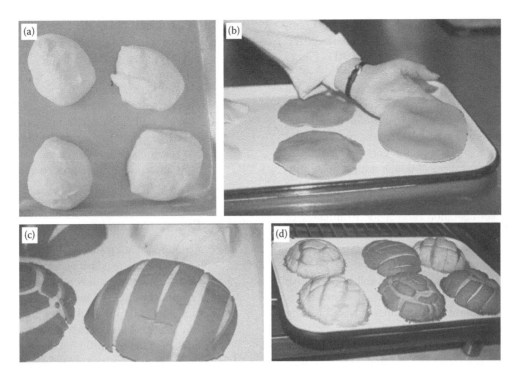

FIGURE 9.11 Production of *conchas*. (a) Fermented dough balls; (b) placing covering on top of the dough patty; (c) proofed *conchas* prior to baking; and (d) baked chocolate and vanilla-flavored *conchas*.

B. *Materials and Equipments*
- Digital scale
- Graduated cylinder (100 mL, 200 mL, or 1 L)
- Dough mixer
- Fermentation cabinet
- Plastic or stainless steel containers
- Baking sheets
- Punching or degassing roll unit

- Deep fat fryer
- Dough cutter
- Rolling pin
- Cutting die for donuts
- Beaker
- Thermometer
- Donut cutter
- Chronometer
- Heat-resistant gloves
- Safety goggles

C. *Procedure*
1. Weigh all ingredients except water listed in Table 9.21 and place them in the dough mixer. Mix dry ingredients for 1 to 2 minutes.
2. Add the predetermined amount of water and blend until the dough is properly developed. Register optimum mix time and dough

TABLE 9.21

Recommended Formulation for the Elaboration of Yeast-Leavened Donuts

Ingredients	Donut (%)
All-purpose flour	100.0
Water	58.0
Sugar	10.0
Shortening	11.0
Whole egg solids[a]	5.0
Nonfat dry milk	4.0
Salt	2.5
Dry yeast	2.0

[a] Fresh eggs could be used instead of egg solids. The formulation should be adjusted according to solid contents. Fresh whole eggs contain 24% solids whereas egg solids contain about 94%. 5% eggs solids are equivalent to 19.6% fresh eggs. The water required if fresh eggs are used is approximately 15% less (43% water absorption).

TABLE 9.22

Recommended Formulation for the Elaboration of Donut Glazing[a]

Ingredients	Amount
Powdered sugar	100.0
Water (80°C)	20.0
High-fructose corn syrup	56.0
Vanilla	14.0

[a] Mix ingredients and heat to 45°C before glazing.

consistency. Then, place the dough inside previously greased containers for 90 minutes of fermentation at 28°C–30°C and 85% RH (Figure 9.12).

3. Dust dough with small amounts of flour in preparation for sheeting. Sheet or laminate the piece of dough through 0.79-cm or 5/16-in. roll spacing. Then with a rolling pin gradually reduce the dough sheet thickness to 1.5 cm. Cut the resulting sheet of dough with a donut cutter. Recover all the scrap dough and round it into one piece of dough. Place the scrap dough in the fermentation cabinet for 10 minutes of proofing. Then repeat the donut forming and cutting procedure.

4. Place donuts on baking sheets for 40–60 minutes of fermentation at 36°C and 60% relative humidity. The higher temperature and lower relative humidity will enhance surface crusting and lower oil uptake during frying.

5. After final proofing, carefully place donuts in a deep fat fryer containing oil at 175°C. Donuts should be fried for 20 seconds on each side or immersed in the frying oil. Make sure to wear safety goggles and protective gloves.

6. Take donuts out of the fryer and allow to drain excess oil for only 10 seconds. Then, immediately glaze (Table 9.22) or flavor the donuts (Figure 9.12).

7. Allow glazed donuts to cool down at ambient temperature for 30 minutes.

8. Upon cooling, calculate raw and glazed donut yield, amount of covering, and finish properties of resulting donuts in terms of crumb texture, oil absorption, moisture content, color, and organoleptic properties.

9.3.6 Research Suggestions

1. Prepare croissants using fresh and dehydrated egg solids. Make sure to adjust water absorption and add the same amount of solids to the two formulations. Determine the effect of adding dehydrated solids on optimum mixing time and water absorption, dough texture, and stickiness, crust color, and organoleptic properties of the two different croissants.

2. Prepare Danish pastries applying two contrasting amounts of *roll-in* fat (130 vs. 260 g/kg dough) and two contrasting laminating-folding procedures (twofold and threefold methods). Compare flaki-

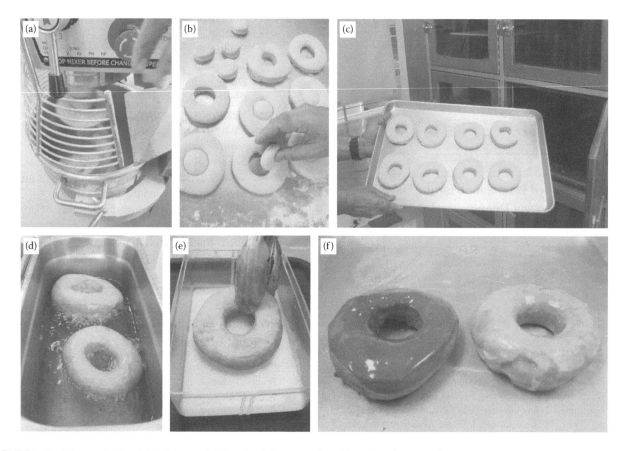

FIGURE 9.12 Yeast-raised and fried donuts. (a) Dough mixing operation; (b) cutting donut configurations; (c) fermented donuts; (d) frying of donuts; (e) glazing donut with vanilla covering; and (f) vanilla and chocolate-covered donuts.

ness, crust color, and organoleptic properties of the four different Danish pastries.

3. Prepare cinnamon rolls applying two different icings suited for cold and hot weather conditions. Compare the viscosity of the two icings, appearance, and color. Then, determine the organoleptic properties of the two different types of cinnamon rolls.

4. Prepare *conchas* using all-purpose or hard wheat flours. Make sure to adjust water absorption and mix times as affected by the type of flour. Determine optimum mixing time and water absorption, dough texture, bread volume and height, and the overall organoleptic properties.

5. Prepare yeast-raised and fried donuts using three contrasting flours (soft, all-purpose, and hard flours) and determine optimum mixing time and water absorption, dough texture, oil uptake during frying, and donut volume.

9.3.7 Research Questions

1. Define the following concepts:
   a. *Roll-in* fat
   b. Book fold dough
   c. Retarding
   d. Make up
   e. Egg wash
   f. Bench time

2. Why are the mixing times of Danish doughs typically short?

3. What is the functionality of the following ingredients used in sweet doughs: potassium bromate, protease, dough conditioners, and egg solids?

4. What are differences among laminating using the envelope, threefold, and fourfold methods?

5. What is the amount of *roll-in* fat commonly suggested per kilogram of Danish dough? What are the ideal properties of the *roll-in* fat? How does the solid fat index affect functionality of *roll-in* fats?

6. What is the main functionality of milk or milk solids in sweet doughs?

7. Compared to most bread doughs, what are the most common additional ingredients used for the manufacturing of sweet doughs?

8. Why is it recommended to use stronger flours when retarding doughs?

9. What is the difference between dough fat and *roll-in* fat?

10. What kind of adjustments in sweet dough formulations should be made when fresh whole eggs are substituted by dehydrated or powdered egg solids?

11. What are the basic ingredients for the production of icings or glazes?

12. What changes in formulation are necessary for the production of sweet roll icings for cold and hot weather conditions?

13. What is the most functional type of wheat flour for yeast-raised donuts?

14. How much oil does a donut usually uptake during frying? What kind of frying oil is recommended for yeast-leavened donuts? What is the typical frying time and oil temperature?

15. What formulation and processing changes would you suggest to avoid excessive oil uptake during the frying process of donuts?

16. What are main differences in formulation and processing between cake and fried donuts?

17. Why are yeast raised and fried donuts allowed to cool for 1 to 2 minutes before applying the glaze?

REFERENCES

American Association of Cereal Chemists. 2000. *Approved Methods of the AACC*. St. Paul, MN: AACC.

Bath, D., and R. Hoseney. 1994. "A Laboratory-Scale Bagel Making Procedure." *Cereal Chemistry* 71:403–408.

Boge, J. A. 1972. "Hard Rolls—Formulation and Production." *The Bakers Digest* December:18–23.

Calvel, R. 1987. *O Pâo Francés e os Productos Correlatos: Tecnologia e Práctica da Panificâo*. Fortaleza, Ceara, Brasil: Fortaleza, J. Macedo S. A. Comercio Administrcâo e Particiacôes.

Cauvain, S. P., and L. S. Young. 1998. *Technology of Breadmaking*. London: Blackie Academic & Professional.

Cross, N. 2007. "Muffins and Bagels." In *Handbook of Food Products Manufacturing. Principles, Bakery, Beverages, Cereals, Cheese, Confectionary, Fats, Fruits, and Functional Foods*, edited by Y. H. Hui, Chapter 15. Hoboken, NJ: Wiley Interscience.

Doerry, W. T. 1995. *Breadmaking Technology*, Chapters 4–6. Manhattan, KS: American Institute of Baking.

Doerry, W. T., and E. Meloan. 1986. "Croissant Technology." *Tech. Bull. Am. Inst. Baking*. VIII (10):1–9.

Esteve, C. C., C. B. De Barber, and M. A. Martinez. 1994. "Microbial Sour Doughs Influence Acidification Properties and Breadmaking Potential of Wheat Dough." *Journal of Food Science* 59:629–633.

Finney, K. F. 1984. "An Optimized Straight-Dough Making Method After 44 Years." *Cereal Chemistry* 61:20.

Finney, K. F., G. Rubenthaler, and Y. Pomeranz. 1963. "Soy Product Variables Affecting Bread Baking." *Cereal Sci. Today* 8 (5).

Huang, S. 1999. "Wheat Products. 2. Breads, Cakes, Cookies, Pastries, and Dumplings." In *Asian Foods Science and Technology*, edited by C. Y. W. Ang, K. Liu, and Y. W. Huang, Chapter 4. Lancaster, PA: Technomic Publishing.

Hui, Y. H., H. Corke, W. H. Nip, I. De Leyn, and N. Cross. 2006. *Bakery Products: Science and Technology*. Ames, IO: Blackwell Publishing.

Kulp, K. 1991. "Breads and Yeast Bakery Foods." In *Handbook of Cereal Science and Technology*, edited by K. J. Lorenz and K. Kulp, Chapter 16. New York: Marcel Dekker.

Kulp, K. 1988. "Bread Industry and Processes." In *Wheat Chemistry and Technology*, edited by Y. Pomeranz, Chapter 6. St. Paul, MN: AACC.

Kulp, K., and K. J. Lorenz. 2003. *Handbook of Dough Fermentation*. New York: Marcel Dekker.

Kulp, K., K. Lorenz, and J. Brummer. 1995. *Frozen and Refrigerated Doughs and Batters*. St. Paul, MN: AACC.

Kulp, K., and R. Loewe. 1990. *Batter and Breading in Food Processing*. St. Paul, MN: AACC.

Kulp, K., and J. G. Ponte. 1981. "Staling of White Pan Bread. Fundamental Causes." *CRC Crit. Rev. Food Sci. Nutr.* 15: 1–48.

Matz, S. A. 1972. *Bakery Technology and Engineering*. 2nd ed. Westport, CT: AVI Publishing.

Matz, S. A. 1987. *Formulas and Processes for Bakers*. McAllen, TX: Pan Tech International.

Pomeranz, Y., and J. A. Shellenberger. 1971. *Bread Science and Technology*. Westport, CT: AVI Publishing.

Pyler, E. J. 1988. *Baking Science and Technology*. 3rd ed., vols. I–II. Merriam, KS: Sosland Publishing.

Quaglia, G. 1991. *Ciencia y Tecnología de la Panificación*. Zaragoza, España: Editorial Acribia.

Quail, K. J. 1996. *Arabic Bread Production*. St. Paul, MN: AACC.

Schunemann, C., and G. Treu. 1988. *Baking: The Art and Science*. Calgary, Alberta, Canada: Baker Tech.

Serna-Saldivar, S. R. O. 2003. *Manufactura y Control de Calidad de Productos Basados en Cereales*. México, Mexico: AGT Editor.

Sultan, W. J. 1983. *Practical Baking*. 3rd ed. Westport, CT: AVI Publishing.

10 Production of Chemical-Leavened Products: Crackers, Cookies, Cakes and Related Products, Donuts, and Wheat Flour Tortillas

10.1 INTRODUCTION

There is a wide array of chemical-leavened wheat products. The main categories are cookies, crackers, coffee donuts, flour tortillas, cakes, and other assorted products such as pancakes, wafers, muffins, and biscuits. Most of these manufactured goods are elaborated from soft wheat or all-purpose flours supplemented with high amounts of sugar and fats such as shortenings, oil, butter, and margarine (Faridi et al. 2000; Manley 1996; Matz 1992). Most of these chemically leavened products also contain large quantities of sugar or sweeteners. In fact, some recipes, such as high-ratio cake mixes and angel cakes, contain more sugar than flour. The high quantities of sugar significantly lower Aw, impeding the growth of microorganisms including yeast. Soft wheat products are easier and faster to produce because they do not need fermentation, and proofing times are nonexistent or normally short.

The basic ingredients for the production of these products are flour, chemical leavening agents frequently formulated into baking powders and water. The baking powder produce the desired leavening effect due to the carbon dioxide generated. The chemical leavening system contains two functional components: a leavening base and an acid. Sodium bicarbonate is the most widely used and is chemically neutralized by acid. During this reaction, these agents generate gas and the rate of gas produced greatly depends on the pH. Generally, the more acidic the pH, the higher rate of gas production. The most common leavening agents are monocalcium phosphate, dicalcium phosphate, sodium acid pyrophosphate, and sodium aluminum sulfate. Chemical leavening agents are classified into three categories: fast, slow, and double acting. Fast-acting such as monocalcium phosphate generates nearly all the gas at room temperature during mixing and proofing. Slow-acting agents such as dicalcium phosphate, sodium aluminum sulfate and sodium aluminum phosphate, require elevated temperatures to produce most of the gas, therefore, are very effective during baking. Double-acting agents are the most popular because they release carbon dioxide at both ambient and baking temperatures. Most baking powders are manufactured from a blend of selected chemical leavening agents, acids, and an inert compound (generally starch). Both the acid and acid salts are the key elements to control the release of carbon dioxide. The use of acids is important

especially in regular or nonchlorinated flours or in those products where the pH is neutral. The most used acids are tartaric and gluco-delta-lactone. The inert or carrier agent is necessary to minimize loss of leavening power because it significantly lowers the interaction between salts and the acid. The most important property of chemical leavening agents is the neutralization value covered in Chapter 8.

10.2 CRACKERS

Crackers represent one of the most important segments of the baking industry because consumers view these products with lower energy density compared to sugar cookies and other related items. Crackers are considered a hybrid product because it uses bread and cookie procedures and are one of the few products that are leavened both with yeast and chemical leavening agents. Saltines or soda crackers are the major cracker category, and they are prepared first following the principles of the sponge dough procedure and then the classic sheeting-forming cookie line. The industrial processes usually last more than 24 hours because the sponge dough is fermented for 12–24 hours. Crackers are formulated with stronger mixing and higher protein flours compared to sweet cookies. In the case of crackers made with the sponge and dough method, the type of mixer commonly is called vertical spindle mixer where the dough is mixed in a trolley and transported to the fermentation room and then back to mix again. This type of mixer also allows the dough to be mixed with less gluten development compared to single or double sigma horizontal mixers. The ideal flour usually contains from 10% to 10.5% protein and is classified as all-purpose flour (Faridi et al. 2000; Matz 1992; Serna-Saldivar 2008).

The industrial manufacturing process starts when batches of blends of hard and soft wheat flours containing about 10.5% protein are mixed with yeast and water to yield sponges that are fermented at 28°C and 85% relative humidity in proof rooms. The sponge usually contains 60% of the total flour used in the manufacturing process. Resulting sponges are left to ferment for approximately 20 hours. During fermentation, natural occurring lactic acid bacteria adhered to the surfaces of the trough develops and contributes to the typical cracker flavor and acid development. The initial sponge pH is around 7 and drops to about 4.2–4.5 during fermentation. Once the sponge is ripe, it is mixed with the rest of the flour (generally 40%), other ingredients, and sodium bicarbonate and other chemical leavening agents to produce a dough adjusted to a pH of 7–7.4. The dough is placed again in the fermentation room for 2 to 5 hours before forming into the typical round or rectangular cracker configurations with the sheeting-cutting-forming equipment. The fermented dough is first passed through a three-roll sheeter and then gradually reduced with two other gauging roll stations. After the first coarse lamination, the dough is lapped/layered and then gradually sheeted to about 2–3 mm. Layering is essential for the final cracker texture and work required to masticate the product. The sheet of dough is finally cut into the typical cracker form and the trim or scrap dough carried back to the dough hopper and recycled. The formed pieces of dough could be salted or treated with toppings such as sesame or poppy seeds on a mash conveyor with a dispenser or egg washed prior to baking. Baking is performed on continuous direct gas-fired ovens equipped with moving bands and different baking zones. The dwell time varies from 2 to 3 minutes at temperatures ranging from 220°C to >240°C. Crackers generally exit the baking oven at moistures of about 2% and are cooled before packaging with materials resistant to the atmospheric moisture. From the microbial viewpoint, crackers are shelf-stable because of their low Aw. The preservation of the characteristic crisp and brittle texture and the prevention of lipid oxidation are fundamental for cracker producers.

Many snack crackers and saltines are oil-sprayed immediately after baking and before cooling. Round-shaped crackers are usually coated with an oil base. The oil is generally applied at a temperature of 65°C–70°C and can be applied from 1% up to 18% or more, based on the weight of the unsprayed crackers. The oil is usually sprayed by nozzles or spinning disks (Moreth 1994; Serna-Saldivar 2008).

Cheese crackers are also classified as a ready to eat foods. The combination of the fermented flavor complements the cheese flavor so they are ideally suited for social events and for snacking at schools. These crackers are generally colored with paprika to intensify the color. Additional flavorings such as cayenne and sage are added to improve sensory properties. The crackers have a distinctive orange-red coloring that is easily recognized by the customer. Fresh or dehydrated aged or regular cheddar cheese is normally used. The preferred method is to incorporate the dry powdered form to achieve a better distribution during the sponge-producing stage (Faridi et al. 2000; Matz 1992).

10.2.1 Production of Crackers

A. Samples, Ingredients, and Reagents
- Refer to Table 10.1
- Flaked or coarse salt

B. Materials and Equipments
- Digital scale
- Dough mixer
- Sheeting rolls
- Proof box or cabinet

TABLE 10.1
Classic Formulations for the Production of Regular Saltines and Cheese Crackers

Ingredients	Saltines (%)	Cheese-Flavored (%)
Sponge		
All purpose wheat flour	58.8	75.0
Water	30.7	25.0
Shortening	8.3	12.0
Fermented dough (seed dough)	2.0	–
Fresh compressed yeast	0.25	0.25
Paprika	–	1.0
Diastatic malt	0.15	–
Dough Stage		
All-purpose wheat flour	41.2	25.0
Aged or regular cheddar cheese	–	25.0
Water	6.0	5.0
Sodium bicarbonate	1.5	0.5
Calcium phosphate	–	0.25
Ammonium bicarbonate	–	0.25
Diammonium phosphate	0.1	–
Salt	1.4	–
High-fructose syrup	1.4	–
Lecithin	0.2	0.2
Sodium stearoyl-2-lactylate	0.1	0.1

- Baking oven
- pH meter with electrode for dough
- Perforated baking sheets
- Graduated cylinders
- Wooden roller pin
- Pipette
- Knife
- Dissection pin
- Thermometer
- Ruler
- Protective gloves (heat-resistant)

C. Procedure
1. Weigh sponge dough ingredients listed in Table 10.1. Place ingredients without water and shortening in a mixing bowl. If dry yeast is used instead of fresh compressed yeast make sure to adjust the concentration (0.8% instead of 0.25%) and dissolve the yeast in water before making the sponge. Melt the shortening, and when its temperature lowers to 40°C, add it to the rest of the sponge dough ingredients.
2. Add water and then mix at low speed for 1 minute or until the formation of the dough. Weigh the sponge and measure the initial pH and internal temperature.
3. Place the dough in a proof cabinet adjusted to 38°C and 85% RH for 20 hours of fermentation.

Construct a curve of dough pH throughout the 20 hours of fermentation. Make sure to sample more frequently during the first 8 hours of fermentation.

4. Weigh and place the rest of the ingredients listed in Table 10.1. Add the sponge and mix first at low speed for 1 minute and then for 3 minutes at medium speed. After dough mixing, immediately measure the dough pH and weight of the dough.

5. Place the dough back in the proof box for 3 hours of fermentation. Measure the dough pH every hour.

6. Sheet the resulting dough using the following steps:

   a. Sheet dough through sheeting rolls adjusted to 0.79 cm, or 5/16 in., and fold the laminated dough so to obtain two layers of dough. Rotate the sheet 90° and repeat it.

   b. Repeat the above procedure twice to produce a multilayered (eight layers) of dough (Figure 10.1).

   c. Laminate the dough through the sheeting rolls adjusted to 0.48 cm, or 3/16 in., and then gradually reduce the thickness to 1 mm to 1.3 mm with a roller pin.

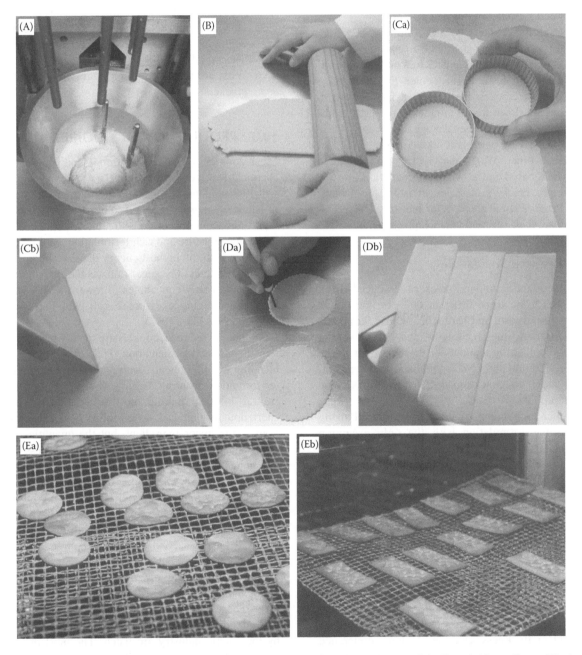

FIGURE 10.1 Procedure for the production of crackers. (A) Mixing the sponge with the rest of the flour and ingredients; (B), sheeting of multilayered cracker dough; (C), cutting sheeted dough with round (Ca) and rectangular (Cb) configurations; (D), docking round (Da) and rectangular (Db) pieces of dough; and (E) baked round (Ea) and rectangular (Eb) crackers.

7. With a rectangular or round die, cut the sheet of dough. If the die does not have pins to mark the typical holes then dock or perforate the dough piece form with a metal pin (6 holes per side in the rectangular-shaped dough or 6 holes evenly distributed in the round forms). Make sure to mark each piece of dough in the same place.

8. Calculate the average thickness of the cut pieces of dough by placing at least 5 pieces on top of each other.

9. For saltines, sprinkle coarse or flaked salt on top of the pieces of dough (0.5 g/100 g dough).

10. Place dough pieces on a perforated baking sheet and then cover with other baking sheet perforated as well.

11. Bake the crackers for 3 to 4 minutes at 175°C, rotate the baking sheet 180° to ensure even baking and bake for another 2 to 4 minutes or until achieving desired golden color (Figure 10.1).

12. Remove crackers from the oven and allow them to cool down for 10 minutes at room temperature. Calculate the average thickness of the crackers by placing at least 5 pieces on top of each other. Weigh the crackers and calculate yield based on the original formulation.

13. Place crackers in sealed moisture proof bags. Reserve some crackers for moisture, color, texture, shelf life, and organoleptic evaluations.

10.2.2 RESEARCH SUGGESTIONS

1. Produce and compare crackers produced from sponges using three different types of flours (i.e., soft, all-purpose, and hard wheat flour), fermented for different times (i.e., 8, 16, and 24 hours), and using contrasting amounts of diastatic malt in the sponge formulation. Make emphasis in determination of pH, dough texture, and characteristics of the final product.

2. Produce and compare crackers produced using the same formulation with the only exception of including (a) amylases, (b) proteases, and (c) sodium bisulfite. Make emphasis in dough texture and handling properties and characteristics of final crackers (color, texture, average height or thickness, etc.).

3. Produce high-protein quality crackers supplemented with 6% defatted soybean concentrate and 6% defatted soybean concentrate supplemented with 1% vital gluten and 0.3% SSL and compare them with the control cracker. Determine optimum water absorption, dough texture, characteristics of the final products (color, texture, average height or thickness, etc.), and hedonic preference by untrained panelists. In addition, calculate the amino acid composition of the three different types of crackers.

10.2.3 RESEARCH QUESTIONS

1. Define the following terms:
   a. Seed dough
   b. Grahams
2. Why are crackers considered as a hybrid product from the formulation and processing viewpoint? What are the optimum flour specifications for crackers and saltines?
3. In a flowchart, detail all the critical steps to produce crackers. Why is the dough multilaminated before final sheeting/forming?
4. What kind of formula and process modifications would need to be made in order to produce an acceptable 100% whole wheat cracker?
5. How are crackers optimally baked and cooled in continuous operations? How do these operations affect quality?
6. What are the essential packaging requirements for crackers?

10.3 PRODUCTION OF COOKIES

Most cookies are manufactured from soft wheat dough chemical-leavened with baking powder and supplemented with high amounts of sugar and shortening. The cookie dough or batter is extensively baked so most of these products contain limited amounts of moisture and low water activity. Due to the low moisture and rich formulation, cookies are among the foods with the highest energy density and considered as shelf-stable items. The sugar imparts the characteristic sweet flavor and greatly contributes to lower the Aw, whereas the shortening the classic texture (Faridi 1994; Faridi et al. 2000; Manley 1996; Matz 1992).

Compared to bread, cookies are rapidly produced because they do not need fermentation. The general process includes blending dry ingredients, water addition, and dough or batter formation, forming, baking, cooling, and packaging. In contrast to bread making, most formulations are made from short doughs that lack extensibility and elasticity. Wheat flour is the major ingredient, but the quantities of fat and sugar added create a plasticity and cohesiveness with minimal gluten formation. Other important change is in terms of water absorption level. Cookie doughs are usually hydrated with relatively low amounts of water and mixing or kneading is minimized. In fact, many processes have two mixing stages, one to cream up the sugar with fat, milk, and eggs followed by the second where the flour is added. During creaming, the ingredients emulsify and air is trapped. Other cookie-manufacturing processes such as sheeting and forming demand slightly higher protein flour and gluten development. These doughs are generally hydrated with more water and mixed to achieve gluten formation. Most mixers used by the cookie industry are batch. The most popular is the horizontal mixer that is usually positioned above the hoppers so the dough is dropped aided by gravity. The different sorts of cookies are classified according to the forming/molding equipment into rotary mold, sheeting/forming, deposit, and wire-cut. Wafers are produced from a batter that is processed and baked on a couple of baking plates commonly known as books (Manley 1996; Matz 1992).

The extruding and depositing equipments are forming machines capable of extruding doughs ranging in consistency from extremely soft to stiff. Most equipments basically consist of a hopper over a system of two or three smooth or grooved rolls that force the soft, smooth, and almost pourable dough into a pressure balancing chamber underneath equipped with a set of piping nozzles. These nozzles are usually cone-shaped and may have patterned ends to give strong relief of the extruded dough. Individual deposits are achieved by raising and lowering the oven conveyor to coincide with intermittent extrusion. The intermittent action may be achieved by activating the feed rollers briefly to push the desired amount of dough through the nozzles and then stopping the rollers while the deposit is completed and the depositing device returned to its original position (Manley 1996, 1998; Matz 1992).

Nearly all cookies formed with these equipments are baked on metal wire mesh bands or traveling ovens. This means that oven conditions such as temperature, movement, and humidity changes during the course of baking. Oven-dwell times range from only a couple to 15 minutes depending on the sort of cookie and oven conditions. During baking, the cookie develops a less dense and open porous structure, the moisture level decreases to 1% to 4% and there are significant changes in surface coloration and flavor development. Chemically the starch gelatinizes, the gluten denatures, the sugar and fat reduce consistency, and setting occurs.

Sugar wafers have unique manufacturing processes, because instead of a dough, a batter is used. The production line yields low density lids that are generally filled with a cream consisting of a mixture of sugar and shortening. Wafers are produced from flour, sweeteners, chemical leavening agents, and colorants mixed with high amounts of water so a batter is obtained. From the mixing tanks the batter with a certain viscosity is first pumped to a supply tank and later dispensed by an accurate metering device onto a couple of metallic wafer plates in the oven. After a certain oven-dwell time, the baked wafer sheets are removed from the plates by takeoff units, and then positioned on a conveyor that feeds the wafer building unit. The cream is continuously deposited as the wafers are being carried under the spreader by a moving belt. The built up large wafer sandwich are passed through a pressing unit and then through a cooling tunnel to a collator in preparation for cutting. The large wafer sandwich is cut with either wire cutters or rotary saws into the desired finished product size (Manley 1996; Matz 1992).

After baking, the cookies have to cool in preparation for packaging. During cooling and equilibration, the cookies keep losing significant amounts of moisture and some types become more rigid. Low-moisture cookies are especially prone to checking or crack formation and breaking during handling and storage. These cracks are the result of stress that develops as the product cools down too fast and the dimensional changes associated with equilibration of moisture within the structure. The cooling time can be controlled by the conveyor velocity and varies among cookies but normally averages from 20 to 25 minutes (Manley 1996).

The most relevant quality tests for cookie flours are the alkaline water retention (Yamasaki 1953) and spread factor assays. The spread factor method (AACC 2000, Method 10-50D) determines the height and diameter of cookies baked following a standard recipe and laboratory manufacturing procedure. The average height or thickness and diameter are measured, respectively, by overlapping and by placing side to side six cookies. The ratio diameter (W)/thickness (T) multiplied by 10 yields the uncorrected spread factor, which is corrected according to altitude or atmospheric pressure. The best quality flours for cookies have high spread factor values.

10.3.1 SPREAD FACTOR

The spread factor functionality test is the most important for soft wheat flours destined for cookies. The spread factor method determines the height and diameter of cookies baked following a standard formula and procedure. Briefly, the test flour (225 g 14% moisture) is blended with fixed amounts of shortening, sugar, salt, sodium bicarbonate, dextrose, and distilled water to produce a dough that is first divided into six equal portions and then sheeted under standard conditions (7 mm height). The dough sheet is cut with a round die (60 mm diameter). The dough discs are baked for 10 minutes at 204°C and allowed to cool down at ambient temperature for 30 minutes. The average height or thickness and diameter are measured, respectively, by overlapping and by placing side to side six cookies. The ratio diameter (W)/thickness (T) multiplied by 10 yields the uncorrected spread factor, which is corrected according to altitude or atmospheric pressure. The best quality flours for cookies have high spread factor values. Generally, the flour protein content is closely related to the average diameter and height. Soft wheat flours, due to the low protein and gluten strength, yield cookies with higher diameter and low height. In addition for flour screening, the test can help processors to decide the type and amount of chlorination and reducing and oxidizing agents required to produce uniform products.

10.3.1.1 Spread Factor Assay (AACC 2000, Method 10-50D)

A. *Samples, Ingredients, and Reagents*
- Refer to Table 10.2

B. *Materials and Equipments*
- Digital scale
- Graduated cylinder (100 mL)
- Pipette (5 mL)
- Spatula
- Hand mixer with flat beaters
- Sieve (1.12 mm)
- Roller cylinder
- Sheeting device
- Round die (60 mm diameter)
- Baking sheets

TABLE 10.2

Recipe Recommended for the Production of Spread Factor Cookies

Ingredients	Amount (g)
Cream	
Shortening	64.0
Sugar (granulated fine)	130.0
Salt	2.1
Sodium bicarbonate	2.5
Dextrose solution[a]	33.0
Water[b]	Refer to Table 10.3
Flour[b]	Refer to Table 10.3

[a] Blend 8.9 g dextrose in 150 mL distilled water.

[b] The amounts of water and flour will vary according to the flour moisture content (Table 10.3).

- Microdough mixer
- Baking oven
- Laboratory clock
- Ruler with mm markings
- Heat-resistant protective gloves

C. *Procedure*

1. With an electric hand mixer equipped with flat beaters, cream the shortening, sugar, salt, and sodium bicarbonate at low speed for 3 minutes. Stop the mixer every minute in order to reincor-porate cream that adhered to the blending bowl (Figure 10.2).

2. Add the dextrose solution and distilled water. Blend for 1 minute at low speed and make sure to reincorporate ingredients adhered to the sides. Add the wheat flour and mix at low speed for 2 minutes.

3. Divide the dough into six equal parts and then sheet each to a constant thickness using the roller cylinder and sheeting device that yields 7-mm-thick pieces of dough. Cut the dough sheet with the round die in order to obtain the 60-mm-diameter and 7-mm-thick piece of dough (Figure 10.2).

4. Place round forms on a greased metallic baking sheet in preparation for baking.

5. Bake cookies at 204°C for exactly 10 minutes.

6. Wearing protective gloves, remove baking sheet from the oven. With the spatula, carefully remove cookies from the baking sheet and allow then to cool down at room temperature for 20 minutes. After cooling, place side to side all the cookies and measure the total length. Overlap he cookies in order to determine total height. Divide the total length and height by the number of cookies (Figure 10.2).

7. Calculate the uncorrected spread factor using the following equation: spread factor = (average diameter/mm thick thickness or height) × 10.

TABLE 10.3

Effect of Flour Moisture on the Recommended Amounts of Wheat Flour and Water Required to Standardize the Spread Factor Test

Flour Moisture Content (%)	Distilled Water (mL)	Amount of Flour (g)	Flour Moisture Content (%)	Distilled Water (mL)	Amount of Flour (g)
9.0	28.4	212.6	12.0	21.1	219.9
9.2	27.9	213.1	12.2	20.6	220.4
9.4	27.4	213.6	12.4	20.1	220.9
9.6	27.0	214.0	12.6	19.6	221.4
9.8	26.5	214.5	12.8	19.1	221.9
10.0	26.0	215.0	13.0	18.6	222.4
10.2	25.5	215.5	13.2	18.1	222.9
10.4	25.0	216.0	13.4	17.6	223.4
10.6	24.6	216.4	13.6	17.1	223.9
10.8	24.1	216.9	13.8	16.5	224.5
11.0	23.6	217.4	14.0	16.0	225.0
11.2	23.1	217.9	14.2	15.5	225.5
11.4	22.6	218.4	14.4	15.0	226.0
11.6	22.1	218.9	14.6	14.6	226.5
11.8	21.6	219.4	14.8	14.1	227.0

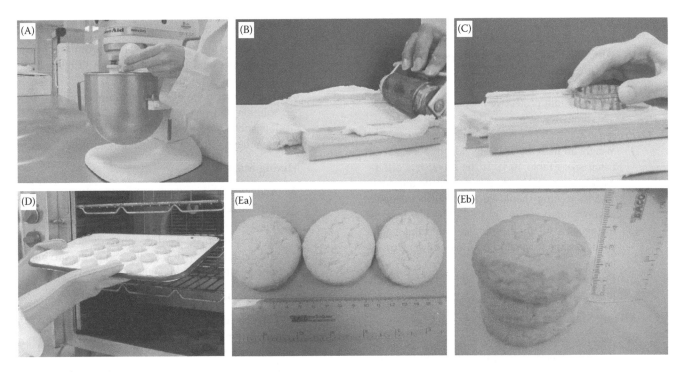

FIGURE 10.2 Sequential steps followed to perform the cookie spread factor test. (A) Creaming and dough mixing; (B) sheeting; (C) die-cutting; (D) baking; and (E) evaluation of average cookie diameter (Ea) and height (Eb).

8. Correct spread factor values according to the altitude or atmospheric pressure using the table detailed in the official AACC (2000) method 10-50D.

10.3.2 Rotary-Molded Cookies

The rotary mold is the simplest and more economical way to produce cookies. The dough is forced through a couple of rolls, one known as forcing and the other as former. The forming roll has molds to form the desired shape of the dough pieces. The dough is forced into molds that are the negative shape of the dough pieces complete with patterns, name, type, and docker holes. Bearing on the forming roll is a blade or steel known as scrapper (Manley 1996, 1998). The rotary mold dough to is formed with a limited amount of water (<20%) and high shortening so the formed piece of dough is adhered to a canvas conveyor and released from the mold, followed to a band transition where is dropped by gravity to the conveying belt that feeds the oven.

10.3.2.1 Production of Rotary-Molded Cookies

A. Samples, Ingredients, and Reagents
- Refer to Table 10.4

B. Materials and Equipments
- Digital scale
- Large bowls
- Small bowls
- Spatula
- Large spoon
- Hand-held flour sifter
- Graduated cylinder
- Chocolate mold

TABLE 10.4
Formulation Recommended for the Production of Rotary-Molded Cookies

Ingredients	Bakers Formulation (%)
Stage 1	
Granulated sugar	23.21
Salt	1.61
Vegetable shortening or butter	21.43
Soy lecithin	0.36
Vanilla extract	0.36
Sodium stearoyl-2-lactylate	0.54
Cocoa powder (sifted)	8.93
Molasses	7.14
Stage 2	
Water	13.57
Ammonium bicarbonate	0.54
Stage 3	
Soft wheat flour	100.00
Sodium bicarbonate	0.71
Sodium acid pyrophosphate	0.18

- Wooden roller
- Dough mixer with flat beaters
- Perforated baking sheets or trays
- Baking oven
- Chronometer
- Heat-resistant protective gloves
- Thermometer

C. *Procedure*

1. Weight all ingredients independently for a 1.5-kg batch size (Table 10.4). If the mixer has different capacity, the batch size should be adjusted. The shortening should be tempered beforehand at room temperature (18°C–25°C). The leavening agents (sodium bicarbonate and sodium acid pyrophosphate) should be sifted and be free of lumps.
2. Preheat the baking oven at 160°C before dough mixing and preparation.

Mixing Stage 1 (Creaming)

3. Add the granulated sugar, salt, vegetable shortening, soy lecithin, vanilla extract, SSL, cocoa powder, and molasses in the mixing bowl.
4. Mix for 1 minute at low speed using the flat beater. After the first minute, stop the mixer and scrape the bowl to make sure all the shortening is incorporated. Mix for one additional minute at high speed. At the end of mixing, the dough should be homogeneous. If lumps remain in the blend, mix for one extra minute until all lumps disappear (Figure 10.3).

Mixing Stage 2

5. Use part of the water to dissolve the ammonium bicarbonate and make sure the resulting solution is free of lumps.
6. Then slowly add the ammonium bicarbonate solution and rest of the water while mixing at low speed for 1 minute. Water may need adjustment depending on the type of flour used.

Mixing Stage 3

7. Add the soft wheat flour, sodium bicarbonate, and start mixer and then add the sodium pyrophosphate. Mix for 30 more seconds. Avoid overmixing because overmixed doughs produce harder and deformed cookies. At the end of the mixing schedule, the dough should look dry and crumbly.

Cookie Forming and Baking

8. Place the dough inside the mold and press it first with your fingers and then with the roller pin (Figure 10.3).
9. Release the cookie from the mold, you may use pressurized air in one end of the cookie or tap on the back of the mold.
10. Place cookies preferably on a perforated baking sheet in preparation for baking.
11. Place baking sheet with cookies in the oven for 6 minutes. Wearing heat resistant gloves, turn the tray 180° to assure an evenly heat treatment. Bake the cookies for 5 additional minutes.

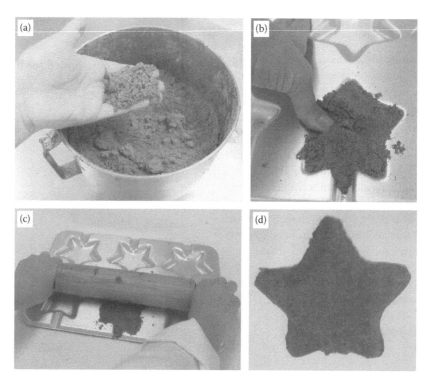

FIGURE 10.3 Sequential steps for the production of rotary molded chocolate flavored cookies. (a) Crumbly dough characteristic of rotary cut cookies; (b) manual pressing of dough into a star-shaped mold; (c) further roller-pressing of dough; and (d) baked cookie.

12. Remove baking sheet with baked cookies from the oven and allow tray to cool down for 5 minutes. Then, remove cookies from baking sheet and allow them to further cool down in preparation for packaging.

13. Determine the yield, the weight of 10 cookies and their average moisture content (2.5–3.5). Evaluate the cookie shape, texture, color, and flavor.

10.3.3 SHEETED AND FORMED COOKIES

The sheeting and forming equipment is one of the most popular systems to manufacture cookies. This universal equipment sheets, compacts, and gauges the dough into a sheet of even thickness and width before cutting. The principle is to progressively sheet the dough to the desired thickness using several pairs of gauging rolls. These systems are capable of producing multilayered cookies because most are provided with a lapper. The dough sheet is usually cut with a rotating interchangeable roll or cutter. Flours used for production of cookies in this system usually contain more protein and require more water to produce fully developed and slack doughs. Doughs are mixed to develop the gluten network capable of producing upon gradual sheeting 2-mm-thick sheets (Faridi 1994; Faridi et al. 2000; Manley 1996, 1998; Matz 1992).

10.3.3.1 Production of Sheeted and Formed Cookies

A. *Samples, Ingredients, and Reagents*
- Refer to Table 10.5
- Eggs
- Whole milk

B. *Materials and Equipments*
- Digital scale
- Graduated cylinder
- Electric hand mixer with beaters

TABLE 10.5
Formulation Recommended for the Production of Sugar Cookies Produced with Sheeting-Forming Equipments

Ingredients	%
All-purpose wheat flour	100.0
Water	54.0
White sugar	20.0
Corn syrup	8.0
Shortening	6.5
Double-acting baking powder	1.5
Nonfat dry milk	1.0
Salt	1.0
Vanilla flavoring	0.5
Lecithin	0.3
Sodium stearoyl-2-lactylate	0.2

- Brush for egg wash application
- Spatula
- Dough mixer with hook attachment
- Sheeting rolls
- Wooden roller pin
- Round die (6 cm diameter)
- Perforated baking sheets
- Baking oven
- Laboratory clock
- Ruler with mm markings
- Heat-resistant protective gloves

C. *Procedure*
1. Weigh or measure all ingredients listed in Table 10.5. Place ingredients without the water, corn syrup, and vanilla flavoring in a dough bowl and mix for 1 minute at slow speed. Add corn syrup, vanilla flavoring, and water and mix at low speed for 1 minute. Switch mixer speed to medium and mix dough until attaining optimum gluten development (dough looks smooth and lustrous or glossy).

2. Weigh the total dough and allow it to rest for 10 minutes.

3. Dust the dough ball and then sheet it through a 0.79-cm, or 5/16 in., opening. Decrease the dough thickness by passing the sheet of dough through smaller gaps.

4. Place sheet of dough on a dusted surface in preparation for final lamination. Allow sheet of dough to rest for at least 5 minutes.

5. With the wood roller pin, gradually sheet the dough until achieving a thickness of 1.5 mm to 2 mm. Make sure to detach dough from the dusted surface before die cutting.

6. Transfer the sheet of dough to a greased baking sheet and readjust the dough thickness with the roller pin. Cut the round forms with the die cutter. Make sure to optimize the number of cuts and minimize the generation of scrap dough. Remove scrap dough and after allowing dough to relax for 5 minutes repeat steps 3 to 5 to produce additional round configurations.

7. If the die does not have pins to mark the typical holes then perforate the round forms with a metal pin (8 holes evenly distributed 1 cm from the perimeter and 5 additional holes 2 cm from the perimeter.

8. With a brush apply an egg wash coating on the surface of the cookies. With the electric mixer equipped with flat beaters prepare the egg wash by whipping eggs with whole milk (1 egg with 10 mL milk). Make sure that the egg is completely beaten, since otherwise chunks of egg may disturb the surface of the finished cookies.

9. Place baking sheets with the formed dough pieces in a baking oven set at 185°C for 13–15 minutes (Figure 10.4).

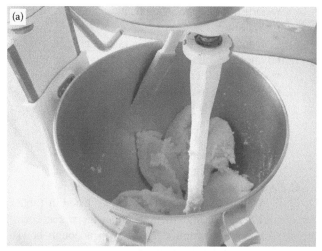

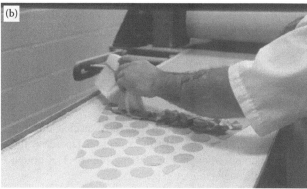

FIGURE 10.4 Sequential steps for the production of sheeted/formed cookies. (a) Dough mixing; and (b) sheeting and forming.

baking oven. This lets the cookies freely spread and rise to give the special texture and flavor.

10.3.4.1 Production of Wire-Cut Cookies
A. *Samples, Ingredients, and Reagents*
- Refer to Table 10.6

B. *Materials and Equipments*
- Digital scale
- Large bowls
- Small bowls
- Spatula
- Large spoon
- Hand-held flour sifter
- Graduated cylinder
- Metal cylinder and wire holder
- Dough mixer with flat beaters
- Baking sheets or trays
- Baking oven
- Chronometer
- Thermometer
- Heat-resistant protective gloves

C. *Procedure*
1. Weight all the ingredients independently listed in Table 10.6 for a 1.5-kg batch size. If the mixer has different capacity, the batch size should be adjusted. The shortening should be tempered beforehand at room temperature (18°C–25°C). The leavening agents (sodium bicarbonate and sodium acid pyrophosphate) should be sifted and be free of lumps. Keep chocolate chips in the refrigerator to avoid melting.
2. Preheat the baking oven at 160°C before dough mixing and preparation.

10. Remove baking sheets with sugar cookies from the oven. After 5 minutes, detach cookies and place them on the counter for 10 minutes cooling. Calculate the average thickness and diameter of the sugar cookies by overlapping and placing side to side 5 cookies. Compare diameters and heights of the cookies before and after baking. Weigh the cookies and calculate yield based on the original formulation.
11. Place cookies in sealed moisture proof bags. Reserve some sugar cookies for moisture, color, texture, shelf life, and organoleptic evaluations.

10.3.4   WIRE-CUT COOKIES

The process of making wire-cut cookies is unique because the dough is soft in consistency for optimum wire cutting. These cookies are normally produced with high-fat and sugar doughs that are extruded and forced through dies and cut with an oscillating wire positioned underneath the set of dies or nozzles (Manley 1996, 1998; Matz 1992). The dough pieces fall on a conveyor that feeds the baking oven infrared

TABLE 10.6
Formulation Recommended for the Production of Wire-Cut Chocolate Chip Cookies

Ingredients	Bakers Formulation (%)
Stage 1	
Granulated sugar	57.80
Salt	1.20
Vegetable shortening or butter	29.60
Soy lecithin	1.00
Vanilla extract	0.20
Stage 2	
Pasteurized liquid egg	7.40
Water	21.00
Stage 3	
Soft wheat flour	100.00
Double-acting baking powder	2.70
Chocolate chips	25.90

Mixing Stage 1 (Creaming)

3. Add the granulated sugar, salt, vegetable shortening, soy lecithin, and vanilla extract in the mixing bowl.

4. Mix for 1 minute at low speed using the flat beater. After the first minute, stop the mixer and scrape the bowl to make sure all the shortening is incorporated. Mix for one additional minute at high speed. At the end of mixing, the dough should be homogeneous. If lumps remain in the blend, mix for one extra minute until all lumps disappear (Figure 10.5).

Mixing Stage 2

5. Add liquid egg and water tempered at room temperature and continue mixing at low speed for 1 minute.

Mixing Stage 3

6. Add the soft wheat flour and double-acting baking powder, and start mixer and mix for 30 seconds. Then incorporate the refrigerated chocolate chips and keep mixing for 20 to 30 seconds. Avoid overmixing because overworked doughs produce harder and deformed cookies and will break chocolate chips.

Cookie Forming and Baking

7. Place the dough inside the die making sure it is evenly distributed across the forming die.

8. Slowly start to press the dough from the wider end of the die so it comes out smoothly from the other end (Figure 10.5). Once the dough is evenly out of the smaller end and with the desired thickness, cut the dough with the wire.

9. Make individual cookies of the same weight and thickness to ensure even baking.

10. Place dough pieces on a baking sheet in preparation for baking. Make sure the round dough pieces are separated at least 2.5 cm in order to make sufficient room for spreading during baking.

11. Place baking sheet with wire-cut cookies in the oven for 6 minutes. Wearing heat-resistant gloves, turn the tray 180° to assure an evenly heat treatment. Bake the cookies for 5 additional minutes.

12. Remove baking sheet with cookies from the oven and allow tray to cool down for 5 minutes. Then, remove cookies from baking sheet and allow them to further cool down in preparation for packaging.

13. Determine the yield, the weight of 10 cookies and their average thickness, height, and

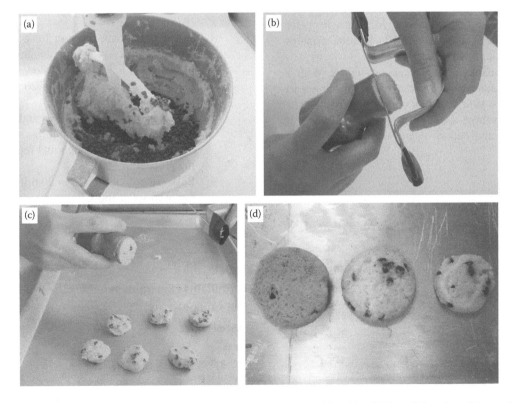

FIGURE 10.5 Sequential steps for the production of wire-cut chocolate chip cookies. (a) Addition of chocolate chips at the end of dough mixing; (b) wire-cutting of dough; (c) wire-cut dough pieces prior to baking; and (d) wire-cut cookies (from right to left, unbaked, external, and internal surfaces of baked cookie).

moisture content. In addition, evaluate texture, color, and flavor.

10.3.5 OTHER SWEET COOKIES

10.3.5.1 Production of Chocolate-Chip Cookies

A. *Samples, Ingredients, and Reagents*
- Refer to Table 10.7

B. *Materials and Equipments*
- Digital scale
- Graduated cylinder
- Spatula
- Hand-held flour sifter
- Electric hand mixer with flat beater
- Dough mixer with hook attachment
- Baking sheets
- Baking oven
- Chronometer
- Heat-resistant protective gloves
- Large spoon
- Thermometer
- Ruler with mm markings

C. *Procedure*
1. Weigh ingredients listed in Table 10.7. Sift the soft wheat flour with a hand-held flour sifter.
2. Place butter and sugar in the blending bowl and cream at medium speed for at least 2 minutes. Then, add eggs and continue blending for 2 additional minutes.
3. Place all ingredients except the chocolate chips in a bowl for dough mixing. Mix ingredients for 1 minute at slow speed and 2 additional minutes at medium speed.
4. Stop mixer and add chocolate chips. With a spoon manually blend chocolate chips or restart mixer at slow speed for only 15 seconds.
5. With a large spoon, grab portions of 35 g of dough and deposit them on a greased baking

sheet. Make sure to leave adequate space among dough portions.
6. Bake at 190°C for approximately 12 minutes.
7. Remove baking sheets with chocolate chip cookies from the oven and allow to cool down for 5 minutes.
8. With a spatula, carefully remove cookies from the baking sheet and cool them for 20 minutes. Weigh cookies and determine yield based on the original formulation. Measure the average diameter and height of the cookies.
9. Place cookies in sealed moisture proof bags. Reserve some cookies for moisture, color, texture, shelf life, and organoleptic evaluations.

10.3.5.2 Production of Oat Cookies

A. *Samples, Ingredients, and Reagents*
- Refer to Table 10.8

B. *Materials and Equipments*
- Digital scale
- Wooden roller pin
- Round die (6 cm diameter)
- Dough mixer with hook attachment
- Baking sheets
- Baking oven
- Refrigerator
- Spatula
- Chronometer
- Heat-resistant protective gloves
- Ruler

C. *Procedure*
1. Weigh ingredients listed in Table 10.8. Place all ingredients in a bowl for dough mixing. Mix ingredients for 3 minutes at slow speed.
2. Place the resulting dough for 20 to 30 minutes in a refrigerator (5°C).
3. With a roller pin, sheet the dough in a greased baking pan. Cut the round forms with the round die. Remove scrap dough and repeat the forming procedure.
4. Bake oat cookies for 15 to 20 minutes in a baking oven set at 160°C.

TABLE 10.7

Formulation Recommended for the Production of Chocolate-Chip Cookies

Ingredients	%
Soft wheat flour	100.0
Chocolate chips	84.8
White sugar	68.3
Butter	57.1
Eggs	39.1
Brown sugar	34.1
Water	1.6
Double-acting baking powder	1.0
Vanilla	0.9
Salt	0.5

TABLE 10.8

Formulation Recommended for the Production of Oat Cookies

Ingredients	%
Oat flour	100.0
Brown sugar	61.5
Vegetable oil	61.5
Ground cinnamon	1.5
Egg	31.0
Salt	1.0

5. Remove baking sheets with oat cookies from the oven and allow cooling down for 5 minutes.

6. With a spatula carefully remove cookies from the baking sheet and allow them to equilibrate at room temperature for 20 minutes. Weigh cookies and determine yield based on the original formulation. Measure the average diameter and height of the cookies.

7. Place cookies in sealed moisture proof bags. Reserve some cookies for moisture, color, texture, shelf life, and organoleptic evaluations.

10.3.5.3 Oat-Chocolate Bars

A. *Ingredients and Reagents*
- Refer to Table 10.9

B. *Materials and Equipments*
- Digital scale
- Spatula
- Electric hand mixer with flat beaters
- Wooden roller pin
- Sheeting rolls
- Baking sheets
- Dough mixer
- Knife
- Baking oven
- Chronometer
- Ruler with mm markings
- Heat-resistant protective gloves

C. *Procedure*
1. Weigh independently ingredients listed in Table 10.9. With an electric mixer equipped with regular flat beaters, cream the butter and sugar at low speed for 3 minutes. Stop the blender every minute in order to reincorporate cream that adhered to the blending bowl. Then add the vanilla flavoring and blend for 15 seconds.

2. In a mixing bowl, blend the cream with the water, flour, cocoa, baking powder, and salt.

TABLE 10.9

Recommended Formulation for the Production of Oat-Chocolate Bars

Ingredients	%
All-purpose wheat flour	100.0
Unsweetened chocolate chips	136.4
Oat meal	118.2
Brown sugar	91.0
Butter	81.8
Water	36.4
Cocoa	4.5
Vanilla	1.8
Double-acting baking powder	1.8
Salt	0.9

After dough mixing, incorporate first the oat meal and then the chocolate chips.

3. With a roller pin laminate the resulting dough into a 25-cm-long × 25-cm-wide × 1-cm-thick piece of dough. With a knife, cut the scrap dough, then cut 5 cm × 2.5-cm bars.

4. Place the bars on previously greased baking pans.

5. Bake for 25 to 30 minutes at 190°C.

6. Remove baking sheets with bars from the oven and allow to cool down for 5 minutes.

7. With a spatula carefully remove bars from the baking sheet and allow them to equilibrate at room temperature for 20 minutes. Weigh cookies and determine yield based on the original formulation. Measure the average length, width, and thickness of bars.

8. Place cookie bars in sealed moisture proof bags. Reserve some cookies for moisture, color, texture, shelf-life, and organoleptic evaluations.

10.3.6 RESEARCH SUGGESTIONS

1. Compare wire-cut cookies produced with different amounts of powdered vs. granulated sugar. Determine differences in average height and diameter, texture, and color.

2. Compare sheeted-formed cookies elaborated with different amounts of wheat bran ground to different particle sizes and inulin or fructoligosaccharides. Optimize formulations in terms of water absorption and determine cookie texture and the organoleptic properties of the cookies.

3. Compare wire-cut cookies produced with half the amount of the shortening and supplemented with extra amounts of emulsifiers (lecithin and SSL). Compare the texture, properties, flavor, and overall organoleptic properties.

4. Compare wire-cut cookies produced with a soft wheat flour and a hard wheat flour. Compare the spread factor, texture, properties, flavor, and overall organoleptic properties.

5. Substitute 50% of the soft wheat flour with 50% oat flour and produce a sheeted-formed cookie. Adjust water absorption and compare properties of the resulting cookies in terms of color, texture, flavor, and chemical-nutritional composition.

6. Produce and compare a regular sheeted-formed cookie with a whole grain counterpart. Remember that the whole grain should contain bran, germ, and even aleurone at the same level commonly observed in the whole grain. Determine the necessary changes in terms of formulation, water absorption, and processing and then compare properties of the resulting cookies especially in terms of color, texture, and organoleptic properties.

10.3.7 Research Questions

1. Define the following terms:
   a. Short dough
   b. Elastic dough
   c. Trans-free shortening
   d. Cookie checking
2. In a table list five industrial technologies to produce cookies indicating differences in formulation and kind of commercial products obtained from each processing line.
3. What are the principles of the spread factor test? Compare the spread factor test of a soft, soft-chlorinated, and all purpose flours.
4. What are differences in color and flavor between a cookie produced with a glucose syrup and a 90 high-fructose corn syrup?
5. Why almost all cookie formulations do not contain antimold agents?
6. What is the common shelf-life of cookies? What are the most common packaging materials used to extend shelf-life?
7. Which cookie technology would you choose to develop a lower fat product?
8. Investigate the ideal processing line to manufacture a filled sandwich cookie. What are the most common ingredients used to produce fillings?
9. What would you expect to happen to the texture of cookies filled with a fruit jelly during the expected shelf life?
10. Describe the general procedure to manufacture filled wafers. What are the most important ingredients and processing steps of this technology?
11. Investigate the possible use of coextrusion to produce a fruit bar.
12. Investigate the types of oven bands and their main uses in the cookie industry.

10.4 PRODUCTION OF BISCUITS, MUFFINS, CHEMICAL-LEAVENED DONUTS, AND CAKES

10.4.1 Biscuits

The term *biscuit* is completely different for people living in the United States or Commonwealth Nations. In the United States, it relates to a small soft chemical-leavened bread, whereas in Commonwealth English countries is used to refer a hard cookie or a cracker. In this book, biscuits refer to the chemically leavened soft bread product.

Regular biscuits are produced from soft wheat flour, baking powder, sugar, fats, and other ingredients. The dough is usually sheeted and then cut with a round die, placed on baking pans, egg washed, and baked.

Cornbread is a generic name for a quick cornmeal-based biscuit leavened with baking powder or chemical leavening agents. This biscuit is widely consumed in the United States,

particularly in the South and Southwest. In rural areas of the southern United States, it was a traditional staple for populations where wheat bread was prohibitively expensive. Today it is produced as a common side dish often served with eggs and fried chicken. There are many formulations and types that differ in volume, apparent density, texture, and flavor. Most formulations are based in a mixture of wheat flour and yellow or white maize meal or flour, baking powder, shortening/lard, and other ingredients that improve texture and flavor. The functional gluten of the wheat flour allows the production of more aerated breads whereas maize flour imparts the characteristic flavor. These ingredients are blended with water to obtain dough that is processed similar to regular biscuits.

10.4.1.1 Production of Biscuits and Cornbread

A. *Samples, Ingredients, and Reagents*
   - Refer to Table 10.10
   - Eggs
   - Whole milk

B. *Materials and Equipments*
   - Digital scale
   - Spatula
   - Electric hand mixer with flat beaters
   - Wooden roller pin
   - Sheeting rolls
   - Baking sheets
   - Dough mixer with hook attachment
   - Round die (6 cm to 8 cm diameter)
   - Electric hand mixer with flat beaters
   - Brush for egg wash application
   - Baking oven
   - Laboratory clock
   - Heat-resistant protective gloves
   - Ruler with mm markings

C. *Procedure*
   1. Weigh ingredients listed in Table 10.10. Place dry ingredients in a bowl for 1 minute blending with the hook attachment. Then add eggs and water and mix the dough for 3 minute at slow speed (Figure 10.6).

TABLE 10.10

Recommended Formulation for the Production of American Regular and Corn Biscuits

Ingredients	Regular (%)	Cornbread (%)
All-purpose wheat flour	100.0	50.0
Refined corn meal or flour	–	50.0
Water	60.0	50.0
Nonfat dry milk	7.2	10.0
Shortening	14.4	15.0
Sugar	14.4	20.0
Eggs	7.2	15.0
Double-acting baking powder	5.4	2.5
Salt	1.0	1.0

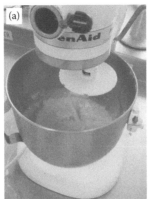
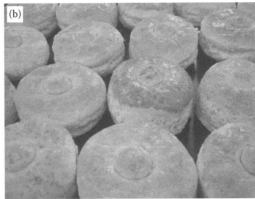

FIGURE 10.6 Sequential steps for the production of biscuits. (a) Dough mixing and (b) baked biscuits.

2. Place the resulting dough for 15 minutes resting on the counter.
3. With a roller pin sheet the dough to 1.5 cm and then cut the round forms with the round die. Remove scrap dough and repeat the forming procedure.
4. Place pieces of formed dough on a greased baking sheet and rest for at least 5 minutes before baking.
5. With a brush, apply an egg wash coating onto the surface of the biscuits (Figure 10.6). With the hand mixer equipped with flat beaters prepare the egg wash by whipping eggs with whole milk (1 egg with 10 mL milk). Make sure that the egg is completely beaten, otherwise chunks of egg may disturb the surface of the finished cookies.
6. Allow egg wash biscuits to rest for at least 10 minutes before baking. Measure the average diameter and height of the biscuits immediately before baking.
7. Bake biscuits for 12–15 minutes in a baking oven set at 185°C.
8. With protective gloves, remove baking sheets with biscuits from the oven and allow cooling down for 20 minutes (Figure 10.6).
9. With a spatula carefully remove biscuits for weighing and determination of yield based on the original formulation. Measure the average diameter and height of the baked biscuits.
10. Place biscuits in sealed moisture proof bags. Reserve some for moisture, color, texture, and organoleptic evaluations.

10.4.2 MUFFINS

A muffin is defined as the type of bread that is baked in small portions. Many forms are somewhat like small cakes or cupcakes in shape, although they usually are not as sweet as cupcakes and generally lack frosting. Muffins are produced similar to low-ratio cakes, but the batter is placed in small cup-shaped molds before baking (Cross 2007). Most are produced from refined soft wheat flour, although whole wheat muffins and batters supplemented with blueberries, raspberries, date, nuts, chocolate chips, raisings, carrots, and other related products are gaining popularity. As in cakes, the type of flour, double-acting baking powder, and batter consistency greatly affects product characteristics. Muffins are often eaten for breakfast or between meals.

10.4.2.1 Production of Muffins

A. *Samples, Ingredients, and Reagents*
   - Refer to Table 10.11

B. *Materials and Equipments*
   - Digital scale
   - Spatula
   - Electric hand mixer with flat beaters
   - Baking sheets
   - Muffin paper cups
   - Muffin baking pans
   - Baking oven
   - Chronometer
   - Heat-resistant protective gloves
   - Ruler with mm markings

C. *Procedure*
   1. Weigh or measure ingredients listed in Table 10.11. In a container, dissolve the sodium bicarbonate with the water for the wheat based muffins and with the buttermilk for the cornbread muffins. Place shortening, salt, dry milk, molasses, baking powder, and cinnamon in the mixer bowl and beat them for 3 minutes at medium speed (Figure 10.7).
   2. Add approximately half of the eggs and mix for 30 seconds at medium speed. Add the rest of the eggs and mix for 30 additional seconds.
   3. Add the flours (wheat and/or cornmeal) and beat contents gradually adding the mix of water and sodium bicarbonate. Keep beating at medium speed for a total of 5 minutes. If raisins or other

TABLE 10.11
Recommended Formulation for the Production of Muffins

Ingredients	Regular Muffins (%)	Whole Wheat Muffin[a] (%)	Cornbread Muffin (%)
All-purpose flour	100.0	64.8	35.0
Whole wheat flour	–	35.2	–
Corn meal	–	–	65.0
Water	100.0	94.0	
Sugar	37.5	35.3	16.5
Eggs	37.5	35.3	35.0
Shortening	37.5	35.3	20.0
Nonfat dry milk	12.5	11.8	–
Buttermilk	–	–	153
Molasses	12.5	11.8	–
Double-acting baking powder	0.65	0.6	5.0
Sodium bicarbonate	0.25	0.15	1.0
Salt	0.25	0.15	2.0
Ground cinnamon	0.08	0.07	

[a] For production of whole wheat muffins with raisins, add 45 g/100 g flour at the end of the batter-producing process.

coarse flavorings are added, make sure to incorporate them at the end of the process by simply mixing with a spoon.

4. Place muffin paper cups in the muffin baking pan and pour fixed amounts of batter. For a 7-cm-above-diameter muffin cup, add from 38 g to 45 g of batter.
5. Bake muffins for 18 minutes in a baking oven set at 205°C (Figure 10.7).
6. With protective gloves, remove baking pans from the oven and allow cooling down for 20 minutes.
7. Carefully remove muffins for weighing and determination of yield based on the original formulation. Make sure to subtract the paper cup weight. Measure the average height of the baked biscuits.
8. Place muffins in sealed moisture proof bags. Reserve some for moisture, chemical, color, crumb texture, and organoleptic evaluations.

10.4.3 PRODUCTION OF CHEMICAL-LEAVENED OR COFFEE DONUTS

Coffee donuts are classified as chemical-leavened products. Compared to yeast-leavened donuts these are of quick preparation and generally produced from a pourable thick batter. The batter can be baked or fried to produce donuts with different oil contents and organoleptic properties. Chemical-leavened donuts are generally produced from all-purpose wheat flours that are mixed with water, a combination of chemical leavening agents, and other ingredients to yield a batter that is formed into the typical donut configuration for frying. The donuts are generally covered with fine sugar or a combination of sugar and ground cinnamon.

10.4.3.1 Production of Chemical-Leavened Donuts
A. *Samples, Ingredients, and Reagents*
- Refer to Table 10.12
- Partially hydrogenated frying oil

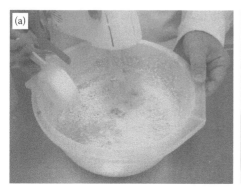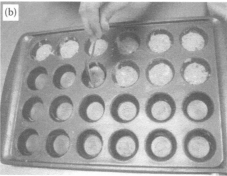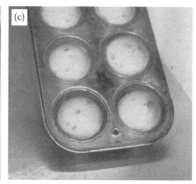

FIGURE 10.7 Sequential steps for the production of muffins. (a) Batter mixing; (b) muffin pan filling; and (c) baked muffins.

TABLE 10.12
Recommended Formulations for the Production of Chemical-Leavened Donuts

Ingredients	Formulation, %	
	A	B
All-purpose wheat flour	100.0	100.0
Water[a]	68.0–72.0	58.0
Sugar	32.0	40.0
Shortening	6.0	–
Butter	–	30.0
Whole egg solids[b]	–	10.0
Egg yolks	8.3	–
Nonfat dry milk	8.3	7.5
Dextrose	2.0	–
Honey	–	4.0
Salt	2.0	1.0
Double-acting baking powder	–	1.8
Sodium acid pyrophosphate	2.0	–
Sodium bicarbonate	1.5	1.3
Ground cinnamon	–	1.0
Ground nutmeg	0.25	0.8
Ground mace	0.15	–
Ground cloves	–	0.2
Vanilla	0.50	–

[a] Adjust water absorption in order to modify the desired viscosity of the batter that varies according to the donut forming machine or depositor.

[b] If fresh eggs are used for formulation B: for 100 g flour and 35.4 g of fresh egg (equivalent to 10 g of egg solids with 8% moisture), reduce water absorption to 33%.

- White powdered sugar
- Ground cinnamon
- Frying oil (partially hydrogenated)

B. Materials and Equipments
- Scale
- Graduated cylinder (100 mL)
- Mixer with regular beaters
- Donut batter depositor
- Baking sheets
- Scraper
- Baking oven
- Deep-fat fryer
- Chronometer
- Thermometer (250°C)
- Heat-resistant protective gloves
- Protective lenses

C. Procedure
1. Weigh individually the ingredients listed in Table 10.12. Place the fat ingredients and the sugar in a mixing bowl and beat contents for 2 minutes at slow speed.
2. Add the flour and keep blending for 5 additional minutes at slow speed. Then, add the rest of the dry ingredients and keep blending for 3 minutes at slow speed.
3. Gradually add the water and mix for 2 minutes at slow speed and then 3 minutes at medium speed. Make sure to scrape solids attached to the sides of the mixing bowl. The resulting batter should be smooth, cohesive, and glossy (Figure 10.8).
4. Place the resulting thick batter in the donut depositor or forming machine. Adjust machine to deliver a certain amount of batter (30 g to

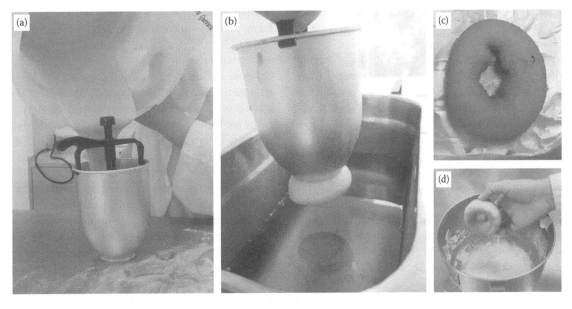

FIGURE 10.8 Sequential steps for the production of donuts. (a) Filling donut batter dispenser; (b) dispensing the batter on the hot oil; (c) fried donuts; and (d) glaced fried donuts with vanilla flavoring.

40 g per donut). After calibrating the depositor machine, weigh the predetermined amount of raw batter. Reserve batter for determination of moisture, fat, and viscosity.

5. For baked donuts, deposit the donuts onto a greased baking pan and allow donuts to proof for 10 minutes. Bake donuts at 185°C for 12 minutes. Determine the average weight, moisture and fat content of the baked donuts.

6. For fried donuts, directly deposit the donut on the frying oil heated to 175°C. Wearing protective gloves and lenses, make sure to deliver the preformed donut batter about 3 to 5 cm above the frying oil (Figure 10.8). Allow donut to fry for 15 seconds on one side, then turn for 15 seconds frying on the other side and then submerge donut in the frying oil for 30 seconds. Remove donut from the fryer and allow donut to drain excess oil for 20 seconds. Determine the average weight, moisture, and fat content of the resulting donuts.

7. Place baked or fried donuts on a bowl containing a mixture of sugar and cinnamon. Determine the average weight of the sugar flavored donuts (Figure 10.8).

8. Determine the average covering of the flavored donuts. Reserve some for moisture, color, texture, and organoleptic evaluations.

9. Compare donuts obtained from the two formulations and two procedures. Place donuts in sealed moisture proof bags.

10.4.4 PRODUCTION OF CAKES AND RELATED PRODUCTS

Cakes and related products are produced from soft wheat flour based batters containing high quantities of sugar and shortening or oils. The starch associated to the batter completely gelatinizes during baking and sets the typical structure. Most cake formulations contain chemical leavening agents, milk solids, emulsifiers, coloring, and flavoring agents. Most wheat flours for cakes are chlorinated after milling in order to bleach and acidify the flour and breakdown disulfide bonds of the gluten structure. Cake flours are usually chlorinated to drop the pH to 4.9 to 5.0. There are two basic categories of cakes: shortened and foam. The most popular shortened cakes also known as pound cakes are made with a batter rich in fat. Foam cakes are made without fat and include angel and sponge cakes. A cake batter is a complex dispersion of foam-oil-water emulsion with air bubbles entrapped in the fat phase. The basic functional ingredients include refined and preferably chlorinated soft wheat flour, water, eggs, shortening or oil, sugar, emulsifiers, and baking powder. Cake making usually includes batter mixing, molding, baking, and cooling. The purpose of the whipping stage is to disperse all ingredients, develop the desired viscosity and to incorporate air into the batter. The type of fat especially in terms of hydrogenation level affects aeration

and cake specific gravity. The emulsifiers aid in the emulsion and improve fat dispersion in the batter. Baking is critically important because it greatly affects volume, appearance, and organoleptic properties. It is generally accepted that the aeration of a cake depends on the expansion of the gases, air, and carbon dioxide if baking powder is used, together with the water vapor pressure. The volume of the cake batter generally increases 3.5 times during baking. During the critical baking step the batter thins and some coalescence of the entrapped bubbles occurs resulting in some loss of gas. The rate of coalescence depends on the batter viscosity and bubble size. The process of coalescence is finally arrested by the thickening of the batter due to starch swelling and to the coagulation of the egg and gluten (Bennion and Bamford 1997; Conforti 2007).

Shortened cakes are divided into two broad categories: high and low ratio. The most popular is the high ratio in which the quantities of sugar is higher than the amount of flour whereas low ratio mixes contain more flour than sugar.

Independent of the type of cake, both cakes are manufactured with refined soft wheat flours mixed with high amounts of water so batters are produced. Due to the high amount of water, the flour starch granules completely gelatinize during baking imparting the typical internal structure. Most cake mixes contain chemical leavening agents and milk solids, flavorings, and emulsifiers that affect texture, color, and flavor and manufactured from chlorinated soft flour. During dough batter mixing, tiny air bubbles are trapped and then enlarged due to the carbon dioxide generated by the baking powder. In almost all cake mixes, double-acting baking powder is used because they release gas during both batter mixing and baking. The egg albumin proteins trap air and improve cake volume and texture. The emulsifiers and tensoactive additives such as propylene glycol lower the aqueous phase surface tension also aiding air incorporation. A good cake batter should have enough viscosity to avoid the settling of denser starch granules that yield defective cakes. High- and low-ratio cakes are usually baked at temperatures of 180°C–190°C for 25 to 35 minutes depending of the size and/or volume.

Sponge or angel cakes differ from high or low ratio cakes because they are very light, almost fluffy, and they do not necessarily contain chemical leavening agents and shortening. These cakes are leavened by trapped air and steam derived from egg whites (Conforti 2007). For this reason, egg whites constitute the most important ingredient. Sugar is the tenderizing agent in substitution of the shortening. The soft wheat flour (regular or chlorinated) is mixed with starch and serves as a vehicle for the incorporation of the other ingredients. The most functional and key ingredient is the egg albumin because this protein traps the air incorporated during batter whipping and retains the air during baking. The addition of emulsifiers such as polyglycerol esters or distilled monoglycerides contributes to cake quality. Benefits include better batter aeration and stability, resulting in a cake with higher volume and better crumb texture. Needless to say, the quality and concentration of the egg albumin is critically important. In addition, angel cakes should be produced by sequentially adding the ingredients in an optimized whipping schedule. Generally, the egg whites are blended with the sugar and tartar cream. This last ingredient reduces the pH and helps to trap air and forms stronger and larger foams. Then, the flour/starch mix is slowly added with the aim of avoiding breaking the foam. Angel cakes are usually baked at a high temperature (190°C–200°C) in ungreased tube style pans, which provide a more efficient heat distribution within the batter that translates into higher expansion rates or cake volume (Conforti 2007).

10.4.4.1 Production of Shortened Low-Ratio Cakes

A. *Samples, Ingredients, and Reagents*
- Refer to Table 10.13
- Wax paper

B. *Materials and Equipments*
- Digital scale
- Hand-held flour sifter
- Graduated cylinder (100 mL)
- Egg yolk separator
- Electric hand mixer with flat beaters
- Round baking pans for cakes
- Baking oven
- Sifter
- Heat-resistant protective gloves
- Scissors
- Ruler for cake evaluation
- Knife for cakes
- Cake volume meter (rapeseed displacement)
- Chronometer

C. *Procedure*
1. Weigh separately ingredients for formulations A or B listed in Table 10.13. Blend the baking powder, salt, and flour and then sift contents with the hand-held sifter.
2. Cream the butter, sugar, and vanilla for 2 minutes on an electric mixer set at medium-high speed. While mixing, gradually pour the egg

and continue mixing until a light and foamy blend is obtained.

3. Add approximately one third of the sifted flour, baking powder, and salt. After stirring the mixture for 30 seconds, add half of the milk and continue blending for 15 more seconds. Then add the second third of the flour mixture and blend for 30 seconds. Add the rest of the milk and blend for 15 seconds and finally add the rest of the flour mixture and blend for 45 seconds.
4. Cut a round piece of wax paper to place it at the bottom of the baking pan. Grease with shortening two round baking pans and then dust with flour. Then place the round piece of wax paper on the bottom of the pan.
5. Tare baking pan and then add exactly 425 g of the batter in preparation for baking.
6. Bake cakes for 25 to 30 minutes in a preheated oven set at 185°C until toothpick inserted in the center comes out clean. In order to prevent the collapsing of the cake, do not open the oven at least during the first 20 minutes of baking.
7. Wearing protective gloves, remove baking pans from the oven.
8. Allow cakes to cool down for 10 minutes. Then carefully remove cakes from baking pans. An adequate way for depanning cakes is first to detach the sides of the cake with a knife, then place a wood or plastic board on top of the cake, turn the pan upside down until the cake detaches and then place other board on the bottom for turning to the right position. Allow cakes to cool down for 30 more minutes. Record the weight of the cake.
9. Evaluate the volume of the cake by rapeseed displacement. The apparatus should be calibrated beforehand. Calculate the apparent density of the cake using the following equation: apparent density = cake weight (g)/cake volume (cm³). With a cake knife, cut the cake through the middle in order to evaluate height at the central and sides. Register measurements with an accuracy of 1 mm. Evaluate subjectively the crumb uniformity and texture.
10. Reserve part of the cake for crust and crumb color, chemical, and sensory evaluations.
11. If desired, a frosting can be prepared beforehand and applied (for frosting formulations refer to Table 10.16).

10.4.4.2 Production of Shortened High-Ratio Cakes

A. *Samples, Ingredients, and Reagents*
- Refer to Table 10.14
- Wax paper

B. *Materials and Equipments*
- Digital scale
- Hand-held flour sifter

TABLE 10.13
Recommended Formulations for the Preparation of Shortened Low-Ratio Cakes

	Formulation A		Formulation B	
Ingredients	g[a]	%	g[a]	%
Soft or chlorinated or cake flour	238.2	100.0	263.0	100.0
White sugar	238.2	100.0	176.2	67.0
Milk	190.4	80.0	210.4	80.0
Butter	88.8	37.3	100.0	38.0
Egg	76.2	32.0	84.2	32.0
Double-acting baking powder	8.6	3.6	9.5	3.6
Vanilla	6.2	2.6	5.3	2.0
Salt	3.1	1.3	1.5	0.6

[a] Amounts required for the production of two cakes.

TABLE 10.14

Recommended Formulations for the Preparation of High-Ratio Cakes

Ingredients	Formulation A		Formulation B	
	g	%	g	%
Soft or chlorinated or cake flour	200.0	100.0	227.0	100.0
White sugar	280.0	140.0	295.0	130.0
Water	162.0	81.0	–	–
Shortening	–	–	113.8	50.0
Milk	–	–	227.0	100.0
Egg whites	150.0	75.0	136.2	60.0
Egg yolk	–	–	11.5	5.0
Butter	100.0	50.0	–	–
Dry milk	24.0	12.0	–	–
Tartar cream	–	–	1.5	0.5
Double-acting baking powder	18.0	9.0	14.4	6.5
Salt	6.0	3.0	7.2	3.0

- Graduated cylinder (100 mL)
- Egg yolk separator
- Electric hand mixer with flat beaters
- Round baking pans for cakes
- Baking oven
- Sifter

- Heat-resistant protective gloves
- Scissors
- Ruler for cake evaluation
- Knife for cakes
- Cake volume meter (rapeseed displacement)
- Chronometer

C. *Procedure*

Formulation A

1. Weigh ingredients for formulation A listed in Table 10.14. Mix all dry ingredients in a bowl and sift them using the hand held flour sifter. Place sifted ingredients in the bowl.
2. Add the butter and approximately 60% of the water and blend at medium speed for 4 minutes.
3. Add the rest of the water and egg whites and mix at low speed for 30 seconds and then at medium speed for 2 minutes.
4. Cut a round piece of wax paper to place it at the bottom of the baking pan. Grease with shortening two round baking pans and then dust with flour. Then place the round piece of wax paper on the bottom of the pan.
5. Tare baking pan and then add exactly 425 g of the batter in preparation for baking.
6. Bake cakes for 30 minutes in a preheated oven set at 190°C (Figure 10.9). In order to prevent the cake from collapsing, do not open

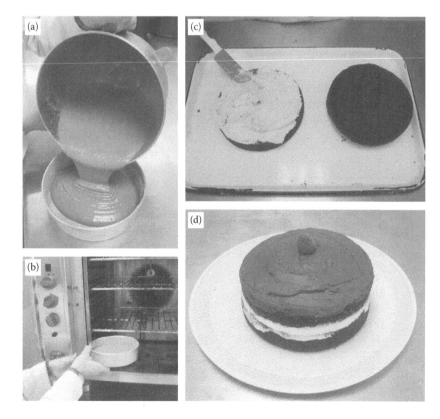

FIGURE 10.9 Sequential steps for the production of high-ratio cake. (a) Filling baking pan; (b) baking; (c) application of frosting; and (d) decorated high-ratio cake.

the oven at least during the first 25 minutes baking.

7. Wearing protective gloves, remove baking pans from the oven.

8. Allow cakes to cool down for 10 minutes. Then, carefully remove cakes from baking pans. An adequate way for depanning cakes is first to detach the sides of the cake with a knife, then place a wood or plastic board on top of the cake, turn the pan upside down until the cake detaches, and then place the other board on the bottom for turning to the right position. Allow cakes to cool down for 20 more minutes. Record the weight of the cake.

9. Evaluate the volume of the cake by rapeseed displacement. The apparatus should be calibrated beforehand. Calculate the apparent density of the cake using the following equation: apparent density = cake weight (g)/cake volume (cm^3). With a cake knife, cut the cake through the middle in order to evaluate height at the central and sides parts. Register measurements with an accuracy of 1 mm. Evaluate subjectively the crumb uniformity and texture (Figure 10.9).

10. Reserve part of the cake for crust and crumb color, chemical, and sensory evaluations.

11. If desired, a frosting can be prepared beforehand and applied (for frosting formulations refer to Table 10.16).

Formulation B

1. Weigh separately ingredients for formulation B listed in Table 10.14. Mix all dry ingredients in a bowl and sift them using the hand held flour sifter. Place sifted ingredients in the bowl.

2. Add the shortening and 60% (136.2 mL) of the milk and blend contents at medium speed for 5 minutes.

3. In other container, blend the rest of the milk, egg whites, and egg yolks. Add approximately half of the milk/egg mix to the batter and mix at low speed for 1 minute.

4. Add the rest of the milk/egg mix and blend at low speed for 1 minute and then 2 more minutes at medium speed.

5. Cut a round piece of wax paper to place it at the bottom of the baking pan. Grease with shortening two round baking pans and then dust with flour. Then place the round piece of wax paper on the bottom of the pan.

6. Tare baking pan and then add exactly 425 g of the batter in preparation for baking.

7. Bake cakes for 30 minutes in a preheated oven set at 190°C. In order to prevent the collapsing of the cake, do not open the oven at least during the first 25 minutes baking.

8. Wearing protective gloves, remove baking pans from the oven.

9. Allow cakes to cool down for 10 minutes. Then, carefully remove cakes from baking pans. An adequate way for depanning cakes is first to detach the sides of the cake with a knife, then place a wood or plastic board on top of the cake, turn the pan upside down until the cake detaches, and then place other board on the bottom for turning to the right position. Allow cakes to cool down for 30 more minutes. Record the weight of the cake.

10. Evaluate the volume of the cake by rapeseed displacement. The apparatus should be calibrated beforehand. Calculate the apparent density of the cake using the following equation: apparent density = cake weight (g)/cake volume (cm^3). With a cake knife, cut the cake through the middle in order to evaluate height at the central and sides. Register measurements with an accuracy of 1 mm. Evaluate subjectively the crumb uniformity and texture.

11. Reserve part of the cake for crust and crumb color, chemical, and sensory evaluations.

12. If desired, a frosting can be prepared beforehand and applied (for frosting formulations refer to Table 10.16).

10.4.4.3 Production of Angel Cakes

A. Samples, Ingredients, and Reagents
- Refer to Table 10.15
- Wax paper

B. Materials and Equipments
- Digital scale
- Hand-held flour sifter
- Graduated cylinder (100 mL)
- Egg yolk separator
- Electric hand mixer with flat beaters
- Baking pans (tube configuration)
- Baking oven

TABLE 10.15

Recommended Formulation for the Preparation of Angel Cakes

Ingredients	Angel Cake Flavored with Maple Syrup	Angel Cake
Egg whites	274.0	230.2
Sugar	171.2	235.0
Chlorinated soft wheat flour	102.7	85.0
Maple syrup	102.7	–
Cream of tartar	3.9	3.4
Salt	3.9	1.0

- Sifter
- Heat-resistant protective gloves
- Scissors
- Ruler for cake evaluation
- Knife for cakes
- Cake volume meter (rapeseed displacement)
- Chronometer

C. *Procedure*

1. Weigh independently ingredients listed in Table 10.15.
2. Place egg whites in the mixing bowl and whip with the electric mixer preferably equipped with whisk beaters until achieving the maximum consistency of the meringue (approximately 5 to 7 minutes at high speed; Figure 10.10).
3. Add maple syrup, cream of tartar, and salt while mixing at medium speed.
4. Lower the hand mixer speed to low and incorporate the flour and sugar and continue mixing for only 20 to 30 seconds. Do not overmix the blend.
5. Weigh and place the batter in an angel cake pan (Figure 10.10).
6. Bake for 40 minutes in a preheated oven set at 160°C (Figure 10.10). Wearing protective gloves, remove baking pan from the oven.
7. Turn baking pan upside down and cool for 30 minutes.
8. Carefully remove cake from baking pan. Record the weight of the angel cake and estimate yield based on the original batter weight.
9. Evaluate the volume of the cake by rapeseed displacement. The apparatus should be calibrated beforehand. Calculate the apparent density of the cake using the following equation: apparent density = cake weight (g)/cake volume (cm^3). With a cake knife, cut the angel cake in order to evaluate height, crumb uniformity, and texture (Figure 10.10). Calculate the apparent density of the cake using the following equation: apparent density = cake weight (g)/cake volume (cm^3).

10. Reserve part of the cake for crust and crumb color, chemical, and sensory evaluations.
11. If desired, a frosting can be prepared beforehand and applied (for frosting formulations refer to Table 10.16).

10.4.5 CAKE FROSTINGS

Frostings or icings complement the flavor, appearance, and overall acceptability of cakes, cupcakes, and related products. In addition, they are used as a way to decorate and increase the image and sales of these products. Frostings are divided into three major categories: plain, creamy or fluffy, and combined. Plain frostings are a sweet sugary mixture that contains powdered sugar, water, syrups, and flavorings. They contain low amounts of fats and oils and yield a relatively dense icing that must be maintained warm (40°C–42°C) in a steamer before its application. The fluffy types are manufactured with shortening, emulsified shortening, and/or butter or margarine, powdered sugar, eggs, dry milk solids, water, and flavorings. These frostings are first creamed and later on eggs are whipped in order to trap air. The water and flavorings are added at the last stage of the process. Needless to say, the quality of the egg is critically important in order to produce the best quality creamed frostings. The combined frostings use the ingredients and principles previously described for plain and creamed frostings (Sultan 1983).

There are other types of frostings, both thick and thin, cooked and uncooked, starting with a simple mixture of powdered sugar and water to beating hot sugar syrup into stiffly beaten egg whites, cooling, and then beating in softened butter to make what is called an Italian butter cream. What is important in deciding what type of frosting to use is to match the icing to the baked good. That is, the icing should complement the flavors and texture of the dessert being frosted. For example, a cinnamon roll is flavored with a simple icing of powdered sugar and milk. A butter cream icing will perfectly complement a butter cake whereas a white butter cake is filled with white butter cream frosting.

A meringue is commonly used as cake frosting. It is made from whipped egg whites, sugar, cream of tartar, and

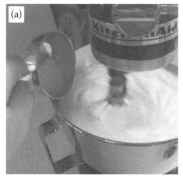
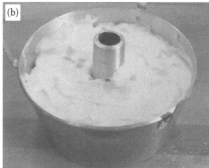
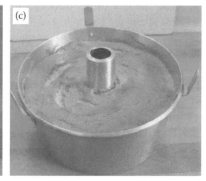

FIGURE 10.10 Sequential steps for the production of angel cake. (a) Beating egg whites with the whisk attachment to obtain the meringue; (b) placing the angel cake batter in the baking pan; and (c) baked angel cake.

cornstarch. Meringues are often flavored with vanilla and a small amount of almond or coconut extract.

It is very important that the frosting be the proper consistency so it spreads easily over the baked goods, yet at the same time adheres to the surface. Frostings should be applied when the baked goods equilibrate to room temperature. Otherwise, the frosting will or become too thin and run. Also, be sure to remove all loose crumbs from the baked good before icing to ensure a smooth finish. Some soft cakes benefit from first covering the cake with a very thin layer of icing, commonly known as crumb coat, letting it dry, and then frosting.

10.4.5.1 Production of Different Types of Frostings
A. Samples, Ingredients, and Reagents
- Refer to Table 10.16

B. Materials and Equipments
- Digital scale
- Electric hand mixer with regular and whisk beaters
- Steamer
- Spatula
- Egg yolk separator
- Hot-plate or stove
- Thermometer
- Hand-held flour sifter

C. Procedure
Royal or Wedding Cake Frosting

1. Weigh ingredients for royal frosting listed in Table 10.16. Sift the powdered sugar with a hand sifter.
2. In the bowl of the electric mixer beat the egg whites with the lemon juice until combined.

Add the vanilla flavoring and continue beating for few seconds.
3. Add the sifted powdered sugar and continue mixing on low speed until attaining a smooth and firm consistency.
4. Transfer the icing to an airtight container because this frosting hardens when exposed to air.

Egg-Vanilla Frosting

1. Weigh ingredients for egg-vanilla frosting listed in Table 10.16. Mix the water, sugar, syrup, and vanilla extract and bring contents to the boil. Avoid overcooking.
2. Place egg whites in the mixing bowl for whipping. Whip egg whites until attaining maximum consistency of the meringue.
3. Slowly add the hot sugary solution and continue mixing until attaining a firm consistency.
4. Finally, incorporate the maple flavoring and keep mixing for only a few seconds.

White-Vanilla Frosting

1. Weigh ingredients for white-vanilla frosting listed in Table 10.16. Preheat the water to boiling.
2. Sift the powdered sugar with a hand sifter.
3. Cream the sugar and shortening until attaining a smooth consistency.
4. Continue mixing and incorporate half of the hot water and after one additional minute mix the rest of the water. Keep mixing until attaining a smooth and consistent frosting.

TABLE 10.16
Recommended Formulations for the Production of Different Types of Frostings[a]

Ingredients	Royal (g)	Egg-Vanilla (g)	White-Vanilla (g)	Chocolate (g)	Butter cream (g)	Meringue (g)
White sugar	–	150.0	–	–	–	–
Powdered sugar	330.0	–	67.3	71.5	48.5	150.0
Shortening	–	–	–	6.0	–	–
Emulsified shortening[b]	–	–	21.0	–	19.0	–
Butter	–	–	–	–	20.0	–
Dry milk	–	–	–	–	1.2	–
Water	–	60.0	10.7	12.0	7.3	–
Corn syrup	–	65.0	–	3.0	–	–
Egg whites	60.0	100.0	–	–	3.7	180.0
Cream of tartar	–	–	–	–	–	4.8
Cocoa	–	–	–	6.0	–	–
Maple flavoring	–	7.0	–	–	–	–
Vanilla extract	1.0	1.0	1.0	1.5	0.6	0.5
Lemon juice	14.0	–	–	–	–	–

[a] The royal, white vanilla, and butter cream frostings can be colored with artificial FD&C coloring agents to produce an assortment of colors.

[b] The emulsified shortening can be produced in the laboratory by blending 1 kg of melted regular shortening with 20 g lecithin and 20 g monoglycerides or diglycerides.

Chocolate Frosting

1. Weigh ingredients for chocolate frosting listed in Table 10.16. Melt the shortening on a hot plate.
2. Sift the powdered sugar with a hand sifter.
3. With the hand mixer, blend the water, sugar, syrup, and cocoa until attaining a smooth paste.
4. While mixing, add the melted shortening and vanilla until a smooth and firm frosting is obtained.

Butter Cream Frosting

1. Weigh ingredients for butter cream frosting listed in Table 10.16. Melt the shortening and butter on a hot plate.
2. Sift separately the powdered sugar and dry milk with a hand sifter.
3. With the electric hand mixer, blend the water and sugar.
4. While mixing, add the dry milk solids, shortening, and butter until attaining a smooth and fluffy consistency.
5. Add the egg whites and vanilla flavoring and continue mixing until a smooth and fluffy frosting is obtained.

Meringue

1. Weigh ingredients for meringue listed in Table 10.16.
2. Place egg whites in the mixing bowl for whipping. Whip egg whites on the fastest speed until attaining maximum consistency of the meringue.
3. Add the cream of tartar and gradually add the sugar and vanilla flavoring and continue mixing until attaining a firm consistency. The optimum whipping time is when the meringue peaks just bend over when pulled up with a spatula.

10.4.6 Production of Waffles, Pancakes, and Crepes

Waffles were first introduced to North America in 1620 by Pilgrims who brought the recipe and used procedures from the Netherlands. A waffle is a sweetened batter with baking powder or yeast baked in a waffle iron patterned to impart the distinctive and characteristic shape. Waffles are mainly consumed as breakfast or dessert in the United States and the Netherlands. After baking, the waffles are usually flavored with butter or margarine, syrups, honey, ice cream, strawberries, blueberries, and other fruits. American waffles are regularly made from a batter leavened with baking powder and may be baked on round, square, or rectangular irons. They are usually served as a sweet breakfast food or dessert. American waffles are generally denser and thinner compared to the Belgian counterparts. Belgian waffles, also known as Brussels waffles, are prepared with a batter supplemented with active yeast. It is generally, but not always, lighter, thicker, and crispier and has larger pockets

compared to other existing varieties. In Belgium, most waffles are served warm by street vendors and dusted with sugar and topped with whipped cream, soft fruits, or chocolate spread. Other important types are the European *Liège*, *Bergische*, and Scandinavian waffles. The Bergische waffles are always heart-shaped, crisp, and less dense compared to the Belgian counterparts and served with cherries and cream or rice pudding as part of the traditional afternoon feast on Sundays. The Scandinavian waffles are also baked in a heart-shaped waffle iron with a batter similar to the other types. They are frequently eaten with sweets, sour cream, and strawberry or raspberry jams, or berries.

Hot pancakes and crepes are similar to low-ratio cakes in terms of formulation but differ because they are baked on a hot griddle instead of a baking pan. Batters do not contain high quantities of sugar because these products are usually flavored with sweeteners, maple syrup, honey, jams, and jellies. The basic difference between pancakes and crepes is that pancakes recipes contain double-acting baking powder that imparts the typical crumb texture. Although most pancakes are leavened with baking powder, some could be leavened with active yeast.

Crepes are considered the national dish of France. They are typically manufactured without baking powder and therefore are thinner and denser compared to pancakes. The crepe-making process consists of the preparation of a pourable thin batter that is baked on a hot flat griddle. After applying some butter over the cooking hot surface, the batter is spread evenly either by leaning the griddle or by distributing the batter with a spatula. Dessert crepes are typically flavored with various sweet toppings such as maple syrup and powdered sugar, lemon juice, whipped cream, fruit spreads, custard, and sliced soft fruits. On the other hand, lunch crepes are usually savored with fillings such as cheese, eggs, various prepared meat products, ham, cooked rice, asparagus, spinach, and mushrooms.

10.4.6.1 Production of Waffles

A. *Samples, Ingredients, and Reagents*
   - Refer to Table 10.17
   - Can of nonstick cooking oil for spraying

B. *Materials and Equipments*
   - Digital scale
   - Graduated Cylinder (100 mL)
   - Egg yolk separator
   - Electric hand mixer with flat beaters
   - Waffle-maker (iron grid) machine
   - Egg yolk separator
   - Measuring cup
   - Wooden tongs
   - Spatula
   - Thermometer
   - Chronometer

C. *Procedure*
   American Waffles (Regular and Whole Wheat)

   1. Weigh ingredients for regular or whole wheat American waffles listed in Table 10.17. Preheat

TABLE 10.17

Recommended Formulations for Waffles, Pancakes, and Crepes

	American Waffles				
Ingredients	Regular (%)	Whole Wheat (%)	Belgian Waffles (%)	Pancakes (%)	Crepes (%)
Soft wheat flour	–	–	–	100.0	100.0
All-purpose flour	100.0	27.5	100.0	–	–
Whole wheat flour	–	72.5	–	–	–
Water	–	55.0	–	–	–
Eggs	45.0	36.0	–	–	60.0
Egg whites	–	–	18.0	–	–
Egg yolks	–	–	11.0	–	–
Regular milk	166.0	55.0	142.0	–	145.0
Sugar	4.0	–	20.0	27.6	20.0
Honey	–	11.0	–	–	–
Butter	–	10.0	34.0	–	12.0
Oil	48.0	–	–	8.3	–
Double-acting baking powder	6.5	7.0	–	8.3	–
Dry active yeast	–	–	1.4	–	–
Salt	0.8	0.8	1.5	2.8	0.8
Sodium stearoyl-2-lactylate	0.1	0.1	0.1	0.7	–
Vanilla extract	1.2	–	2.0	–	–
Maple flavoring	–	–	–	0.5	–

waffle making machine (approximately 80°C to 85°C).

2. With the electric hand mixer, beat eggs in a large bowl until fluffy. While mixing, add flour, milk, vegetable oil, sugar, baking powder, salt, and vanilla. Continue to blend all ingredients until the batter is homogenous, smooth, pourable, and lump-free (Figure 10.11).

3. Before baking, spray some nonstick cooking oil on the iron grid. Pour a constant volume (i.e., 200 mL) or weight of the batter on the hot grid of the waffle machine. Then, close the lid and bake for 4 to 5 minutes.

4. After baking, immediately remove the waffle with the aid of a wooden tong (Figure 10.11).

5. Weigh waffles and estimate yield based on the original formulation.

6. Reserve waffles for crust color, chemical, and sensory evaluations.

Yeast-Leavened Belgian Waffles

1. Weigh ingredients for Belgian waffles listed in Table 10.17. Warm the milk and melt the butter.

2. In a small container, dissolve and activate the dry yeast in 12 mL warm milk (37°C). Let stand for 10 minutes.

3. In a large bowl, whisk together egg yolks, 12 mL warm milk, and melted butter. Then add and mix the yeast/milk solution, sugar, salt, and vanilla. After about 1 minute of blending, gradually add the remaining warm milk and the flour. Make sure the resulting batter is homogenous, smooth, pourable, and lump-free.

4. Finally, add the egg whites and blend until they are fully incorporated into the batter. Measure the pH of the batter. Cover the bowl tightly with plastic wrap and allow the batter to ferment for at least 1 hour in a warm place. Determine the pH of the batter before baking.

5. On a preheated waffle-maker, spray nonsticky cooking oil on the surface of the iron. Pour a constant volume (i.e., 200 mL) or weight of the fermenting batter on the grid of the waffle machine. Then close the lid and bake for 4 to 5 minutes.

6. Open the maker machine and with wooden tongs remove waffle.

7. Weigh waffles and estimate yield based on the original formulation.

8. Reserve waffles for crust color, texture, chemical, and sensory evaluations.

10.4.6.2 Production of Pancakes

A. Samples, Ingredients, and Reagents
- Refer to Table 10.17
- Can of nonstick cooking oil for spraying

B. Materials and Equipments
- Scale
- Graduated cylinder (100 mL)
- Egg yolk separator
- Electric hand mixer with flat beaters

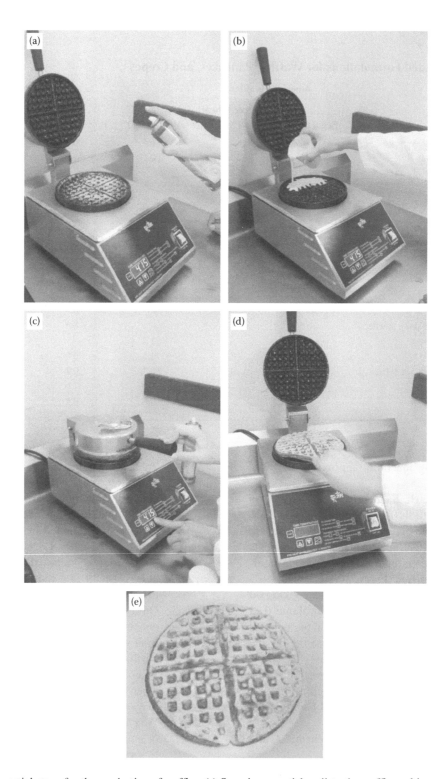

FIGURE 10.11 Sequential steps for the production of waffles. (a) Spraying nonsticky oil to the waffle-making machine; (b) addition of batter onto the surface of the iron grid; (c) baking of waffle batter; (d) waffle at the end of baking; and (e) waffle.

- Hot griddle
- Stove with gas-fired heater
- Measuring cup
- Spatula
- Thermometer
- Chronometer

C. *Procedure*

1. Weigh ingredients for pancakes listed in Table 10.17.
2. With the electric hand mixer, blend all ingredients in a bowl 1 minute at low speed and 2 minutes at medium speed. Make sure the resulting

batter is homogenous, smooth, pourable, and lump-free (Figure 10.12).

3. Preheat griddle and place a teaspoon of butter or margarine on the cooking surface. Then, immediately pour a constant volume or weight (i.e., one third of a cup) of the batter to form a 10-cm to 13-cm-diameter round form onto the hot griddle or surface.

4. Bake (approximately 2 minutes) until the observation of bubbles on the perimeter of the pancake. Then, with a spatula, carefully turn pancakes for baking on the other side (1 additional minute).

5. Remove pancakes from the hot griddle and allow pancakes to cool down for 10 minutes.

6. Weigh pancakes and estimate yield based on the original formulation. Measure the average diameter and height of the pancakes (Figure 10.12).

7. Reserve pancakes for crust and crumb color, chemical, and sensory evaluations.

10.4.6.3 Production of Crepes

A. *Samples, Ingredients, and Reagents*
- Refer to Table 10.17
- Can of nonstick cooking oil for spraying

B. *Materials and Equipments*
- Scale
- Graduated cylinder (100 mL)
- Egg yolk separator
- Electric hand mixer with flat beaters
- Crepe making machine
- Egg yolk separator
- Measuring cup
- Wooden tongs
- Spatula
- Thermometer
- Chronometer

C. *Procedure*
1. Weigh ingredients for crepes listed in Table 10.17. Preheat crepe making machine.
2. With the electric hand mixer, blend all ingredients in a bowl 1 minute at low speed and 2 minutes at medium speed. Make sure the resulting batter is homogenous, smooth, pourable, and lump-free (Figure 10.13).

3. Pour a constant volume or weight of the batter on the hot round surface of the crepe machine. If a crepe machine is not available, alternatively preheat griddle and place a teaspoon of butter or margarine on the cooking surface. Then, immediately pour 20 mL of the crepe batter on the Teflon-coated hot griddle.

4. Bake crepes until they turn golden (approximately 15 seconds). Then, with a spatula carefully remove crepes and allow them to cool down for 10 minutes.

5. Weigh crepes and estimate yield based on the original formulation. Measure the average diameter of the crepes (Figure 10.13).

6. Reserve crepes for crust color, chemical, and sensory evaluations.

10.4.7 Pies

There is a great tradition of serving pies on special occasions and parties. The production of pies dates back to the Middle Ages and the European settlers introduced them to the New World. A pie is constituted by at least two major parts, although many also contain one third element. All pies contain a crust and a fruit paste or custard-like filling, which, in many instances, is covered by frosting or whipped cream. The custard-like filling is made with fruit puree, eggs, cream or milk, sugar, and spices. The crust can be baked before placing the filling or baked along the filling. This last class is commonly named "soft" pie.

The pie crust plays an important role because it holds the filling and contributes to the flavor and texture. In addition, the crust should be formulated and baked to minimize the transfer of moisture from the filling to the crust, which leads to a corresponding loss of texture (soggy). Crusts are usually made with pastry flour and other ingredients and should not be mixed too vigorously. The resulting crust is pressed onto the pan. The sweet filling is the most important part of the pie. Most fillings are fruit-based (apple, peach, blueberry, strawberry, pumpkin, cherry) and flavored with various types

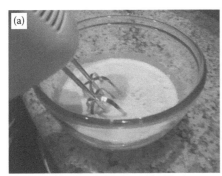 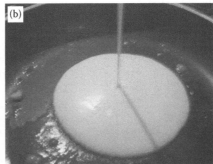 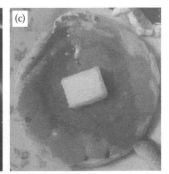

FIGURE 10.12 Sequential steps for the production of pancakes. (a) Mixing; (b) pouring the batter on a hot griddle; and (c) baked pancake.

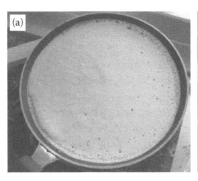
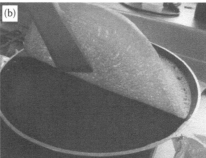
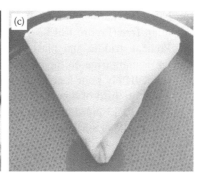

FIGURE 10.13 Sequential steps for the production of crepes. (a) Baking crepe batter on hot round griddle; (b) finished crepe; and (c) folded crepe.

of syrups, sugar, and other flavorings, such as vanilla. In some instances, the filling is prepared with modified starches (refer to Chapter 13) to enhance the formation of a clear paste. Then, the pie is baked at 175°C to 190°C for around 30 to 40 minutes. After cooling, the pie can be decorated with whipped cream.

10.4.7.1 Production of Pies

A. *Samples, Ingredients, and Reagents*
  - Refer to Tables 10.18, 10.19, and 10.20

B. *Materials and Equipments*
  - Digital scale
  - Graduated cylinder
  - Dough mixer with hook attachment
  - Wooden roller pins
  - Cooking pot
  - Refrigerator
  - Wire whisk
  - Fruit peeler
  - Electric hand mixer with flat beaters
  - Blender
  - Beakers
  - Colander
  - Whipped cream applicator (various tips/nozzles)
  - Fork
  - Knife

  - Baking oven
  - Pie pans (25 cm diameter)
  - Pipette
  - Thermometer
  - Spatula
  - Chronometer
  - Refractometer
  - Heat-resistant protective gloves

TABLE 10.18

Recommended Formulation for the Production of Butter-Flavored, Regular, and Mealy Pie Crusts[a]

Ingredients	Butter-Flavored Crust (%)	Regular Crust (%)	Mealy Crust (%)
Pastry flour	100.0	100.0	100.0
Shortening	–	70.0	65.0
Butter	43.0	–	–
Water	16.0	28.0	28.0
Dextrose	–	1.0	
Salt	0.7	2.0	2.0

[a] The pastry flour, shortening, butter, and water should be placed in a refrigerator for cooling.

TABLE 10.19

Recommended Formulation for the Production of Peach, Apple, and Blueberry Pie Fillings[a]

Ingredients	Peach Filling (%)	Apple Filling (%)	Blueberry Filling (%)
First Stage			
Apple juice	–	29.3	–
Blueberries	–	–	18.0
Lemon juice	–	0.4	–
Sugar	14.0	5.5	14.8
Dextrose	–	–	8.0
Corn syrup	5.5	3.5	–
Cinnamon	–	0.2	–
Salt	0.4	0.4	0.5
Instant starch	4.5	–	–
Water	–	–	27.0
Second Stage			
Modified starch	–	3.5	4.5
Peach puree	2.5	–	–
Peach juice	34.5	–	–
Water	–	7.5	11.0
Third Stage			
Peaches (drained)	39.0	–	–
Sliced-peeled apple	–	39.5	–
Frozen blueberries	–	–	16.1
Lemon juice	0.3	–	0.1
Cinnamon	0.05	–	0.05
Butter	–	1.0	–
White sugar	–	9.4	–

[a] Prepare the filling formulation according to the number of pies. One regular size pie is usually filled with 560 g.

TABLE 10.20

Recommended Formulation for the Production of Strawberry Cream Cheese Pie

Ingredients	Amount (1,000 g)
Filling	
Condensed milk	298.4
Cheese cream	142.8
Eggs	139.1
Vanilla extract	4.2
Covering	
Strawberries	370.1
Water	50.0
Corn syrup	18.8
Sugar	15.0
Acid-modified starch	11.3
Salt	0.15
Citric acid	0.1
Potassium sorbate	0.03
Whipped cream[a]	–

[a] The necessary amount needed for decoration.

10.4.7.1.1 Crust Production

1. Weigh or measure the crust ingredients listed in Table 10.18. In a dough mixer equipped with a hook attachment, mix for 1 minute at low speed the pastry flour with the shortening or butter. Then, dissolve the dextrose or salt in the water and add the predetermined amount of water and mix for one more minute at slow speed. It is very important to use cold flour, water, and shortening for the optimum preparation of the crust and not to overmix the dough.
2. Measure the temperature of the pie dough place it in a closed container and retard the dough overnight in the refrigerator.
3. Divide the dough into 210-g pieces and hand roll the dough into a round form of approximately 28 cm diameter (Figure 10.14).
4. Place the preformed dough sheet on the pie baking pan making sure to form the characteristic crusted cup. Remove excess crust with a knife.
5. With a fork, press the crust located at the top part of the pan perimeter and then mark small holes on the bottom in order to prevent blistering during baking.
6. Bake the crust for 8 minutes at 175°C.
7. Remove baked crust from the oven and allow it to cool down for at least 10 minutes.

10.4.7.1.2 Procedures for Production of Fruit Pies

Peach Pie

1. Weigh independently peach pie ingredients listed in Table 10.19. Make sure to calculate the total amount ingredients according to the number of pies. Each pie will need about 560 g filling. In a mixing bowl, dry blend stage 1 ingredients (sugar, salt, corn syrup solids, and instant or pregelatinized starch) for 30 seconds. If pregelatinized starch is not available, gelatinize the starch to at least 80°C with the peach juice of step 2.
2. In a blender, mash peaches into puree and then add the predetermined amount of peach juice (stage 2) obtained from the can.
3. Add gradually the ingredients of step 2 to the mixing bowl containing the dry ingredients. Make sure to scrape the sides of the mixing bowl. Determine the °Brix of the solution with the refractometer.
4. With a spoon, mix the peach pieces and ingredients of stage 3 to the blend obtained in step 3. Place the resulting filling (560 g/pie) on the prebaked crust (refer to procedure in Section 10.4.7.1.1).
5. Place peach pie in the refrigerator.

Apple Pie

1. Weigh independently apple pie ingredients listed in Table 10.19. Make sure to calculate the total amount ingredients according to the number of pies. Each pie will need about 560 g filling. Make sure to peel the apple just before preparation in order to avoid browning. Cut the peeled apple into small square pieces (approximately 1.5 cm × 1.5 cm × 1.5 cm).
2. In a cooking pot, bring to boil the apple and lemon juices, sugar, corn syrup, cinnamon, and salt (stage 1 ingredients).
3. Mix the instant starch and water and then add the starch dispersion (stage 2 ingredients) to the cooking pot containing the contents of step 1. Continue heating to 80°C and stir continuously the mixture with a wire whisk for 3 more minutes.
4. While still heating, add the sugar and butter (stage 3 ingredients) until reboil. Determine the °Brix of the solution with the refractometer.
5. Add the peeled dices of apple and stir with a spoon.
6. Place (560 g/pie) the resulting apple filling on the prebaked crust (refer to procedure in Section 10.4.7.1.1)
7. Place pie in a refrigerator.

Blueberry Pie

1. Weigh independently blueberry pie ingredients listed in Table 10.19. Make sure to calculate the total amount ingredients according to the number of pies. Each pie will need about 560 g filling.
2. In a cooking pot bring to boil the sugar, dextrose, salt, water, and blueberries (stage 1 ingredients). Stir with a metal whisk.
3. Mix the modified starch and water and then add the starch dispersion (stage 2 ingredients) to the cooking pot containing the contents of step 2. Continue heating to 80°C and stir continuously the mixture for 2 to 3 more minutes. Determine the °Brix of the solution with the refractometer.

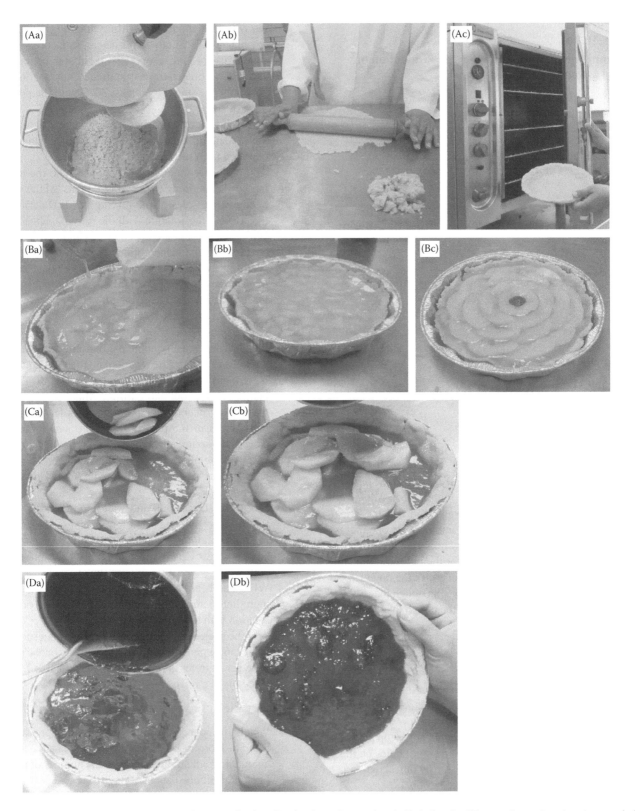

FIGURE 10.14 Production of pies. (A) Crust production: Production of crust dough (Aa), hand-rolling, and panning the characteristic crusted cup (Ab) and baking of crust (Ac); (B) peach pie: filling the baked crust (Ba), peach pie before refrigeration (Bb), and decorated and refrigerated peach pie (Bc); (C) apple pie: filling the baked crust (Ca); (D) blueberry pie: filling of baked crust (Da), appearance of refrigerated blueberry pie; (E) strawberry cream cheese pie: pouring cream cheese filling onto the baked crust (Ea), baking of cream cheese filling (Eb), application of starch slurry over baked pie (Ec), and appearance of refrigerated strawberry decorated pie (Ed); (F) pecan: filling of baked crust (Fa), baking of pecan pie filling (Fb), and final appearance of pecan pie (Fc).

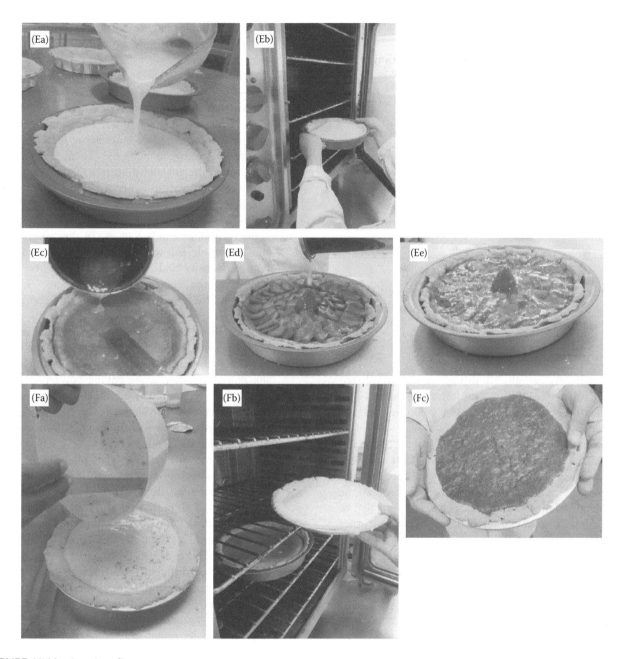

FIGURE 10.14 (*continued*)

4. Add the individual quick frozen blueberries, lemon juice, and cinnamon and stir with a spoon.
5. Place (560 g/pie) the resulting blueberry filling on the prebaked crust (refer to procedure in Section 10.4.7.1.1). Place pie in a refrigerator.

10.4.7.1.3 Procedure for Strawberry Cream Cheese Pie

Filling Production

1. Weigh all filling ingredients listed in Table 10.20 and place them in the blender jar. Blend contents at high speed for 2 minutes.
2. Pour the filling on the baked crust (refer to procedure in Section 10.4.7.1.1).
3. Bake for 25 to 30 minutes at 175°C (Figure 10.14).

Covering Production

1. Sanitize strawberries with 1% chlorine solution for 30 minutes. Wash strawberries and then cut them transversally to produce strawberry halves.
2. In a beaker, place the starch, corn syrup, sugar, citric acid, and potassium sorbate. Stir contents and place beaker on a hot plate. Heat contents to 85°C until the starch gelatinizes and produce a viscous slurry. Make sure to frequently stir contents while cooking.
3. Pour the starch slurry over the pie filling and carefully place strawberry halves over the surface.
4. Place pie for at least one hour in the refrigerator in order to enhance retrogradation and gelation.

TABLE 10.21

Recommended Formulation for the Production of Pecan Pie Filling

Ingredients	Amount (g)
Sugar	100.0
Eggs	86.0
Corn syrup	79.0
Pecan pieces	46.5
Pecan halves	6.0
Whipped cream	41.9
Butter	4.7
Vanilla	1.3
Salt	0.7

5. Take pie out of the refrigerator and apply whipped cream with a frosting applicator (Figure 10.14).
6. Place pie back in the refrigerator.

10.4.7.1.4 Production of Pecan Pie

1. Separately weigh all filling ingredients listed in Table 10.21. With a knife cut the pecans into small pieces. In a heat resistant container melt the butter.
2. With the electric hand mixer, beat the eggs, sugar, salt, melted butter, honey, and cream for 1 minute at low speed and another minute at high speed.
3. Add the vanilla extract and the pecan pieces to the blend and mix for only 10 seconds.
4. Pour the resulting filling on the prebaked crust (refer to procedure in Section 10.4.7.1.1). Then, distribute evenly the pecan halves on top of the filling.
5. Bake for 25 to 30 minutes at 175°C until a brown coloration on the surface of the filling is attained (Figure 10.14).
6. Remove pecan pie from the oven, and allow it to cool down for at least 10 minutes.

10.4.8 RESEARCH SUGGESTIONS

1. Prepare biscuits or muffins using the same formulation only varying in the type of flour used (soft or all-purpose flour or hard wheat). Determine optimum water absorption, dough, or batter consistency. After baking, evaluate the average height and volume of the resulting products, the texture (softness), crumb grain distribution, and organoleptic properties.
2. Prepare biscuits or muffins using the same formulation only varying in the type and amounts of baking powder used (compare two types of contrasting baking powders at two concentrations). Determine dough or batter pH and consistency. After baking, evaluate the average height and volume of the resulting products, the texture (softness), crumb

grain distribution, and organoleptic properties especially in terms of off flavors possible caused by the baking powders.
3. Prepare two different types of pancakes using the same formulation. One pancake will be produced from soft damaged flour whereas the other with regular soft wheat flour. Determine batter viscosity and bake same amounts of batter under the same baking conditions. Then, determine the average height and diameter of the resulting pancakes, the texture (softness), crust color, and organoleptic properties.
4. Prepare two different types of waffles using the same formulation only varying in the concentration of double-acting baking powder. Determine batter viscosity and bake same amounts of batter under the same baking conditions. Then, determine the quality properties of the resulting waffles.
5. Prepare three different types of low-ratio cakes using the same formulation only varying in the type of baking powder (prepared with double-acting baking powder or slow-acting baking powder or fast-acting baking powder. Determine differences in batter viscosity, cake volume and structure, crumb texture, apparent density, crumb grain uniformity, and other defects (symmetry).
6. Prepare three different types of high-ratio cakes using the same formulation only varying in the type of flour used (regular soft flour, chlorinated soft flour, and all purpose flour). Determine differences in batter viscosity, cake volume and structure, crumb texture, apparent density, crumb grain uniformity, and other defects (symmetry).
7. Prepare three different types of high-ratio cakes varying in the amount of egg whites added to the formulation. Determine differences in batter viscosity, cake volume, and structure, crumb texture, apparent density, crumb grain uniformity, and other defects (symmetry).
8. Prepare three different types of high-ratio cakes using the same formulation only varying in the mixing time (one half, regular, and twice as long). Determine differences in batter viscosity, cake volume and structure, crumb texture, apparent density, crumb grain uniformity, and other defects (symmetry).
9. Prepare a high-moist high-ratio cake by supplementing the basic formulation with gums and modified starches. Determine the necessary amount of extra water needed to optimize the cake batter viscosity and cake quality.
10. Prepare six different types of angel cakes using the same formulation only varying in the type of egg whites used (fresh egg whites, dehydrated egg white powder reconstituted to the same moisture level, and egg whites from old eggs). In addition,

process the same batters overmixing the egg whites. Determine differences in meringue volume, angel cake volume and structure, crumb texture or grain uniformity, and other defects (symmetry).

11. Prepare two different types of angel cakes using the same formulation with the exception of including the cream of tartar. Determine differences in batter pH, batter viscosity, angel cake volume and structure, crumb texture or grain uniformity, and other defects (symmetry).

12. Produce and compare pie dough from soft wheat and pastry flours varying in the amount of fat and test its functionality in a strawberry cream cheese pie.

10.4.9 RESEARCH QUESTIONS

1. What is the main role of the following ingredients used to produce muffins?
   a. Milk
   b. Shortening
   c. Eggs
   d. Sugar
   e. Double-acting baking powder
   f. Salt
   g. Sodium bicarbonate

2. What kind of recipe and process modifications would need to be made in order to produce an acceptable 100% whole wheat biscuit?

3. Explain how the level of fat and water influences tenderness, volume, and diameter of pancakes.

4. What are the components of an egg? What is the chemical composition of each component?

5. Describe differences between fresh and deteriorated eggs. How does the freshness affect functionality especially for cake making?

6. Describe the principle of the Haugh unit test used to determine egg freshness.

7. What are the effects of heat, amount of protein, acid, salts, and quality of eggs on the coagulation temperature and air trapping properties?

8. What is the main role of the following ingredients used to produce cakes?
   a. Cream of tartar
   b. Propylene glycol
   c. Egg whites
   d. Sugar
   e. Double-acting baking powder
   f. Emulsifiers
   g. Modified starch

9. Why are chlorinated soft wheat flours preferred to manufacture cakes?

10. What is a chiffon type of cake and what are its general manufacturing steps?

11. What is a pastry flour? What are the basic ingredients needed for pastry formulations?

12. How is a puff pastry leavened?

13. What changes in formulation are needed in order to produce a high-ratio moistened (high moist) cake?

14. What are the differences between an angel and a high-ratio cake?

15. Outline the steps involved in the preparation of shortened cakes indicating the main reason of each step.

16. What effects can be observed when the levels of egg or fat are increased in the production of shortened cakes?

17. How critical is the baking temperature for a cake? What would happen if the baking temperature is significantly decreased or increased?

18. What method and ratio of ingredients would result in the best stirred and baked custard?

19. Does freezing affect baked custards prepared with yolks and albumin or whites? If so, in what manner?

20. What factors contribute to making and stability of an egg white foam? What kind of beater is recommended to produce egg white foams? Why?

21. What are the desired characteristics of an excellent quality angel cake? What are the characteristics of angel cakes made with egg whites that are clearly unbeaten, beaten correctly, and overbeaten? What temperature is best for baking an angel cake?

22. What are the main reasons why a cake undergoing the first stage of baking collapse if the oven is open?

23. What are the optimum conditions for producing a meringue?

24. Why are acid or dextrinized starches used for the preparation of refrigerated pies?

25. Describe at least one functional ingredient used for cake manufacturing that affects cake structure, cake tenderness, cake moisture content, and cake flavor.

26. What are the major defects of cakes? How can you prevent each defect?

27. What is the typical formulation of a pie dough? Investigate the types of crust flakiness used to prepare these crusts or shells.

10.5 PRODUCTION OF WHEAT FLOUR TORTILLAS

Wheat flour tortillas is one of the fastest growing baking goods worldwide because they are fundamental in the elaboration of many Mexican type dishes widely sold by fast food restaurants. Wheat tortillas are considered the fastest growing market in the United States. In 2000, U.S. sales at wholesale prices totaled more than 4 billion dollars representing a growth rate of 57% over the previous four years. Wheat flour tortillas are the second highest selling product in the packaged bread category surpassing bagels, croissants, muffins, and pita breads (Dally and Navarro 1999). Tortillas are mainly used as wraps to produce tacos filled with shredded meats, beans, vegetables, cheeses, and other fillings.

A flour tortilla can be defined as a circular-shaped chemical-leavened flat bread. Flour tortillas are mainly produced from refined flours, although whole wheat flour tortillas are gaining popularity. Generally, tortillas are 2 mm thick and have diameters that vary from 15 cm to 33 cm. Most wheat tortillas are industrially manufactured by hot-press, die-cut, or hand-stretch procedures (Serna-Saldivar et al. 1988; Serna-Saldivar and Rooney 2003). Each operation requires different flour specifications, dough preparation, and baking conditions, which result in various tortilla characteristics.

Hot-pressed tortillas are slightly off-round, elastic, resistant to tearing, have a smooth surface texture, and resist moisture absorption from fillings. They are consumed as gourmet table tortillas and soft tacos. Die-cut tortillas are perfect circles and have lower moisture content and are less resistant to cracking. Most have dusting flour on the surface and are mainly used in *burritos*, frozen Mexican foods, and fried products (i.e., taco salad bowls, and taco shells). Hand-stretched tortillas are irregular in shape, elasticity, moderately resistant to tearing, and usually have leftovers of dusting flour on the surface. These tortillas are mainly consumed as table tortillas, *burritos*, and some fried products (Serna-Saldivar et al. 1988; Serna-Saldivar and Rooney 2003).

All wheat tortillas contain flour, water, fat, and salt. However, in the United States, tortillas may contain several others ingredients to improve flavor, softness, rollability, and shelf-life expectations. These ingredients include chemical leavening agents, emulsifiers, antimicrobial agents, acidulants, gums, and reducing agents (Serna-Saldivar et al. 1988; Serna-Saldivar and Rooney 2003).

Wheat flour, the most important ingredient, is preferably enriched, bleached, and should have intermediate protein content. Equipment limitations and processing conditions determine the functionality of the flour. Flours for hot-pressed and hand-stretched tortillas generally require less protein and gluten strength compared to flours for die-cut tortillas. Dough mixing time and dough properties are modified by reducing agents (sodium sulfites or cysteine), emulsifiers (lecithin, monoglyceride, diglycerides, sodium stearoyl lactylate), salt, hydrocolloids, fats, water content, and dough temperature. Water (45%–55% of flour weight) is needed to form the gluten complex. In some bakeries, water is warmed (35°C–45°C) before mixing. Solid or liquid fats (5%–15% of flour weight) are added to improve dough properties, retard staling, and produce a softer and more flexible tortilla. Salt (1%–2%) is added for taste and to strengthen the gluten complex. Baking powder (1.0%–2.5%) gives whiter, less dense, and fluffy products. Various natural and modified cellulose gums are added at 0.1%–10.5% levels to improve dough machinability and decrease stickiness of baked tortillas. Antimicrobial agents (propionates, sorbates) and acidulants (citric and fumaric acids) limit fungal growth and extend shelf-life. Wheat tortilla dough is mixed to incorporate the dry ingredients, fat, and water and to form a pliable, viscous dough. Tortilla dough is optimally mixed and varies in temperature from 26°C to 38°C. The dough is divided and rounded into dough balls in the hot-pressed and

hand-stretched procedures. The dough balls are proofed in a warm and humid environment for 5–20 minutes to relax the gluten complex. Rested dough balls machine easier and form better tortillas (Adams and Waniska 2002; Serna-Saldivar et al. 1988; Serna-Saldivar and Rooney 2003; Waniska et al. 2004).

Hand-stretching operations require more labor, sanitation, and maintenance. The preformed and proofed dough balls are forced to pass through a pair of rolls; the first pair of rolls presses the dough ball into an ellipsoidal tortilla while the second positioned perpendicularly further compresses into a semiround configuration. The preformed tortillas fall onto a hot surface where operators manually stretch into round forms. That is the reason this method is named hand-stretched (Serna-Saldivar et al. 1988; Serna-Saldivar and Rooney 2003).

In die-cut operations, the dough is pumped and shaped into a sheet that is further thinned by a series of cross-rollers on a moving belt. The thin sheet of dough (about 0.5 mm) is cut by a circular die, which forms the shape. The scrap dough is returned to the dough pump and processed. Regardless of the process, the formed tortilla are baked (190°C–260°C for 30–50 seconds) in gas-fired ovens that generally have three tiers. Oven conditions vary depending upon tortilla thickness, type of conveyor (slat or wire), and forming operation. Puffing of tortilla occurs near the end of baking and is more common in hot-pressed and hand-stretched tortillas. Tortillas are cooled to lower than 32°C on cooling conveyors before placing into plastic bags for distribution. Improper cooling causes the tortilla to stick together and increase microbial problems. Most processors manufacture both white and different versions of whole wheat flour tortillas (Friend et al. 1992; Serna-Saldivar et al. 1988). Wheat flour tortilla producers have recently developed low-fat, fat-free, and zero–trans fat products (Bejosano et al. 2006).

Bello et al. (1991) developed and standardized a laboratory procedure to prepare and evaluate hot-pressed tortillas. Equipment conditions and quality parameters emulate commercial operations. The laboratory technique allows testing the functionality of flour and key ingredients such as chemical leavening agents and shortenings and the optimization of water absorption, mixing time, and the necessary proof time for dough ball resting. The pilot plant procedure consists of first mixing dry ingredients including shortening. Next, warm water is added to dry ingredients and mixed until the dough is fully developed. The resulting dough is divided into uniform pieces and rounded into balls with a divider/rounder. Resulting dough balls are rested for different times (10–30 minutes) in a proof cabinet set at 32°C and 85% relative humidity. After proofing, the dough balls are pressed into tortilla discs in between the hot platens (200°C–218°C) of a press and then immediately baked on a three-tier gas-fired oven for 40 seconds at temperatures ranging from 230°C to 270°C. The hot tortillas are allowed to cool down for further evaluations. The tortilla weight and yield, thickness, diameter, rollability, appearance, texture (rollability and firmness with a texturometer), color, and sensory properties can be determined in fresh tortillas and tortillas stored under different conditions. The resulting tortillas are optimally produced for determining chemical composition and microbial and textural shelf-life studies.

10.5.1 Wheat Flour Tortillas

10.5.1.1 Production of Hot-Press Tortillas

A. Samples, Ingredients, and Reagents
- Refer to Table 10.22

B. Materials and Equipments
- Digital scale
- Dough mixer with hook attachment
- Dough cutting and rounding machine
- Proof box
- Hot-press
- Three-tier baking oven
- Stove
- Teflon-coated hot griddle
- Cooling rack
- Wooden roller pin
- Graduated cylinder
- 10-cm or 12-cm diameter round cutter
- Infrared spot thermometer (300°C)
- pH meter with dough electrode
- Baking sheets
- Thermometer (0°C–100°C)
- Ruler with mm markings
- Laboratory clock
- Plastic bags

TABLE 10.22

Recommended Formulation for the Production of Regular and Whole Wheat Flour Tortillas

Ingredients	White Regular Tortillas (%)	Whole Wheat Tortillas (%)
All-purpose wheat flour	100.0	50.0
Whole wheat flour	–	50.0
Water	48.0–52.0	48.0–52.0
Shortening	10.0–15.0	10.0–15.0
Salt	1.5–2.0	1.5–2.0
Nonfat dry milk	1.0–2.0	1.0–2.0
Double-acting baking powder	1.5–2.0	1.5–2.0
Emulsifiers[a]	0.3–1.0	0.3–1.0
Gums[b]	0.2–0.5	0.2–0.5
Antimold agents[c]	0.1–0.2	0.2–0.3
Acidulant[d]	0.2–0.3	0.2–0.3
Reducing agents[e]	10–20 ppm	0
Corn syrup or honey	–	2.0

[a] CMC, guar, and xanthan gums are commonly used.

[b] Lecithin, monoglycerides, diglycerides, and sodium stearoyl lactylate are commonly used.

[c] Calcium propionate and/or potassium sorbate are frequently used.

[d] Fumaric and citric acids are the most common acidultants used to drop pH to 5.4–5.9.

[e] Sodium bisulfite and cysteine are the most common reducing agents.

C. Procedure

1. Weigh ingredients listed in Table 10.22. Warm the water to 40°C.

2. Place all dry ingredients and shortening in the dough bowl and mix with the hook attachment for 1 minute (Figure 10.15). Add the warm water and continue mixing for 1 minute at low speed. Next, switch speed to medium and keep mixing until attaining optimum gluten development (dough should be smooth and lustrous and when stretched produce a thin gluten film). Weigh the resulting dough and measure its pH.

3. If a dough cutting and rounding machine is available, then place dough in the hopper and adjust cutting rate to yield 35-g dough balls. Make sure to recheck dough ball weights. If a batch type of cutting-rounding machine (36 dough balls) is available then scale 1.26 kg of dough, spread it on the cutting plate in preparation for cutting and rounding. Make sure to spread the dough evenly so to produce uniform dough balls (Figure 10.15). If a dough cutter is not available, then manually cut and weight equal portions of dough (i.e., 35 g) and hand round. The recommended hand rounding process consists of placing the dough piece on a smooth surface in preparation for applying pressure with the hand palm with circular movements for about 7–10 seconds.

4. Place dough balls in a greased baking sheet for proofing at 28°C and 80%–85% RH for 20–25 minutes. If a proofing time vs. tortilla diameter test will be run, then sample the unrested dough balls and proof balls after 3, 5, 8, 10, 15, 20, 25, and 30 minutes. The interpretation of these results will determine optimum proof time.

5. Preheat hot-press at least 20 minutes before pressing. With the infrared spot thermometer determine the surface temperature of the platens and adjust to the desired temperature (190°C–225°C). If a manual hot-press is available make sure to check the turn on the press at least 20 minutes before pressing and check the temperature (Figure 10.15). Make sure to recheck and readjust temperatures when hot pressing at a steady state because dough balls slightly decreases temperature.

6. Hot-press dough balls at the predetermined temperature (210°C for automatic hot presses and 180 for manual presses) (Figure 10.15). Measure the average weight, diameter, and thickness of the tortillas. For average diameter measure the diameter on two different places and for average thickness overlap at least 5 tortillas and measure thickness.

7. Preheat three-tier baking oven at least 20 minutes before baking. With the infrared spot thermometer, determine the surface temperature of

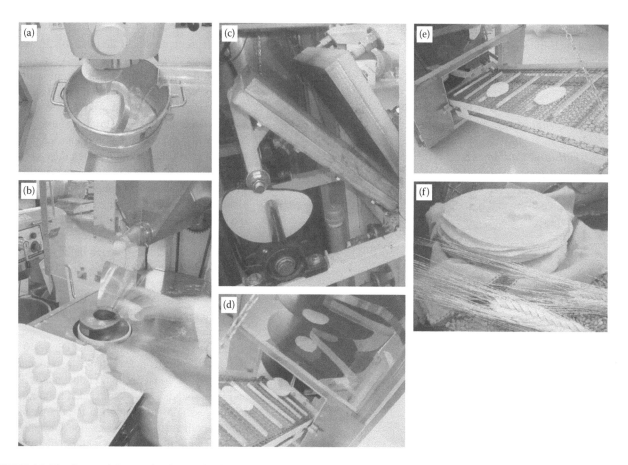

FIGURE 10.15 Sequential steps for the production of hot-press wheat flour tortillas. (a) Dough mixing; (b) dough cutting and rounding; (c) hot-pressing dough balls into tortilla rounds; (d) baking of tortillas; (e) cooling of tortillas; and (f) stack of ready to eat tortillas.

the three moving tiers and adjust the gas flame to the desired temperature (190°C–210°C). If the oven has control adjustments of dwell time make sure to regulate it to 40–50 seconds. If a continuous oven is not available, prepare baking on a hot griddle. Turn on the stove at least 5 minutes before baking and adjust surface temperature to 185°C (Figure 10.15).

8. Bake tortillas at 190°C–210°C for 40–50 seconds (Figure 10.15) in the three-tier baking oven. Alternatively, bake tortillas on the Teflon-coated hot griddle adjusted to 185°C for 20 seconds. Then flip the tortilla and bake the raw side for 20 to 30 seconds and turn over again to the original side for 15 seconds. Generally, during this last baking stage of the tortilla puffs. Measure the average weight, diameter, and thickness of the tortillas. For average diameter, measure the diameter on two different places and for average thickness overlap at least 5 tortillas and measure thickness.

9. Allow baked tortillas to cool down in the cooling rack or place them on a sanitized surface for 10 minutes cooling on one side and 10 additional minutes on the other side. Sample tortillas

for moisture, chemical, textural, and microbial shelf life and organoleptic evaluations.

10. Pack rest of the tortillas in sealed plastic bags.

10.5.1.2 Laminated and Formed Tortillas

1. Weigh ingredients listed in Table 10.22. Add two percent more water to the formulation so to produce slack dough. Warm the water to 40°C.

2. Place all dry ingredients and shortening in the dough bowl and mix with the hook attachment for 1 minute. Add the warm water and continue mixing for 1 minute at low speed. Next, switch speed to medium and keep mixing until attaining optimum gluten development (dough should be smooth and lustrous and when stretched produce a thin gluten film). Weigh the resulting dough and measure its pH.

3. If a dough cutting and rounding machine is available then place dough in the hopper and adjust cutting rate to yield 35 g dough balls. Make sure to recheck dough ball weights. If a batch type of cutting-rounding machine (36 dough balls) is available then scale 1.26 kg of dough, spread it on the cutting plate in preparation for cutting and rounding. Make sure to spread evenly the dough so to produce uniform dough balls. If a dough cutter is not available then

manually cut and weight equal portions of dough (i.e., 35 g) and hand round. The recommended hand rounding process consists of placing the dough piece on a smooth surface table in preparation for applying pressure with the palm of the hand with circular movements for about 7–10 seconds.

4. Place dough balls in a greased baking sheet for proofing at 28°C and 80%–85% RH for 30 minutes.

5. Take relaxed dough balls from the proof box in preparation for sheeting. Dust dough balls with small amounts of flour. Next, sheet the dough ball through a set of sheeting rolls set at 0.48 cm, or 3/16 in. Recuperate the ovoid-shaped pressed dough and place it on the counter. Change the setting of the sheeting rolls to 0.32 cm, or 1/8 in., and sheet again the ovoid-shaped tortilla. Make sure to press the ovoid form wide wise. Place preformed tortilla on a flour dusted smooth surface and with the wooden roller pin manually press the tortilla into its round configuration making sure to produce a round tortilla with approximately 20 cm diameter and 1.5 mm thick.

6. Preheat three-tier baking oven at least 20 minutes before baking. With the infrared spot thermometer, determine the surface temperature of the three moving tiers and adjust the gas flame to the desired temperature (190°C–210°C). If the oven has control adjustments of dwell time, make sure to regulate it to 40–50 seconds. If a continuous oven is not available, bake on a hot griddle. Turn on the stove at least 5 minutes before baking and adjust surface temperature to 185°C.

7. Make sure to sheet and form at least 20 tortillas before baking. Bake tortillas at 190°C–210°C for 40–50 seconds in the three-tier baking oven. Alternatively, bake tortillas on the Teflon-coated hot griddle adjusted to 185°C for 20 seconds. Then flip the tortilla and bake the raw side for 20 to 30 seconds and turn over again to the original side for 15 seconds. Generally, during this last baking stage the tortilla puffs. Measure the average weight, diameter and thickness of the tortillas. For an average diameter, measure the diameter on two different places and for average thickness overlap at least 5 tortillas and measure thickness.

8. Allow baked tortillas to cool down in the cooling rack or place them on a sanitized surface for 10 minutes cooling on one side and 10 additional minutes on the other side. Sample tortillas for moisture, chemical, textural, and microbial shelf-life and organoleptic evaluations.

9. Pack rest of the tortillas in plastic bags.

10.5.2 Sweet Flour Tortillas

10.5.2.1 Production of Sweet Tortilla Pancakes

A. Samples, Ingredients, and Reagents
- Refer to Table 10.23

TABLE 10.23

Recommended Formulation for the Production of Sweet Flour Tortillas or Pancakes

Ingredients	%
All-purpose flour	100.0
Water	38.0
White sugar	21.5
Shortening	20.0
Double-acting baking powder	2.5
Salt	1.5
Nonfat dry milk	1.5
Lecithin	0.5
Sodium stearoyl-2-lactylate	0.3

B. Materials and Equipments
- Digital scale
- Dough mixer with hook attachment
- Dough cutting and rounding machine
- Proof box
- Hot-press
- Three-tier baking oven
- Stove
- Teflon-coated hot griddle
- Cooling rack
- Wooden roller pin
- Graduated cylinder (100 mL)
- 10-cm or 12-cm-diameter round cutter
- Infrared spot thermometer (300°C)
- pH meter with dough electrode
- Baking sheets
- Thermometer (0°C–100°C)
- Ruler with mm markings
- Chronometer
- Plastic bags

C. Procedure
1. Weigh separately ingredients listed in Table 10.23.

2. Place all dry ingredients and shortening in the dough bowl and mix with the hook attachment for 1 minute. Add the water and continue mixing for 1 minute at low speed. Next switch speed to medium and keep mixing until attaining optimum gluten development (approximately 4 minutes). Weigh the resulting dough.

3. If die-cut tortillas will be produced place dough in a proof box for 25 minutes at 28°C to 30°C and 80 to 85% RH. If pressed tortillas will be produced first cut and then hand-round dough pieces of 50 g of weight. Allow resulting dough balls to relax in the proof box.

4. Take dough or dough balls from the proof box for patty forming. For die-cut tortillas, laminate the dough with sheeting rolls or with the wooden roller pin to a thickness of 1 cm. Then, with the 10-cm or 12-cm round cutter, cut the round formed patties. For press tortillas, place

the 50-g dough ball in a manual press operating at room temperature and pressed with sufficient force to obtain a 10-cm diameter by 1-cm-thick dough patty.

5. Prepare baking on a hot griddle. Turn on the stove at least 5 minutes before baking and adjust surface temperature to 185°C.

6. Preheat hot griddle at least 5 minutes before baking and adjust surface temperature with the infrared spot thermometer to 190°C–200°C. Place butter on the hot surface and bake sweetened pancakes on the Teflon-coated hot griddle adjusted to 190°C–200°C for 40 seconds. Then flip the pancake and bake the raw side for 60 seconds and turn over again to the original side for 30 additional seconds. Measure the average weight, diameter, and thickness of the tortillas. For average diameter, measure the diameter on two different places, and for average thickness overlap at least 5 baked pancakes and measure thickness.

7. Allow baked sweet tortilla pancakes to cool down on a sanitized surface for 10 minutes cooling on one side and 10 additional minutes on the other side. Sample tortillas for moisture, chemical, textural, and microbial shelf life and organoleptic evaluations. Place rest of the pancakes in plastic bags.

10.5.3 RESEARCH SUGGESTIONS

1. Determine and compare the making properties of hot-pressed tortillas produced from soft, all-purpose, and hard refined flours. Compare optimum water absorptions, dough textures, tortilla bending capacities throughout 5 days storage at room temperature and design a organoleptic test (refer to Chapter 3) aimed toward determining differences in color, texture, flavor, and overall preference.

2. Prepare wheat flour tortillas from a given lot of all purpose flour following the hot-press procedure. Using the same basic formulation vary the amounts of the supplement additives: (1) 0.2% fumaric acid and 0.2% potassium sorbate; (2) 0.2% lecithin, 0.1% SSL (sodium stearoyl 2-lactylate and 0.2% CMC [carboxy methyl cellulose]); (3) 0.1% fumaric acid, 0.1% potassium sorbate, 0.2% lecithin, 0.1% SSL (sodium stearoyl 2-lactylate) and 0.2% CMC. Determine the dough consistency or texture, pH, and optimum dough ball relaxing time and average press tortilla diameter. Process the control and supplemented flours into tortilla packages and then determine differences in terms of pH, microbial stability throughout 10 days at room temperature, tortilla bending or folding capacity, and preference with a sensory evaluation panel. The objective is to determine which tortilla system is the best in terms of overall acceptability and shelf life.

3. Produce whole grain wheat flour tortillas using hard red winter or hard white winter wheats. Compare properties of these two tortillas with a regular tortilla in terms of color, nutritional attributes, texture throughout 10 days of storage at room temperature (tortilla folding, bending, and firmness), and organoleptic properties.

4. Produce a low-fat and fat-free white flour tortillas and compare it with a regular tortilla containing 12% to 15% shortening. Determine optimum formulations, supplemented additives to counteract the positive effect of shortening (i.e., emulsifiers, gums, etc.), optimum water absorptions, dough texture, and dough relaxation times. Then, determine the reheatability of the tortillas after 5 days storage, the quality of the tortillas and the energy density based on 100 g of product.

10.5.4 RESEARCH QUESTIONS

1. What are the three industrial processes to produce flour tortillas? Which one is the most adequate to obtain flour tortillas for the elaboration of frozen products?

2. What ingredients are necessary to produce a long shelf-life wheat flour tortilla with adequate reheatability properties?

3. What are optimum flour characteristics for hot-pressed, hand-stretched, and die-cut tortillas?

4. What are the ingredients commonly used to reduce dough proofing or resting times before tortilla forming?

5. What are the differences in formulation and processing of regular and whole wheat flour tortillas?

6. What are the best approaches to produce a long microbial shelf life tortilla (i.e., 21 days at room temperature) from the formulation, processing, and packaging view points?

7. What are the best approaches to produce a long textural shelf life tortilla (i.e., 21 days at room temperature) from the formulation, processing, and packaging view points? Which microorganisms are in the main responsible for tortilla spoilage?

8. What kinds of additives are recommended for tortillas that will stand freezing-thawing cycles?

9. What is the comparative caloric value of flour tortillas vs. table bread? Why do flour tortillas contain a higher calorific value?

10. What are the major chemical changes that occur to gluten and starch during tortilla baking?

11. What are the main quality control parameters used in wheat flour tortilla plants?

12. Investigate novel technologies to produce low-fat and trans-free tortillas.

13. Define two strategies to enhance tortilla texture (better folding or bending and decreased cracking) and reheatability. Which texture studies will effectively detect differences between tortillas stored for different periods of time at different temperatures and supplemented with different amounts of antistaling agents?

REFERENCES

Adams, J. L., and R. D. Waniska. 2002. "Effects of the Amount and Solubility of Leavening Compounds on Flour Tortilla Characteristics." *Cereal Foods World*, 47:60–64.

American Association of Cereal Chemists. 2000. *Approved Methods of the AACC*. St. Paul, MN: AACC.

Bejosano, F. P., J. Novie Alviola, and R. D. Waniska. 2006. "Reformulating Tortillas with Zero Trans Fat." *Cereal Foods World* 51(2):66–68.

Bello, A., S. O. Serna-Saldivar, R. D. Waniska, and L. W. Rooney. 1991. "Methods to Prepare and Evaluate Wheat Flour Tortillas." *Cereal Foods World*. 36:315–322.

Bennion, E. B., and G. S. T. Bamford. 1997. *The Technology of Cake Making*, edited by A.J. Bent. 6th ed. London, UK: Blackie Academic & Professional.

Conforti, F. D. 2007. "Fundamentals of Cakes." In *Handbook of Food Products Manufacturing. Principles, Bakery, Beverages, Cereals, Cheese, Confectionary, Fats, Fruits, and Functional Foods*, edited by Y.H. Hui, Chapter 16. Hoboken, NJ: Wiley Interscience.

Cross, N. 2007. "Muffins and Bagels." In *Handbook of Food Products Manufacturing. Principles, Bakery, Beverages, Cereals, Cheese, Confectionary, Fats, Fruits, and Functional Foods*, edited by Y.H. Hui, Chapter 15. Hoboken, NJ: Wiley Interscience.

Faridi, H. 1994. *The Science of Cookie and Cracker Production*. New York, NY: Chapman & Hall.

Faridi, H., C. S. Gaines, and B. L. Strouts. 2000. "Soft Wheat Products." In *Handbook of Cereal Science and Technology*, edited by K. J. Lorenz and J. G. Ponte, chapter 18. 2nd ed. New York, NY: Marcel Dekker.

Friend, C., S. O. Serna-Saldivar, R. D. Waniska, and L. W. Rooney. 1992. "Increasing the Fiber Content of Wheat Tortillas." *Cereal Foods World* 37:325–328.

Habighurst, A. B. 1969. "Quality Factors in Wire-Cut Cookie Production." *Bakers Digest*. February 57–59.

Harvey Lang, J. 1990. "Crepas." In *Larousse Gastronomique*, pp. 332–335. 1st ed. New York, NY: Crown Publishers.

Howard, N. B. 1972. "The Role of Some Essential Ingredients in the Formation of Layer Cake Structures.' *Bakers Digest* October: 28–37.

Manley, D. 1996. *Technology of Biscuits, Crackers and Cookies*. 2nd ed. Cambridge, UK: Woodhead Publishing.

Manley, D. 1998. *Biscuit Dough Piece Forming. Manual 3*. Cambridge, UK: Woodhead Publishing.

Matz, S. A. 1992. *Cookie and Cracker Technology*, 3rd ed. Westport, CT: AVI Publishing.

Matz, S. A. 1972. *Bakery Technology and Engineering*, 2nd ed. Westport, CT: AVI Publishing.

Matz, S. A. 1987. *Formulas and Processes for Bakers*. McAllen, TX: Pan Tech International.

Moreth, N. 1994. "Engineering and Processing." In *Cookie Chemistry and Technology*, edited by K. Kulp (ed.), chapter 13. Manhattan, KS: American Institute of Baking.

Pizzinatto, A., and R. C. Hoseney. 1980. "A Laboratory Method for Saltine Crackers." *Cereal Chem.* 57:249–252.

Serna-Saldivar, S. O. 2008. "Manufacturing of Wheat-Based Baked Snacks." In *Industrial Manufacture of Snack Foods*, Chapter 9. London, UK: Kennedys Publication.

Serna-Saldivar, S. O., L. W. Rooney, and R. D. Waniska. 1988. "Wheat Flour Tortilla Production." *Cereal Foods World* 33:857–863.

Serna-Saldivar, S. O., R. D. Waniska, and L. W. Rooney. 1993. "Wheat and Corn Tortillas." In *Encyclopedia of Food Science, Food Technology and Nutrition*, edited by R. MacRae, R. Robinson, and M. Sadler. London, UK: Academic Press.

Sultan, W. J. 1983. *Practical Baking*. 3rd ed. Westport, CT: AVI Publishing.

Waniska, R. D., et al. 2004. "Effects of Flour Properties on Tortilla Qualities." *Cereal Foods Word*. 49(4):237–244.

Yasmasaki, W. T. 1953. "An Alkaline Water Retention Capacity Test for the Evaluation of Cookie Baking Potentialities of Soft Winter Wheat Flours." *Cereal Chem.* 30:242.

11 Production of Pasta Products and Oriental Noodles

11.1 INTRODUCTION

Western pasta and Asian noodles are nonleavened products manufactured from durum semolina and soft wheat flour, respectively. The Italian pasta, widely consumed in Europe and America, still dominates the world market, although Asian noodles have increased sales during the past years. Oriental noodles, also known as Chinese or Japanese noodles, have traditionally been staple for Asian countries for more than 1,000 years. Asian noodles are usually made from common wheat flour using a process of sheeting and cutting, as opposed to pasta products that are generally cold-extruded using durum semolina. Asian noodles are usually softer but more elastic and range from white to creamy white to moderately yellow in appearance. Asian noodles are alternatively produced from other cereals such as rice.

11.2 PASTA PRODUCTS FROM DURUM SEMOLINA

Pasta is one of the simplest products in terms of raw materials because is produced from semolina that, in some instances, is supplemented with salt and eggs. Pasta products are classified according to shape and size into two broad categories, short and long, and according to processing method into extruded, sheeted/formed and precooked microwaveable. Nowadays, the market is still dominated by dry pasta although fresh pasta is gaining popularity. There is still controversy about the origin of pasta. Some believe that Marco Polo brought pasta from China to Italy and others that the Etruscans were the first people who consumed a product similar to spaghetti. The early Romans developed the first machines to elaborate pasta and Marco Polo imported from the kingdom of Kublai Khan a new technology to manufacture pasta that complemented the existing Italian technologies developed around year 1200 A.D.

For pasta production, amber durum wheats are preferred. Durum is milled into refined semolina, which has larger granulation compared to conventional wheat flour. Semolinas generally have a particle size distribution that vary from −60 to 100 U.S. mesh and yellow color due to the presence of β-carotenes, lutein, and zeaxanthin in the endosperm. Some pastas are supplemented with egg products to impart a stronger yellow color and improve flavor, nutritional value, and texture or mouth feel of the cooked pasta. Eggs may be added in either liquid or dehydrated forms. Liquid pasteurized egg is the preferred choice but requires proper control of microorganisms. Liquid egg with approximately 20%–25% solids is usually added at the rate of 160 g/kg. Spray-dried egg products are also used. The advantage is that they have longer shelf life, less microbial risk, and are easier to incorporate into semolina before production.

The manufacturing of most pasta products consists of three major steps: hydration of the semolina, mixing–forming, and drying (Ambrogina Pagani et al. 2007) to lower the moisture to approximately 10%. There are two basic manufacturing procedures: sheeting-cutting and extruding. The first process was the one that originated pasta and the second is the most commonly used today.

The fresh pasta with Aw of 0.92 to 0.95 and moisture contents of about 30% can be packaged in modified atmosphere (20%–50% CO_2 and 50%–80% N_2) and refrigerated. The advantage is that the hydrated pasta is viewed as natural and is more convenient because it requires less cooking compared to dry pasta. Fresh pasta is usually mixed with spinach, tomato, chlorophyll, and/or other coloring agents or used for the production of Italian filled pastas. Dehydrated spinach and tomato are primarily used to impart green and red colorations, respectively. Normally, 2% and 4% dry powder forms are mixed with the semolina before processing. Shelf-life expectations of fresh pasta are 30–45 days at refrigeration temperatures (Ambrogina Pagani et al. 2007; Kruger et al. 1996).

Drying is considered the most critical unit operation for dry pasta. The aim is to gradually and cautiously remove water from 31% to 10% moisture of the preformed pieces of dough. The dehydration rate is related to the dough vapor pressure and the available water on the surface of the piece of dough. The rate of water diffusion within the product is closely related with the temperature and air humidity. Commonly, one third of the moisture is removed in a short period (30 minutes) because the fresh pasta is plastic and elastic and possesses capillary porosity. After that, the pasta enters a second drying phase, called equilibration, where the dough pieces are subjected to a low temperature and a high relative humidity (90%) program. The aim of this drying stage is to achieve water equilibration within the pasta (2–3 hours) and avoid the formation of a surface crust that will impede water migration during the rest of the drying program. The final drying stage consists of the lengthy dehydration (45°C for 8–12 hours) until the target moisture of 10%–12% is achieved. There are innovations in pasta drying where the dehydration time is greatly reduced due to the use of elevated temperatures These dehydration regimes apply temperatures and controlled relative humidities ranging from 60°C–84°C and 74%–82% RH, respectively. The very high temperature regime known as THT applies temperatures higher than 84°C and drying time is significantly reduced to only 2 to 5 hours. Better control systems and more sophisticated dryers are used for the fast-high temperature pasta drying. The THT drying is preferable for better pasta color because lipooxygenase and peroxidases are inactivated and the reduction of microorganisms due to the higher temperature and lower residence time (Kruger et al. 1996).

Pasta products are generally inspected in terms of color, specks, texture, and strength/flexibility. Color is mainly affected by the amount of carotenoid/xantophylls pigments in the semolina and polyphenol oxidase and lipooxigenase activities. The cooking characteristics of pasta are the most relevant for consumers, therefore of greatest importance to processors. The semolina proteins are in the main responsible for cooking qualities. Cooking quality is generally assessed in terms of minimum, optimal, and maximum cooking times, which correspond to the moment at which the starch is gelatinized, the time required to give the pasta the desired texture, and the time beyond which the product disintegrates, respectively (Feillet and Dexter 1996). The water uptake is easily measured by determining the weight of the pasta before and after cooking (100 g pasta generally absorbs 160 g to 180 g of water). Cooking loss can be also determined by weighing the residue of cooking water after evaporation or after freeze drying or by measuring amylose with the iodine assay (Matsuo et al. 1992). The texture of the cooked product, which generally includes firmness, cohesiveness, elasticity and stickiness, can be determined by sensory evaluation or by instrumental texture measurements.

11.2.1 Sheeted and Cut Pasta

Sheeted or laminated pasta is used to produce short cut pasta noodles, folded, or even presented to a noodle nesting machine. The semolina is first dampened with limited amounts of water to increase the moisture from 29% to 32% and then subjected to mixing with water tempered to 35°C–40°C. The coarser semolina takes longer to hydrate so some equilibration is required. During kneading the gluten network develops reducing dough adhesion in preparation for optimum sheeting. The resulting dough is gradually sheeted to the desired thickness using mechanical sheeters and cut with rolls (Kill and Turnbull 2001; Ambrogina Pagani et al. 2007).

11.2.1.1 Production of Pasta by Sheeting and Cutting

A. Samples, Ingredients, and Reagents
- Semolina from durum wheat
- Distilled water
- Salt
- Dehydrated or fresh eggs

B. Materials and Equipments
- Digital scale
- Graduated cylinder (100 mL)
- Mixer with hook or paddle
- Plastic bags
- Pasta cutter
- Perforated drying sheets
- Colander
- Hot plate or stove
- Cooking vessels (5 L)
- Convection drier
- Thermometer
- Chronometer
- Electric or manual pasta machine with steel rollers

C. Procedure
1. Place in a mixing bowl equipped with a hook or paddle attachment 1000 g of durum semolina (14% mb), 250 g of whole eggs, 80 mL water, and 5 g salt. The eggs should be beaten with a fork before addition.
2. Mix contents at low speed for 1 minute and then switch to medium for two more minutes. If the pasta dough is too dry or crumbly add small quantities of water (Figure 11.1).
3. Place dough ball in a plastic bag for 10 to 15 minutes resting. This will enhance water distribution and equilibration.
4. If making pasta strands, roll out the dough using a roller pasta machine, dusting lightly with flour to prevent from sticking. Fold up and roll a second time or continue to roll each sheet until the surface of the dough becomes smooth. Once the pasta sheets begin to smooth out, decrease the roller setting gradually until achieving the desired thickness (Figure 11.1).
5. After achieving the desired sheeted dough thickness (1.5–2 mm), cut the pasta with any of pasta cutters designed for spaghetti, tagliatelle, capelli d'angelo, trenette, or fettuccine.
6. Divide the resulting extruded pasta into two lots: one for fresh pasta and the other for production of dry pasta. Determine moisture content of fresh pasta, color, and cooking characteristics (texture of the cooked pasta that generally includes firmness, cohesiveness, elasticity and stickiness, water uptake, and cooking loss). The pasta cooking method is described in procedure in Section 11.2.2.2.
7. Place a weighed amount of fresh pasta in a perforated sheet in convection oven set at 40°C for first stage drying. Construct a drying curve by graphing the pasta moisture content vs. drying time. Remove pasta from the dryer when it decreases its moisture to 20%. For instance, 1 kg of fresh pasta with 31% moisture will lose 137.5 g water. Place partially dehydrated pasta

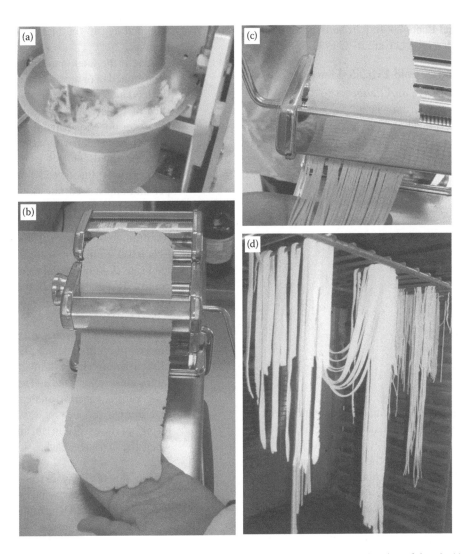

FIGURE 11.1 Production of sheeted and cut pasta. (a) Semolina dough mixing; (b) progressive sheeting of dough; (c) cutting of pasta; and (d) pasta drying.

for 2 hours in an environmental chamber at 30°C and 80% relative humidity for equilibration. Then place pasta again in the drying oven set at 32°C for dehydration until the pasta drops its moisture to 10%. Construct a drying curve by graphing the pasta moisture content vs. drying time. Remove pasta from the dryer when it decreases its moisture to 10%. For instance, 1 kg of fresh pasta with 31% moisture will yield 766.6 g of 10% moisture pasta.

8. Allow pasta to cool down and equilibrate at room temperature for 30 minutes and determine its moisture content (procedure in Section 2.2.1.1), color (Chapter 3), checking, and cooking characteristics (procedure in Section 11.2.2.2).

11.2.2 EXTRUDED PASTA

Most pasta products are produced by cold extrusion. In this process, the semolina is first hydrated and then kneaded into

a dough that in its plastic stage is forced to continuously pass through a die at relatively high pressure. Optimally, the extruder is furnished with a vacuum system with the purpose of reducing the formation of tiny air bubbles that lower color, texture, and acceptability. The removal of air, specifically oxygen, avoids the enzymatic oxidation of carotenoids by lipooxygenases that demerit color. Pasta are extruded at relatively low temperatures (<45°C) because the heat generated by friction is dissipated with water jackets located on the barrel. If the dough temperature exceeds 55°C, adverse changes can occur such as denaturing of the gluten proteins and starch gelatinization. Pastas produced under these conditions have poor cooking qualities. In addition, the extruder screw is designed to cause low shear rate and the inside barrel surface grooved to aid in the movement of the dough minimizing starch damage. The screw basically has two zones, dough intake-pressure build up and kneading. Then, the extruded dough is continuously cut by rotating knives positioned after the die in preparation for packaging if fresh pasta is desired or dehydration if dry pasta is produced (Ambrogina Pagani et al. 2007; Donnelly and Ponte 2000; Kill and Turnbull 2001; Kruger et al. 1996; Mercier and Cantarelli 1986).

11.2.2.1 Production of Cold-Extruded Pasta

A. *Samples, Ingredients, and Reagents*
- Semolina from durum wheat
- Dehydrated spinach
- Distilled water
- Salt
- Dehydrated or fresh eggs

B. *Materials and Equipments*
- Pasta extruder
- Pasta dies
- Digital scale
- Graduated cylinder
- Mixer with paddle
- Perforated drying sheets
- Colander
- Hot plate or stove
- Cooking vessels (5 L)
- Convection drier
- Thermometer
- Chronometer

C. *Procedure*
1. Determine the semolina moisture content and its particle size distribution and color (refer to procedures in Sections 2.2.1.1, 5.3.1.1, and 3.2.1).
2. Prepare the extruder in the mode of pasta production. The extruder should optimally have a low shear screw, barrel temperature control (<45°C), air vacuum system, the proper die plate, and the cutting device with sharp knives.
3. In a mixer place dry ingredients listed in Table 11.1 and blend at low speed for 5 minutes. For the fresh egg formulation, gradually add the whipped egg to the blend and mix for 5 more minutes.
4. Decide if the feed material will be hydrated or conditioned in or outside the extruder. Condition the feed material with the amount of water specified in Table 11.1 if the extruder does not have the water injection capability.
5. Start the extruder without material and set the predetermined controls (screw rpm and barrel temperature). Place feed material in the hopper and adjust feed rate (kg/hours). Make sure to recuperate the feed material before entering the barrel. Then, calculate the amount of water required to increase the moisture content to 31% [(100 − initial moisture/100 − 31%) − 1] × feed rate (kg/hours) and set the injection water control. If possible, check the amount of water/ hours being injected to the extruder.
6. Allow feed material to enter the extruder when the feed and water rates are controlled and set. Turn on the cutting device and control the speed of the rotating knifes to obtain the desired configurations. Adjust feed and water rates, extruder temperature, vacuum, and cutting knives speed to optimize product quality. Record the time history of the extrusion run and sample products when the extruder reaches steady state (Figure 11.2).
7. Divide the resulting extruded pasta into two lots: one for fresh pasta and the other for production of dry pasta. Determine moisture content of fresh pasta, color, and cooking characteristics (texture of the cooked pasta that generally includes firmness, cohesiveness, elasticity and stickiness, water uptake, and cooking loss). The pasta cooking method is described in the next procedure.
8. Place a known amount of fresh pasta in a perforated sheet in convection oven set at 40°C for first stage drying (Figure 11.2). Construct

---

TABLE 11.1
Formulations Recommended for the Production of Durum Wheat Pasta Products

Ingredients	Regular Pasta	Regular Pasta with Spinach	Pasta with Fresh Eggs	Pasta with Dried Eggs
	%	%	%	%
Durum semolina	100.0	100.0	100.0	100.0
Fresh eggs	–	–	16.0	3.8
Dried whole eggs	–	–	–	3.8
Distilled water	24.8	24.8	14.4	26.4
Salt	0.16	0.16	0.16	0.16
Dehydrated ground spinach	–	3.0	–	–

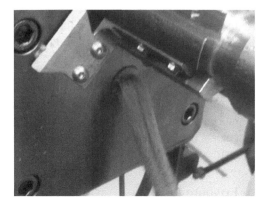

FIGURE 11.2 Production of extruded pasta. The picture depicts fettuccini extruded fresh pasta.

a drying curve by graphing the pasta moisture content vs. drying time. Remove pasta from the dryer when it decreases its moisture to 20%. For instance, 1 kg of fresh pasta with 31% moisture will lose 137.5 g water. Place partially dehydrated pasta for 2 hours in an environmental chamber at 30°C and 80% relative humidity for equilibration. Then place pasta again in the drying oven set at 32°C for dehydration until the pasta drops its moisture to 10%. Construct a drying curve by graphing the pasta moisture content vs. drying time. Remove pasta from the dryer when it decreases its moisture to 10%. For instance, 1 kg of fresh pasta with 31% moisture will yield 766.6 g of 10% moisture pasta.

9. Allow pasta to cool down and equilibrate at room temperature for 30 minutes and determine its moisture content (procedure in Section 2.2.1.1), color (procedure in Section 3.2.1), checking (visual observations of stress cracks), and cooking characteristics as described in the next procedure.

11.2.2.2 Cooking Quality of Pasta

The cooking quality of pasta is generally regarded as the capacity of the product to maintain good texture after cooking. Aroma and taste are also important to the consumer. The cooking quality depends essentially on the intrinsic characteristics of the durum wheat, the extraction rate of the semolina, and the pasta making process (Cubadda 1988). There is not a standard method for cooking quality evaluation. However, Cubadda (1988) suggests a method based on the evaluation of the cooked pasta in terms of stickiness, firmness, resistance to flattening, and bulkiness. The method is performed on spaghetti having a diameter of 1.6 to 1.65 or 1.7 to 1.75 mm, cooked under standard conditions for 10–11 minutes and examined by a trained sensory evaluation panel. The panelists evaluate stickiness, firmness, and bulkiness using a scoring scale of 0 to 100. The overall value of the cooking quality is determined by summing the score obtained for each characteristic, multiplying the sum by 33.3 and dividing by 100. Value of <40, 40 to 50, 50 to 70, 70 to 80, and >80 are considered poor, unsatisfactory, fair, good, and excellent, respectively.

The test can be performed with optimally and overcooked pasta. Normal cooking is considered the minimum cooking time plus 1 or 2–3 minutes depending on the spaghetti diameter. Minimum cooking time is attained when the central white line of the spaghetti strand disappears. Overcooking is obtained by adding 11 minutes to the normal cooking time or by doubling the minimum or regular cooking time (Cubadda 1988).

A. Samples, Ingredients, and Reagents
- Dry pasta
- Water
- Salt
- Desiccant (activated alumina)

B. Materials and Equipments
- Digital scale
- Cooking vessels or pots
- Graduated cylinder (2 L)
- Aluminum dishes
- Convection oven
- Airtight desiccator
- Tongs or pincers
- Colander
- Thermometer
- Chronometer

C. Procedure (Pasta Cooking Quality and Organic Matter Loss, Cubadda 1988)

1. Weigh 2 lots of 100 g of dry pasta, one for optimum cooking and the other for overcooking. Determine the pasta moisture content (procedure in Section 2.2.1.1), color (procedure in Section 3.2.1), checking or stress cracks, and chemical composition including starch (refer to Chapter 2).

2. In two separate cooking vessels preheat 1,000 mL water to gentle boiling (100°C). Add 1 g salt per 100 g dry pasta.

3. Add the pasta (i.e., spaghetti) to the boiling water of cooking vessel one and after 7 minutes start evaluating the white line commonly observed at the center of the spaghetti strand. Keep evaluating the white line until it disappears. Register this time as the minimum cooking time. Keep cooking for two additional minutes (optimum cooking). The spaghetti of cooking vessel two will be overcooked for 10 more minutes.

4. After cooking, immediately place the cooked spaghetti in a colander making sure to recuperate all the cooking water. Allow hot spaghetti to drain excess water for 1 minute and then cool down the spaghetti with running water for 1 minute. Allow excess water to drain and after weighing the spaghetti evaluate firmness, stickiness, and bulkiness. Score the spaghetti based on Table 11.2.

5. Calculate cooked pasta yield (weight of cooked pasta/weight of dry pasta) and the overall value

TABLE 11.2

Sensory Evaluation of the Quality of Cooked Pasta

Score	Firmness	Stickiness	Bulkiness
0	Absent	Totally	Totally
20	Rare	Very high	Very high
40	Insufficient	High	High
60	Sufficient	Rare	Rare
80	Good	Almost absent	Almost absent
100	Excellent	Absent	Absent

Source: Cubadda, R., *Durum Chemistry and Technology*, Chapter 11, AACC, St. Paul, MN, 1988.

of the cooking quality by summing each of the organoleptic scores, multiplying the sum by 33.3 and dividing by 100.

6. Measure the exact volume of the drained cooked water and after stirring sample a known volume for determination of total solids. Place sample on weighed aluminum dishes for at least 8 hours drying at 100°C. After drying, cool samples in a dessicator and calculate the amount of solids per milliliter of sample. Multiply the amount of solids by the total cook water volume and estimate loss of solids based on the original dry pasta weight.

11.2.2.3 Determination of Pasta Texture with the Texture Analyzer

The TAXT2 analyzer is used to test texture of experimental and commercial pasta and noodles products. A texture profile analysis consisting of a two-bite compression test is done to determine adhesiveness, cohesiveness, firmness, springiness, and other important parameters associated to cooked pasta characteristics. The texture analyzer technique is used for quality control purposes and is sensitive to raw material quality (i.e., particle size distribution, starch gluten content, starch damage, etc.) and processing conditions (extrusion and drying). The sample preparation procedure is critical to assure acceptable sensitivity of the test.

A. *Samples, Ingredients, and Reagents*
- Different types of cooked pasta or noodles
- Plastic shortening

B. *Materials and Equipments*
- Digital scale
- Hot plate or stove
- Cooking pots
- Large spoon
- Thermometer
- Chronometer
- Colander
- Texture analyzer TAXT2
- Caliper
- Heat-resistant protective gloves
- Knife
- Graduated cylinder (1 L)
- Acrylic mold (1.5-in. diameter 1.5-in. deep)
- Acrylic plunger to fit 1.5-in. mold
- 4-lb weight

C. *Procedure*
1. Prepare and calibrate the texture analyzer. Equip the instrument with the special plastic tooth. Standardize or calibrate the equipment to compress 70% of the average thickness of the cooked pasta or noodle strand.
2. Cook 100 g sample of pasta or noodles in 1 L of boiling water for a predetermined fixed period (refer to procedure in Section 11.2.2.2). It is

recommended to establish the optimum cooking time for samples. Gently stir contents every other minute during cooking.

3. Wearing protective gloves, pour the contents onto a colander so to discard the hot cooking water. Allow hot water to drain and then rinse the cooked pasta or noodles with cool tap water for 20–30 seconds. Allow excess water to drain.

4. Choose five pasta or noodle strands randomly and cut them into 7-cm-long pieces.

5. Lay side by side, the five pasta or noodle pieces on the TAXT2 Texture Analyzer instrument platform.

6. Run the two-bite compression test to 70% of the pasta or noodle thickness.

7. The computer will determine hardness, springiness, cohesiveness, and chewiness.
   a. Hardness. Gives an indication of the pasta or noodle bite.
   b. Springiness. Gives an indication of the degree of recovery after the first bite.
   c. Cohesiveness. Related to cooked pasta or noodle structure.
   d. Chewiness. Is a single parameter that incorporates firmness, cohesiveness, and springiness.

11.2.3 Research Suggestions

1. Prepare and compare pasta products produced from regular yellow semolina and a refined hard wheat flour. Determine differences in color and rheological properties of the raw materials and then compare the pasta products in terms of machinability, color, texture, water absorption during cooking, and cooking losses.

2. Prepare and compare pasta products produced from regular and damaged (heat damaged or high in diastatic activity) semolina. Determine the color and functionality of the semolina with a rheological instrument. Compare the pasta in terms of machinability, color, texture, water absorption during cooking, and cooking losses.

3. Prepare and compare pasta products produced with and without egg solids. Compare the fresh and dry pasta products in terms of machinability, color, texture, optimum cooking, water intake at optimum cooking, and cooking losses.

11.2.4 Research Questions

1. What are the ideal characteristics of durum semolina for pasta products?
2. What is pasta checking? What are main reasons of this defect? How can you prevent checking?

3. What are the main advantages of using egg solids in the manufacturing of pasta products?

4. What is the most critical operation in pasta production? Why is vacuum usually applied during pasta extrusion?

5. What are the potential risks of using fresh egg solids in the production of pasta or noodles?

6. Explain differences between conventional and fast pasta drying procedures. Regardless of the drying operation, what are the different drying phases?

7. Investigate two methods to produce precooked or microwavable durum wheat pasta products.

11.3 ORIENTAL NOODLES

11.3.1 ORIENTAL NOODLES FROM WHEAT FLOUR

Wheat flour noodles represent a dominant usage of refined wheat flour in Asia and thus are considered a major staple of the Southeast Asian diet with alkaline Chinese or Cantonese noodles having the dominant market share. It is believed that noodles originated in north China as early as 5000 B.C. Present-day noodles (*mian*) were a unique contribution to the Chinese culinary art by the Han dynasty (206 B.C. to 220 A.D.). According to Hatcher (2001), wheat-based noodles account for 30% to 40% of the cereal diet in most Asian countries, second only to rice dishes. Asian wheat noodles are made from wheat flour instead of durum semolina. The product is blended with water, sheeted, and cut from a low moisture dough (Corke and Bhattacharya 1999). Wheat noodles exist in two distinct types based on the use or not of alkaline salt: white salted and yellow alkaline. The other major type is the white salted noodles widely consumed in Japan. Alkaline noodles are made from flour, other ingredients, and alkaline salts such as sodium or potassium carbonates and less commonly sodium hydroxide. The alkali affects color, flavor, and texture. Noodles supplemented with high alkali levels have stronger flavor and coloration because flavones react with the alkaline salts (Hatcher and Anderson 2007). There are many sorts of alkaline noodles. The most popular are the fresh (Cantonese), partially boiled (*Hokkien* stype), and fresh or steamed with whole egg or egg whites (wonton) noodles. White salted noodles are divided in fresh (ramen) and high moisture steamed noodles (yakisoba) (Fu et al. 2006). Oriental noodles are commercialized in dried and fresh forms.

Wheat noodles can be produced from hard, intermediate, or soft wheat flours. Flours for yellow alkaline and savory noodles (containing shrimp, eggs, dried meats, tomato sauce, chili powder, and other foods) should contain higher protein (10%–12%) compared to white salted noodles (Nip 2007). The preferred flour is milled from medium protein wheats that yield intermediate gluten properties. High-quality Chinese noodles are also produced from partial waxy wheats that upon cooking yields noodles with distinctive textural properties. Oriental wheat noodles are produced by mixing with 33%–37% water, 2%–3% salt, and 0.05%–0.2% alkali (sodium potassium carbonate or sodium hydroxide). The alkali reagents influence starch gelatinization, cooking properties, and stiffness of raw noodles. The blend is mixed for 5–10 minutes and the resulting dough allowed to rest for gluten relaxing. The relaxed dough is then formed into noodles with a sheeting/cutting or extruder devices. The most popular method used in Asia is sheeting and cutting. The resulting fresh noodles can be dehydrated for the production of regular noodles or first steam-cooked and later on dried for the production of instant dried noodles. Fresh noodles have a limited shelf life of only 1 to 3 days, whereas dehydrated products have several months. Typically, noodles uptake from 0.83 g to 0.9 g water/g raw product. The percent cooking loss varies from 8% to 13%, the sodium hydroxide noodles being the ones with the highest losses. Cooked sodium potassium carbonate noodles are firmer and more resilient compared to counterparts produced with sodium hydroxide (Hatcher 2001; Hatcher and Anderson 2007; Hatcher et al. 2008).

The use of eggs for Asian noodles has been practiced for many decades in Hong Kong and parts of China because they contribute to the color, textural properties, and organoleptic properties (Nip 2007).

11.3.1.1 Production of Wheat-Based Oriental Noodles

A. *Samples, Ingredients, and Reagents*
- Refer to Table 11.3
- Peanut oil

B. *Materials and Equipments*
- Digital scale
- Sheeting rolls
- Mixer with paddle
- Noodle testing machine
- Graduated cylinders
- Stove
- Perforated drying sheets
- Hot plate or stove

TABLE 11.3
Formulations Recommended for the Production of Asian Noodles

Ingredients	Egg (%)	Japanese (%)	Chinese (%)	Hokkien (%)
Soft wheat flour	100.0	–	–	
Hard wheat flour	–	100.0	100.0	100.0
Distilled water	34.0	34.0	32.0	31.0
Fresh eggs	12.0	–	–	–
Salt	2.0	2.0	1.0	1.0
Sodium carbonate	–	–	0.4	0.9
Potassium carbonate	–	–	0.6	0.1
Sodium stearoyl-2-lactylate	0.2	–	–	–

- Wire-basket
- Steamer or aluminum pot for boiling
- Colander
- pH meter
- Convection drying oven
- Wooden roller pin
- Deep-fat fryer
- Cutting knives
- Ruler with millimeter markings
- Thermometer
- Chronometer

C. *Procedure*

1. Mix and beat the eggs, salt, and/or carbonates in the water.
2. Mix flour with the solution. Mix for 1 minute at low speed and then change to medium speed until attaining dough development. The resulting dough is stiff due to the low water absorption (Figure 11.3). Record the weight and pH of the dough.
3. Place the dough in a proof box set at 28°C–30°C and 75%–85% RH for 5 minutes.
4. Progressively laminate the dough using a pair of sheeting rolls. Start laminating using a roll gap of 3/8 in. and then gradually decrease the gap until achieving the minimum dough thickness (3 mm). Fold the resulting dough sheet in half and pass the two-layered dough through the rolls with a 3-mm gap setting. If necessary, allow sheet of dough to relax for at least

5 minutes. Then, gradually reduce the thickness to about 1.7 mm to 2 mm. If the sheeting roll unit is not capable, use a wooden pin roll.

5. Pass the dough sheet through a pair of cutting rolls with square grooves to produce the noodle strands (25 cm long × 3 mm wide × 1.7 to 2.5 mm thick). Alternatively, and if the noodle testing machine is not available, cut the sheet of dough with a sharp knife. Make sure to cut strips of the same sizes (Figure 11.3). For Hokkien noodles, place noodles in a wire basket and immerse them for 40 seconds in boiling water, then rinse with tap water, and after draining the water, apply 1% of peanut oil.
6. Divide the resulting noodles into two equal lots: one for fresh cooked noodles and the other for production of cooked instant noodles.
7. For fresh noodles cooking in an aluminum pot, boil 10 times the amount of water based on the fresh noodle weight. Bring water to boiling and then place fresh noodles in a wire basket for cooking. Immerse the basket in the pot and cook for 20 to 24 minutes. Heating should be maintained to keep the noodles in a gentle rolling boil (Figure 11.3).
8. After cooking, immediately remove noodles from the basket, place them in a plastic colander and wash noodles with plenty of running water. Allow excess water to drain and then pat five times the colander. Weigh the resulting

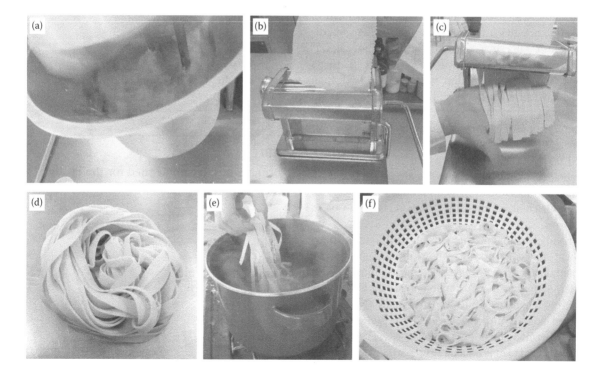

FIGURE 11.3 Production of wheat-based oriental noodles. (a) Dough mixing; (b) progressive sheeting of dough; (c) cutting of oriental noodles; (d) fresh noodle nest; (e) noodle cooking test; and (f) cooked and drained noodles for estimation of yield.

cooked noodles and estimate yield based on the uncooked weight.

9. Determine moisture content of fresh and cooked noodles, and the color and texture of cooked noodles (firmness, cohesiveness, elasticity and stickiness, water uptake, and cooking loss).

10. For instant noodles, first immerse noodles for 180 seconds in boiling water and then immediately rinse noodles with running tap water. Allow excess water to drain and place a known amount of cooked noodles in a perforated sheet in a convection oven set at 40°C for drying. Construct a drying curve by graphing the noodle moisture content vs. drying time. Remove dry noodles from the dryer when they contain a moisture content of 13%. If fried noodles are desired, then place a known amount of precooked noodles in a deep fat fryer containing palm oil at 160°C for 3 minutes. Allow excess oil to drain and then weigh the fried noodles for calculation of weight loss during frying.

11. Allow instant dried or fried noodles to cool down and equilibrate at room temperature for 30 minutes and determine its moisture and oil contents, color, cooking, and organoleptic characteristics.

11.3.2 Production of Rice Noodles

Rice noodles are also staple foods in Asia and are commercialized and merchandized in wet and dry forms. In China, rice noodles are named *mi fen*, whereas in Japan, they are called *harusame* (Luh 1999). Mi fen is only made from rice, whereas the Japanese counterpart is also produced from mung bean, starch, and blends. There are other types of Asian rice noodles. One of the most consumed is the *shahe fen* which is believed to have originated in the town of Shahe in the city of Guangzhou, China. *Shahe fen* is typical of southern Chinese cuisine, although similar noodles are also prepared in nearby nations such as Vietnam, Thailand, Cambodia, Philippines, Malaysia, Indonesia, and Singapore. *Shahe fen* is often stir fried with meat and vegetables in a dish called *chao fe*. Rice vermicelli is particularly prominent in the cuisines of People's Republic of China, Hong Kong, South India, and Sri Lanka. Due to the lack of functional gluten, the rice meal or flour should be gelatinized in order to produce a cohesive dough that is further formed and cut into noodles or vermicelli forms and steamed or regularly cooked in excess water. The fresh product has a limited shelf life.

Rice noodles are manufactured from two basic ingredients: rice flour and water. The raw material for making *mi fen* is nonglutinous rice because this allows easy extrusion of the pregelatinized dough (Lu 1999). The traditional process starts when nonglutinous rice is soaked in excess water for 2 to 4 hours, ground and mashed into a paste that is then pressed in a bag to force out excess water. Then, the starch-rich paste is steamed for 50–80 minutes to achieve about 80% gelatinization. The cooked paste is then kneaded and extruded into the typical configurations. Finally, the extruded product is steamed for 30 additional minutes, dipped into a seasoning, and placed on racks for dehydration (sun or artificial) or alternatively fried. The properly packaged dehydrated product can be kept for 1 to 2 years at room temperature. Rice noodles are frequently supplemented with maize or tapioca starch in order to improve the transparency and improve texture. Rice noodles are most commonly used in the cuisines of East and Southeast Asia and are available fresh, frozen, or dried, in various shapes and thicknesses. Rice noodles are usually freshly prepared at home and tend to be more tender, with distinctive texture compared to the dried form of Chinese noodles. Rice noodles are being viewed as an alternative to wheat flour-based noodles for individuals who are allergic or gluten intolerant. Rice noodles are more delicate than wheat noodles because they lack gluten that gives wheat noodles a structure that stands up to the onslaught of heat and liquids. Therefore, rice noodles soon pass from an adequate chewy to a mushy undesirable texture. The most recommended way to use rice noodles is at the end of the dish preparation so to avoid overcooking. The main advantage of rice noodles is that they easily absorb the flavors of a dish's liquids.

11.3.2.1 Production of Rice-Based Noodles
A. Samples, Ingredients, and Reagents
- Nonglutinous or regular white polished rice
- Distilled water
- Tapioca starch

B. Materials and Equipments
- Digital scale
- Tempering device
- Container with lids
- Hammer or roller mill
- Thermoplastic extruder
- Large pot for boiling water
- Chronometer
- Wire-basket
- Colander
- Thermometer
- Convection oven
- Perforated drying pans
- Heat-resistant protective gloves

C. Procedure
1. Temper 1 kg of white polished rice with 20 mL water in preparation for roller milling. Place the rice and the water in a container and shake contents to distribute the water. If rice is milled in a hammer mill do not condition the rice. Roller or hammer mill the rice to produce particles lower than 60 U.S. mesh and higher than 100 U.S. mesh (−60 to 100 U.S. mesh sieves). Determine the rice moisture content and particle size distribution of the rice meal.

2. In a large container, boil water and keep it at gentle boiling.

3. Mix rice with 3% tapioca starch and place contents in the hopper of a thermoplastic extruder equipped with a high shear screw and 1 mm round die orifices (vermicelli) or 1 cm × 1 mm slits for noodle production. Regulate the temperature of the three zones of the extruder barrel at 70°C, 120°C, and 140°C. Regulate the flow rate of the water to produce a feedstock with 34% to 36% moisture and the cutter to yield 25-cm-long vermicelli or noodle strands. Start collecting extruded noodles when the extruder enters to a steady state. Collect some of the extruded noodles for moisture, color, degree of starch gelatinization, and other chemical analyses.

4. Immerse known amounts of vermicelli or noodle strands in the boiling water for exactly 2 minutes. Collect the precooked noodles with the wire basket and place contents in a colander for washing with running tap water for approximately 30 seconds. Allow excess water to drain and weigh the rice noodles. Calculate the water absorption during the cooking process. Determine color, moisture, degree of starch gelatinization, and chemical composition of the precooked noodles.

5. Place a known amount of noodles on a perforated drying pan in a convection oven set at 40°C for drying. Dehydrate noodles to a moisture content of approximately 10%–12%. Allow dry noodles to equilibrate at room temperature for 1 hour. Determine moisture, color, degree of starch gelatinization, and chemical composition of the dried noodles.

6. Cook a known amount of dried noodles in 10 parts boiling water for 2 to 3 minutes. Remove noodles from cooking pot and place them in a colander for excess water draining and cooling with tap water. After cooling, allow excess water to drain and weigh the cooked noodles for calculation of water absorption during cooking. Reserve cooked rice noodles for sensory evaluations.

11.3.3 RESEARCH SUGGESTIONS

1. Prepare and compare regular noodles produced from refined soft, all-purpose, and hard wheat flours. Determine differences in color and rheological properties of the raw materials and then compare noodles in terms of machinability, color, texture, water absorption during cooking, and cooking losses.

2. Prepare and compare oriental noodles produced with and without alkaline compounds. Compare the noodle dough in terms of machinability, color, and texture, and then the cooked noodles in terms of water absorption during cooking, color, texture, and sensory properties.

3. Prepare and compare oriental noodles produced without and with 5% waxy starch. Compare the noodle dough in terms of machinability (stickiness), color, and texture, and then the cooked noodles in terms of water intake during cooking, cooked noodle texture, and sensory properties.

4. Compare pregelatinzed-extruded oriental rice noodles prepared with semolina obtained from long (regular starch), short (waxy), and a combination or regular and short white polished rices. Compare the cooked rice noodles in terms of texture (stickiness), water intake during cooking, and sensory properties.

11.3.4 RESEARCH QUESTIONS

1. Investigate two methods to produce precooked or microwavable noodles.

2. Why is it necessary to pregelatinize the starch of nonwheat milled fractions before the noodle forming operation?

3. What are differences in terms of raw materials and processing between oriental noodles and pasta? What is the functionality of waxy wheat, or starch in oriental noodles?

4. What are the major differences between alkali and regular wheat noodles? Describe the process to produce instant cup noodles seasoned with dried seasoning and ingredients such as vegetables and shrimp.

5. What are processing differences between wheat and rice noodles?

REFERENCES

Ambrogina Pagani, M., M. Lucisano, and M. Mariotti. 2007. "Traditional Italian Products from Wheat and Other Starchy Cereals." In *Handbook of Food Products Manufacturing. Principles, Bakery, Beverages, Cereals, Cheese, Confectionary, Fats, Fruits, and Functional Foods*, edited by Y. H. Hui, Chapter 17. Hoboken, NJ: Wiley Interscience.

Corke, H., and M. Bhattacharya. 1999. "Wheat Products. 1. Noodles." In *Asian Foods Science and Technology*, edited by C. Y. W. Ang, K. Liu, and Y. W. Huang, Chapter 3. Lancaster, PA: Technomic Publishing.

Cubadda, R. 1988. "Evaluation of Durum Wheat, Semolina and Pasta in Europe." In *Durum Chemistry and Technology*, edited by G. Fabriani and C. Lintas, Chapter 11. St. Paul, MN: AACC.

Donnelly, B. J., and J. G. Ponte. 2000. "Pasta: Raw Materials and Processing." In *Handbook of Cereal Science and Technology*, edited by K. Kulp and J. G. Ponte, Chapter 20. 2nd ed. New York, Marcel Dekker.

Feillet, P., and J. E. Dexter. 1996. "Quality Requirements of Durum Wheat for Semolina Milling and Pasta Production." In *Pasta and Noodle Technology*, edited by J. E. Kruger, R. B. Matsuo, and J. W. Dick, pp. 95–131. St. Paul, MN: AACC.

Fu, B. X., E. G. Assefaw, A. K. Sarkar, and G. R. Carson. 2006. "Evaluation of Durum Wheat Fine Flour for Alkaline Noodle Processing." *Cereal Foods World* 51(4):178–183.

Hatcher, D. W. 2001. "Asian Noodle Processing." In *Cereals Processing Technology*, edited by G. Owens, pp. 131–157. Cambridge, UK: Woodhead Publishing.

Hatcher, D. W., and M. J. Anderson. 2007. "Influence of Alkaline Formulation on Oriental Noodle Color and Texture." *Cereal Chemistry* 84:253–259.

Hatcher, D. W., N. M. Edwards, and J. E. Dexter. 2008. "Effect of Particle Size and Starch Damage of Flour and Alkaline Reagent on Yellow Alkaline Noodle Characteristics." *Cereal Chemistry* 85(3):425–432.

Kill, R. C., and K. Turnbull. 2001. *Pasta and Semolina Technology*. Oxford, UK: Blackwell Science.

Kim, S. K. 1996. "Instant Noodles." In *Pasta and Noodle Technology*, edited by J. E. Kruger, R. B. Matsuo, and J. W. Dick, pp. 195–225. St. Paul, MN: AACC.

Kruger, J. E., R. B. Matsuo, and J. W. Dick. 1996. *Pasta and Noodle Technology*. St. Paul, MN: AACC.

Luh, B. S. 1999. "Rice Products." In *Asian Foods Science and Technology*, edited by C. Y. W. Ang, K. Liu, and Y. W. Huang, Chapter 2. Lancaster, PA: Technomic Publishing.

Matsuo, R. R., L. J. Malcolmson, N. N. Edwards, and J. E. Dexter. 1992. "A Colorimetric Method for Estimating Spaghetti Cooking Losses." *Cereal Chemistry* 69:27–29.

Mercier, C., and C. Cantarelli. 1986. "Pasta and Extrusion Cooked Foods. Some Technological and Nutritional Aspects." *Tecnoalimenti Food Technology and Nutrition Series*, No.1. New York: Elsevier.

Miskelly, D. M. 1996. "The Use of Alkali for Noodle Processing." In *Pasta and Noodle Technology*, edited by J. E. Kruger, R. B. Matsuo, and J. W. Dick, pp. 227–273. St. Paul, MN: AACC.

Nagao, S. 1996. "Processing Technology of Noodle Products in Japan." In *Pasta and Noodle Technology*, edited by J. E. Kruger, R. Matsuo, and J. W. Dick, pp. 169–194. St. Paul, MN: AACC.

Nip, W. K. 2007. "Asian (Oriental) Noodles and Their Manufacture." In *Handbook of Food Products Manufacturing. Principles, Bakery, Beverages, Cereals, Cheese, Confectionary, Fats, Fruits, and Functional Foods*, edited by Y. H. Hui, Chapter 23. Hoboken, NJ: Wiley Interscience.

12 Production of Breakfast Cereals and Snack Foods

12.1 INTRODUCTION

One of the chief uses of dry-milled fractions of cereal grains is for the manufacturing of breakfast cereals and snacks. The new trend of these industries is the production of highly nutritious foods rich in dietary fiber, nutraceuticals, and micronutrients. Both families of products are obtained following similar operations but differ in formulation. Breakfast cereals are usually flavored with sugars or sweeteners and enriched with vitamins and minerals, whereas snacks are usually salty and rich in fat. The fat is absorbed by the base product during frying and flavoring. This is the main reason these foods are considered as empty. Snacks usually contain a high energy density and sodium and are, in most cases, low in protein and micronutrients. Regardless of the process and bad image among dietitians, snacks are increasing in popularity due to their flavor, convenience, and change of food habits.

The snack food industry also produces an array of ready-to-eat (RTE) and convenient foods high in oil and flavored with salt or salty flavorings. From the processing viewpoint, snacks can be manufactured by a wide array of processes ranging from simple to sophisticated/complex. The simpler snacks are those produced from popcorn and the most complex are those obtained by thermoplastic extrusion. Snacks are classified into first-, second-, and third-generation items. The first generation is the easiest to produce and consists of natural products used for snacking such as popcorn. Most snacks produced today fall into the category of second generation. These include simple formed products mainly obtained after direct extrusion processes (i.e., corn chips, puffed, or expanded corn products) or by sheeting/forming such as tortilla chips and pretzels. The most elaborate category in terms of ingredients and processing is the third-generation snacks produced by extrusion processes aimed toward the production of pellets or half-products. Extrusion commonly consists of two sequential steps: cooking and forming. The forming extruder yields dense pellets that require further processing to reach the consumer. Frying the pellets produces most third-generation snacks, although conventional baking or microwaving fabricates a number of low-calorie items. The most recent and modern category is the production of snacks by coextrusion. In this process, the extruder is equipped with a special type of die that allows the coextrusion of two types of materials: an outer covering generally produced from cereals and an inner filling that contains salty based flavorings (Serna-Saldivar 2008).

One of the major types of snacks is the so-called nixtamalized items. These are obtained from fresh or dry *masa*

flour that is hydrated and further processed into corn and tortilla chips. These products are usually produced from coarse *masa* or flours in order to avoid pillowing or blistering during frying. Corn chips are produced by directly deep-fat frying of preformed pieces of *masa*, whereas tortilla chips are manufactured from baked tortilla pieces that are further fried. Most snacks contain low-moisture and high-fat contents and are packed inside multilaminated polyethylene or aluminum bags that present a good barrier against environmental moisture and solar light, which acts as a prooxidant (Serna-Saldivar 2008; Serna-Saldivar et al. 1998).

The quality of breakfast cereals and snacks greatly depends on the characteristics of the raw materials and on the various manufacturing steps used throughout processing. The quality of raw materials described in Chapters 1–3 is critically important because this also affects processing conditions. Moisture, ash, particle size distribution, starch damage, and color are important quality attributes of raw materials. For starches, the viscoamylograph assay is very useful because it predicts pasting, retrogradation, and other important functionalities imparted by the starch (Shuey and Tipples 1982). For oils, the stability, acidity, and fatty acid composition are important factors to consider.

The most important quality control parameters used in these industries are summarized in Table 12.1. The breakfast cereal industry relies on quality control parameters previously discussed for whole grains (Chapter 1), dry and wet-milled products (Chapters 5 and 6), and wheat quality tests (Chapter 5). Quality greatly depends on the characteristics of the various types of raw materials and on the manufacturing steps used throughout processing. For all breakfast cereals, the qualities of refined grits and starches are critically important because they affect organoleptic properties, product expansion, and processing conditions. Moisture, ash, particle size distribution, starch damage, and color are important quality attributes. For starches, the viscoamylograph assay is very useful as it predicts pasting, retrogradation, and other important functionalities (Table 12.1).

The most important quality attributes of breakfast cereals are bulk density, texture, color, sweetness, and sensory properties. For direct extruded products or puffs the radial expansion rate is almost always evaluated by simply dividing the extrudate diameter by the die orifice diameter. There are different ways to assess the bulk density of flakes, oven-puffed rice, extruded puffs, and pellets. Most processors subjectively evaluate the bulk density by determining the weight of a certain volume. This simple nondestructive and quick procedure is commonly employed in processing lines.

TABLE 12.1

Quality Control Parameters Most Commonly Used to Assess Quality of Breakfast Cereals and Snack Foods

Quality Control	Equipment Instrument	Importance
Moisture (refer to Chapter 2)	NIRA, microwave, moisture meters/balances, air oven method (AACC 2000, Method 44-15A)	The moisture content of raw materials, tempered-equilibrated blends, extrudates, and finished products affects processing, product quality, and texture of breakfast cereals and snacks.
Water activity (refer to Chapter 3)	Water activity meter	The determination of the A_w is critically important for low-moisture breakfast cereals snack foods. These products are manufactured to reach certain or given A_w level. Water activity affects microbial growth, enzyme activity and product texture.
Bowl-life test	Texture analyzer TAXT2	The bowl-life test is widely used to test the loss of texture of breakfast cereals after blending with milk. The texturometer equipped with the Ottawa cell and a watertight base is used to perform the test.
Expansion rate or radial expansion	Diameter or extrudate/ diameter of die orifice	Test widely used to monitor in plant expansion of extrudates. Many factors affect the expansion rate: quality of raw materials (refer to Chapter 1), tempering, extrusion conditions (temperature-pressure gradient), and pressure release valves or vents prior to die forming.
Bulk density (refer to Chapter 1)	Winchester bushel meter (AACC 2000, Method 55-10) or measurement of weight/volume	Bulk density is important because it is closely related to the extrudate expansion rate and extrusion conditions. The advantage of this simple test is that it can be rapidly determined.
Density (refer to Chapter 1)	Pycnometer (nitrogen or air displacement)	True density is important because it is closely related to the quality of pellets or half-products. The advantage of this simple test is that it can be rapidly determined.
Starch content (refer to Chapters 2 and 6)	NIRA, analytical determination of total starch (AACC 2000, Method 76-11)	This is the most important single component of dry milled fractions, extrudates, and finished products. Starch greatly affects functionality and expansion rate of breakfast cereals and snacks.
Starch gelatinization (refer to Chapter 6)	Birefringence with microscope equipped with polarized filters	Microscopic technique used to determine the relative amount of gelatinized vs. native starch granules (starch granules are shaped like the Maltese cross).
	Glucoamylase method with subsequent measurement of glucose (AACC 2000, Method 76-16)	Chemical analysis in which the *masa* is subjected to amyloglucosidase hydrolysis followed by the determination of glucose with glucose oxidase. The ESS assay correlates with degree of cooking and starch gelatinization.
Starch properties (refer to Chapter 6)	Viscoamylograph (Shuey and Tipples 1982)	One of the most important functional tests because after analyzing the viscoamylograph curve it could be the determined temperature at start of gelatinization, peak viscosity, shear thinning, and set back viscosity (retrogradation). These properties greatly influence processing characteristics and quality of end products.
Water absorption and solubility indexes (refer to Chapter 7)	Centrifugation of slurry (Anderson et al. 1969)	These parameters are greatly affected by the degree of starch gelatinization affected by extrusion conditions.
Oil content (refer to Chapter 2)	NIRA	The most important chemical determination for snacks. This is generally determined via near infrared analysis. When properly calibrated, NIRA instruments determine fat in several seconds. However, instrument calibration and recalibration are critical for reliable analyses.
	Hydraulic press (Rooney 2007)	The hydraulic or carver press is widely used to determine oil for quick quality control purposes. A ground sample is placed in a chamber for mechanical-pressing extraction. After the pressing cycle is completed, the free oil or the partially defatted snack sample is weighed. The instrument should be calibrated for each type of snack because they leave different amounts of residual oil (around 12% oil). Values should be correlated to solvent extraction values.
	Solvent extraction Goldfisch or Soxhlet Extractor (AACC 2000, Method 30-25)	The ether extraction technique is the official method of fat analysis. It consists of extracting oil using petroleum ether, followed by removal of the solvent and weighing of the oil. The main disadvantage of ether extraction is that it takes several hours to perform the test.
Peroxide value (refer to Chapter 2)	AOCS (2009) Method Cc8-53; AACC 2000 Method 58-16	It is the most widely used quality control parameter to estimate rancidity of snack foods. The main oxidation products of oils are hydroperoxides, which can be quantitatively measured by the amount of iodine liberated by its reaction with potassium iodide.
Active oxygen method (AOM) (refer to Chapter 2)	AOCS (2009) Method Cd12-57; AACC (2000), Method 58-54	Most common rapid method to determine oxidative stability of oil-laden products. The method predicts the resistance of the extracted heated oil (97.8°C) to oxidation by bubbling air into the sample.

(continued)

TABLE 12.1 (Continued)
Quality Control Parameters Most Commonly Used to Assess Quality of Breakfast Cereals and Snack Foods

Quality Control	Equipment Instrument	Importance
Hexanal content	Gas chromatography (Pike 1994)	Hexanal is a volatile closely related to extent of lipid oxidation and rancidity. It is determined in the headspace of the package and correlates with peroxide values.
Hardness (refer to Chapter 3)	Instron or TAXT2 Texturometer	Extrudates are compressed at a constant rate in order to obtain a force-deformation curve. The hardness affects the texture and overall acceptability of the extrudates.
Color value (refer to Chapter 3)	Color meters (Hunter Lab, NIRA, and others)	The color of the extrudates is one of the most important attributes affecting the acceptability of breakfast cereals and snacks. The color of the extrudate is affected by the color of the raw materials, percent reducing sugars, baking and frying temperatures, and percentage and type of covering.
Salt (refer to Chapter 2)	AACC (2000), Methods 40–60 ($AgNO_3$ method) or 40–61 (total chloride method); Rooney (2007)	Added salt can be determined by estimating the amount of sodium or chloride. The salt is extremely important in extruded products because it is closely related to the amount added as flavoring, or as an indicator of the percentage of covering. Sodium is also important from the nutritional label.
Laboratory pretzel procedure	Serna-Saldivar (2003)	The yield and quality of pretzels can be determined in the laboratory using a standardized procedure where flour is mixed to obtain dough that is manually shaped into pretzel forms, fermented, NaOH washed, salted, and baked.
Sensory evaluation	Triangular tests (Meilgaard et al. 1991)	Ideally suited for comparison of two different samples. The trained or untrained panelist tries to identify the odd and paired samples among the three samples in the set and then is asked why she/he considered the odd sample different.
	Hedonic preference test (Meilgaard et al. 1991)	Trained or untrained panelists evaluate the color, aroma, flavor, texture, and overall acceptability of the products in a sensory evaluation laboratory. Products are usually evaluated using a 9 point hedonic scale where 4 = like extremely, 0 = neither like nor dislike, and –4 dislike extremely.

Source: American Association of Cereal Chemists, *Approved Methods of the AACC*, St. Paul, MN: AACC, 2000; Anderson et al., 1969; AOCS, *Official Methods and Recommended Practices of the AOCS*, 6th ed., Danvers, MA: The Society, 2009; Meilgaard et al., 1991; Pike, O.A., *Food Analysis*, edited by S.S. Nielsen, pp. 225–228, 2nd ed., Gaithersburg, MD: Aspen Publishers, 1994; Rooney, 2007; Shuey, W.C., and Tipples, K.H., *The Amylograph Handbook*, St. Paul, MN: AACC, 1982; Snack Food Association, *Corn Quality Assurance Manual*, Alexandria, VA: SFA, 1992.

Analytical approaches that are frequently used to study textural properties of extrudates are the Instron or texture analyzer shear force or compression tests. The final moisture and sugar contents are continuously monitored in most breakfast cereals because they affect texture or crispness and flavor, respectively. Moisture can be determined by NIRA and the use of gravimetric methods using the air–oven technique.

For extruded breakfast cereals and snacks, the frequent monitoring of the extrusion process is required to adjust settings for the greatest product uniformity. The most important factors to control are moisture in the tempered raw materials, feed rate, temperatures/pressure in the different zones of the extruder and die, and the extrudate expansion rate and moisture. It is also important to monitor the degree of covering that usually correlates with the sugar content (Stauffer 1990).

The bowl-life test was developed to study the susceptibility of the breakfast cereal to lose texture after hydration with milk. The loss of texture throughout time (usually after 5 minutes) is determined with a texturometer.

Since most breakfast cereals are enriched or fortified with selected vitamins and minerals, the determinations of these nutrients are of upmost importance for the industry and for labeling purposes (refer to Chapter 2).

12.2 PRODUCTION OF BREAKFAST CEREALS

The breakfast cereal industry is one of the most versatile in terms of products and technology. Products are convenient and practical because most do not need cooking and preparation and have a long shelf life. Breakfast cereals are divided into two broad categories: hot or RTE. Undoubtedly, most are categorized as RTE because they do not need any further cooking at home. Breakfast cereals are crucial because they constitute the first meal of the day and are considered highly nutritious because they do not contain significant amounts of fat and do contain important quantities of essential vitamins and minerals and are almost always served with milk, which complements their nutritional value. These products are normally flavored with sugar or sweeteners and nondiastatic malt. In some instances dehydrated fruits and nuts are blended with finished products.

The manufacturing of breakfast cereals needs the appropriate selection and combination of raw materials, highly sophisticated production steps, and stringent quality control programs. Breakfast cereals do not contain significant amounts of moisture in order to preserve the texture and guarantee their microbial stability. Packaging materials and technologies play an important role in keeping the typical characteristics of finished products.

The general manufacturing process starts with the combination of ingredients that are cooked, formed, baked, flavored-enriched, and packaged. Cooking is necessary in order to gelatinize the starch and produce doughs that can be mechanically sheeted, shaped, or formed. It is generally performed in pressure cookers, open-steam jacketed cookers, or with continuous extruders. Pressure and steam-cookers are usually used to process grains or large grits, whereas extruders are used to process smaller grits, semolinas, meals, and even flours. Cooking is aimed toward the gelatinization and pasting of starch granules accompanying water diffusion into the raw material. The moisture and starch modification is required for adequate sheeting, shaping, and forming (Caldwell et al. 2000; Fast 2001; Fast and Caldwell 2000; Valentes et al. 1991). Extrusion is used to manufacture two major categories of products: puffs or pellets. Pellets are also called half or intermediate products because they are shelf-stable and require additional processes in order to reach the consumer. They are generally flaked or expanded in puffing guns or special ovens. The preformed configurations are usually baked in continuous ovens to enhance flavor, texture, and color. Baking greatly affects the sensory properties of breakfast cereals. Texture and bowl-life is achieved during this critical step. Baked or toasted cereals are commonly flavored and/or sweetened with topical coatings of liquid sprays or dry powders on-line or applied inside coating drums. The coating usually contains part of the enrichment premix (Fast and Caldwell 2000). Packaging is essential for the preservation of breakfast cereals especially in terms of texture.

Breakfast cereals are classified according to their manufacturing process into traditional processed flakes, extruded flakes, oven-puffed cereals, gun-puffed whole grains, extruded expanded, cofilled extruded expanded, shredded whole grains, extruded shredded products, filled bite-size shredded wheat, baked cereals, granolas, compressed flake biscuit, and muesli type products (Fast and Caldwell 2000; Fast 2001; Serna-Saldivar 2010; Valentes et al. 1991). The market distribution is dominated by flaked (traditional and extruded) and puffed (oven, extruded, and gun-puffed) products. Most breakfast cereals were born by a traditional process that later on evolved into extrusion. Extrusion offers the advantage of more versatility, faster production rate, lower investment and energy, and personnel savings. Flakes that are shredded or oven-puffed are typical examples of products that can be manufactured following the traditional process or from extrusion.

12.2.1 Corn Flakes

Corn flakes are still the most popular breakfast cereal in the world. Dr. Kellogg developed the traditional process at the beginning of the last century. More than 100 years later, this breakfast cereal is still manufactured following the same basic steps. The process starts with the selection of degermed large grits (U.S. No. 3.5-6) from yellow maize that are pressure-cooked in rotating cookers positioned horizontally at approximately 1 kg/cm² or 15 psi for 1 to 2 hours with flavorings and limited amounts of water. The typical formulation consists of 100 kg of grits, 6 kg sugar, 2 kg malt syrup, and 2 kg salt. Water is added to increase moisture content to approximately 31%. Sugar and salt are sometimes added in water whereas malt syrup is sometimes substituted by nondiastatic malt flour. The aim of cooking is to achieve the proper starch gelatinization and the development of flavor and color. The optimum cooking time varies according to the size and grit hardness. The cooked grits have a translucent appearance and tend to aggregate in lumps. Cooked grits are then conveyed to a lump breaking machine that separates agglomerated grits into single units. Subsequently, the cooked grits are partially dried at approximately 65°C to reduce the moisture to 20% followed by equilibration in tempering bins for 6 to 24 hours. During this time, the internal grit moisture equilibrates throughout the grit structure. The tempered hard and dark-cooked grits are flaked with a pair of counter rotating rolls that apply a pressure of approximately 234 tons/cm². The plastic, light-colored, and soft flakes are toasted with hot air in cylindrical rotary ovens where flakes are evenly toasted on suspended hot air. The toasting time varies from 50 seconds to 3 minutes depending on the temperature profile. Flakes are generally toasted at temperatures of 288°C–302°C. Toasting dehydrates the flakes, develops a crisp texture and the characteristic flavor and color. The golden color is mainly due to Maillard reactions. After toasting, flakes are immediately covered with flavorings, sweeteners, and the enrichment mix. A heavy sugar coating is applied during this step for the production of sugar coated or frosted flakes. Optimally, the minimum moisture to preserve crispiness is less than 2% (Fast and Caldwell 2000; Fast 2001; Rooney and Serna-Saldivar 2003; Serna-Saldivar 2010; Tribelhorn 1991; Whalen et al. 2000).

12.2.1.1 Production of Corn Flakes

A. *Samples, Ingredients, and Reagents*
- Refer to Table 12.2
- Aluminum foil

B. *Materials and Equipments*
- Digital scale
- Close container for tempering
- Pressure cooker with stand
- Stove
- Graduated cylinder (1 L)

TABLE 12.2

Recommended Formulation for Corn Flakes

Ingredients	Amount (g)
Refined maize yellow flaking grits (No. 6)	1,000
Sugar	60
Malt syrup	20
Salt	20
Water	Sufficient to increase grit moisture to 30%

- Aluminum foil
- Beaker (2 L)
- Chronometer
- Air-forced convection oven
- Glass bottle with lid
- Flaking roll unit
- Caliper
- Perforated metal sheets
- Protective gloves
- Protective lenses

C. Procedure

1. Determine the refined grit and malt syrup moisture contents (refer to Chapter 2).
2. Weigh independently the ingredients listed in Table 12.2. Calculate the water required to increase the grit moisture content to 30%. Use the following equation [(100 − grit moisture)/(100 − 30%) − 1] × amount of grits. Mix the water with the sugar, malt syrup, and salt. Place flaking grits in a closed container and incorporate the water and other ingredients. Manually agitate contents until all the solution is absorbed by the grits. This will require at least 1 hour (Figure 12.1). After all the solution has been absorbed, place the tempered grits in a beaker and cover with aluminum foil. Discard excess solution if it remains in the beaker.
3. Place about 3 cm of water and the internal stand in the pressure cooker and turn on the heat source. When the water starts to boil, place the beaker with the corn flake formulation. Then, set and seal the pressure cooker lid.

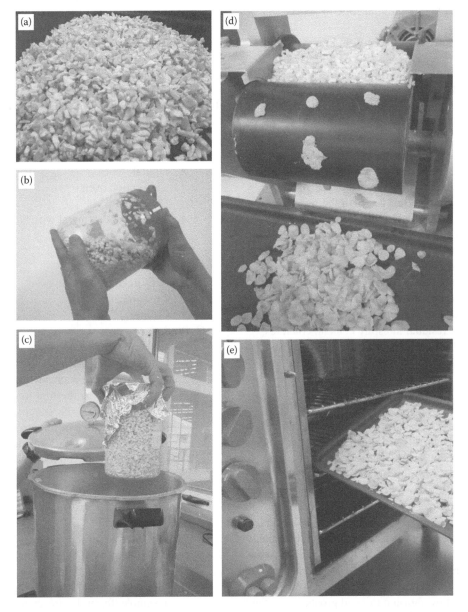

FIGURE 12.1 Sequential steps for the production of maize flakes. (a) Flaking grits; (b) tempering grits with flavorings before pressure cooking; (c) pressure cooking of grits; (d) flaking cooked grits; and (e) toasting of flakes.

4. Register the time required to achieve 0.84 kg/cm^2 to 1.05 kg/cm^2 (12 psi to 15 psi) and pressure cook for 60 more minutes. Suspend heat and allow pressure cooker to cool down for 20 minutes. Then, carefully release the pressure until the pressure cooker mark returns to zero. Do not open the pressure cooker until you are completely sure that it does not have pressure.

5. With protective gloves and lenses take out cooked grits, weigh them, and place them on a clean surface in order to manually delump the grits. According to the initial formulation and cooked weights calculate the moisture content of the cooked grits.

6. Place grits on a tray for partial dehydration. Dehydrate (50°C) grits to lower their moisture to 20%–22%. Weigh grits every 5 minutes in order to estimate optimum time to achieve the target moisture.

7. Place partially dehydrated grits in a glass container for tempering for at least 8 hours. Make sure to seal the container (Figure 12.1).

8. Pass cooked grits through a set of properly adjusted flaking rolls. Measure the dimensions of at least 10 of the resulting flakes. Register the average length, width, and thickness.

9. Place flakes in between two perforated metal sheets in preparation for air-forced oven toasting. Preheat oven to a temperature of 280°C before placing baking sheets in the oven. Toast flakes to lower their moisture content to 2% (approximately 2 to 3 minutes).

10. Remove toasted flakes from baking sheets and allow flakes to cool down for 15 minutes at room temperature.

11. Weigh toasted flakes and immediately place them in sealed high density polyethylene bags. Determine residual moisture content, color, texture, bowl-life, and sensory properties of resulting corn flakes.

12.2.2 Rolled or Flaked Oats

Rolled or flaked oats are considered the most popular breakfast food produced from this cereal grain. The oat process is different from others because flakes are not extensively cooked nor toasted. As a result, oat flakes have quite different texture compared to toasted corn flakes. The basic process starts when whole oat kernels are heat-treated or steamed to inactivate lipases and lipoxygenase (refer to procedure in Section 5.2.4.1). These enzymes catalyze undesirable rancidity reactions that cause off-flavors and odors. Needless to say, this is considered the most critical operation because it greatly influences flavor, aroma, and shelf life. The husked caryopses are then dehulled by abrasion to yield groats. Groats are then cut into large pieces or flaked as whole kernels. The final product requires cooking before consumption because

the grain only receives the heat treatment to inactivate lipolytic enzymes. Generally, regular oat flakes require 5 to 15 minutes cooking (Doehlert and Moore 1997; Doehlert et al. 1999; Doehlert and McMullen 2000; Serna-Saldivar 2010).

To produce instant flakes, the groats are conditioned and steamed before flaking. The steaming at atmospheric pressure softens the groat, gelatinizes the starch, and allows flakes to be rolled with a minimum of breakage. The most common commercial steamer consists of a column in which nozzles inject steam. The dwell time in the steamer is approximately 12–15 minutes during which time the oat pieces increase the temperature to about 100°C and the moisture to 10%–12%. Then the steamed pieces pass directly into the flaking unit consisting of two rolls that rotate at 250 rpm to 450 rpm. The gap between the rolls and nip pressure are hydraulically controlled by oil or compressed air pressure. Following the flaking unit, the rolled oats are passed to a sifter where fines are removed. Last, the flakes are cooled to remove moisture and temperature in columns or band-type coolers (Deane and Commers 1986). The flakes are generally packaged in carton boxes so the internal headspace gases rich in oxidative volatile compounds can easily dissipate through the cardboard barrier (Serna-Saldivar 2010).

12.2.2.1 Production of Rolled Oats

A. Samples, Ingredients, and Reagents
- Different lots of groats

B. Materials and Equipments
- Digital scale
- Convection oven
- Drying pans
- Steamer with a metal wire basket
- Stove
- Flaking rolls
- Baking sheets
- Air forced convection oven
- Chronometer
- Caliper

C. Procedure
1. Weigh a sample of groats obtained following procedure in Section 5.2.4.1.
2. Place groats in a steamer for heat treatment for 15 minutes. This thermal treatment softens the groat, gelatinizes the starch, and allows flakes to be rolled with a minimum of breakage.
3. Allow steamed groats to equilibrate at room temperature and then flake them through the set of flaking rolls.
4. Place flaked or rolled oats onto a perforated pan for 10 minutes toasting in a convection oven set at 140°C–150°C.
5. Measure the average thickness with a caliper, and dimensions (length and width) of at least 10 randomly selected flakes.
6. Calculate the yield of flaked groats and reserve a sample for moisture content determination. Determine color, degree of starch gelatinization, bowl-life, shelf life, and sensory analyses.

12.2.3 OVEN-PUFFED RICE

Oven-puffed rice has been one of the most important breakfast cereals for more than 100 years. This product is manufactured with the same unit operations applied for traditional corn flakes. Generally, white polished rice kernels expand 2 to 5 times their original volume. The preferred rice is medium or short white polished rice with intermediate amylose content (15%–20%) that is pressure cooked at approximately 1 kg/cm² for 60–90 minutes. A typical formula based on 100 kg of rice is 6–10 kg sugar, 2 kg salt, 2 kg of malt extract or its equivalent of nondiastatic malt, and enough water to increase the grain moisture to 28%. The agglomerated cooked rice is lump break, and dried in two stages. The first drying is aimed toward the reduction of the grain moisture from 28% to 17% in preparation for bumping whereas the second to optimize expansion during the critical step of oven-puffing. The cooked and partially dehydrated rice is equilibrated in bins for 4–30 hours in order to allow internal moisture equilibration. After tempering, the rice is bumped through rolls operating with a gap of approximately the thickness of the grain. During bumping, kernels are slightly flattened to improve their expansion during subsequent baking. Next, the bumped rice is dehydrated for a second time to drop its moisture to 10%, which is ideal for maximizing puffing. The rice expands in continuous rotary ovens operating at temperatures of up to 340°C. Finally, the oven-puffed rice is sprayed in a tumbler with selected vitamins and minerals, cooled, and packaged.

12.2.3.1 Production of Oven-Puffed Rice

A. Samples, Ingredients, and Reagents
- Refer to Table 12.3
- Aluminum foil

B. Materials and Equipments
- Digital scale
- Graduated cylinder (1 L)
- Pressure cooker with stand
- Stove
- Beaker (2 L)
- Chronometer
- Air-forced convection oven
- Glass bottle with lid
- Flaking roll unit

TABLE 12.3
Recommended Formulation for Manufacturing Oven-Puffed Rice

Ingredients	Amount (g)
White-polished rice	1,000
Sugar	60
Malt syrup	20
Salt	20
Water	Sufficient to increase rice moisture to 28%

- Caliper
- Perforated metal sheets
- Protective gloves
- Protective lenses

C. Procedure

1. Determine the white rice moisture content, test weight, 1000 kernel weight, and average length, width, and thickness (refer to Chapters 1 and 2).

2. Weigh independently the ingredients listed in Table 12.3. Calculate the water required to increase the rice moisture content to 28%. Use the following equation [(100 − grit moisture)/(100 − 28%) − 1] × amount of rice. Mix the water with the sugar, malt syrup, and salt. Place rice in a closed container and incorporate the water and other ingredients. Manually agitate contents until all the solution is absorbed by the rice (Figure 12.2). This will require at least 1 hour. After all the solution has been absorbed, place the tempered rice in a beaker, and cover with aluminum foil. If solution remains in the beaker discard it.

3. Place about 3 cm of water and the internal stand in the pressure cooker and turn on the heat source. When the water starts to boil place the beaker with the corn flake formulation. Then, set and seal the pressure cooker lid.

4. Register the time required to achieve 0.84 to 1.05 kg-force/cm² (12 psi to 15 psi) and pressure cook for 60 more minutes. Suspend heat and allow pressure cooker to cool down for 20 minutes. Then, carefully release the pressure until the pressure cooker mark returns to zero. Do not open the pressure cooker until you are completely sure that it does not have pressure.

5. With protective gloves and lenses, take out the cooked rice, weigh it, and place it on a clean surface in order to manually delump the cooked kernels. Based on the initial formulation and cooked weights, calculate the moisture content of the cooked rice.

6. Place rice on a tray for partial dehydration. Dry (50°C) grits to lower their moisture to 17%. Weigh rice every 5 minutes in order to estimate optimum time to achieve the target moisture (Figure 12.2).

7. Place partially dehydrated rice in a glass container for tempering for at least 8 hours. Make sure to seal the container.

8. Pass cooked rice through a set of properly adjusted flaking rolls for bumping (Figure 12.2). The gap between the rolls is opened in order to slightly compress kernels. Measure the dimensions of at least 10 of the resulting kernels. Register the average length, width, and thickness.

9. Place rice on a tray for a second dehydration step. Dry (50°C) rice to further lower the

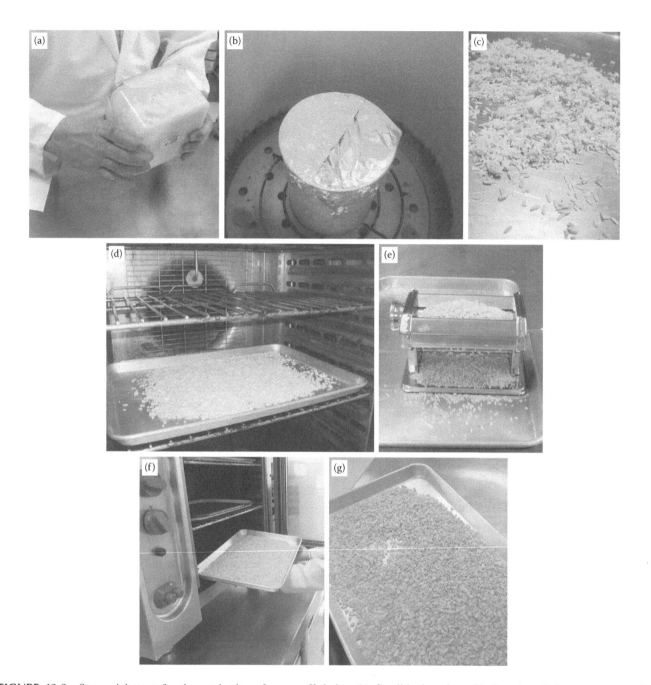

FIGURE 12.2 Sequential steps for the production of oven-puffed rice. (a) Conditioning rice with flavorings before pressure cooking; (b) pressure cooking of rice; (c) pressure cooked rice; (d) first dehydration step of cooked rice kernels; (e) bumping of rice kernels; (f) toasting–puffing operation; and (g) oven-puffed rice.

moisture to 10%. Weigh rice every 5 minutes in order to estimate optimum time to achieve the target moisture.

10. Place rice with 10% moisture in between two perforated metal sheets in preparation for air-forced oven toasting. Preheat oven to a temperature of 280°C before placing baking sheets in the oven. Toast rice to lower their moisture content to 2% (approximately 2–3 minutes).

11. Remove toasted and partially puffed rice from baking sheets and allow to cool down for 15 minutes at room temperature.

12. Weigh oven-puffed rice and immediately place them in sealed high density polyethylene bags. Determine average length, width, thickness, and residual moisture content, test weight, 1000 kernel weight, color, texture, bowl-life, and sensory properties.

12.2.4 Extruded Corn Puffs

Corn puffs are manufactured by gun puffing or direct expansion extrusion. Extruders for direct expanded products cook, expand, and form the extrudate, which is subsequently sized, dried or toasted, flavored with liquid or solid mixes, and packaged. Refined yellow maize grits (Nos. 40 to 60) is the major ingredient in the formulation of corn puffs. This raw material is usually mixed with nonfat dry milk, sugar, and other flavorings that do not compromise puffing or radial expansion (extrudate diameter/die orifice diameter). The best expansion rates are obtained from refined grits low in fat, fiber, and starch damage (refer to Chapter 5). Operationally, the extruder should be equipped with a screw that increases mechanical shear and a die that restricts flow rate. The most frequent used refined grits have an average particle size of 40 to 60 U.S. mesh. These grits are mixed with the other formula ingredients (Table 12.4) and conditioned to approximately 16%–19% before extrusion. The tempered grits are introduced into the inlet of the barrel or screw feeding zone. In this particular place, the distances between flights are longer and deeper compared to the subsequent zones. The pitch or flight angle favors the movement of the feedstock. The flow channel of the screw is typically filled with grits. In this area the incoming material is slightly compressed and trapped air expelled. In some extruders water is injected into the first part of the feeding zone. The temperature of the barrel in the feeding zone is the lowest, generally 60°C–80°C. The conditioned grits enter the kneading or transition zone that is characterized to contain a higher barrel temperature (90°C–120°C) and a screw design that favors compression by lowering the distance between flights and the flight height so the flow channels achieve a higher degree of fill. The starch-rich extrudate starts to lose its granular structure, and gelatinize due to the temperature and pressure. The combination of heat and pressure converts the grits into plastic dough. When the dough reaches the last zone it melts and becomes a viscous fluid due to the high temperature (140°C–180°C) and shear. In this particular area, the screw flights are closer, shallower, and in some instances interrupted. In short, the starch subjected to direct extrusion cooking suffers the phenomena of melting and gelatinization. At the very instant that the viscous fluid exits the die orifice, it will instantaneously equilibrate with the external atmospheric pressure causing the expansion and setting the puff structure. During this moment, most moisture vaporizes so the extrudate drops its moisture to about 5%–8%. The puffed collet is cut and sized to the proper length with a rotating knife. Most of these extrudates have expansion rates of 5 to 8. The puffs are

conveyed into a rotary dryer or oven to drop their moisture to around 1%–2%. The driers, set to approximately 150°C, dehydrate the low density collets in only 4–6 minutes. The dried/toasted collets are finally flavored in a rotary tumbler or bands generally with sweet flavorings, vitamins, and minerals that are dispensed in liquid or dried forms. The product is finally cooled and immediately packaged to avoid loss of texture or crispiness.

12.2.4.1 Production of Extruded Corn Puffs

A. Samples, Ingredients, and Reagents
- Refer to Table 12.4
- Powdered sugar
- Maltodextrin
- Red No. 40 dye

B. Materials and Equipments
- Twin or single thermoplastic extruder equipped with high shear screws and 2-mm die orifice
- Digital scale
- Graduated cylinder (1 L)
- Mixer with paddle attachment
- Rotary tumbler
- Air-forced convection oven
- Drying trays
- Caliper
- Chronometer
- Protective gloves
- Protective lenses

C. Procedure
1. Determine the moisture content of the maize grits (refer to Chapter 1).
2. Weigh the ingredients listed in Table 12.4 and place them in the mixing bowl. Calculate the water required to increase the rice moisture content to 18%. Use the following equation [(100 − grit moisture)/(100 − 18%) − 1] × amount of grits.
3. For extruders that do not have controlled water injection the feedstock has to be tempered before extrusion. Mix dry ingredients at low speed, and then, while mixing gradually, incorporate the water necessary to increase the moisture to 18%. Keep mixing contents at low speed for 5 minutes (Figure 12.3).
4. Fit the extruder with a high shear screw(s), 2-mm die orifice(s), and the extrusion conditions which enhances radial expansion. Generally, the first, second, and third segments of the extruder are set to 70°C, 100°C, and 130°C, respectively. Start the extruder and adjust the speed (in rpm; generally, the extruder is set from 150 to 300 rpm). Adjust the feed rate of the extruder and if the extruder has water injection capabilities adjust the water injection rate using the equation of step 2.
5. To prevent the extruder from getting stuck or jammed, the first stage of the process should be done with excess water (i.e., twice as much).

TABLE 12.4

Recommended Formulation for Manufacturing Extruded Corn Puffs

Ingredients	%
Yellow maize grits (Nos. 40 to 60)	100
Sugar	6.25
Salt	1.25
Vegetable oil	0.63
Monoglycerides	0.38
Nondiastatic malt	0.20

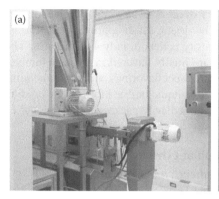 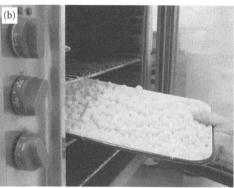 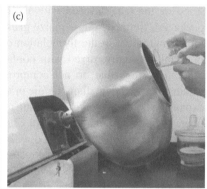

FIGURE 12.3 Sequential steps for production of corn puffs. (a) Thermoplastic twin extruder used to produce round puffs; (b) extruded corn puffs after toasting; and (c) application of flavorings to toasted corn puffs.

Place feedstock in the hopper of the extruder, and then start the extrusion process, making sure to inject more water. Turn on the extruder cutting unit and allow feedstock to run with excess water and then gradually decrease the water injection until achieving the targeted tempering moisture content of 18%. Allow extruder to achieve steady conditions and adjust the size and length of the extrudates by adjusting the speed of the cutting device. This product usually has a round configuration. Then, determine the feedstock residence time by placing a pinch of Red No. 40 dye directly into the inlet. With a chronometer determine the time (seconds) required for the exiting extrudate to stain red. In addition, register the temperatures of the different extruder zones, the rpm of the screw(s), and the cutter (Figure 12.3).

6. Collect the extrudates and measure the average diameter or size and determine their average moisture content.
7. Place extrudates in a convection oven set at 120°C for 20 to 30 minutes. The objective is to decrease the moisture content to 1.5%. Do not overdehydrate the extrudates.
8. Weigh a fixed amount of the dry-toasted extrudates and place them in a rotary tumbler. Turn on the tumbler, and for each kilogram of extrudate, gradually add 550 g of powdered sugar supplemented with 2% maltodextrin. Allow covering to adhere to the extrudates.
9. Remove flavored corn puffs from the tumbler and immediately place them in moisture-proof or aluminized bags.
10. Determine average diameter of the corn puffs, residual moisture content, volumetric weight, color, texture, bowl-life, and sensory properties.

12.2.5 GRANOLA

Granolas are gaining popularity because they are viewed as convenient and nutritious. The major raw material used to make granola is rolled oats mixed with other breakfast cereals such as puffed rice, wheat, nut pieces, coconut, brown sugar, honey, malt extract, dried milk, dehydrated fruits such as raising and dates, soybean products, and sometimes spices such as cinnamon and nutmeg. The water, oil, and syrups are made into a suspension where the dry materials are blended. The resulting wet mass is then spread in a uniform layer on a conveyor of a continuous oven-dryer. Baking takes place at temperatures in the range of 150°C to 220°C until the mat is uniformly toasted and moisture reduced to about 3%. Some granolas are produced by breaking the toasted mat into chunky pieces (Fast and Caldwell 2000). Fat-free, reduced fat, high fiber, and nutraceutical bar granolas are gaining sales and popularity especially among adolescents and young adults.

12.2.5.1 Production of Fermented Baked Granola

A. *Samples, Ingredients, and Reagents*
- Refer to Table 12.5
- Honey or high-fructose corn syrup
- Raisins/dehydrated fruits
- Pecan nut pieces

B. *Materials and Equipments*
- Digital scale
- Dough mixer with hook attachment
- Graduated cylinder (1 L)

TABLE 12.5

Formulation Recommended for Production of Fermented Baked Granola

Ingredients	Amount (%)
Whole wheat flour[a]	100.0
Water	38.0
Fresh compressed yeast	5.0
Sugar	6.5
Salt	1.0
Diastatic malt	0.5

Note: Five percent of the whole wheat flour can be substituted from fines obtained in previous batches. Refer to step 5 of the given procedure.

- Stainless steel containers for proofing
- Fermentation cabinet or proof box
- pH meter fitted with dough electrode
- Punching or degassing roll unit
- U.S. mesh sieve No. 6 and collection pan
- Baking pans
- Baking oven
- Spatula
- Chronometer
- Protective gloves

C. Procedure

1. Weigh independently the ingredients listed in Table 12.5.
2. Place all dry ingredients in the mixing bowl and mix them for 1 minute at low speed. Then add the water and blend contents for 1 minute at low speed and then several minutes at intermediate speed. The objective is to produce a crumbly and stiff dough (Figure 12.4).
3. Place the taut and crumbly dough onto greased baking sheets for 4 hours of fermentation at 28°C and 85% relative humidity. Make sure to distribute the crumbly dough into a 2.5-cm to 3-cm-thick mat. Register the dough pH at the beginning and end of fermentation.
4. Remove baking sheet from the fermentation box and immediately bake the fermented dough pieces for 15 minutes at 220°C.
5. Wearing heat-resistant gloves, remove baking sheets from the oven. Allow baked granola to cool down at ambient temperature for 20 minutes. Then, manually disaggregate the granola mat into pieces and place them back on the baking sheet for further toasting or drying.

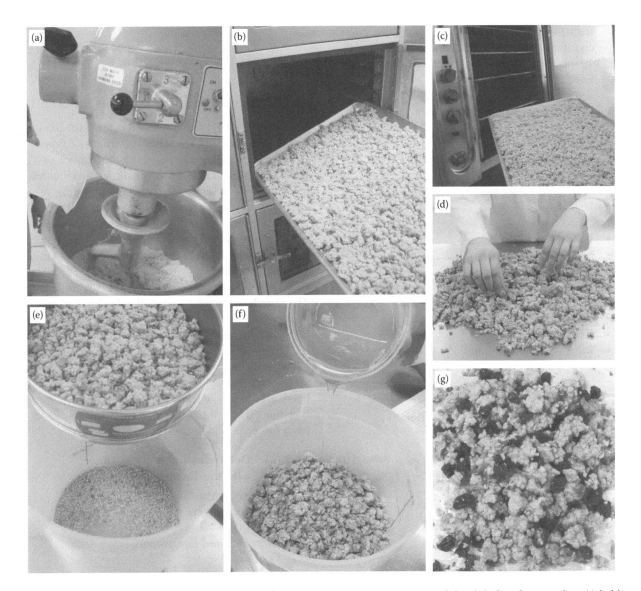

FIGURE 12.4 Production of baked-fermented granola. (a) Dough mixing; (b) appearance of dough before fermentation; (c) baking of fermented granola dough; (d) manual separation of toasted granola pieces; (e) removal of fines from coarse pieces of granola; (f) addition of honey or sweeteners to granola; and (g) granola appearance after addition of raisins and pecans.

6. Place baking sheets with pieces of granola back in the baking oven set at 120°C for 15–20 minutes toasting. With a spatula stir contents every 5 minutes.

7. Remove fines of the granola using a No. 6 U.S. mesh sieve. Collect and weigh the fines. The fines are usually incorporated into the original formulation (<5% of the formulation).

8. Remove baking sheet from the oven, place pieces of granola in a container and then add 40% of honey or high-fructose corn syrup. Distribute the sweetener on the baked granola and spread it on the baking sheet for drying (Figure 12.4).

9. Set the oven at 80°C and dehydrate the flavored granola for 20 minutes (the moisture content of the toasted and sweetened pieces of granola should drop to less than 4%). Stir the granola with a spatula after 10 minutes drying.

10. Remove granola from the dryer and allow it to equilibrate at room temperature (approximately 10 minutes). Mix 1000 g of the dehydrated and sweetened granola with 350 g raisins and/or dehydrated fruits and 100 g pecan nut pieces.

11. Place granola mix in moisture proof bags.

12.2.5.2 Production of Granola Bars

A. *Samples, Ingredients, and Reagents*
  • Refer to Table 12.6

B. *Materials and Equipments*
  • Digital scale
  • Wooden pin
  • Baking sheets
  • Spatula
  • Cooking pot
  • Large spoon
  • Oven
  • Beaker (1 L)
  • Baking sheets
  • Ruler with mm markings

TABLE 12.6
Formulation Recommended for Production of Granola Bars

Ingredients	Amount (g)
Brown sugar and molasses syrup[b]	150
Milk	100
Amaranth	100
Rolled oats	250
Puffed rice	100
Chocolate flavored puffed rice	100
Maple syrup	150
Chocolate chips	100

Note: Mix 150 g brown sugar and 50 g molasses with 500 mL water.

  • Chronometer
  • Protective gloves
  • Protective lenses

C. *Procedure*

1. Preheat oven to 100°C and lightly grease baking sheets with shortening.

2. In a cooking pot, blend the water and molasses, and heat in order to obtain a syrup.

3. Weigh the rest of the ingredients of Table 12.6 and blend them with a spatula.

4. Add 15 g of the molasses syrup and blend until all ingredients stick.

5. Extend the resulting mix with the wooden pin in order to form a 1-cm thick mat. Then with a knife cut rectangles of 10 × 4 cm. Place resulting rectangles on a greased baking sheet.

6. Bake for 20 minutes at 100°C. Wearing protective gloves, remove baking sheet from the oven and allow granola bars to cool for 25 minutes at room temperature.

7. Upon cooling, immediately place granola bars in moisture proof bags.

12.2.6 DETERMINATION OF BOWL-LIFE

The TAXT2 analyzer is used to test the bowl-life of breakfast cereals. The test evaluates the length of time a breakfast cereal retains its crispness after the addition of a certain volume of milk. This instrumental measurement has many advantages over sensory techniques, including repeatability, objectivity, and low cost. The texture analyzer technique is used for quality control purposes and is sensitive to raw material quality (i.e., particle size distribution, starch gluten content, starch damage, etc.), supplemented additives and processing conditions including packaging. The texture analyzer is fitted with an Ottawa cell and a watertight base plate. The sample is immersed into a fixed volume of milk, and at known time intervals, the milk is rapidly drained from the cell and compressed by a plunger. The instrument registers the force, distance, and time data, which are automatically analyzed by the computer software. The bowl-life instrumental method is simple to use and has the main advantage of being able to follow texture changes as a function of hydration time. Thus, this assay is now a valuable asset to the breakfast cereals industry.

12.2.6.1 Determination of Bowl-Life with the Texturometer

A. *Samples, Ingredients, and Reagents*
  • Different types of breakfast cereals
  • Milk

B. *Materials and Equipments*
  • Digital scale
  • Texture analyzer TAXT2
  • Ottawa cell
  • Watertight base plate
  • Knife

- Graduated cylinder (1 L)
- Thermometer
- Chronometer

C. *Procedure*

1. Prepare and calibrate the texture analyzer. Fit the textrurometer with the Ottawa load cell and the special water tight base plate. Standardize or calibrate the equipment to compress at 5 mm/s.
2. Weigh 30 g of the breakfast cereal and place it into the cell. Pour 125 mL of cold milk (8°C) into the watertight based plate. At known time intervals (i.e., 1, 3, 5, and 10 minutes) drain the milk from the cell and compress the wet cereal with the plunger at 5 mm/s.
3. Register the force, distance, and time data.
4. Compare bowl-life results with a sensory panel.

12.2.7 RESEARCH SUGGESTIONS

1. Produce rice and wheat flakes following the same procedure recommended for corn flakes. Use regular white polished rice and white wheat. Compare the physical, chemical, and organoleptic properties of the three different types of toasted flakes.
2. Produce oven puffed rice with three different types of white polished rices: short-waxy, regular, and parboiled. Compare their expansion rate, color, and organoleptic properties of the different oven-puffed kernels.
3. Decorticate white sorghum following the procedure described in Chapter 5. Then mill the sorghum into grits and process sorghum grits and maize grits into flavored puffs. Compare their radial expansion, color, texture, bowl-life, and sensory properties.
4. Produce fermented baked granolas with three different types of flours: (1) whole wheat flour, (2) 50% wheat flour + 50% oat flour, 50% wheat flour + 25% rye flour + 15% amaranth + 10% defatted soybean flour. Compare their final color, texture, and organoleptic properties.

12.2.8 RESEARCH QUESTIONS

1. Define the following terms used in breakfast cereal industries:
   a. Flaking
   b. Shredding
   c. Bumping
   d. Puffing gun
   e. Half-product
   f. Collets
   g. Impingement oven
2. What are the new breakfast cereal industry trends in terms of product development and characteristics?
3. What are the basic operations required to produce any breakfast cereal? What happens to the starch and proteins associated to cereal products during these operations?
4. What is the main classification of major types of breakfast cereals?
5. List at least four types of breakfast cereals that are industrially processed using traditional and extrusion technologies. What are advantages and disadvantages of traditional and extrusion processes?
6. Compare flowcharts for the production of maize, wheat, and rice flakes via traditional processes. What are the ideal properties of these raw materials for toasted flakes?
7. Compare flowcharts for the production of maize flakes via traditional and extrusion processes. What are the advantages and disadvantages of each process? How can you recognize flakes made via extrusion?
8. Describe the general process for producing fermented baked granola.
9. How are instant oat flakes produced? Why are oats heat treated with steam before dehulling and milling? Why are flaked oats usually packaged in carton boxes?
10. Compare traditional and extrusion processes to manufacture shredded wheat.
11. List at least five quality control tests with its main use and principle used to evaluate breakfast cereals.
12. What is thermoplastic extrusion? Give at least two examples of breakfast cereals produced by direct and pellet forming technologies.
13. Describe technologies used to minimize moisture migration from dehydrated fruits (raisins, dates, etc.) and other products to processed crisp cereals.
14. What are the differences between enrichment and fortification programs? What are the common nutrients used in most enrichment programs? What is the main nutritional rationale of adding each of these nutrients?

12.3 CEREAL-BASED SNACKS

Snack foods have always been an important part of life and these products represent an important segment of the food industry worldwide, especially in developed countries. Nowadays, the snack food market is continually changing and adapting to the new consumers needs. Snacking is increasing from factors such as increases in one-person households, higher proportion of working mothers, and more school-age children obtaining their own meals, a highly mobile population, and the availability of RTE snack foods in vending machines and convenience stores (Riaz 2000, 2004). Processors classify snack foods into three main broad categories: first-, second-, and third-generation snacks. First-generation snacks are natural products such as almonds, peanuts, tree nuts, and popcorn. Second-generation snacks are the most important category in terms of commercial snacks manufactured. These are simple shaped products like corn and tortilla chips, puffed curls, and all directly expanded snacks generally produced via thermoplastic extrusion. Third-generation snacks are also called half-products or pellets. This category included all intermediate or half products made via extrusion. The resulting pellets are usually fried or baked and flavored before packaging and reaching the consumer (Serna-Saldivar 2008).

12.3.1 Popcorn

Popcorn has become a favorite traditional snack for more than a century (Ziegler 2000). Popcorn is produced from a special kind of flint maize with a vitreous endosperm texture that contains tightly, packed starch granules. The major traits that distinguish popcorn from other kinds of maizes are the size and shape of the kernels and the ability of the sound grains to explode and produce large puffed flakes when heated (Ziegler 2003). The germ, endosperm, and pericarp commonly consist of 12%, 81%, and 7% of the dry kernel weight. The integrity and soundness of the pericarp is vitally important to optimize popping volume because it acts as the cap of a pressure cooker (Serna-Saldivar 2008). In order to produce the best quality popcorn, farmers should harvest kernels when they reach full maturity and contain approximately 17% moisture. In addition, the harvesting operation should be aimed to minimize kernel damage. After harvesting, kernels are cleaned and dried to lower the moisture to around 13% to 13.5%. Kernels must be dried slowly to prevent the formation of stress cracks or fissures (Metzger et al. 1989). Kernels should not be dried below 11% moisture otherwise the popping expansion will not be realized. The effect of mechanical damage on popcorn seems to be twofold. First, the damaged site acts as a major pathway for the escape of water vapor from the endosperm during the heating of the kernels. Second, the damage weakens the pericarp (Singh et al. 1997).

Expansion volume is the most critical quality factor for popcorn. The popped volume is important because the commercial buyer purchases the popcorn by weight and sells it by volume. In addition, popcorn texture (tenderness and crispness) is positively correlated with popping volume. Most commercial popcorn has a 30- to 40-fold expansion.

Popping occurs at about 177°C, which is equivalent to a steam pressure of 9.45 kg/cm^2 (135 psi) inside the kernel. The water in the grain is superheated and, at the moment of popping, converts to steam, which provides the driving force for expanding the endosperm after the kernel ruptures (Hoseney et al. 1983). Popping occurs when the internal vapor pressure exceeds the sum of the burst pressure of the pericarp and atmospheric pressure. This occurs at internal temperatures in the range of 180°C to 190°C. When the pericarp ruptures, the superheated water rapidly expands in less than 1/15 seconds causing the molten starch to expand resulting in the typical flake (Byrd and Perona 2005). The pericarp and outer layers of the kernel participate directly in the popping action by serving as a pressure vessel (Pordesimo et al. 1990).

Essentially there are two types of popcorn configurations: mushroom or butterfly. Popped kernels with a spherical shape are called mushroom or ball type. Due to its configuration, it is preferred in the confection industry because it is less susceptible to breakage, more resistant to handling and more efficiently coated with flavorings and confectionery syrups. The butterfly type has a higher expansion or lower apparent bulk density and better mouth feel; it is preferred for on-premises popping where it is sold by volume. The popping expansion of the mushroom type is lower than the butterfly because the individual flakes fit closer together. For production of the mushroom or ball popcorn, more heat should be applied during popping. Temperatures of 215°C and 235°C are recommended to favor the production of butterfly- and mushroom-shaped flakes, respectively. The highly expanded or butterfly-shaped popcorn is more tender and contains fewer partially popped kernels that are hard to chew (Snack Food Association [SFA] 1992; Serna-Saldivar 2008).

There are basically two types of popping methods: wet and dry (Table 12.7). Most processors employ the wet-popping method because it produces popcorn with better flavor. However, dry-popping is ideally suited for the production of low-fat products. Dry-popping requires about 25% less oil compared to wet popping. Oil added to dry-popped corn is often the vehicle for addition of other flavors and colors.

Popcorn quality is usually assessed by the quality of raw kernels and quality of flakes. The quality of raw kernels is assessed by moisture, test weight, dockage or foreign material, broken/damaged kernels, thousand kernel weight, and analysis of mycotoxins (Table 12.8). The quality of flakes is determined after expansion in the metric weight volume tester (MWVT), which is considered as the official testing method for the industry. The current MWVT features a solid-state digital temperature control, adjustable power input with a digital watt meter so to maintain exactly 1400 watts in the popping chamber or kettle. The equipment has a large diameter tube to avoid the bridging of the popcorn (SFA 1992). The device measures popping expansion as cubic centimeters of popped maize/g raw kernels. The MWVT power is set to 1,400 watts and a temperature of 260°C. When the pan temperature is reached, 250 g popcorn and 63 g oil are added. The main advantage of this equipment is the consistency of popping expansion volume and the low variability regardless of the operator. A similar volume/expansion test has been especially devised for microwave popcorn. The method was developed by the Technical Committee of the Popcorn Institute (1989). At the completion of popping, the volume is measured in a 13 cm diameter cylinder. Expansion volume is calculated by measuring the total popped volume (mL) divided by the original sample weight (g) and flake size or individual kernel expansion by measuring the popped volume (mL)/number of popped kernels. The percentage of unpopped kernels is determined by measuring the number of unpopped kernels/original number of kernels) × 100 (Mohamed et al. 1993).

12.3.1.1 Popcorn Popping

A. *Samples, Ingredients, and Reagents*

- Popcorn
- Cottonseed oil
- Salt

TABLE 12.7
Advantages and Disadvantages of the Wet- and Dry-Popping Procedures

Wet Popping		Dry Popping	
Advantages	**Disadvantages**	**Advantages**	**Disadvantages**
Animation of the popping	Requires about 25% more oil than dry popping	Requires about 25% less oil than wet popping	More expensive equipment
Better aroma and flavor	The heat of popping is detrimental to oil quality	Low labor cost especially when automatic equipments are used	Less cleaning problems compared with wet popping
Adapted to popping at point of sale	Cleaning problems on the kettles	Ideally suited for production of flavored popcorn, caramel popcorn, popcorn balls, and molded figurines	More fire hazard when hand-fed batch types are used
Relatively inexpensive equipment	Loss of popping volume if the a corn/oil ratio is higher than 4:1	Better distribution of the oil because it is generally sprayed	
Small space process requirement	The resulting popcorn is higher in energy or calorie density	Popcorn usually lower in calories ideally suited for low reduction programs	

Source: Snack Food Association, *Corn Quality Assurance Manual*, Alexandria, VA: SFA, 1992.

- • Water
- • Dessicant (activated alumina)

B. *Materials and Equipments*
- • MWVT
- • Graduated cylinder (13 cm diameter)
- • Graduated cylinder (100 mL)
- • Tempering containers or glass bottles with lids
- • Regular and analytical scales
- • Airtight dessicator
- • Aluminum dishes
- • Convection oven
- • Winchester bushel meter
- • Automatic seed counter
- • Laboratory tweezers
- • Razor blade or scalper

C. *Procedure*
1. Determine moisture, test weight, thousand kernel weight, and amount of foreign material of the popcorn (refer to procedures detailed in Chapter 1). Remove dockage.
2. Divide the lot of popcorn into 6 different samples.
   a. Leave the original lot sample as control. Label as control.
   b. Damage the pericarp of the popcorn with a razor blade or scalper, making two longitudinal 3-mm cuts on opposite sides of the kernel. Label as damaged popcorn.
   c. Dry one lot for 2 hours at 35°C, and after 5 minutes cooling at room temperature, place it in a tempering container or sealed glass bottle. Allow popcorn to equilibrate for 12 hours. Determine the residual moisture content of the sample, thousand kernel weight and the volume of 250 g popcorn.
   d. According to the original moisture content of the popcorn adjust the moisture of the second sample to 14% using the following

equation $[(100 - \text{popcorn moisture})/(100 - 14\%) - 1] \times$ amount of popcorn. Add the tempering water, close the container, and shake contents for at least 5 minutes in order to distribute the water evenly. After 3 minutes of rest, shake contents for 2 additional minutes or until all the water has been absorbed by the kernels. Allow tempered popcorn to equilibrate for 12 hours and determine moisture content, thousand kernel weight, and the volume of 250 g popcorn. Label sample as 14% popcorn.
   e. According to the original moisture content of the popcorn adjust the moisture of the third and fourth samples to 15% and 16%. Repeat the procedure described above. Label samples as 15% and 16% popcorns.
3. Set the MWVT power to 1,400 watts, and a temperature of 260°C. When the pan temperature is reached add 250 g popcorn and 63 g oil.
4. At the completion of popping, measure the volume in a 13-cm-diameter cylinder and the number of unpopped kernels (Figure 12.5). Expansion volume is calculated by measuring the total popped volume (mL) divided by the original sample weight (g) and flake size or individual kernel expansion by measuring the popped volume (mL)/number of popped kernels. The percent unpopped kernels is determined by measuring the number of unpopped kernels/original number of kernels) × 100.

$$\text{Expansion volume} = \text{popcorn flake volume (mL)/popcorn weight (g)}$$

$$\text{Percent unpopped kernels} = (\text{Number unpopped kernels/original number kernels}) \times 100$$

TABLE 12.8

Quality Control Parameters Generally Applied to Popcorn

Quality Control Parameter	Equipment or Technique	Importance
	Raw Popcorn	
Moisture	NIRA, electric conductivity moisture meters, moisture balances	Moisture is one of the most important parameters because it affects yields and stability during storage. Popcorn stored out of their optimum moisture (<14%) has more heat and insect/mold damage. The moisture content of popcorn is one of the most important parameters related to expansion.
Dockage test	Dockage test meter	The amount of foreign material affects yields. Popcorn with a high amount of foreign material is usually more prone to insect and mold damage and requires costly precleaning actions.
Test weight	Winchester bushel meter	Indicates grain condition and hardness. Hardness is associated with expansion volume.
Density	Air pycnometer	Indicates hardness and is associated with endosperm texture. Both parameters are associated with expansion volume.
Stress cracks and fissures	Observation on light box	Stress cracks are created due to faulty harvesting and rapid drying. Stress cracked kernels tend to produce higher incidence of unpopped kernels and less flake volume.
1000 kernel weight	Seed counter	Relates to the average size of the grain. Generally lower-sized kernels produce less expansion volume than larger kernels. The range of 1,000 kernel weight for the large, medium, and small popcorn kernels are 149–152, 133–147, and 95–131 g, respectively.
Damaged kernels: insect, mold, and sprouted	Visual observation	Any kind of damage to the kernels negatively affects popping volume and amount of unpopped kernels. Insect damaged seeds are recognized by punctures or holes in the grain or the presence of a web-like material. Mold damage seeds are recognized because of the darker coloration and dirty appearance of the grain. Several types of molds can produce high levels of mycotoxins that are harmful for humans and domestic animals.
Aflatoxins/mycotoxins	Aflatest/solvent extraction, ELISA separation followed by fluorescence detection	From the food safety viewpoint, this is the most important measurement because aflatoxins are regulated by most governmental food agencies. Aflatoxins are known carcinogens. Popcorn is less affected by molds than regular dent maizes.
Expansion volume	MWVT	Most important quality control parameter. This determines expansion volume = total popped volume (mL)/original sample weight (g), flake size or individual kernel expansion = popped volume (mL)/number of popped kernels and % unpopped kernels = (number of unpopped kernels/original number of kernels) × 100 (Mohamed et al. 1993).
	Popping in the microwave	Method developed by the Technical Committee of the Popcorn Institute (1989).
	Popped Corn	
Moisture	NIRA, moisture meters/balances	Affects texture of popcorn. Popcorn must be consumed at moistures lower than 1.5%.
Oil	NIRA, ether extraction	Affects texture and caloric density of the product. The fat content should be declared in the food label.
Salt	Volhard method ($AgNO_3$); titration of AgCl with $FeNH_4(SO_4)_2$ and NH_4SCN)	Gives an indication of degree of covering. The sodium content should be declared in the food label.
Popcorn or flake form	Visual observation	It can be mushroom or butterfly. Mushroom is used for confectionery purposes and butterfly for conventional use. The mushroom type has higher bulk density than the butterfly.
Peroxide value	AOCS (2009) Cc8-53. Amount of iodine liberated by its reaction with potassium iodide	This is the most analytical method to determine the stability or oxidation of the oil associated with the product. It is a very important attribute in RTE's long shelf-life packaged products because it is closely related to rancidity and organoleptic properties.

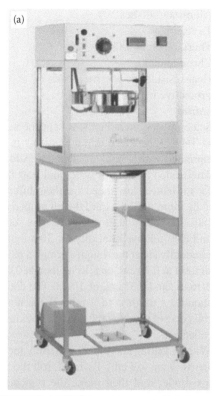

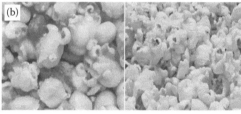

FIGURE 12.5 Popcorn. (a) MWVT used to study expansion volume and properties of popcorn (Courtesy of C. Creators & Company); and (b) illustration of butterfly and mushroom types of popcorns.

$$\text{Flake size} = \text{popcorn flake volume (mL)/number of popped kernels.}$$

7. Tabulate results and determine the effects of popcorn damage and moisture content on expansion volume, percent of unpopped kernels, and flake size.

12.4 WHEAT-BASED SNACKS

Wheat is used for the production of many snacks around the globe. It is mainly used for the production of shelf-stable toasted bread, named crisps in England, crackers/saltines, pretzels, and snack bars. In the United States, sales of crackers and pretzels in 2003 exceeded 1.5 and 1.2 billion dollars, respectively (Anonymous 2004). The processing of saltines and crackers is described in Chapter 10. The industrial manufacturing process to obtain toasted or crispbread is practically identical to the production of fresh bread with the additional operation of bread toasting or drying (refer to Chapter 9). There are many bread formulations generally produced form refined wheat flour, whole wheat flour, or composite flours produced from mixtures of wheat flour with oat, rye, or various crushed grains. Sesame is frequently used as a topping. Typical formulations to obtain French, white pan, whole wheat oat, pumpernickel, and rye breads are described in Chapter 9.

The quality of wheat-based snacks greatly depends on the characteristics of the wheat flour and other formula ingredients. The quality of wheat and flour is covered in Chapter 5. The quality of the gluten forming wheat flour is extremely important because it affects processing conditions and end-product quality.

12.4.1 PRODUCTION OF PRETZELS

Pretzels are wheat-based snacks with 800 years of history and are especially prevalent in the European community and the United States. Among salty snacks it is the one that contains fewer energy density and fat. Pretzels are manufactured from fermented wheat flour dough that is treated with a covering of a sodium hydroxide or other alkali salt before baking. Pretzels are unique because the flavor and color are due to this lye wash. The typical flavor profile is also affected by the products yielded during fermentation, nondiastatic malt, and salt. Soft wheat flour is recommended for hard pretzels. The flour is mixed with water, small amounts of shortening, sugar, and yeast to form a coarse dough that is rested for 20 minutes before mechanical rolling and forming into cylinders that are molded into traditional hard pretzel forms such as bow tie or other configurations. Pretzels are fermented with yeast, formed, and washed for 25–30 seconds with a 1% sodium hydroxide solution heated to approximately 93°C. The aim of the short time proofing is to activate the yeast so to produce carbon dioxide and flavor compounds. The carbon dioxide is necessary to slightly increase the pretzel volume and form the typical crumb structure and the generation of fermented flavor compounds contributes to the pretzel flavor profile and pH. For hard pretzels, baking is performed in three sequential steps with different time-temperature profiles (Seetharaman et al. 2004; Serna-Saldivar 2008). Pretzels are first baked and then kilned to drop the moisture content and produce the typical texture. Baking is continuously performed in wire mesh, gas-fired, and automated ovens that have at least three recognized temperature areas. The common oven conditions to manufacture hard pretzels are 288°C, 260°C, and 260°C for 2.5 to 3 minutes. A good pretzel should have a dark brownish outer crust and a white inner crumb with small and homogenously distributed gas cells or *loci*. Pretzels are usually only flavored with coarse or flaked salt because they are formulated to be low or no fat. Pretzels are cooled and generally packaged in a form-fill-seal machine with laminated or coextruded materials. Hard pretzels are usually packaged with an inert gas to protect the flavor and decrease the rate of product breakage during handling.

A. *Samples, Ingredients, and Reagents*
* Refer to Table 12.9
* Distilled water
* Sodium hydroxide (NaOH)

TABLE 12.9

Recommended Formulation for the Production of Hard Pretzels

Ingredients	Amount (%)
Soft wheat flour	100.0
Water absorption	46.7
Shortening	2.5
Nondiastatic malt	2.5
Dry yeast	0.3
Ammonium bicarbonate	0.15
Flaked or coarse salt[a]	1.5

[a] The flaked or coarse salt is sprinkled onto the pretzel before baking.

B. *Materials and Equipments*

- Digital Scale
- Spatula
- Microdough mixer or Hobart mixer
- Dough sheeter
- Roller pin
- Beaker (2 L)
- Knife
- Baking sheets
- Fermentation cabinet
- Hot plate
- Glass pot
- Stirrer
- Baking oven
- Stove
- Aluminum dishes
- Tweezers
- Thermometer (100°C)
- Chronometer
- Heat-resistant protective gloves
- Protective lenses

C. *Procedure*

1. Scale all dry ingredients, except the salt, listed in Table 12.9. Place dry ingredients in a mixer equipped with a hook attachment. Add the predetermined amount of water and start the mixer for 1 minute at low speed and then shift the speed to medium until the hard dough properly forms.
2. Introduce the dough in a proof box set at 28°C and 85% relative humidity for 30 minutes.
3. Gradually sheet the dough through a pair of rolls first set at 0.79 cm, or 5/16 in. then at 0.48 cm, or 3/16 in., and 0.31 cm, or 1/8 in. The dough sheet should be thinned to 2 mm. If the mechanical rolls do not produce the desired thickness, use a roller pin.
4. With a knife, cut the dough into rectangular strips (7 cm × 2 cm). By hand, roll the strip into a cylinder and then make the typical tie bow configuration.
5. Place tie bow forms in the proof box for 20–30 minutes.
6. Immerse pretzel dough forms for 10 to 25 seconds in a 1.25% NaOH (12.5 g/L) bath previously heated to 90°C (Figure 12.6). Remove

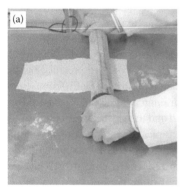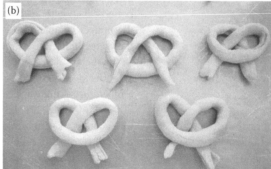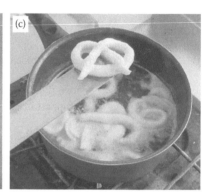

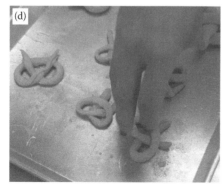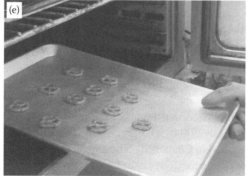

FIGURE 12.6 Pretzels. (a) Sheeting the pretzel dough; (b) forming the typical pretzel configuration; (c) fermented pretzel forms being immersed in hot NaOH solution; (d) addition of coarse or flaked salt; and (e) baked pretzel.

7. Place pretzel forms on perforated baking sheet and then add 1.5% coarse salt. Remove unstuck salt from the baking sheet.

8. Bake pretzels for 3 minutes at 225°C and then lower the temperature to 170°C for 10 minutes or until the product lowers its moisture content to approximately 2.5% (Figure 12.6).

9. Remove pretzels from the oven for 15 minutes cooling at room temperature.

10. Place pretzels in laminated or coextruded bags that have a good barrier against air humidity and gases.

12.4.2 Alkaline-Cooked Snacks

Alkaline-cooked maize snacks are considered the fastest growing market within the category. There are basically three types of snacks produced from alkaline-cooked maize: parched *nixtamal*, corn chips, and tortilla chips. Most parched *nixtamal* is manufactured from Cuzco or *cacahuacintle* kernels that are alkaline cooked and then deep-fat fried and seasoned (Rooney and Serna-Saldivar 2003; Serna-Saldivar 2008). Extruded corn chips are produced from coarsely ground *masa* (refer to Chapter 5) that is formed and deep-fat fried whereas tortilla chips, taco shells, and *tostadas* are produced from pieces or whole baked tortillas that are deep-fat fried. Baking of tortillas prior to frying greatly affects organoleptic properties and nutritional value of these snacks. Tortilla chips have a stronger alkaline-cooked flavor and a crispier texture than corn chips. In addition, tortilla chips are less energy dense because they absorb about 12% units less oil during frying (Rooney and Serna-Saldivar 2003; Serna-Saldivar and Rooney 2003; Serna-Saldivar 2008).

12.4.2.1　Production of Alkaline-Cooked Parched Corn

Parched corn is a popular salty snack item produced from alkali-cooked kernels that are deep-fat fried. The preferred maize for this product is Cuzco that was developed from the Giant Peruvian Cuzco race. The 8-rowed ears produce the largest known maize kernel. Cuzco maize cultivars grow at high altitudes and produces white kernels with a soft endosperm texture and bland flavor. The first Cuzco derived hybrid adapted to the Unites States was introduced in 1964 after 9 years of painstaking breeding work. Several new hybrids have been developed since then. Kernels are harvested when the moisture content of the grain is less than 30%. The kernels are cleaned, sized, and dried to reduce moisture to less than 15% (Rooney and Serna-Saldivar 2003; Serna-Saldivar 2008).

The commercial manufacture of parched corn starts when kernels are alkali-cooked in excess water and washed to remove the pericarp. The chemical decorticated kernels are transferred into steep tanks where it is blanched for a few hours in warm water. After draining the alkaline solution, the cooked kernels are deep-fat fried to develop the

characteristic texture, flavor, and color and immediately flavored, cooled, and packaged (Rooney and Serna-Saldivar 2003; Serna-Saldivar 2008). The final product contains about 14%–15% oil and approximately 440–450 kcal/100 g.

A. *Samples, Ingredients, and Reagents*
- *Cuzco* or *cacahuacintle* maize
- Food-grade lime
- Distilled water
- Partially hydrogenated frying oil
- Salt
- Powdered seasoning mixes

B. *Materials and Equipments*
- Digital scale
- Graduated cylinders (100 mL, 200 mL, or 1 L)
- Dough mixer (hook or paddle attachments)
- Cooker (steam or conventional)
- Deep-fat fryer
- Cooling rack
- Rotary tumbler
- Thermometer (300°C)
- Chronometer

C. *Procedure*
1. Weigh a fixed amount of cleaned Cuzco or *cacahuacintle* kernels and add three times as much water and 1% food-grade lime based on grain weight to the cooking vessel. Keep the maize kernels separated from the lime solution.

2. Adjust the temperature of the cooking solution (most processes cook at near boiling or between 85°C and 100°C). When the cooking solution reaches the proper temperature, add the kernels and register temperatures throughout cooking. Make sure to stir contents frequently (i.e., every 5 minutes). Cook the maize kernels for the predetermined cooking time (refer to mini lime cooking trial of Chapter 7), suspend heat and leave kernels to steep for at least 8 hours (optimally 12–14 hours). Register temperatures during steeping.

3. Drain the cooking liquor or *nejayote* and wash the *nixtamal* with water. Make sure to remove excess lime and adhered pericarp tissue. Collect the *nejayote* and wash waters and measure the volume and solids. Obtain a sample of the cleaned *nixtamal* for moisture analysis.

4. Weigh the cleaned *nixtamal* and place alkali cooked kernels on a baking sheet for 4 hours equilibration at room temperature (Figure 12.7).

5. Wearing protective lenses, preheat frying oil to 175°C and then deep-fat fry the tempered kernels for 1.5 minutes (Figure 12.7).

6. Remove parched kernels form the fryer and allow kernels to drain excess oil during 10 seconds. Then, weigh the fried or parched kernels and place them in a rotary tumbler. Apply salt or a powdered seasoning mix.

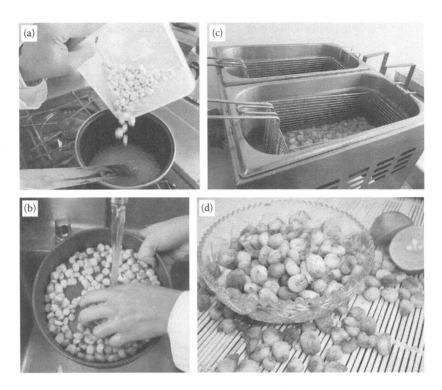

FIGURE 12.7 Parched fried maize. (a) Addition of cacahuacintle or Cuzco maize to hot lime solution; (b) washing of alkaline cooked kernels; (c) frying of tempered alkaline cooked kernels; and (d) flavored parched fried corn.

7. Removed the seasoned kernels from the rotary tumbler and cool for 10 minutes at room temperature.
8. After cooling, place parched and seasoned kernels in moisture-proof bags and sample for moisture, fat, and other analyses.
9. Determine the yield of the parched and flavored corn snack based on the original grain weight. In addition, determine the color, texture, shelf life, peroxide value, and sensory properties.

12.4.2.2 Production of Corn Chips

Corn chips are made from coarsely ground *masa* either from fresh *nixtamal* or dry *masa* flour (refer to Chapter 7), which is extruded and cut into *masa* chips with different configurations, deep-fat fried, and salted/seasoned. The *masa* extruder commonly consists of a horizontal hydraulic piston that forces the *masa* with at least 52% moisture to pass through a 90° forming die or head. Extrusion starts automatically after *masa* is manually loaded and the cylinder is locked into position. Easily interchangeable dies for forming custom shapes are available. A rotary cutoff assembly cuts *masa* into uniform pieces. When the cylinder is empty, the piston retracts for refilling. The extruded *masa* pieces varying in forms and sizes are directly deposited in a deep fat fryer for approximately 1.5 minutes. During frying, the *masa* exchanges water for oil and the product exits the fryer at moisture and oil contents of about 1.5% and 36%, respectively. Resulting chips are usually seasoned with 2% salt and various types of

seasoning mixes containing cheese, citric acid, or chili flavorings (Serna-Saldivar 2008).

A. *Samples, Ingredients, and Reagents*
- Food-grade dent maize
- Food-grade lime
- Distilled water
- Dry *masa* flour tailored for corn chips

B. *Materials and Equipments*
- Digital scale
- Graduated cylinders (100 mL, 200 mL, or 1 L)
- Dough mixer (hook or paddle attachments)
- Cooker (steam or conventional)
- Stone grinder
- Deep-fat fryer
- Cooling rack
- Rotary tumbler
- Dough mixer with hook attachment
- Graduated cylinder (1 L)
- Thermometer (300°C)
- Chronometer
- Protective lenses

C. *Procedure*
Wet *masa*
1. Weigh a fixed amount of cleaned maize kernels and add three times as much water and 1% food-grade lime based on grain weight to the cooking vessel. Keep the maize kernels separated from the lime solution.

2. Adjust the temperature of the cooking solution (most processes cook at near boiling or between 85°C and 100°C). When the cooking solution reaches the proper temperature, add the grain and register temperatures throughout cooking. Make sure to stir contents frequently (i.e., every 5 minutes). Cook the maize kernels for the predetermined cooking time (refer to mini lime cooking trial described in Chapter 7), suspend heat, and leave kernels to steep for at least 8 hours (optimally 12 to 14 hours). Register temperatures during steeping.

3. Drain the cooking liquor or *nejayote* and wash the *nixtamal* with water. Make sure to remove excess lime and adhered pericarp tissue. Collect the *nejayote* and wash waters and measure the volume and solids. Obtain a sample of the cleaned *nixtamal* for moisture analysis.

4. Weigh the cleaned *nixtamal* and place it in the hopper of the stone mill. The stone mill should be calibrated beforehand to produce a coarse *masa* ideally suited for corn chips. Calculate the amount of water to add during the milling procedure. The amount of water to grind 1 kg of *nixtamal* for chips is approximately 150 mL/kg.

5. Start the stone grinder and adjust the pressure between the grinding stones so to obtain the proper *masa* texture (refer to particle size distribution of fresh *masa* procedure in Section 7.2.2.3). Grind all the *nixtamal* making sure to gradually add the water. Measure the temperature of the *masa*, collect it, and place it in a plastic bag to prevent dehydration. Disassemble the stone grinder and collect and weigh all the unground *nixtamal* and *masa* particles.

6. Place *masa* in a forming extruder and set controls to cut *masa* pieces (cylinder or strips) of approximately 5 cm to 7 cm long.

7. Weigh *masa* pieces and immediately deep-fat fry for 60 to 80 seconds at a temperature of 175°C to 180°C. Remove corn chips from the fryer and allow draining of excess oil. Weigh corn chips and determine moisture content, color, texture, and oil uptake.

8. Add salt and flavorings immediately after draining. Make sure to add a predetermined amount of seasoning per weight of corn chips.

9. Place seasoned corn chips on a counter for equilibration at room temperature (approximately 20 minutes).

10. Place corn chips in sealed polyethylene or aluminum bags.

Dry *masa* flour

1. For every kilogram of dry *masa* flour, add 1 L to 1.1 L water. Blend the *masa* flour with the water for 3 minutes at low speed. Make sure to scrap the *masa* from the sides of the mixing bowl.

2. Place the resulting dough in a plastic bag for 10 minutes resting.

3. Proceed from step 6 of the previous procedure.

12.4.2.3 Production of Tortilla Chips

Tortilla chips are usually manufactured from coarsely ground *masa* that is molded into the typical triangular configuration in preparation for baking and frying. In contrast to table tortillas, the maize kernels are cooked for less time and/or quenched immediately after cooking. In addition, the *nixtamal* is ground into a coarse *masa*. For tortilla chips, *masa* pieces are baked before frying to reduce the moisture content so that they absorb less oil and have a firmer texture and a stronger alkaline flavor compared to corn chips. The most common tortilla chip configuration is triangular followed by round and strip forms. Tostadas, taco shells, and baskets are tortillas produced from coarse *masa* fried flat, folded, or in a basket, respectively. Restaurant-style tortilla chips are produced similarly, but fine *masa* is formed and baked into thin tortillas. Baked tortillas are equilibrated for a long time at ambient or refrigeration temperature and cut into 4 pie-shaped pieces before frying. The baking of table tortillas and tortilla chips also differs greatly. Table tortillas are usually baked to retain more moisture and enhance puffing at the last stages of baking, whereas tortilla chips are baked to remove moisture and the oven temperature is regulated to avoid puffing or blistering (Serna-Saldivar et al. 1990; Serna-Saldivar 2008).

Alternatively, tortilla chips can be manufactured from dry *masa* flour (refer to Chapter 7). Manufacturing snacks from dry *masa* flour facilitates the process because processors do not have to be concerned about selection and storage of the maize, lime-cooking, and grinding. In addition, the use of dry *masa* flour greatly reduces processing time, labor, capital investment for processing equipment and wastewater treatment. Disadvantages include the comparatively higher price of dry *masa* and the subtle differences in flavor and texture in favor of fresh *masa* products (Serna-Saldivar 2008).

Tortilla chips are usually examined in terms of oil, moisture and salt contents, and texture and color. Color, crispness, texture, and the amount of oil absorbed are influenced by the baked tortilla moisture content, thickness of the chips, frying temperature, and residence time. The amount of salt and the percentage of seasoning in fried products can be analyzed by procedures suggested by the SFA (1992). Chips are usually analyzed for peroxide value, active oxygen stability, and hexanal with gas chromatography (refer to Chapters 2 and 3). These assays are excellent indicators of lipid oxidation and correlate with the consumer's preference and shelf-life expectations of packaged products (Serna-Saldivar 2008).

A. *Samples, Ingredients, and Reagents*
- Maize
- Food-grade lime
- Distilled water
- Dry *masa* flour tailored for tortilla chips

B. *Materials and Equipments*

- Digital scale
- Graduated cylinders (1 L)
- Dough mixer (hook or paddle attachments)
- Cooker (steam or conventional)
- Stone grinder
- Three-tier baking oven
- Tortilla chip forming machine
- Deep-fat fryer
- Cooling rack
- Rotary tumbler
- Dough mixer with hook attachment
- Thermometer (300°C)
- Chronometer
- Protective lenses

C. *Procedure*

Wet *masa*

1. Weigh a fixed amount of cleaned maize kernels and add three times as much water and 1% food-grade lime based on grain weight to the cooking vessel. Keep the maize kernels separated from the lime solution.

2. Adjust the temperature of the cooking solution (most processes cook at near boiling or between 85°C and 100°C). When the cooking solution reaches the proper temperature, add the grain and register temperatures throughout cooking. Make sure to stir contents frequently (i.e., every 5 minutes) (Figure 12.8). Cook the maize kernels for the predetermined cooking time (refer to mini lime cooking trial described in Chapter

7), suspend heat, and leave kernels to steep for at least 8 hours (optimally 12 to 14 hours). Register temperatures during steeping.

3. Drain the cooking liquor or *nejayote* and wash the *nixtamal* with water. Make sure to remove excess lime and adhered pericarp tissue. Collect the *nejayote* and wash waters and measure the volume and solids. Obtain a sample of the cleaned *nixtamal* for moisture analysis.

4. Weigh the cleaned *nixtamal* and place it in the hopper of the stone mill. The stone mill should be calibrated beforehand to produce a coarse *masa* ideally suited for corn chips. Calculate the amount of water to add during the milling procedure. The amount of water to grind 1 kg of *nixtamal* for chips is approximately 150 mL/kg (Figure 12.8).

5. Start the stone grinder and adjust the pressure between the grinding stones so as to obtain the proper *masa* texture (refer to particle size distribution of fresh *masa* procedure in Section 7.2.2.3). Grind all the nixtamal making sure to gradually add the water. Measure the temperature of the *masa*, collect it, and place it in a plastic bag to prevent dehydration. Disassemble the stone grinder and collect and weigh all the unground *nixtamal* and *masa* particles.

6. Furnish the sheeting rolls with the desired cutter and adjust settings of the cutting wires. Then, place *masa* and adjust the settings to produce triangular or round pieces with the proper

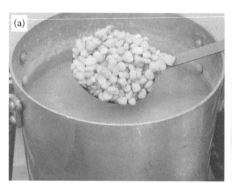 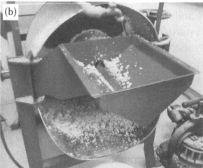 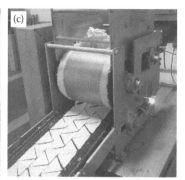

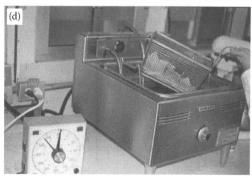 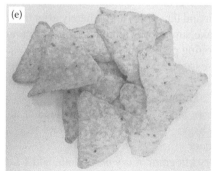

FIGURE 12.8 Sequential steps for the production of tortilla chips. (a) Lime-cooked kernels or *nixtamal*; (b) stone grinding of *nixtamal* into a coarse *masa*; (c) sheeting and forming of triangular tortilla chips; (d) deep-fat frying of baked tortilla; and (e) flavored tortilla chips.

thickness (approximately 1 mm) (Figure 12.8). When the sheeting and cutting device is properly adjusted, weigh 10 *masa* pieces and reserve sample for other analyses (moisture, color, texture, starch gelatinization).

7. Bake *masa* pieces into in a preheated three-tier gas fired baking oven for 60 seconds at an average temperature of 280°C. The temperature of the third tier should be lower in order to prevent blistering due to water vapor formation. Weigh 10 tortilla pieces and reserve sample for other analyses (moisture, color, texture, starch gelatinization).

8. Allow tortilla pieces to cool down for at least 30 minutes before frying. Weigh 10 tortilla pieces and reserve the sample for other analyses (moisture, color, texture, starch gelatinization).

9. Weigh equilibrated tortilla pieces and immediately deep-fat fry for 60 to 80 seconds at a temperature of 175°C to 180°C (Figure 12.8). Remove tortilla chips from the fryer and allow draining of excess oil. Weigh tortilla chips and determine moisture content, color, texture, and oil uptake.

10. Add salt and flavorings immediately after draining excess oil. Make sure to add a predetermined amount of seasoning per weight of tortilla chips.

11. Place flavored chips on a counter for equilibration at room temperature (approximately 20 minutes).

12. Place tortilla chips in sealed polyethylene or aluminum bags.

Dry *masa* flour

1. For every kilogram of dry *masa* flour add 1.1 L to 1.2 L water. Blend the *masa* flour with the water for 3 minutes at low speed. Make sure to scrap the *masa* stuck to the sides of the mixing bowl.

2. Place the resulting dough in a plastic bag for 10 minutes resting.

3. Proceed from step 6 of the previous procedure.

12.4.3 EXTRUDED SNACKS

The history of extruded snacks is traced back to the 1930s to the 1940s after the Second World War. Corn chips were introduced in the early 1930s, while puffed fried and baked products were introduced just after the Second World War. The first extruder used consisted of a rotor, stator, and a screw that produced irregular shaped collets ready for frying. Fried collets were almost always flavored with a salty cheese oil slurry (SFA 1987; Burtea 2001). C. Heigl, an engineer from Adams Corporation, developed an extruder designed to produce less dense extrudates or puffs suitable for drying or baking. The lighter and smoother collets were produced by a short barrel, high shear extruder equipped with a die to form the gelatinized corn extrudate into various regular shapes. Resulting puffs were cut to a predetermined length by a rotating knife. After drying or baking, collets are flavored with cheese slurry, similar to deep-fat fried curls (SFA 1987; Burtea 2001).

Today, extruded snacks are the category with the greatest potential for growth because this technology still offers the greatest flexibility and innovation. Most of the second- and third-generation snacks are produced by extrusion cooking. Differences between the two contrasting processes are detailed in Table 12.10. Extrusion can also be implemented to produce analogs of traditionally manufactured snacks. Coextrusion offers the advantage of creating new and innovative products with fillings. Production of snacks with cooking and forming extruders save space in the processing plant, offers more versatility, adapts to highly productive continuous plants, and saves labor and energy when compared with expenditures of traditional processes.

TABLE 12.10
Comparison between High-Shear and High-Pressure Forming Extrusion Processes

	High Shear or Direct Extrusion	High-Pressure-Forming Extrusion (Pellets)
Product	Direct expanded, puffs, or second-generation snacks	Pellets, half products, or third-generation snacks
Feed moisture	Low (12%–19% moisture)	High (25%–36% moisture)
Extrudate moisture before further processing	2%–6%	20%–25%
Maximum barrel temperature	110°C–180°C	20°C–100°C
Temperature gradient	Increasing	Homogenous or decreasing
Shear rate and energy input	High	Relatively low
Screw design	Produce high shear	Produce low shear
Screw rpm	150–400 rpm	Less than 100 rpm
Screw L/D ratio	<4:1	6–10:1
Pressure at die	High	Low medium
Product or extrudate	Expanded, low density with 5%–10% moisture	Pellet, high density, >20% moisture
Drying	150°C to lower moisture to <2%	70°C to lower moisture to about 8%–10%
Flavorings	After extrusion	Before extrusion

There are basically two families of snack items obtained with thermoplastic extruders. The direct expanded snacks and the third-generation snacks produced from pellets or half products obtained after sequential cooking and forming extrusion steps (Table 12.10). The direct extruded types are subdivided into bake puffs and fried puffs (Rooney and Serna-Saldivar 2003; Serna-Saldivar et al. 2008).

The quality of extruded snacks greatly depends on the characteristics of the raw materials and on the various manufacturing steps used throughout processing. The qualities of raw materials described in Chapters 2 and 3 are critically important because they also affect processing conditions. Moisture, ash, particle size distribution, starch damage, and color are important quality attributes of raw materials (refer to Chapter 2). For starches, the viscoamylograph assay is very useful because it predicts pasting, retrogradation, and other important functionalities imparted by the starch (Shuey and Tipples 1982). For oils, the stability, acidity, and fatty acid composition are important factors to consider.

The most important factor to control during extrusion cooking is the extrudate density. There are different ways to assess the density of puffs and pellets. Most processors subjectively evaluate the bulk density by determining the weight of a certain volume of extrudates. The air displacement pycnometer can be used to determine the density more accurately. Analytical approaches that are commonly used to study textural properties of extrudates are the Instron or texture analyzer shear force or compression tests. As in most snack food products, the final moisture content and fat content are continuously monitored. Moisture can be determined with near-infrared instruments and the use of gravimetric methods using the air–oven technique. The amount of fat can be rapidly determined via the use of near-infrared instruments or the carver press and analytically assayed via solvent extraction in a Soxhlet or Goldfisch apparatus. The near-infrared instruments can also be used to monitor plant color of extruded products.

Frequent monitoring of the extrusion process is required to adjust settings for the greatest product uniformity. The most important factors to control are moisture in the tempered raw materials, feed rate, temperatures/pressure in the different zones of the extruder and the die, the extrudate expansion rate, and moisture and the degree of covering that correlates with the salt content.

For frying operations, the type of oil, the frequency of filtration, and frying practices greatly affect the shelf life of both the oil and the finished product. The free fatty acid (FFA) content, peroxide value, AOM, and smoke and flash points are widely used to determine the condition and stability of oil and fried products (SFA 1992). Rapid methods for evaluating FFA, oxidation, and polar materials have been developed and are frequently used by the snack industry (Serna-Saldivar 2008).

The amount of salt and the percentage of seasoning in fried products can be analyzed by procedures suggested by SFA (1992). Sensory evaluation tests are used to determine the consumer preference of finished products. Tests more widely practiced are the triangular and preference tests; triangular tests are ideally suited to identify the consumer's preference between two samples because panelists try to identify the odd and paired samples among the three samples in a set. The triangular test is widely used for product development purposes. In the preference test, trained or untrained panelists evaluate the color, aroma, flavor, texture, and overall acceptability of the products using a hedonic scale (refer to Chapter 3). This test is used for product development purposes, shelf-life studies, and to study the functionality of additives/technologies.

12.4.3.1 Production of Baked Cheese-Flavored Corn Puffs

Baked corn puffs are typically manufactured with high shear or friction extruders. These extruders are called dry extruders because raw materials are not conditioned or, if conditioned, are tempered to low-moisture contents. Most extruders used to produce puffs are single screw and short barreled (L/D of 4 or less). The major difference between baked and fried collets is that the baked expanded products are expanded in a high shear extruder and then baked or toasted to impart the desired crispy texture. The oil content of these snacks is provided through the liquid or powdered seasonings that are applied onto the product before packaging. On the other hand, fried expanded collets are obtained with a special type of extruder that produces denser and irregular shaped extrudates that are further fried and seasoned or simply seasoned with an oil base (Serna-Saldivar 2008).

In order to produce good quality extrudates or collets, the raw material should be highly refined and properly conditioned. In most instances, refined grits conditioned to moisture contents from 14% to 19% produced the best quality products. The screw is the main part of the extruder because it transports the material and its design greatly affects shear rate. The main screw characteristics are distance between flights, depth of the flight, angle of the flight, and type of flight (full radius or square cut). More shear is produced when the distance between flights are shorter and the depth of the flights are shallow. High-shear extruders produce the greatest shear and compression at the exit end of the screw so as to increase pressure and enhance expansion rate. Higher expansion rates are obtained when pressure differential between the end of the screw and the atmospheric pressure is elevated. The expansion rate is calculated by measuring the average collet diameter divided by the diameter of the die orifice. At the very instant that the viscous fluid exits the die orifice, it will instantaneously equilibrate with the external atmospheric pressure, causing the expansion and setting of the collet structure. During this point in time, most of the moisture instantaneously vaporizes so the extrudate drops its moisture to about 5%–8%. The puffed collet is cut and sized to the proper length with a rotating knife. The collet expansion rate is generally between 6 and 8 and the bulk density is 50 g/L–65 g/L. Resulting puffs are conveyed into a rotary dryer or oven to drop their moisture to around 1%–2%. The driers, set to approximately 150°C, dehydrate the low density collets in only 4–6 minutes. The dehydration rate is fast due to the low collet density and porosity. The baked expanded collets are finally flavored in a rotary tumbler generally with salt-oil-cheese slurry that is sprayed onto the extrudates. The amount of coating applied ranges from 34% to 42% based on the final puff weight. The product is finally cooled and immediately packaged to avoid loss of texture or crispiness. The puffs generally contain from 27% to 36% oil and about 2% salt (Serna-Saldivar 2008).

A. *Samples, Ingredients, and Reagents*
- Maize grits (Nos. 40 or 60)
- Powdered cheese-based seasoning
- Liquid oil-based cheese seasoning
- Red No. 40 dye

B. *Materials and Equipments*
- Twin or single thermoplastic extruder equipped with high shear screws and 2-mm die orifice
- Digital scale
- Graduated cylinder (1 L)
- Mixer with paddle attachment
- Rotary tumbler
- Air-forced convection oven
- Drying trays
- Liquid sprayer
- Caliper
- Chronometer
- Protective gloves
- Protective lenses

C. *Procedure*
1. Determine the moisture content of the maize grits (refer to Chapter 1).
2. Weigh maize grits and place them in the mixing bowl. Calculate the water required to increase the moisture content to 18%. Use the following equation [(100 − grit moisture)/(100 − 18%) − 1] × amount of grits.
3. For extruders that do not have controlled water injection the feedstock has to be tempered before extrusion. Mix dry ingredients at low speed and then while mixing gradually incorporate the water necessary to increase the moisture to 18%. Keep mixing contents at low speed for 5 minutes.
4. Fit the extruder with a high shear screw(s), 2-mm die orifice(s), and the extrusion conditions that enhances radial expansion. Generally, the first, second, and third segments of the extruder are set to 70°C, 110°C, and 140°C, respectively. Start the extruder and adjust the speed (in rpm; generally, the extruder is set from 150 rpm to 300 rpm). Adjust the feed rate of the extruder and if the extruder has water injection capabilities adjust the water injection rate using the equation of step 2 (Figure 12.9).
5. To prevent the extruder from being stuck or jammed, the first stage of the process should be done with excess water (i.e., twice as much).

Place feedstock in the hopper of the extruder and then start the extrusion process making sure to inject more water. Turn on the extruder cutting unit and allow feedstock to run with excess water and then gradually decrease the water injection until achieving the targeted tempering moisture content of 18%. Allow extruder to achieve steady conditions and adjust the size and length of the extrudates by adjusting the speed of the cutting device. This product usually is cut into 4-cm-long cylindrical forms. Then, determine the feedstock residence time by placing a pinch of Red No. 40 dye directly into the inlet of the extruders barrel. With a chronometer determine the time (seconds) required for the exiting extrudate to stain red. In addition, register the temperatures of the different extruder zones, the rpm of the screw(s), and the cutter.

6. Collect the extrudates and measure the average diameter or size and determine their average moisture content (Figure 12.9).
7. Place extrudates in a convection oven set at 120°C for 20 to 30 minutes. The objective is to decrease the moisture content to 1.5%. Do not overdehydrate the extrudates.
8. Weigh a fixed amount of the dry-toasted extrudates and place them in a rotary tumbler. Turn on the tumbler and for each kilogram of extrudates gradually add 550 g of powdered cheese flavoring or an oil-based liquid seasoning. If a liquid seasoning is used, it is recommended to heat the mix to 130°C before spraying. Allow covering to adhere to the extrudates.
9. Remove flavored corn puffs from the tumbler and immediately place them in moisture proof or aluminized bags.
10. Determine average diameter of the corn puffs, residual moisture content, volumetric weight, color, texture, and sensory properties.

12.4.3.2 Production of Fried Cheese-Flavored Corn Puffs

Fried expanded curls are still widely accepted among snack consumers because they possess a different flavor and configuration. These snacks have been produced for more than 60 years and are manufactured using a special type of extruder that generates most of the heat by friction. Technically, this extruder falls into the medium-shear category and works similarly as the direct expanded high-shear extruders. The major difference is that the fry-type snack extruder does not extrude the product through a typical die. Instead, it uses a set of plates: one rotating and the other stationary. These plates shape and expel the extrudate that is internally cut by rotor fingers (Moore 1994; Burtea 2001).

Tempered or nonconditioned maize grits, rice grits, and starches are introduced and transported into the barrel section of the stator and the shear applied by the screw movement

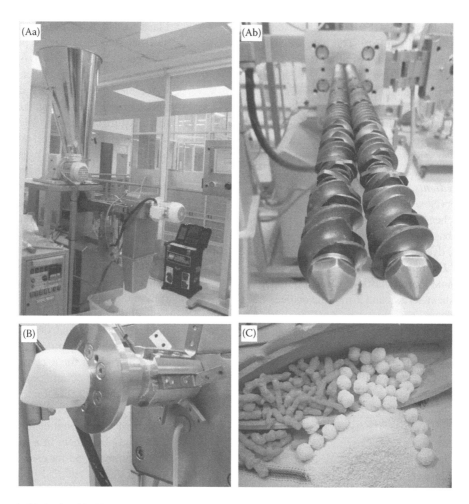

FIGURE 12.9 Extruded baked puffs. Thermoplastic extruder used to produced corn puffs (Aa) and close view of the screws that produce high shear necessary for production of direct expanded products (Ab); (B) view of the extrudates before cutting and achieving optimum expansion; and (C) extruded corn puffs (clockwise baked maize puffs, maize grits, and fried and flavored corn puffs.

increases both the pressure and internal temperature (more than 120°C) so the starch gelatinizes, melts, and plasticizes. The rotor fingers cut the extruding material, which are then immediately extruded radially between the two plates. The main way of controlling this extruder is by adjusting the gap between the rotors. According to Moore (1994), three things occur in this special die: the maize meal or grits are subjected to high shear and pressure, which generates most of the heat to cook the raw material, a rapid pressure loss causes the superheated water to turn into steam, which expands the extrudates and the flow of the raw material between the plates twists and forms the extrudates. Without this special die assembly, the curls would not have the characteristic shape and texture. As the material exists from between the plates the pressure drops from 48 atm to atmospheric and the water superheats and vaporizes expanding the extrudate (Burtea 2001). However, lower expansion rates are obtained in contrast with direct extruded baked products. The higher density curls make these extrudates suitable for a short frying schedule. The extrudates are generally fried to reduce the moisture level from around 8% to 1.5% for texture and stability and the fried curls pick up from 20% to 25% oil (Moore 1994). After frying, the collets are seasoned with a

two-stage seasoning system where an oil-based slurry is first applied followed by a dry seasoning generally consisting of cheddar cheese. The extremely porous surface of extruded snacks enhances oil absorption and adherence. Ten to 15% of seasoning containing 10% to 15% of salt are usually applied onto the extrudates. This brings the total fat content to a level of around 30%–35%. Fry-type extrudates are easily recognized because of their higher density and especially due to their irregular rough-shaped forms varying in lengths. One disadvantage is that the extruder produces more fines than products extruded through die orifices (Serna-Saldivar 2008).

A. *Samples, Ingredients, and Reagents*
- Maize grits (Nos. 40 or 60)
- Frying oil (partially hydrogenated)
- Powdered cheese-based seasoning
- Oil-based cheese seasoning

B. *Materials and Equipments*
- Digital scale
- High-shear extruder
- Graduated cylinder (1 L)
- Mixer with paddle attachment

- Deep fat fryer
- Air-forced convection oven
- Liquid sprayer
- Rotary tumbler
- Thermometer (200°C)
- Chronometer
- Protective gloves
- Protective lenses

C. Procedure

1. Determine the moisture content of the maize grits (refer to Chapter 1).
2. Weigh maize grits and place them in the mixing bowl. Calculate the water required to increase the moisture content to 17%. Use the following equation [(100 – grit moisture)/(100 – 17%) – 1] × amount of grits. Mix grits at low speed, and then, while mixing gradually, incorporate the water necessary to increase the moisture to 17%. Keep mixing contents at low speed during 5 minutes. Allow tempered grits to equilibrate for at least 15 minutes before extrusion.
3. Extrude the feedstock in an adiabatic high-shear extruder designed for the production of curls. Adjust the gap between the rotors in order to control the size and density of the irregular shaped extrudates. After adjusting the settings, allow the extruder to achieve steady conditions.
4. Collect the extrudates and determine its average moisture content and bulk density.
5. Fried the extruded curls in a deep fat fryer containing oil at 175°C. The residence time varies from 15 to 45 seconds depending on the size of the extrudates. The objective is to decrease the moisture content of the curls to 1.5%. Do not overfry the extrudates.
6. Weigh a fixed amount of the dry-toasted extrudates and place them in a rotary tumbler. Turn on the tumbler and for each kilogram of extrudates gradually add 550 g of powdered cheese flavoring or an oil-based liquid seasoning. If a liquid seasoning is used, it is recommended to heat the mix to 130°C before spraying. Allow covering to adhere to the extrudates.
7. Remove flavored corn curls from the tumbler and immediately place them in moisture proof or aluminized bags.
8. Determine average diameter of the corn curls, residual moisture content, volumetric weight, color, texture, and sensory properties.

12.4.3.3 Production of Third-Generation Snacks

Third-generation snacks are also referred to as half-products or pellets. Following extrusion cooking and forming, the pellets are carefully dried to yield a shelf-stable product that could be stored for long periods of time. Pellets are called half-products because they require additional processing to reach the consumer. For snacks, the key additional process is

frying and less frequently conventional or microwave baking. During these heat treatment operations, pellets usually puff or expand and loose moisture so a crisp snack is produced.

Half-products are obtained by cooking and forming in two or one special extruder. The first extruder conditions clearly differ from the second extruder. Pellets, in contrast to the directly expanded puffs, offer the advantage of being distributed with high weight and low volume. Therefore, they can be available at any time and placed for further processing into finished snacks. The basis for the wide variety of these snacks is their shape imparted by the die design and configuration. Most common shapes are flat (for production of pork skin analogs), tube, shell, ring, screw, and wheels weighing from 250 mg to 750 mg each piece (Meuser and Wiedmann 1989).

Most pellets are manufactured from mixtures of starch-rich raw materials that include dehydrated potato products and/or potato starch, wheat flour, and refined grits. The starch content of the blends approximates 90% of the dry matter (Meuser and Wiedmann 1989). The starch, which conforms approximately 90% of the total formulation, is the most important chemical component because it imparts most of the functionality during extrusion and greatly affects the product expansion rate during the subsequent operation of frying. The plastification attained during the thermoplastic extrusion is stopped by the dehydration process and the gelatinized starch plays an important role during deep-fat frying or baking expansion. Key operations for the production of third-generation snacks are extrusion, half-product drying and frying. The first step of the manufacturing process is the mixing of raw materials. The amount of water and mixing rate are important quality control parameters because the aim is to homogenously distribute the water into the blend of raw materials. In contrast to direct extruded products, pellets are usually tempered to moistures from 25% to 35%. The higher tempering enhances starch gelatinization and decreases the expansion of the extrudate. Third-generation snacks are usually extruded in two sequential steps or with only one special extruder that performs cooking and forming in the same equipment. Extruders for these applications usually have a long length/diameter, or L/D ratio, and a vent to depressurize the extrudate before die forming. The first extruder is commonly named cooker because it heats and gelatinizes the starchy materials mixed with texture improvers such as emulsifiers, salt, and flavorings. The inlet barrel section is cooled with water to facilitate feeding and the subsequent barrel zones heated to achieve starch gelatinization (Meuser and Wiedmann 1989). In the cooking stage, it is essential that the raw materials are fully gelatinized unless the formulation contains pregelatinized or modified starches. The typical extrusion cooking processing conditions includes temperatures ranging from 100° to 150°C, 25%–35% moisture and 15–20 seconds residence time. The screw design does not produce high mechanical energy as in high-shear extruders. Most of the energy required to gelatinize the starch is supplied by the barrel usually heated with steam or water vapor. The most common setups are configured to provide a moderate to low shear input. The cooked dough exiting the cooking extruder is fed into the former extruder, which works at totally different conditions. This extruder cools and densifies the cooked plasticized dough before forming the pellets. In order to achieve this, the screw is designed to provide low shear and pressure. Most of the pressure in the forming extruder is produced by the die restriction. The forming zone moves forward and cools down the extrudate to a temperature of 90°C–110°C. The viscoelastic plastic material is continuously shaped by the die into the desired pellet configuration. Some forming extruders are equipped with a pressure release device or vent located immediately before the die or forming zone. This prevents the expansion of the extrudate and enhances the formation of a high dense pellet. The cooked, formed pellet exits the extruder with moisture contents varying from 20% to 25%. In most instances the material existing in the die is cut into thin pieces by a cutter blade, which is riding around the external die face. In some cases the die is a thin slot, which makes a continuous ribbon that is cut into uniform pieces with a rotary cutter (Moore 1994). According to Meuser and Wiedmann (1989) approximately 3%–4% moisture is loss in extruders equipped with vents at the discharge end. These extruders are relatively easy to operate and maintain and are designed to produce up to 25 tons/hour (Serna-Saldivar 2008).

Pellets are immediately dehydrated to lower their moisture content to about 10%–12%. The drying process is a critical step because water should be carefully removed from the pellet by evaporation is a manner such that the quality characteristics of the fried pellets will be controlled. Optimally drying should be performed in two sequential steps (predrying and drying) (Meuser and Wiedmann 1989). Control of moisture removal is achieved by adjusting the temperature-relative humidity residence time profile. Most plants use continuous belt or drum driers set at temperatures around 45°C–90°C. The temperature and relative humidity of the dryer should be carefully controlled to prevent blistering and cracking of the pellet. The residence time required to lower the moisture to 12% or less is between 1 and 8 hours depending on the pellet size, density, and initial moisture content. It is recommended to equilibrate or temper the dried pellets for at least 1 day before frying or baking (Serna-Saldivar 2008). Frying or baking of recent dried pellets yield products with less expansion rate because moisture is not properly equilibrated in the pellet configuration. Snack pellets are usually expanded in deep-fat fryers or microwave ovens. Frying is usually performed at an oil temperature of 170°C–175°C for 10 to 40 seconds depending on the pellet size. The expanded snacks exit the fryer onto a mesh belt for oil draining. During the deep-fat frying operation, heat is transferred from the hot oil onto the product surface by convection and from the surface into the center of the pellet by conduction. The water moves from the inside to the evaporation zone, leaving the product surface as vapor. Some of this vapor remains trapped within the intracellular pores due to restrictive diffusion. The vapor will expand distorting the pore walls and contributing to the internal porosity. Most of the water is released

and oil is absorbed during the first 10 seconds of frying. The result is production of an expanded product having suitable cell structure and desirable texture or mouthfeel. The bulk density of these expanded products fluctuates from 40 g/L to 100 g/L (Moore 1994). During this critical operation the extrudate drops its moisture to less than 2%, and also develops the characteristic texture and flavor and color due to Maillard reactions. Baking is the other common alternative for expanding pellets. Air impingement ovens are suggested because of their high rate of heat transfer. The development of products for microwaving and production of low-fat items is gaining popularity.

Third-generation snacks are usually seasoned with powdered flavorings generally applied with a belt type flavor depositor or in a rotary tumbler. The first equipment has an adjustable dispenser to promote uniform application of dry seasonings and a wire mesh belt that moves and sifts the flavorings to eliminate lumps (Serna-Saldivar 2008). Alternatively, salt and flavorings are also applied in revolving tumblers fitted with liquid sprayers or electrostatic powder dispensers. After the application of the flavorings, snacks are cooled and immediately packaged in moisture proof bags to avoid rancidity and loss of crispiness due to moisture uptake (Serna-Saldivar 2008).

A. Samples, Ingredients, and Reagents
- Refer to Table 12.11
- Powdered seasoning
- Liquid oil-based seasoning
- Red No. 40 dye

B. Materials and Equipments
- Single or twin cooking extruder
- Single or twin forming extruder
- Digital scale
- Mixer with paddle attachment
- Rotary tumbler
- Air-forced convection drier
- Drying trays
- Liquid sprayer
- Caliper
- Thermometer (200°C)
- Chronometer
- Protective gloves
- Protective lenses

TABLE 12.11
Basic Formulation for the Production of Third-Generation Snack Pellets

Ingredients	Amount (%)
Wheat flour	74.0
Potato flour	15.0
Corn starch	10.0
Lecithin	1.0

C. *Procedure*

1. Weigh the ingredients listed in Table 12.11 and place them in the mixing bowl. Calculate the water required to increase the moisture content to 27%. Use the following equation [(100 − grit moisture)/(100 − 27%) − 1] × amount of ingredients. For instance if the average moisture content of the ingredients is 12%, 20.7 L water needs to be added to 100 kg of the ingredient mix.

2. For extruders that do not have controlled water injection, the feedstock has to be tempered before extrusion. Mix dry ingredients at low speed and then while mixing gradually incorporate the water necessary to increase the moisture to 27%. Keep mixing contents at low speed for 5 minutes. For extruders that have water injection capabilities calculate the water flow rate according to the ingredient feed rate.

3. Extrude the tempered or conditioned ingredients through a cooking extruder fitted with a high shear screw(s) (Figure 12.10). The three successive zones of the barrel should be set at 100°C, 120°C, and 150°C (positive temperature gradient). In addition, adjust the speed of the extruder from 100 rpm to 200 rpm. To determine the feedstock residence time in the first extruder add a pinch of Red No. 40 dye directly into the inlet of the cooking extruder and with a chronometer determine the time (seconds) required for the exiting extrudate to stain red. In addition, register the temperatures of the different extruder zones, the rpm of the screw(s), and the torque (amp). When the cooking extruder reaches steady state, sample the extruded dough for moisture, color, gelatinization, and other chemical analysis.

4. Extrude the cooked dough from the first extruder through the forming extruder. This extruder should be fitted with a forming screw(s), adjusted to 70°C–90°C and a depressurization vent or valve so to enhance the formation of a dense pellet. Generally, the extruder operates at a relatively low rpm. Make sure that the cutting system of the second extruder is properly adjusted in order to obtain uniform-shaped pellets. To determine the feedstock residence time, add a pinch of Red No. 40 dye directly into the inlet of the extruders barrel. With a chronometer, determine the time (seconds) required for the exiting pellet to stain red. In addition, register the temperatures of the different extruder zones, the rpm of the screw(s) and the cutter (Figure 12.10).

5. Collect the pellets and measure the average diameter or size and determine their average moisture content.

6. Place pellets in a convection drier set at 60°C to 70°C for 45 minutes to 3 hours. The drying time will change according to the size of the pellets and drier conditions (temperature, relative humidity, air velocity, etc.). The objective is to decrease the moisture content of the pellet to 10%. It is extremely important to not overdehydrate the pellets.

7. Allow dehydrated half products to equilibrate its moisture for at least 24 hours.

8. Weigh a fixed amount of the pellets and fry them in a deep-fat fryer containing partially hydrogenated oil at 175°C. Determine the optimum frying time (varies from 15 to 45 seconds) for the extruded and dehydrated pellets (Figure 12.10).

9. With a ruler and caliper determine the average dimensions of the fried pellets. Reserve expanded pellets for moisture, oil, texture, color, and other analysis.

10. Place a known amount of expanded and fried pellets in the rotary tumbler or drum and for each kilogram of product gradually add 40 g of salted powdered flavorings supplemented or spray it with an oil-based liquid seasoning. If a liquid seasoning is used, it is recommended to heat the mix to 130°C before spraying. Allow covering to adhere to the third-generation snack.

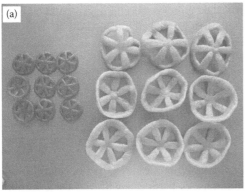

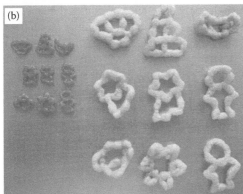

FIGURE 12.10 Third-generation pellets before and after frying. Wheels (a) and other configurations (b) before and after deep-fat frying.

11. Remove flavored snacks from the tumbler and immediately place them in moisture proof or aluminized bags.

12. Determine residual moisture content, oil content, color, percent covering, texture, and sensory properties of the flavored snacks.

12.4.4 RESEARCH SUGGESTIONS

1. Compare expansion rates, texture, and organoleptic properties of dry and wet-popped popcorn.

2. Adjust the moisture content of a given lot of popcorn to 10%, 12%, 14%, and 16% moisture. Split each of the four treatments into two lots. One lot will serve as control whereas the other will be purposely damaged with a razor blade by cutting a 3-mm mark on the pericarp of each kernel. Using the MWVT test, determine the expansion rate, percentage of unpopped kernels, and flake size of the eight different treatments.

3. Produce corn chips following the same procedure except for the substitution of the frying oil for olestra. Compare the color, texture, oil uptake, energy or caloric density, and organoleptic properties of the two different types of corn chips.

4. Produce pretzels with three different types of refined flours: soft, all purpose, and hard. Compare their color, crumb texture, and organoleptic properties of the different finished products.

5. Produce pretzels with three different types of alkaline baths or treatments: 1.25% NaOH, 2% sodium bicarbonate, and 1.25% KOH. Treat the pretzel dough for 30 seconds, 1 minute, and 2 minutes with the hot bath solution (90°C) and then proceed with the manufacturing process. Compare the color, crumb texture, and organoleptic properties of the nine different types of pretzels.

6. Determine and compare the parched corn making properties of two contrasting maizes (i.e., Large soft-textured Cuzco kernels vs. white with intermediate endosperm texture) cooked with lime or calcium hydroxide or potassium hydroxide. Compare the four different treatments in terms of oil uptake, texture, color, and sensory properties.

7. Determine and compare the tortilla chip making properties of three contrasting maizes (i.e., white with intermediate endosperm texture, yellow with soft texture, and soft blue maize). Compare yields, oil uptake, incidence of blistering, tortilla chip texture, color, and design a sensory evaluation test (refer to Chapter 3) aimed toward determining differences in color, texture, flavor, and overall acceptability.

8. Determine and compare the tortilla chip making properties of a white dent maize processed via traditional fresh coarse *masa* process or using a coarse dry *masa* flour. Compare *masa* textures, incidence of blistering or pillowing, tortilla chip texture, and design a triangular evaluation test (refer to Chapter 3) aimed toward determining differences in color, texture, flavor, and overall preference.

9. Determine and compare the tortilla chip-making properties of a white dent maize and a white food-grade sorghum used as whole and decorticated to remove 20% of the external layers. First determine the optimum cooking times using the nylon lab technique and then process the coarsely ground maize, whole sorghum, or decorticated sorghum *masa* into tortillas and chips. Compare color of baked tortillas and fried chips, oil uptake during frying, tortilla chip texture, and organoleptic properties.

10. Produce regular, light, and fat-free tortilla chips from the same lot of white dent maize. Light tortilla chips will be produced by flash frying (5 seconds frying) followed by oven toasting and fat-free tortilla chips by toasting of baked tortilla pieces preferably in an impingement oven. Compare color, texture, oil content, and sensory properties of the three contrasting chips. Based on their chemical composition determine their caloric or energy density.

11. Produce pretzels with three different types of flours: (1) refined all purpose wheat flour a, (2) 50% wheat flour + 50% oat flour, and (3) 75% whole wheat flour + 25% rye flour. Compare their final crust and crumb color, texture, and organoleptic properties.

12. Decorticate white sorghum following the procedure described in Chapter 5. Then, mill the sorghum into grits and process sorghum grits and maize grits into extruded baked puffs flavored with cheese. Compare their radial expansion, color, texture, and sensory properties.

13. Decorticate white sorghum following the procedure described in Chapter 5. Then, mill the sorghum into grits and process sorghum grits and maize grits into extruded fried curls flavored with cheese. Compare their oil uptake, color, texture, and sensory properties.

14. Compare the properties of pellets and third-generation snacks produced with the basic formulation with the only difference of using a damaged refined wheat flour (high falling number or high starch damage). Compare the color of the pellets and properties and processability of the fried snacks in terms of color, expansion rate, oil uptake, texture, and flavor.

12.4.5 RESEARCH QUESTIONS

1. Define the following terms:
   a. Second-generation snack
   b. Third-generation snack
   c. Oil turnover rate
   d. Half-product
   e. Corn chip
   f. Tortilla chip

g. Collet
h. Coextrusion
i. Blistering or pillowing
j. Compound die

2. What are differences among first-, second-, and third-generation snacks?

3. What are the ideal popcorn kernel properties? What are the differences and uses of mushroom and butterfly popcorn? Which is the most critical and important equipment to test popcorn? Briefly describe its principle.

4. How does popcorn moisture affect expansion rate?

5. What are the differences between corn chips and tortilla chips in terms of processing and product characteristics?

6. Why is maize for lime cooked snacks less cooked compared to soft tortillas? Why is the *nixtamal* commonly ground into a coarse instead of a fine *masa*?

7. Describe the flowchart of the alkaline parched corn manufacturing process. What is the ideal kernel for this application?

8. Describe at least one process alternative to produce low-fat corn chips.

9. Describe at least two process alternatives to produce low-fat tortilla chips and one to produce fat-free (no added fat) tortilla chips.

10. What is thermoplastic extrusion? What are the five basic parts of the extruder? What are the main advantages of using extrusion cooking instead of traditional processes?

11. Compare direct and pellet-forming extrusion processes in terms of equipment, raw materials, and product characteristics.

12. Compare the direct-baked expanded and fried extrusion processes used to produce puffs.

13. Describe the water–oil exchange phenomena that occur during frying operations.

14. What are the key and most critical operations for the manufacturing of pretzels? What is the main functionality of the NaOH treatment in terms of organoleptic properties of pretzels?

15. Investigate at least three different procedures to measure crunchiness of snack foods.

16. Why are most snack foods salted with coarse or flaked salt? What is usually done in snack operations to enhance the adherence of the salt and seasonings?

17. What is the chemical composition of hard pretzel? How does it compare with corn chips and potato chips especially in terms of energy density?

18. What is the optimum packaging material for most snacks?

19. Why are hard pretzels dark on the outside and white in the inside?

20. Using mass balance, calculate the yield of fried tortilla chips containing 24% oil and 1.7% moisture manufactured from 750 g of triangular cut tortillas that contained 44% moisture and 1.2% oil.

21. Define the term oil turnover rate (OTR) widely used in snack operations. If you are operating a fryer containing 1600 kg oil that is producing corn chips with 36% oil at a rate of 500 kg/hour, what is the OTR?

22. What are the three primary ways oil breaks down during frying? What are the most common quality control procedures to determine oil deterioration in frying operations?

23. List at least five quality control tests with its main use and principle used to evaluate snack foods.

REFERENCES

American Association of Cereal Chemists. 2000. *Approved Methods of the AACC*. St. Paul, MN: AACC.

Anderson, R. A., H. F. Conway, V. F. Pfeifer, and E. I. Griffin. 1969. Roll and Extrusion Cooking of Grain Sorghum Grits. *Cereal Science Today* 14: 372–375.

Anonymous. 2004. "State of the Industry Report." *Snack Food and Wholesale Bakery* 93(5):SI1–SI64.

AOAC International. 1998. *Official Methods of Analysis of AOAC International*. 16th ed. Gaithersburg, MD: AOAC International.

AOCS. 2009. *Official Methods and Recommended Practices of the AOCS*. 6th ed. Danvers, MA: The Society.

Bawa, A.S. 1993. "Snack Foods." In *Encyclopedia of Food Science, Food Technology and Nutrition*, edited by R. Macrae, R. K. Robinson, and M. J. Sadler, pp. 4167–4172. Vol. 6. London, UK: Academic Press.

Byrd, J. E., and M. J. Perona. 2005. "Kinetics of Popping of Popcorn." *Cereal Chemistry* 82(1):53–59.

Caldwell, E. F., R. B. Fast, J. Ievolella, C. Lauhoff, H. Levine, R. C. Miller, L. Slade, B. S. Strahm, and P. J. Whalen. 2000. "Cooking of Ready to Eat Breakfast Cereals." *Cereals Foods World* 45(6):244–252.

Deane, D., and E. Commers. 1986. "Oat Cleaning and Processing." In *Oats: Chemistry and Technology*, edited by F. H. Webster, Chapter 13. St. Paul, MN: AACC.

Doehlert, D. C., and W. R. Moore. 1997. "Composition of Oat Bran and Flour Prepared by Three Different Mechanisms of Dry-Milling." *Cereal Chemistry* 74:403–406.

Doehlert, D. C., M. S. McMullen, and R. R. Baumann. 1999. "Factors Affecting Groat Percentage in Oat." *Crop Sci.* 39:1858–1865.

Doehlert, D., and M. S. McMullen. 2000. "Genotypic and Environmental Effects on Oat Milling Characteristics and Groat Hardness." *Cereal Chemistry* 77(2):148–154.

Faridi, H., V. F. Rasper, and B. Launay. 1987. *The Alveograph Handbook*. St. Paul, MN: AACC.

Fast, R. B. 2001. "Breakfast Cereals." In *Cereals Processing Technologies*, edited by G. Owens, Chapter 8, pp. 158–172. Cambridge, UK: CRC Press, Woodhead Publishing.

Fast, R. B., and E. F. Caldwell. 2000. *Breakfast Cereals and How Are They Made*, 2nd ed. St. Paul, MN: AACC.

Hoseney, R. C., K. Zeleznak, and A. Abdelrahman. 1983. "Mechanism of Popcorn Popping." *J. Cereal Sci.* 1:43.

Meilgaard, M., G. A. Civille, and B. T. Carr. 1991. Sensory Evaluation Techniques. 2nd ed., Boca Raton, FL: CRC Press.

Lin, Y. E., and R. C. Anantheswaran. 1988. "Studies in Popping of Popcorn in a Microwave Oven." *J. Food Sci.* 53:1746–1749.

Metzger, D. D., K. H. Hsu, K. E. Ziegler, and C. J. Bern. 1989. "Effect of Moisture Content on Popcorn Popping Volume for Oil and Hot Air Popping." *Cereal Chem.* 66:247–248.

Mohamed, A. A., R. B. Ashman, and A. W. Kirelis. 1993. "Pericarp Thickness and Other Kernel Physical Characteristics Relate to Microwave Popping Quality of Popcorn." *J. Food Sci.* 58(2): 342–346.

Mohamed, S. 1990. "Factors Affecting Extrusion Characteristics of Expanded Starch-Based Products." *J. Food Proc. Preserv.* 14:437–452.

Moore, G. 1994. "Snack Food Extrusion." In *The Technology of Extrusion Cooking*, edited by N.D. Frame, Chapter 4, pp. 110–143. Glasgow, UK: Blackie Academic & Professional.

Pike, O. A. 1994. "Fat Characterization." In *Food Analysis*, edited by S. S. Nielsen, pp. 225–228. 2nd ed. Gaithersburg, MD: Aspen Publishers.

Popcorn Institute. 1989. *Test for Evaluating Popcorn Hybrids in a Microwave Oven.* Chicago, IL: Technical Committee Popcorn Institute.

Pordesimo, L. O., R. C. Anantheswaran, A. M. Fleischmann, Y. E. Lin, and M. A. Hanna. "Physical Properties as Indicators of Popping Characteristics of Microwave Popcorn." *J. Food. Sci.* 55(5):1352–1355.

Pordesimo, L. O., R. C. Anantheswaran, and P. J. Mattern. 1991. "Quantification of Horny and Floury Endosperm in Popcorn and Their Effects on Popping Performance in a Microwave Oven." *J. Cereal Sci.* 14:189–198.

Pringle, F. E., E. J. Monhahan, and E. F. Caldwell. 2000. "Packaging of Ready to Eat Breakfast Cereals." *Cereal Foods World* 45(6): 255–260.

Riaz, M. N. 2000. "Introduction to Extruders and Their Principles." In *Extruders in Food Applications*, edited by M. N. Riaz, Chapter 1. Lancaster, PA: Technomic Publishing.

Riaz, M. N. 2004. "Snack Foods, Processing." In *Encyclopedia of Grain Science*, edited by C. Wrigley, C. Walker, and H. Corke, pp. 98–108. 1st ed. Oxford, UK: Elsevier.

Rooney, L. W. 2007. *Corn Quality Assurance Manual.* 2nd ed. Arlington, VA: SFA.

Rooney, L. W., and S. O. Serna-Saldivar. 2003. "Food Uses of Whole Corn and Dry Milled Fractions." In *Corn Chemistry and Technology*, edited by P. White and L. Johnson, Chapter 13. 2nd ed. St. Paul, MN: AACC.

Serna-Saldivar, S. R. O. 2003. *Manufactura y Control de Calidad de Productos Basados en Cereales.* S.A. México, D.F., México: AGT Editor.

Serna-Saldivar, S. O. 2008. *Industrial Manufacture of Snack Foods.* London, UK: Kennedys Publications.

Serna-Saldivar, S. O. 2010. "Manufacturing of Breakfast Cereals." In *Cereal Grains: Properties, Processing and Nutritional Attributes,* Chapter 11. Boca Raton, FL: CRC Press (Taylor & Francis Group).

Serna-Saldivar, S. O., H. D. Almeida-Dominguez, L. W. Rooney, M. H. Gómez, and A. J. Bockholt. 1991. "Method to Evaluate Ease of Pericarp Removal on Lime-Cooked Corn Kernels." *Crop Sci.* 31:842–844.

Serna-Saldivar, S. O., Gomez, M. H., Almeida-Dominguez, H. D., Islas Rubio, A., and Rooney, L. W. 1993. "A Method to Evaluate the Lime Cooking Properties of Corn (*Zea mays*)." *Cereal Chemistry* 70:762–764.

Serna-Saldivar, S. O., M. H. Gomez, and L. W. Rooney. 1990. "The Technology, Chemistry and Nutritional Value of Alkaline-Cooked Corn Products." In *Advances of Cereal Science and Technology*, edited by Y. Pomeranz, pp. 243–307. Vol. X. St. Paul, MN: AACC.

Shuey, W. C., and K. H. Tipples. 1982. *The Amylograph Handbook.* St. Paul, MN: AACC.

Singh, V., N. L. Barreiro, J. McKinstry, P. Buriak, and S. R. Eckhoff. 1997. "Effect of Kernel Size, Location and Type of Damage on Popping Characteristics of Popcorn." *Cereal Chemistry* 74(5):672–675.

Snack Food Association. 1992. *Corn Quality Assurance Manual.* Alexandria, VA: SFA.

Song, A., and S. R. Eckhoff. 1994. "Optimum Popping Moisture Content for Popcorn Kernels of Different Sizes." *Cereal Chemistry* 71:458–460.

Song, A., and S. R. Eckhoff. 1994. "Individual Kernel Moisture Content of Preshelled and Shelled Popcorn and Equilibrium Isotherms of Popcorn of Different Sizes." *Cereal Chemistry* 71:461–463.

Song, A., and S. R. Eckhoff, M. Paulsen, and J. B. Litchfield. 1991. "Effects of kernel size and genotype on popcorn popping volume and number of unpopped kernels." *Cereal Chemistry* 71:464–467.

Tribelhorn, R. E. 1991. "Breakfast Cereals." In *Handbook of Cereal Science and Technology*, edited by K. J. Lorenz and K. Kulp, Chapter 18. New York, NY: Marcel Dekker.

Valentes, K. J., L. Levine, and J. P. Clark. 1991. "Ready to Eat Breakfast Cereals." In *Food Processing Operations and Scale Up*, Chapter 6. New York, NY: Marcel Dekker.

Whalen, P. J., J. L. DesRochers, and C. E. Walker. 2000. "Ready-to-Eat Breakfast Cereals." In *Handbook of Cereal Science and Technology*, edited by K. Kulp and J. G. Ponte, Chapter 19. New York, NY: Marcel Dekker.

White, P. J. 1991. "Methods for Measuring Changes in Deep Fat Frying Operations." *Food Technology* 45(2):75–83.

Ziegler, K. E. 2000. "Popcorn." In *Specialty Corns*, edited by A. R. Hallauer, pp. 199–234. Boca Raton, FL: CRC Press.

Ziegler, K. E. 2003. "Popcorn." In *Corn Chemistry and Technology*, edited by P. E. White and L. A. Johnson, Chapter 22. 2nd ed. St. Paul, MN: AACC.

13 Production of Modified Starches, Syrups, and Sweeteners

13.1 INTRODUCTION

Native starches, obtained by the various wet-milling processes described in Chapter 7 of the textbook, are industrially transformed by physicochemical processes into modified starches or bioenzymatic processes into an array of syrups with different degrees of sweetness and properties. Most of these products are obtained from maize starch although wheat, rice, potato (*Solanum tuberosum*), and tapioca (*Mandioca suculenta*) starches are also used. Modified starches have specific functional properties for special applications in the food industry. They are widely used as thickeners for the canning industry, as a base for batters and breadings, emulsifiers, and as adhesives or glues in nonfood-related industries (Table 13.1).

Starches are also used as raw materials for the production of an array of syrups being the most widely produced glucose and fructose rich sweeteners. Undoubtedly, the most popular syrup is the high fructose. The transformation of starch into syrups consists in the hydrolysis of the starch components by specific enzymes into soluble sugars. Alternatively, starch can be hydrolyzed into dextrins with the use of an acid conversion. Independently of the process the dextrins are further hydrolyzed into maltose, glucose, and fructose with the use of specific enzymes such as α-amylase, β-amylase, amyloglucosidase, and glucose isomerase (Bemiller and Whistler 2009). This last enzyme isomerizes glucose into fructose for the industrial production of fructose syrups. These syrups are widely used for the production of soft drinks.

13.2 MODIFIED STARCHES

Native starches are physically and chemically transformed into an array of modified starches. The most common physical modification yields the thermal-treated or pregelatinized starches. These instant starches are hydrosoluble even in cold water and are frequently used as thickeners in foods that receive minimal heat processing Pregelatinization methods include drum drying, spray cooking, solvent-based processing, and extrusion.

On the other hand, the chemical modified starches are industrially produced to satisfy or meet special functionalities. Modifications are aimed toward altering the starch granule characteristics and therefore the susceptibility to gelatinization, cooking, retrogradation, and/or gelling. Chemical modifications can be hydrolytic, oxidative, ester forming, or ether forming. The most widely used types of modified starches are acid thinning, oxidized/bleached, molecular cross-bonded, and chemically substituted or derivatized (Table 13.1; Johnson 2000; Mauro et al. 2003; Thomas and Atwell 1999).

Most manufacturing technologies consist of treating native starches in a reactor with temperature and agitation controls. Generally, a starch slurry with approximately 35% solids and adjusted to a certain pH is treated with chemicals to promote the desired reactions. In most instances, gelatinization and starch solubilization is avoided so to prevent the disruption of the starch granule.

13.2.1 PREGELATINIZED STARCHES

The pregelatinized or instant starches are soluble even in cold water and therefore are commonly used as thickeners in foods or beverages that receive minimal heat treatments. Pregelatinization methods include drum drying, spray cooking, solvent-based processing, and extrusion (Thomas and Atwell 1999). Drum drying is the most common manufacturing method. Spray cooking consists of first heating a starch slurry in a jet cooker followed by spray drying. This manufacturing process is not frequently used in the industry due to the comparatively high costs (Mauro et al. 2003). Drum drying is the most common industrial manufacturing method of pregelatinized starches.

13.2.1.1 Production of Pregelatinized Starches

A. *Samples, Ingredients, and Reagents*
  - Native starch
  - Distilled water

B. *Materials and Equipments*
  - Digital scale
  - Stirring rod
  - Drum dryer
  - Graduated cylinder (2 L)
  - Container (15 L)
  - Roller mill
  - Rotap (U.S. Nos. 60, 80, 100, and 120 sieves and collection pan)

C. *Procedure*
  1. Determine the native starch moisture content (refer to procedure in Section 2.2.1.1).
  2. In a container, blend 3.5 kg of native starch with 6.5 L distilled water. Make sure to thoroughly mix the starch with the water avoiding the formation of lumps.

TABLE 13.1

Properties and Major Uses of Modified Starches

Type of Starch	Process	Uses and Applications
Pregelatinized	Heat treatment in the presence of water to enhance starch gelatinization	Instant starches or cold water dispersible Used in beverages and puddings
Acid	Treatment with acids in order to random hydrolyze starch molecules	Known as acid-thinning starches are mainly used for confectionary products (fillings for candies) and paper coatings Produce firmer gels
Dextrinized	Dry heat with acid or alkaline catalyst	Improved water solubility and reduced viscosity Similar to acid-treated counterparts
Oxidative	Treatment with sodium hypochlorite in order to oxidize hydroxyl groups to carboxyl or carbonyl groups	Oxidative starches have reduced viscosity, gelling, and retrogradation and yield clear pastes Used as additive for batters and breadings
Bleached	Treatment with hydrogen peroxide, peracetic acid, ammonium persulfate, potassium permanganate, and sodium chlorite or hypochlorite to oxidize pigments such as carotenoides/xantophylls	Used as fluidizing agent for dry powders such as confectioner's sugar
Phosphated	Treatment with monosodium orthophosphate or sodium tripolyphosphate	Starch with higher viscosity and produce stable and clear gels Used as flocculants, emulsifiers, and adhesives in the food and paper industries
Hydroxyethyl and hydroxypropylated	Treatment with ethylene oxide and propylene oxide, respectively	They have reduced gelatinization temperature and produce more clear and stable pastes Used in food gravies, pie fillings, and salad dressings
Acetate derivative	Treatment with acetic anhydride	The introduction of acetyl groups reduces gelatinization temperature, increases hot peak viscosity, reduces cold paste viscosity, and prevents retrogradation Used as food thickeners and stabilizers in gravies, fruit pies, salad dressings, and filled cakes
Succinate derivatives	Succinic anhydride	Used as food thickeners and for encapsulation Also used as textile sizings and adhesives
Cross-bonded, distarch phosphate	Phosphorus oxychloride, trimetaphosphate	Reduce swelling and loss of viscosity due to temperature, shear, and acid
Cross-bonded, distarch adipate	Adipic and acetic acids	Used as retortable thickener (canning industry), salad dressings, and baby foods Functional ingredient in the production of thermoplastic extruded foods

Source: Johnson, L. A., *Handbook of Cereal Science and Technology*, Chapter 2, Marcel Dekker, New York, 2000; Mauro, D. J., Abbas, I. R., and Orthoefer, F. T., *Corn Chemistry and Technology*, Chapter 16, American Association of Cereal Chemists, St. Paul, MN, 2003; Thomas, D. J., and Atwell, W. A., *Starches*, Eagan Press, St. Paul, MN, 1999.

3. Heat the resulting starch slurry in a drum dryer consisting of an applicator roll and a heated drum equipped with a blade. During this operation, most of the water evaporates and the resulting pregelatinized and dried starch film is removed from the drum with a blade.

4. Weigh the resulting pregelatinized starch and determine its residual moisture. Calculate the starch yield based on the original dry native starch weight.

5. Grind the pregelatinized starch preferably with a roller mill or alternatively with a hammer mill into the desired granulation. Determine the particle size distribution of the ground pregelatinized starch using a Rotap furnished with sieves U.S. Nos. 60, 80, 100, 120, 150, and collection pan.

6. Determine birefringence, Congo red test, color, water solubility, and viscoamylograph properties of both native and pregelatinized starches (refer to Chapter 6).

13.2.2   Chemically Modified Starches

Modified starches are commercially produced to fulfill special uses. Modifications are aimed toward altering the starch granule, which in turns affects the gelatinization, retrogradation, and gelling behavior. These chemical modifications modify the viscoamylograph properties in terms of water affinity, pasting, viscosity, retrogradation, and gelling (Johnson 2000; Mauro et al. 2003; Thomas and Atwell 1999).

13.2.2.1   Production of Acid-Treated or Dextrinized Starches

The acid-treated starches, also known as dextrinized, are obtained after treating the starch slurry with acid at temperatures below gelatinization. These acid thinning starches are mainly used as confectionary filling. The chemical process consists of treating the starch slurry with 1% to 3% aqueous hydrochloric or sulfuric acid. Most reactions are carried on slurries containing 35% solids at temperatures of approximately 50°C. The acid causes the random hydrolysis of both α 1-4, and α 1-6 glycosidic bonds yielding dextrinized starch. These starches maintain their granular structure and birefringence. The depolymerization mainly occurs in the amorphous concentric areas of the starch granule. When the desired viscosity is achieved the solution is generally neutralized and the starch filtered out. Acid-treated starches need higher temperature for gelatinization, have reduced granule swelling capacity and primarily reduced paste viscosity. These starches are water soluble and produce weaker pastes and strong and clear gels upon gelatinization and cooling. This is because the lower molecular weight dextrins are more prone to retrogradation (Rohwer and Klem 1984; Sharp and Sharp 1994).

A. *Samples, Ingredients, and Reagents*
- Native starch
- Distilled water
- Hydrochloric or sulfuric acids
- Sodium hydroxide (NaOH)
- Standard solutions for pH meter

B. *Materials and Equipments*
- Digital scale
- Beakers (2 L)
- Stirring rod
- Thermoregulated water bath
- Filtering cloth
- Filter paper
- Aluminum foil
- Pipette (10 mL)
- Graduated cylinder (1 L)
- Air-forced convection dryer
- Roller mill
- pH meter
- Thermometer
- Chronometer
- Rotap (U.S. Nos. 60, 80, 100, and 120 sieves and collection pan)

C. *Procedure*
1. Determine the native starch moisture content (refer to procedure in Section 2.2.1.1).
2. In a beaker, mix 350 g of native starch with 650 mL water. Make sure to thoroughly mix the starch with the water avoiding the formation of lumps. Add 7 mL hydrochloric acid, stir contents, and heat the resulting slurry in a shaking water bath to 50°C for 30 minutes. Cover the beaker with aluminum foil.
3. Neutralize the acid-treated slurry with 0.1 N NaOH.
4. Filter the acid-treated starch first though a cloth and then through filter paper. Dehydrate the resulting starch cake in a convection oven set at 60°C. Weigh the resulting acid-treated starch and determine its residual moisture. Calculate the acid-starch yield based on the original dry native starch weight.
5. Grind the starch preferably with a roller mill or alternatively with a hammer mill into the desired granulation. Determine the particle size distribution of the ground pregelatinized starch using a Rotap furnished with sieves U.S. Nos. 60, 80, 100, 120, and 150 and a collection pan.
6. Determine birefringence, color, water solubility, and viscoamylograph properties of both native and acid-treated starches (refer to Chapter 6).

13.2.2.2   Production of Oxidized/Bleached Starches

The oxidation of native starches is aimed toward bleaching and modifying functional properties. The main purpose of bleaching is to improve the whiteness of the starch powder by oxidizing the impurities such as carotenes and xanthophylls. Bleaching is generally accomplished by using oxidizing agents at relatively low concentrations. The alkaline hypochloride is the reagent most utilized for this purpose. Hypochlorite oxidation primarily involves carbons 2, 3, and 6. Other compounds used are hydrogen peroxide, paracetic acid, ammonium persulfate, and potassium permanganate. The sodium hypochlorite treatment oxidizes hydroxyl groups to carboxyl or carbonyl groups. The oxidation mainly occurs in the amorphous regions of the starch granule where starch chains depolymerize due to breakage of glycosidic bonds. In addition, the hydroxyl group oxidizes into carboxyl and carbonyl groups. Similarly to acid-treated starches, oxidized counterparts had a comparatively lower viscosity at peak of gelatinization and after retrogradation. This starch is used to improve adhesiveness of batters and breadings, in the textile industry, and as a surface paper coating (Table 13.1). The oxidixing treatment also reduces significant bacterial and mold counts (Johnson 2000; Mauro et al. 2003; Rutenberg and Solarek 1984; Sharp and Sharp 1994; Thomas and Atwell 1999).

A. *Samples, Ingredients, and Reagents*
- Native starch
- Distilled water

- Sodium bisulfite
- Sodium hypochlorite
- Standard solutions for pH meter

B. *Materials and Equipments*
- Digital scale
- Beakers (2 L)
- Stirring rod
- Thermoregulated water bath
- Filtering cloth
- Filter paper
- Aluminum foil
- Pipette (10 mL)
- Graduated cylinder (1 L)
- Air-forced convection dryer
- Roller mill
- pH meter
- Thermometer
- Chronometer
- Rotap (U.S. Nos. 60, 80, 100, and 120 sieves and collection pan)

C. *Procedure*
1. Determine the moisture content of the native starch (refer to procedure in Section 2.2.1.1).
2. In a beaker, mix 350 g of native starch with 650 mL water. Make sure to thoroughly mix the starch with the water avoiding the formation of lumps. Adjust the pH of the starch slurry to pH 7.5 to 8 with 0.1 N sodium hydroxide solution.
3. Place the slurry in a thermoregulated water bath adjusted to 30°C and gradually add during few minutes with stirring 3% sodium hypochlorite based on the starch weight. Incubate and continue stirring the slurry for 120 minutes.
4. Adjust the treated slurry to pH 6.8 with 0.1 N sodium bisulfite.
5. Filter the oxidized starch first through a cloth and then through filter paper. Dehydrate the resulting starch cake in a convection oven set at 50°C. Weigh the resulting starch and determine its residual moisture. Calculate the oxidized starch yield based on the original dry native starch weight.
6. Grind the starch preferably with a roller mill or alternatively with a hammer mill into the desired granulation. Determine the particle size distribution of the ground oxidized starch using a Rotap furnished with sieves U.S. Nos. 60, 80, 100, 120, and 150 and a collection pan.
7. Determine starch color before and after oxidation, water solubility, and viscoamylograph properties of both native and oxidized starches (refer to Chapter 6).

13.2.2.3 Production of Cross-Bonded Starches

Cross-linking is one of the most common types of chemical modifications because the resulting starches have a relatively constant viscosity during heating and cooling cycles and reduced granular swelling and loss of viscosity due to temperature, shear, and acid. In fact, highly modified cross-bonded starches do not gelatinize with regular cooking or even with pressure cooking in retorts (Rutenberg and Solarek 1984). Briefly, the process consists of treating the starch with phosphorus oxychloride, trimetaphosphate or epichlorohydrin, and adipic/acetic acid. After achieving the desired degree of cross-linking, the slurry is neutralized, filtrated, washed, and dried. These modified starches are mainly used as thickeners in the canning industry (i.e., soups, gravies, infant foods), in batter and breading recipes, for the preparation of dressings, and as a functional ingredient in the production of thermoplastic extruded foods (Johnson 2000; Mauro et al. 2003; Sharp and Sharp 1994; Thomas and Atwell 1999).

A. *Samples, Ingredients, and Reagents*
- Native starch
- Distilled water
- Hydrochloric or sulfuric acids
- Sodium hydroxide
- Standard solutions for pH meter

B. *Materials and Equipments*
- Digital scale
- Beakers (2 L)
- Stirring rod
- Thermoregulated water bath
- Filtering cloth
- Filter paper
- Aluminum foil
- Pipette (10 mL)
- Graduated cylinder (1 L)
- Air-forced convection dryer
- Roller mill
- pH meter
- Thermometer
- Chronometer
- Rotap (U.S. Nos. 60, 80, 100, and 120 sieves and collection pan)

C. *Procedure*
1. Determine the moisture content of the native starch.
2. Mix 400 g of native starch with 600 mL water. Make sure to thoroughly mix the starch with the water avoiding the formation of lumps.
3. Adjust the pH of the starch slurry to pH 9 with sodium sulfate.
4. Place the slurry in a thermoregulated water bath adjusted to 35°C and gradually add during few minutes with stirring 5% sodium tripolyphosphate and 2.5% sodium trimetaphosphate based on the starch weight. Incubate and continue stirring the slurry for 80 minutes.
5. Remove beaker from the incubator and heat the phosphate cross-linked starch slurry time for 1.5 hours at 100°C. Make sure to cover the beaker with aluminum foil.

6. Filter the cross-linked starch first though a cloth and then through filter paper. Dehydrate the resulting starch cake in a convection oven set at 60°C. Weigh the resulting starch and determine its residual moisture. Calculate the cross bonded starch yield based on the original dry native starch weight.

7. Grind the starch preferably with a roller mill or alternatively with a hammer mill into the desired granulation. Determine the particle size distribution of the ground cross-linked starch using a Rotap furnished with sieves (U.S. Nos. 60, 80, 100, 120, and 150 and a collection pan).

8. Determine color, water solubility, water holding capacity, and viscoamylograph properties of both native and cross-bonded starches (refer to Chapter 6).

13.2.2.4 Production of Derivatized and Substituted Starches (Acetylated, Propionylated, and Butyryated)

The chemical substitution of starch hydroxyl groups with functional units yields modified starches with distinctive functionalities and applications. Acetylated and hydroxypropylated starches are produced after treatment with anhydrous acetic and propylene oxide under an alkaline pH, respectively, in order to yield starches less prone to retrogradation, that produce weaker and clearer gels (Mauro et al. 2003; Thomas and Atwell 1999). Other relevant categories are the esterified starches produced after reaction with acetate, phosphate, or succinates. Acetylated starches are manufactured from anhydrous acetic, which reacts with hydroxyl groups forming methyl esters. These sorts of starches require lower temperatures to gelatinize and to achieve peak viscosity (approximately 10°C less compared to regular maize starch) and are less prone to retrogradation. Thus, they are mainly used as thickeners in the canning industry and in refrigerated or frozen food products (Rutenberg and Solarek 1984). On the other hand, the hydroxyalkylated starches are obtained after treatment with alkylane oxide under alkaline conditions. The hydroxyl groups located in the second position of glucose units are the preferred sites of substitution. Hydroxypropylation increases freeze–thaw stability, decreases gelatinization and pasting temperatures, and improves paste clarity.

Phosphate-substituted starches are manufactured by treating native starch with orthophosphate at a slightly acidic pH (5–6.5) at temperatures of 120°C–160°C. These starches form a phosphate ester that imparts distinctive functionalities such as production of clear and stable, high viscosity, and cohesive gels that resist retrogradation. Additionally, they are used as emulsifiers due to the high polar capacity of the phosphate ester.

A. Samples, Ingredients, and Reagents
- Native starch
- Distilled water
- Dimethyl sulfoxide (DMSO)
- 1-Methylimidazole
- Acetic anhydride
- Propionic anhydride
- Butyric anhydride
- Ethanol
- Standard solutions for pH meter

B. Materials and Equipments
- Digital scale
- Large container (50 L)
- Stirrer for large tank
- Filtering cloth
- Filter paper
- Air-forced convection dryer
- Roller mill
- pH meter
- Thermometer
- Chronometer
- Rotap (U.S. Nos. 60, 80, 100, and 120 sieves and collection pan)

C. Procedure (Annison et al. 2003)
1. Determine the moisture content of the native starch.
2. Mix 500 g of native starch with 30 L DMSO and heat contents with continuous stirring to 80°C.
3. Add 600 g of starch to the hot DMSO through a domestic sieve to prevent clumping. Stir constantly for 1 hour until a clear and viscous solution is achieved. Then, add 110 mL of 1-methylimidazole as catalyst.
4. For production of acetylated, propionylated, or butyrylated derivatized starches, add 115, 180, or 230 mL of acetic, propionic, or butyric anhydride and incubate for 4 hours.
5. After incubation, add 6 L distilled water to decompose remaining anhydride. Then, precipitate the starch with 24 L of ethanol.
6. Recover the modified starch and wash it four times with 1 L of ethanol to remove DMSO and leftovers of the reagents.
7. Filter the derivatized starch first though a cloth and then through filter paper. Dehydrate the resulting starch cake in a convection oven set at 50°C. Weigh the resulting modified starch and determine its residual moisture. Calculate the modified starch yield based on the original dry native starch weight.
8. Grind the starch preferably with a roller mill or alternatively with a hammer mill into the desired granulation. Determine the particle size distribution of the ground cross-linked starch using a Rotap furnished with sieves (U.S. Nos. 60, 80, 100, 120, and 150).
9. Determine the degree of substitution, color, water solubility, and viscoamylograph properties of the native and the three different types of modified or derivatized starches (refer to Chapter 6).

13.2.3 Research Suggestions

1. Produce pregelatinized starches following two contrasting procedures the drum drying process described herein and an alternative process in which the starch slurry is gelatinized through a jet cooker and then spray dried. Compare the properties of the resulting instant starches especially in terms of viscoamylograph behavior (refer to procedure in Section 6.4.1.1 or 6.4.1.2), solubility, and color.

2. Produce two acid-treated starches following exactly the same procedure with the only difference of using hydrochloric or sulfuric acid. Compare the properties of the resulting acid-treated starches especially in terms of viscoamylograph behavior (refer to procedure in Section 6.4.1.1 or 6.4.1.2), solubility, and gel appearance.

3. Investigate alternative methods to produce oxidized/bleached starches and compare them with the sodium hypochlorite process described before. Compare the properties of the modified starches especially in terms of viscoamylograph behavior (refer to procedure in Section 6.4.1.1 or 6.4.1.2), solubility, and gel appearance.

4. Investigate the use of thermoplastic extrusion to produce cross-linked and derivatized starches.

13.2.4 Research Questions

1. Define the following terms widely used in starch:
   a. Native starch
   b. Instant starch
   c. Gelatinization
   d. Birefringence
   e. Retrogradation
   f. Synerisis
   g. Dextrin
   h. Dextrose
   i. Degree of substitution
   j. Starch amorphous zone
   k. Hydroxy-methyl-furfural
   l. Shear-thinning
2. What are the characteristic behaviors of native and instant or pregelatinized starches in terms of viscoamylograph properties?
3. Why are some of the starches chemically modified?
4. Indicate the main characteristic and food use of the following modified starches:
   a. Pregelatinized
   b. Acid-treated
   c. Oxidized/bleached
   d. Cross-bonded
   e. Derivatized
5. Investigate the positive health implications or nutraceutical properties of acetylated, butyryted, and propionylated starches.

13.3 PRODUCTION OF SYRUPS

Cereal-based sweeteners are mainly produced to substitute crystallized sugar or sucrose produced from cane sugar (*Saccharum officinarum*) or sugar beet (*Brassica* sp.) and to provide an array of other products such as thickeners and flavorings demanded by the food industry. These syrups and sweeteners are biotechnologically produced with the use of selective microbial enzymes such as α-amylase, β-amylase, amyloglucosidase, pullulanase, and glucose isomerase. These products are refined with carbon and ion-exchange technologies that improve the sensory and color attributes and concentrated in order to minimize microbial contamination. The major category of sweeteners produced nowadays are the high fructose corn syrups produced from glucose syrups treated with glucose isomerase that substitutes crystallized sugar, especially for the production of soft drinks. Syrups are generally divided into two classes: maltodextrins and sweeteners. Maltodextrins are manufactured from acid or enzyme hydrolyses. These processes yield products with low sweetness due to the low reducing power or dextrose (D-glucose) equivalents. The sweetener class is subdivided into maltose, glucose, and high-fructose (HFCS) syrups. These are produced from maltodextrins with specific enzymes. Key enzymes for the production of maltose and fructose syrups are β-amylase and amyloglucosidase, respectively. HFCS are produced from glucose syrups that are treated with immobilized glucose isomerase. The 90 HFCS is produced after the chromatographic separation of glucose and fructose using a sophisticated technique named moving bed technology. The 90 HFCS imparts 1.4 times more sweetness compared to sucrose at equivalent concentrations.

13.3.1 Low-Dextrose Equivalent (DE) Syrups (Maltodextrins)

The low DE or maltodextrin-rich syrups are industrially produced by acid hydrolysis or by α-amylase conversion. These syrups are the easiest to manufacture and are the first step for the production of maltose, glucose, and HFCS. The acid hydrolysis is performed in 35%–40% starch suspensions using a 0.02- to 0.2-N HCL solution in a pressurized reactor. A higher acid concentration or longer process time can yield undesirable compounds such as methyl-furfural, formic acid, and/or off-flavors and colors. That is the reason why the use of this technology is now limited. The most popular way to convert starch into maltodextrins is by the utilization of α-amylases. Today, heat-stable α-amylases are used because they require shorter incubation and save processing time and energy. Their optimum activity is achieved at a pH of 6.5 and temperatures of 90°C–100°C. Regular corn starch produces haze formation, whereas utilization of waxy starch produces more stable syrups.

The syrups with 10–20 DE are very viscous, rich in maltodextrins, and low in sweetness; therefore, they are mainly used as thickeners. After refining, most maltodextrin rich syrups are commonly dehydrated using spray-drying technology (Johnson 2000; Hoobs 2003). All syrups are refined in order to remove protein, pigments, and other contaminants that affect color, flavor, and overall acceptability. After acid, acid-enzyme, or enzyme–enzyme conversions, the hydrolyzates contain residual protein from the starch. This protein may interfere with enzyme reactions, foul the other refining operations and produce off-colors. In most processes, the protein is removed after the hydrolysis step and consists of passing the hydrolyzate through continuous centrifuges. In order to remove the protein more efficiently, the pH of the slurry is adjusted to 4.7 because at this acidity proteins become insoluble. After centrifugation, syrups are usually vacuum-filtered in rotary filters coated with a 10-cm to 15-cm layer of diatomaceous bleaching earth. The outer layer of the coat rich in insoluble materials is continuously removed by a knife as the drum rotates. Following filtration, hydrolyzates are treated with granular active carbon to remove important contaminants such as amino acids, peptides, and hydroxyl-methyl-furfural. These compounds are known to form undesirable flavors and colors. The typical carbon unit consists of a pulsed bed column through which the syrup is pumped at a temperature of 70°C–80°C. The carbon columns have to be refurnished with fresh regenerated carbon. Spent carbon is regenerated through heating in a series of hearths. This refining step is important in preparation for isomerization and other refining steps of demineralization and absorption. Ion-exchange systems are used to further remove colored compounds and other impurities. Typically, sweeteners are first passed through a demineralization step consisting of anion and cation columns packed with resins. In addition to removing salts, these columns are very effective protein and colored compounds. The resins more commonly used are strong acid cation and weak base anion either in combination or in separated reactors designed for upward or down-flow operations. As in carbon columns, the resins become exhausted so they are commonly used in tandem so the exhausted unit could be regenerated without interrupting the refining process. The ion exchange reactors have a longer life when syrups are refined with active carbon. Refined syrups are taken to a certain solids in multiple-effect and falling-film vacuum evaporators. These evaporators are ideally suited to minimize undesirable color development. Most syrups are concentrated to 65%–72% solids.

13.3.1.1 Production of Low-DE Syrups via Acid Hydrolysis

A. *Samples, Ingredients, and Reagents*
- Native starch
- Distilled water
- Hydrochloric acid (HCl 0.03 N)
- Sodium hydroxide (NaOH)
- pH meter standard solutions
- Granular active carbon
- Ion-exchange resin
- Diatomaceous bleaching earth
- Aluminum foil

B. *Materials and Equipments*
- Digital scale
- Beaker (2 L)
- Stirring rod or magnetic stirrer
- Graduated pipette (5 mL)
- Volumetric flask (1 L)
- Hot plate
- pH meter
- Pressure cooker with stand
- Stove
- Buchner filters (3)
- Kitasato flasks
- Filter cloth
- Rotavapor with vacuum pump
- Refractometer
- Thermometer (0°C–100°C)
- Chronometer
- Protective gloves
- Protective glasses

C. *Procedure*
1. Determine the moisture content of the native starch (refer to procedure in Section 2.2.1.1).
2. Prepare 1 L of a 20% starch slurry with a solution containing 0.03 N HCl (2.44 mL concentrated HCl/L distilled water). Make sure to completely dissolve the starch with the stirring rod. Check the slurry pH before and after acid addition.
3. Add about 5 cm water (underneath the stand) to the pressure cooker and preheat the water to boiling.
4. At the same time, on a hot plate, heat the acid-treated starch slurry to 85°C in order to gelatinize the starch. Make sure to agitate contents with the magnetic stirrer or glass rod. Wearing heat-resistant gloves and protective lenses, cover the beaker with aluminum foil, and transfer it to the pressure cooker.
5. Close the preheated pressure cooker and keep heating. Register the time required to reach 1.05 kg/cm^2 or 15 psi. Allow contents to cook at this pressure for an additional 15 minutes. Discontinue heat and allow pressure to drop to zero.
6. Open the pressure cooker carefully and filter the acid-treated starch slurry through the filter cloth. Adjust the pH with a NaOH solution (0.1 N).
7. Determine the volume of the slurry, the amount of solids, degrees Brix, reducing sugars, color, viscosity at 25°C, protein, and hydroxyl-methyl-furfural (refer to Chapters 2 and 3).
8. Heat the slurry to 70°C in preparation for bleaching. Pass the starch slurry first through a Buchner filter containing a 2-cm ionic resin, then through another filter containing a 2-cm layer of diatomaceous bleaching earth followed by another filtration step through a 2-cm granular active carbon.

9. Place the starch slurry in the rotavapor in order to concentrate solids to 68%. Operate the rotavapor under vacuum at a temperature of about 50°C.

10. Determine the volume of the concentrated acid-treated and bleached syrup, the amount of solids, degrees Brix, reducing sugars, color, *Aw*, viscosity at 25°C, residual protein, and hydroxyl-methyl-furfural (refer to Chapters 2 and 3).

13.3.1.2 Production of Low-DE Syrups via Hydrolysis with Heat-Stable α-Amylase

A. *Samples, Ingredients, and Reagents*
- Native starch
- Distilled water
- Heat-stable α-amylase
- Aluminum foil
- HCl solution 0.1 N
- NaOH solution (0.1 N)
- Calcium hydroxide
- pH meter standard solutions
- Granular active carbon
- Ion-exchange resin
- Diatomaceous bleaching earth

B. *Materials and Equipments*
- Digital scale
- Beaker (2 L)
- Stirring rod or magnetic stirrer
- Graduated pipette (5 mL)
- Volumetric flask (1 L)
- Thermoregulated water bath
- Hot plate
- pH meter
- Buchner filters (3)
- Kitasato flasks (3)
- Filter cloth
- Rotavapor with vacuum pump
- Refractometer
- Thermometer (0°C–100°C)
- Chronometer
- Protective gloves
- Protective glasses

C. *Procedure*
1. Determine the moisture content of the native starch.

2. In a 2-L beaker, prepare 1 L or 1.5 L of a 35% starch slurry with distilled water. Make sure to completely dissolve the starch with the stirring rod. If necessary, adjust slurry pH to 6.5 and add 0.1 g of calcium oxide (just in case the α-amylase is calcium dependent).

3. Add 0.13 mL of the heat-stable α-amylase/100 starch (the recommended enzyme concentration can change according to the supplier) and place beaker on a hot plate. Make sure to agitate contents with the magnetic stirrer or stirring rod and cover the beaker with aluminum foil. Allow contents to heat to 85°C.

4. Transfer the beaker to a water bath adjusted to 85°C for 120-minute incubation. Make sure to turn on the agitation system.

5. Filter the low-DE syrup through a filter cloth.

6. Determine the volume of the syrup, the amount of solids, degrees Brix, reducing sugars, pH, color, viscosity at 25°C, and hydroxyl-methyl-furfural.

7. Heat the slurry to 70°C and adjust its pH to 7 in preparation for bleaching. Pass the starch slurry first through a Buchner filter containing a 2-cm ionic resin, then through another filter containing a 2-cm layer of diatomaceous bleaching earth followed by another filtration step through a 2-cm granular active carbon.

8. Place the starch slurry in the rotavapor in order to concentrate solids to 68% solids. Operate the rotavapor under vacuum at a temperature of 50°C.

9. Determine the volume of the low DE and bleached syrup, the amount of solids, degrees Brix, reducing sugars or dextrose equivalents, pH, color, *Aw*, viscosity at 25°C, residual protein, and hydroxyl-methyl-furfural (refer to Chapters 2 and 3).

13.3.2 MALTOSE SYRUPS

Regular and high-maltose corn syrups are manufactured starting with a low-DE syrup that is further treated with β-amylase or a combination of pullulanase and β-amylase. β-Amylase works best at pH 5 and 55°C. The utilization of only β-amylase yields syrups with 50%–55% maltose whereas the additional use of pullulanase syrups with approximately 70%–80% maltose. Regular and high-maltose syrups are widely used as flavorings for breakfast cereals, beverages, and other food products (Hoobs 2003).

13.3.2.1 Production of Regular and High-Maltose Syrups

A. *Samples, Ingredients, and Reagents*
- Native starch
- Distilled water
- Heat-stable α-amylase
- β-Amylase
- Maltogenase (β-amylase + pullulanase)
- Aluminum foil
- HCl solution 0.1 N
- NaOH solution (0.1 N)
- Calcium hydroxide
- pH meter standard solutions
- Granular active carbon
- Ion-exchange resin
- Diatomaceous bleaching earth

B. *Materials and Equipments*
- Digital scale
- Beaker (2 L)
- Stirring rod or magnetic stirrer

- Graduated pipette (1 mL)
- Volumetric flask (1 L)
- Thermoregulated water bath
- Hot-plate
- pH meter
- Buchner filters (3)
- Kitasato flasks (3)
- Filter cloth
- Rotavapor with vacuum pump
- Refractometer
- Thermometer (0°C–100°C)
- Chronometer
- Protective gloves
- Protective glasses

C. Procedure

1. Determine the moisture content of the native starch.
2. In 2-L beakers, prepare two 1-L or 1.5-L slurries with distilled water containing 35% starch slurry. One is for the production of regular maltose syrup, while the other for the manufacturing of a high-maltose syrup. Label the beakers. Make sure to completely dissolve the starch with the agitator. If necessary, adjust slurry pH to 6.5 and add 0.1 g of calcium hydroxide (just in the case that the α-amylase is calcium dependent) to each beaker.
3. Add 0.13 mL/100 starch of the heat stable α-amylase and place beakers on a hot plate. Make sure to agitate contents and cover beakers with aluminum foil. Allow contents to heat to 85°C.
4. Transfer beakers to a water bath adjusted to 85°C for 120-minute incubation. Stir contents frequently.
5. Allow liquefied slurry to lower the temperature to 45°C, adjust pH to 5.5, and add 0.02 to 0.05 mL/100 g original starch of β-amylase to one beaker and a combination of β-amylase and pullulanase (maltogenase) at the rate of 0.05 to 0.1 mL/100 g starch to the other. Check the recommended amounts of enzymes suggested by the suppliers.
6. Transfer beakers to a water bath adjusted to 50°C for 90-minute incubation.
7. Filter the resulting hydrolyzates through a filter cloth.
8. Determine the volume of the syrup, the amount of solids, degrees Brix, reducing sugars, maltose content, pH, color, Aw, and viscosity at 25°C (refer to Chapters 2 and 3).
9. Heat syrups to 70°C and adjust pH to 7 in preparation for bleaching. Pass syrups first through a Buchner filter containing a 2-cm ionic resin, then through another filter containing a 2-cm layer of diatomaceous bleaching earth followed by another filtration step through a 2-cm granular active carbon.

10. Place syrups in the rotavapor in order to concentrate solids to 68%. Operate the rotavapor under vacuum at a temperature of 50°C.
11. Determine the volume of the maltose and bleached syrups, the amount of solids, degrees Brix, reducing sugars or dextrose equivalents, HPLC sugar composition, pH, color, Aw, and viscosity at 25°C (refer to Chapters 2 and 3).

13.3.3 GLUCOSE SYRUPS

For production of glucose syrups the low-DE syrups (refer to procedure in Section 13.3.1) are treated with amyloglucosidase (formerly named glucoamylase) or saccharifying enzyme at pH 4.6–5.2 and a temperature of 55°C–60°C. The sweetener is refined and clarified through columns of activated carbon and ionic resins with the aim of removing minerals, pigments, soluble protein, fat, and enzyme-resistant starches. Glucose syrups are utilized as sweeteners for soft drinks, baking formulations, and as a source of fermentable carbohydrates for light beer, alcohol production, and bakery products. Crystallized dextrose can be produced by concentrating the syrup to 75% solids, adding glucose and gradual cooling to drop the temperature to 20°C–30°C for several days (Hoobs 2003; Lloyd and Nelson 1984).

13.3.3.1 Production of Glucose Syrups

A. Samples, Ingredients, and Reagents

- Native starch
- Distilled water
- Heat-stable α-amylase
- Amyloglucosidase
- Aluminum foil
- HCl solution 0.1 N
- NaOH solution (0.1 N)
- Calcium hydroxide
- pH meter standard solutions
- Granular active carbon
- Ion-exchange resin
- Diatomaceous bleaching earth

B. Materials and Equipments

- Digital scale
- Beaker (2 L)
- Stirring rod or magnetic stirrer
- Graduated pipette (1 mL)
- Volumetric flask (1 L)
- Thermoregulated water bath
- Hot plate
- pH meter
- Buchner filters (3)
- Erlenmeyer flasks (3)
- Filter cloth
- Rotavapor with vacuum pump
- Thermometer (0°C–100°C)
- Chronometer
- Protective gloves
- Protective glasses

C. Procedure

1. Determine the moisture content of the native starch.
2. In a 2-L beaker prepare 1 L or 1.5 L of a 35% starch slurry with distilled water. Make sure to completely dissolve the starch with the agitator. If necessary, adjust slurry pH to 6.5 and add 0.1 g of calcium hydroxide if the α-amylase is calcium-dependent.
3. Add 0.13 mL/100 starch of the heat stable α-amylase and place beaker on a hot plate. Make sure to agitate contents and cover beaker with aluminum foil. Allow contents to heat to 85°C.
4. Transfer beakers to a water bath adjusted to 85°C for 120-minute incubation.
5. Allow contents to lower the temperature to 60°C, adjust pH to 4.6 with diluted HCl acid and add 0.6 mL/100 g starch of the amyloglucosidase enzyme solution.
6. Transfer beaker to a water bath adjusted to 60°C for 4- to 8-hour incubation.
7. Filter the resulting hydrolyzate through a filter cloth.
8. Determine the volume of the syrup, the amount of solids, degrees Brix, glucose, pH, color, Aw, and viscosity at 25°C.
9. Heat syrups to 70°C and adjust pH to 7 with 0.1 N NaOH in preparation for bleaching. Pass syrups first through a Buchner filter containing a 2-cm ionic resin, then through another filter containing a 2-cm layer of diatomaceous bleaching earth followed by another filtration step through a 2-cm granular active carbon.
10. Place syrups in the rotavapor in order to concentrate solids to 68%. Operate the rotavapor under vacuum at a temperature of about 50°C.
11. Determine the volume of the bleached glucose syrup, the amount of solids, degrees Brix, reducing sugars or dextrose equivalents, glucose, residual protein, pH, color, Aw, and viscosity at 25°C (refer to Chapters 2 and 3).

13.3.4 High-Fructose Corn Syrups

HFCS are manufactured starting from a glucose (90 DE) hydrolyzate described in procedure in Section 13.3.3.1 that is additionally treated with glucose isomerase (Carasik and Carroll 1983). The conversion of glucose into fructose in most instances occurs in a column or reactor packaged with the immobilized enzyme. The refined glucose syrup is deaerated and treated with magnesium sulfate so to assure oxygen removal and the sequestration of calcium that lowers enzyme activity and half-life. There are three major types of HFCS syrups: 42, 55, and 90. Both the 55 and 90 HFCS are produced from the 42 HFCS. The optimum operating conditions are pH 7.5 to 8.2 and 55°C–60°C. The substrate flow rate is controlled to convert 42%–45% of the glucose into fructose. The 90 HFCS is obtained after separating fructose and glucose in a moving bed chromatography system that produces two syrups with approximately 90% of each sugar. If desired, the glucose rich syrup can be converted into 42 and 90 HFCS as explained before. The 55 HFCS is manufactured by mixing 73 parts of 42 and 27 parts of 90 HFCS. The 90 HFCS imparts approximately 1.2 to 1.6 times more sweetness than the others HFCS and crystallized sugar. HFCS are used as substitutes of table sugar especially in soft drinks and confectionary industries. The main advantage of using HFCS is that they readily dissolve in water, are easily flavored, and impart a fruit sweet flavor to beverages and foods (Bernetti 1990; Hoobs 2003; Lloyd and Nelson 1984).

13.3.4.1 Production of Fructose Syrups (HFCS)

A. Samples, Ingredients, and Reagents
- Native starch
- Distilled water
- Heat-stable α-amylase
- Glucose isomerase (Sweetzyme)
- Sodium sulfite (Na_2SO_3)
- Sodium acetate buffer
- Magnesium sulfate ($MgSO_4 \cdot 7H_2O$)
- Sodium carbonate (Na_2CO_3)
- HCl solution 0.1 N
- NaOH solution (0.1 N)
- Sulfuric acid (H_2SO_4)
- Cotton balls
- Calcium hydroxide
- pH meter standard solutions
- Granular active carbon
- Ion-exchange resin
- Diatomaceous bleaching earth
- Aluminum foil

B. Materials and Equipments
- Digital scale
- Beaker (2 L)
- Stirring rod or magnetic stirrer
- Graduated pipette (1 mL, 5 mL, and 10 mL)
- Volumetric flask (1 L)
- Thermoregulated water bath
- Hot plate
- pH meter
- Buchner filters (3)
- Erlenmeyer flasks (3)
- Filter cloth
- Rotavapor with vacuum pump
- Glass columns (13 cm × 1.5 cm)
- Peristaltic pump
- Sonicator
- Refractometer
- Thermometer (0°C–100°C)
- Chronometer
- Protective gloves
- Protective glasses

C. *Procedure*

1. Produce a glucose syrup following the steps 1–9 of the glucose syrup procedure in Section 13.3.3.1.

2. Inactivate the amyloglucosidase enzyme by heat treatment at 80°C for 20 minutes. Then adjust the pH of the glucose syrup to 7.5 with Na_2SO_3 at 25°C.

3. Determine the degrees Brix and calcium content of the glucose syrup by titration with ethylendiamino-tetraacetate (change color from red-orange to purple). The calcium inhibits the isomerization reaction. Concentrate the glucose syrup to a 40–45°Brix in a rotavapor operating under vacuum at 45°C–50°C.

4. Adjust the pH of the glucose syrup to 7.5 with Na_2SO_3 at 25°C.

5. Preparation of the immobilized glucose isomerase column.
   a. Prepare the glucose substrate by blending 530 g anhydrous glucose, 1 g $MgSO_4$ $7H_2O$, 0.21 g Na_2CO_3, 0.18 g $Na_2S_2O_5$, and 700 mL distilled H_2O. Heat the resulting solution to 70°C, adjust pH to 7.5 with 0.5 M H_2SO_4, and add more water to produce 1 L. Eliminate the air by vacuum and measure the degrees Brix.
   b. Mix 6 g of glucose isomerase (Sweetzyme®) and 30 mL glucose substrate.
   c. Stir contents gently every 5 minutes for the first 15 minutes and occasionally during the next 30 minutes.
   d. Fill the column with the immobilized enzyme avoiding trapping air.
   e. Prepare two cotton balls of approximately 0.5 g and immerse them in a 0.1% $MgSO_4$ solution. Place the cotton balls 1 cm apart from the column head. These cotton balls will trap air and calcium.

6. With the peristaltic pump feed the refined glucose syrup to the column at a flow rate of approximately 0.7 mL/min. Determine the Brix, sugar composition, viscosity at 25°C, color, and pH of the syrups before and after reaction with glucose isomerase.

7. Filter the HFCS through a filter cloth.

8. Heat HFCS to 70°C and adjust pH to 7 with 0.1 N NaOH in preparation for bleaching. Pass syrups first through a Buchner filter containing a 2-cm ionic resin, then through another filter containing a 2-cm layer of diatomaceous bleaching earth followed by another filtration step through a 2-cm granular active carbon.

9. Place HFCS in the rotavapor in order to concentrate solids to 68%. Operate the rotavapor under vacuum at a temperature of 50°C.

10. Determine the volume of the bleached HFCS syrup, the amount of solids, fructose, glucose, residual protein, pH, color, Aw, and viscosity at 25°C (refer to Chapters 2 and 3).

13.3.5 Research Suggestions

1. Produce a 20 DE syrup and then investigate the enzyme and processing conditions needed to convert it into cyclodextrins (alpha, beta, and gamma). At equivalent solids, compare the properties (i.e., viscosity, color, etc.) of the two types of syrups (refer to Chapter 3).

2. Produce a 20 DE, glucose, and fructose syrups concentrated to 68% solids using as raw materials starches from maize, sorghum, and wheat. Determine the properties of the resulting syrups in terms of viscosity, sugar composition, Aw, pH, and color (refer to Chapters 2 and 3).

3. Produce a 20 DE, glucose, and fructose syrups concentrated to 68% solids using regular, and waxy maize starches. Determine the properties of the resulting syrups in terms of viscosity, sugar composition, Aw, pH, and color (refer to Chapters 2 and 3).

4. Produce glucose and fructose syrups concentrated to 68% solids using regular starch and a starch rich in resistant starch. Determine the properties of the resulting syrups in terms of viscosity, sugar composition, Aw, pH, and color (refer to Chapters 2 and 3).

5. Produce a glucose syrup from previously liquefied starch (35% solids treated with heat resistant α-amylase). Install an ultrafiltration unit to separate glucose from dextrins and develop a continuous process to convert the 20 DE syrup into a 90 DE glucose syrup. Compare the resulting sweeteners concentrated to 68°Brix of the traditional batch and UF processes in terms of viscosity, glucose concentration (glucose oxidase or HPLC determination), color, and Aw (refer to Chapters 2 and 3).

13.3.6 Research Questions

1. Define the following terms:
   a. Dextrose equivalents
   b. Degree of polymerization
   c. Cyclodextrins
   d. Maltodextrins

2. What are the two major industrial processes to produce 20 DE (low) syrups? Investigate the way to produce dehydrated maltodextrins.

3. Describe the industrial process to convert a 20 DE syrup into a glucose sweetener with more than 90 DE.

4. When producing maltose syrups, why the addition of pullulanase or debranching enzyme significantly increases maltose content? What are the major food uses of regular and high-maltose syrups?

5. Why the production of HFCS has clearly increased during the past decades? What are differences in terms of properties and industrial production among HFCS 42, 54, and 90?

6. What is an immobilized enzyme? What kinds of materials are used to immobilize glucose isomerase? What kind of elements can inactivate commercially used glucose isomerase systems? What are the processing steps used to prevent inactivation and enhance the half-life of the enzyme?

7. How many liters of 90-HFCS and 42-HFCS are needed in order to obtain a 55-HFCS? Why the food industry demands high quantities of 55-HFCS?

8. Compare enzyme hydrolyses for production of glucose syrups and sweet worts for grain bioethanol production.

9. For the following enzymes investigate the main source (microbial, GMO, extracted from grains, etc.), preferred substrate, mode of action, optimum pH and temperature conditions, and products formed.
   a. α-Amylase
   b. β-Amylase
   c. Pullulanase
   d. Amyloglucosidase
   e. Glucose Isomerase
   f. CGT'ase

10. How are liquid syrups and sweeteners generally refined? What kind of bleaching materials are generally used?

11. What are the main quality control measurements applied to sweeteners?

REFERENCES

Annison, G., R. J. Illman, and D. L. Topping. 2003. "Acetylated, Propionylated or Butyrylated Starches Raise Large Bowel Short-Chain Fatty Acids Preferentially When Fed to Rats." *J. Nutr.* 133:3523–3528.

Bemiller, J. N., and R. L. Whistler. 2009. *Starch: Chemistry and Technology.* 3rd ed. Orlando, FL: Academic Press.

Bernetti, R. 1990. "From Corn Syrup to Fructose." *Cereal Foods World.* 35(4):390–393.

Carasik, W., and J. O. Carroll. 1983. "Development of Immobilized Enzymes for Production of High-Fructose Corn Syrup." *Food Technology* 37(10):85–91.

Hoobs, L. 2003. "Corn Sweeteners." In *Corn Chemistry and Technology*, edited by P. J. White and L. A. Johnson, Chapter 17. St. Paul, MN: American Association of Cereal Chemists.

Johnson, L. A. 2000. "Corn: The Major Cereal of the Americas." In *Handbook of Cereal Science and Technology*, edited by K. Kulp and J. Ponte, Chapter 2. 2nd ed. New York: Marcel Dekker.

Lloyd, N. E., and W. J. Nelson. 1984. "Glucose and Fructose Containing Sweeteners from Starch." In *Starch: Chemistry and Technology*, edited by R. L. Whistler, J. N. Bemiller, and E. F. Paschall, Chapter 21. 2nd ed. Orlando, FL: Academic Press.

Mauro, D. J., I. R. Abbas, and F. T. Orthoefer. 2003. "Corn Starch Modification and Uses." In *Corn Chemistry and Technology*, edited by P. J. White and L. A. Johnson, Chapter 16. St. Paul, MN: American Association of Cereal Chemists.

Rohwer, R. G., and R. E. Klem. 1984. "Acid Modified Starch: Production and Uses." In *Starch: Chemistry and Technology*, edited by R. L. Whistler, J. N. Bemiller, and E. F. Paschall, Chapter 17. 2nd ed. Orlando, FL: Academic Press.

Rutenberg, M. W., and D. Solarek. 1984. "Starch Derivatives: Production and Uses." In *Starch: Chemistry and Technology*, edited by R. L. Whistler, J. N. Bemiller, and E. F. Paschall, Chapter 10. 2nd ed. Orlando, FL: Academic Press.

Sharp, R. N., and C. Q. Sharp. 1994. "Food Applications for Modified Rice Starches." In *Rice Science and Technology*, edited by W. J. Marshall and J.I. Wadsworth, Chapter 17. New York: Marcel Dekker.

Thomas, D. J., and W. A. Atwell. 1999. *Starches.* St. Paul, MN: Eagan Press.

14 Production of Malt, Beer, Distilled Spirits, and Fuel Ethanol

14.1 INTRODUCTION

Cereal grains, especially barley, are extensively used to produce beers, distilled alcoholic beverages, and fuel ethanol. Beer is the main alcoholic beverage consumed in the world and has been enjoyed for more than 8,000 years. The use of cereals as raw materials by the brewing industry can be divided into two main categories: malt and adjuncts. Malt is usually produced from barley because this husked kernel produces high diastatic activity and aids during the critical step of mash filtration. The most common brewing adjuncts are grits from maize and rice and starch from the wet-milling process of maize (refer to Chapters 5 and 6). Adjuncts provide the necessary carbohydrates that upon mashing are hydrolyzed into dextrins and fermentable carbohydrates.

Malting is defined as the controlled germination of the grain followed by kilning or drying. The aim is to generate the maximum amounts of starch degrading enzymes. The malt is mainly used for brewing beers and production of distilled spirits such as whiskeys. The malt hydrolyzes the starch into fermentable sugars that are further metabolized by the fermenting yeast into ethanol and other organic compounds.

Among cereals, barley possesses the highest diastatic activity when it is properly germinated. The final diastatic activity is the result of the grain quality and malting conditions. The grain activates during soaking due to the synthesis of gibberellic acid in the germ. This hormone controls germination and the different enzymes produced mainly in the germ and multilayered aleurone. The enzymes break down lipids, proteins, and carbohydrates, yielding the necessary energy for germination. The enzymes are sequentially produced first in the germ and afterward in the aleurone. Generally, the first enzymes produced are lipolytic (lipases and lipoxigenases), followed by fibrolitic (celullases, β-glucanases, xylanases, hemicellulases), proteases, and amylases. Both α- and β-amylases are produced by the aleurone cells and start degrading from the outer to the inner endosperm (MacGregor and Batthy 1993).

The preferred barley for brewing is the two-rowed bred to produce upon germination high diastatic activity. The supreme malting barley is relatively low in protein and yields sound and uniform kernels that upon germination at temperatures higher than 5°C develop high amounts of both α- and β-amylases. Furthermore, the malt should not produce off-flavors due to polyphenols present in glumes and bran.

A high-quality malting barley should have good and uniform germination (higher than 90%) and keep the grain structure after malting. Maltsters select barley based on moisture, amount of foreign material, test weight, protein content, and germ viability (refer to Chapters 1 and 2).

The most critical step in beer and distilled spirits production is fermentation because during this step the fermentable sugars and other components of the wort are transformed into ethanol and other alcohols and metabolites that impart the characteristic organoleptic properties to finished products. Most processes use common yeast (*Saccharomyces cerevisiae*) for fermentation.

One of the fastest growing industries is the one that transforms the starch associated to cereals into fuel ethanol. Anhydrous ethanol has been used as a fuel since the early 1900s. During the past 10 years, the interest and use of fuel ethanol has dramatically increased because ethanol is a renewable fuel, it has positive proven environmental benefits compared to the combustion of fossil fuels, and there is an escalation of petroleum prices. Brazil and the United States are the two main producers of fuel ethanol. Brazil produces most of the ethanol from sugar cane (*Saccahrum officinarum*) stalks whereas the United States, from maize. Today, about half of the world's ethanol is produced from sugar cane and the other half from cereals. Among cereals, maize is the preferred feedstock because of its high availability, relatively low cost, and high starch content (Coble et al. 1981). The basic principles of fuel ethanol production are based on production of distilled spirits with two major modifications, use of microbial enzymes instead of malt and a third step in the distillation to obtain pure ethanol.

Among cereal-based foods or beverages, beer has many quality control measurements due to its processing complexity and the ample array of raw materials used for its manufacture. Furthermore, beer is unique for the reason that has important biochemical changes during storage and expected shelf life.

Several laboratory assays are crucial to follow the progress of fermentation and determine the final beer properties. The most common and useful measurement is the specific gravity made with a hydrometer (ASBC 2009, method wort 4) or more accurately by the measurement of mass and volume (ASBC 2009, method wort 2). As fermentable carbohydrates are consumed and alcohol produced, the specific gravity falls. One indication of the end of carbohydrate fermentation is that the specific gravity stops declining. The real degree of fermentation (ASBC 2009, method beer 6B) measures the percent of the extract that was fermented (Munroe 2006). The quantification of yeast cells during fermentations is relevant because counts strongly reproduce during the aerobic stage of fermentation. Dead cells can be quantitated by staining with methylene blue and counting with a hemacytometer (ASBC 2009, method yeast 3A). Other important parameters are color (refer to Chapter 3), bitterness, haze, pH, dissolved oxygen, and carbon dioxide.

After bottling, the quality of beer starts to decrease depending on storage temperature, exposure to light, and other environmental factors. Beer stability involves a wide range of chemical processes that can be subdivided into physical, flavor, foam, gushing, and light. The physical stability is mainly dictated by the colloidal stability that can produce haziness and opaqueness. Although there are a number of types of haze, primarily it is the polymerization of polyphenols and their binding with soluble proteins. Haze formation is increased by a number of factors of which storage temperature has the greatest influence as an increase in temperature increases the rate of haze formation. The thermal process of pasteurization and oxidation accelerate haze formation. Haze determination is based on the principle of nephelometry in which light reflected from particles in solution is measured. It is also possible to rate beer haze visually by comparing the sample with standards prepared with different concentrations of formazin. The flavor stability of beer depends primarily on the oxygen content of beer. It is critically important to control the oxygen level in the bottled beer because it enhances the development of off-flavors such as unsaturated aldehydes, *trans*-2-nonenal, nonadenial, decadienal, and others. Foam stability is also of paramount importance in the acceptability of beer. There are many foam-promoting compounds such as protein, *iso*-α-acids from hops and polysaccharides, with proteins being the most relevant (Steward 2006). Foam stability is measured in terms of head retention and lacing properties. Excess foaming, commonly known as gushing, is also viewed as a defect. The main reasons for gushing are increased levels of carbonation and the presence of hydrophobin proteins from contaminating fungi. Beer is sensitive to light especially in the wavelength range of 350–500 nm. The beer is said to be sunstruck and skunky due to formation of MBT (3-methyl-2-butene-1-thiol. The formation of this compound is minimized by using brown glass bottles or by selecting hops that fail to produce significant quantities of MBT (Steward 2006). The sensory evaluation of beer is the result of a complex mix of qualities and defects in terms of color, aroma, clarity, foam, carbonation, and mouthfeel or body. As a result, most breweries have developed procedures that enable sensory analysis based on difference, descriptive, preference, and drinkability tests usually performed with highly trained panelists.

The same quality control parameters described for beer ingredients, enzymes, and the various processing steps are applied for alcoholic spirits and fuel ethanol. Since most distilled beverages are aged, the quantification of flavorful compounds via gas chromatography is even more relevant (refer to Chapter 2). The fusel alcohols and volatiles are the most important products to evaluate because they could be partially or totally removed during distillation and they greatly affect the *bouquet* and acceptability of final products.

14.2 PRODUCTION OF EUROPEAN BEERS AND SAKE

14.2.1 PRODUCTION OF BARLEY MALTS

Among cereal grains, barley possesses the highest diastatic activity when it is properly germinated. The final diastatic activity is the result of the grain quality and malting conditions. The grain activates during soaking due to the synthesis of gibberellic acid in the germ. This hormone controls germination and the different enzymes produced mainly in the germ and aleurone layer. The enzymes break down lipids, proteins, and carbohydrates, yielding the necessary energy for germination. The enzymes are sequentially produced first in the germ and afterward in the multilayered aleurone. Generally, the first enzymes produced are lipolytic (lipases and lipoxigenases), followed by cell wall degrading (celullases, β-glucanases, xylanases, hemicellulases), proteases, and amylases. Both α- and β-amylases are produced by the aleurone cells and start degrading from the outer to the inner endosperm (MacGregor and Batthy 1993; Palmer 1989; Briggs 1998; Hardwick 1995; Hough et al. 1993).

Barely is generally classified as malting or feed and winter or summer. The classes are subdivided into two: two- or six-rowed (refer to Chapter 1). For brewing, the two-rowed malting and summer barley is preferred. Two-rowed barleys yield larger kernels, thinner glumes or husks, and more starch in the endosperm. The ideal malting barley is relatively low in protein and yields sound and uniform kernels that upon germination at temperatures higher than 5°C develop high amounts of both α- and β-amylases. In addition, the resulting malt should not have off-flavors produced by polyphenols associated to the husks and bran. The chemical composition of barley and malt is greatly affected by the physiological and biochemical events that occur during germination.

A high-quality malting barley should have good and uniform germination (higher than 90%) and keep the grain structure after malting. Maltsters select barley based on moisture, amount of foreign material, test weight, protein content, and germ viability. The last test is performed in cut kernels with exposed germ that are treated with tetrazolium (refer to procedure in Section 1.2.9.2). Viable embryos have dehydrogenases that reduce the tetrazolium coloring the germ. The most relevant tests for malting barley are germination capacity, diastatic activity, and dry matter losses incurred during malting.

14.2.1.1 Production of Diastatic Malts
A. *Samples, Materials, and Reagents*
- Different types of barleys
- Formaldehyde
- Sodium hypochlorite

B. *Materials and Equipments*
- Digital scale
- Winchester bushel meter
- Dockage tester with sieves to clean barley
- Air pump (aquarium)
- Germinator

- Stainless steel sheets
- Colander
- Beaker (2 L and 5 L)
- Roller or hammer mills
- Air-convection drier
- Aluminum dishes
- Desiccator
- Plastic bottle with sprayer
- Spatula
- Petri dishes

C. Procedure

1. Clean the lot of barley using the dockage test meter and record the percentage of foreign material.
2. Determine the test weight and 1,000 kernel weight of the clean barley grain (refer to procedures in Sections 1.2.1.1 and 1.2.7.1).
3. Sample the barley and determine its moisture content (refer to procedure in Section 2.2.1.1). Keep sample for other determinations (chemical composition, diastatic activity, color, etc.).

4. Weigh exactly three lots of 500 g of the cleaned barley in preparation for steeping. Place kernels in 2-L beakers and then add 1 L distilled water previously tempered to 15°C. Label the three samples as A, B, and sampling beaker. Place the three beakers in a germinator set at 15°C. Turn on the aquarium pump, making sure that the tubing is immersed in the water to aerate samples during steeping.
5. Allow samples to steep under aeration for at least 24 hours and preferably for 48 hours. The optimum moisture level in the soaked kernels is >42%. Make sure to sample the soaked barley placed in the sampling beaker for moisture analysis. The recommended sampling frequency is 0.5, 1, 2, 4, 8, 16, 24, 32, 40, and 48 hours (Figure 14.1).
6. Discard the steep water by placing kernels in a colander. Then, place kernels for 10 minutes in a 2% sodium hypochlorite wash solution. Discard

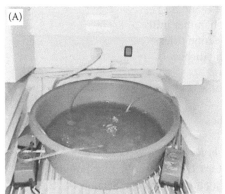
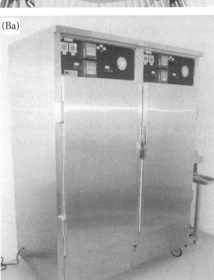
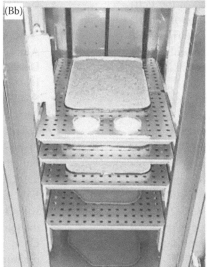
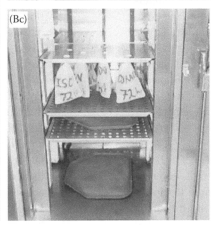
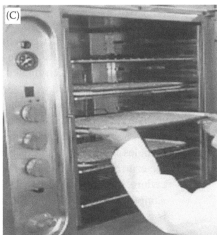
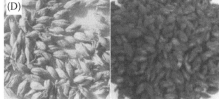

FIGURE 14.1 Sequential steps for the production of barley malt. (A) Soaking of barley kernels with aeration; (B) germination cabinet with temperature and relative humidity controls (Ba) germination of soaked barley on trays (Bb) and germination of different types of barley kernels in nylon bags (Bc); (C) kilning or drying of germinated barley; and (D) regular and chocolate barley malts.

the wash solution using the colander. Repeat the procedure for each beaker.

7. Place three lots of 100 soaked and disinfected kernels from the sampling beaker in three Petri dishes containing moistened filter paper for percent germination analyses.

8. Place steeped kernels on a baking sheet for malting in a germinator set at 15°C and 85% to 90% relative humidity. Make sure to manually stir the sample every 4 to 6 hours. To avoid dehydration, samples can be covered with a moistened paper towel or spray small amounts of water. Make sure to avoid addition of excess water.

9. Sample the malting barley placed in the sampling baking sheet for chemical, dry matter loss, and diastatic analyses. The recommended sampling frequency is 6, 12, 24, 36, 48, 60, 72, 84, 96, 108, and 120 hours. After each sampling time, record the average size of the acrospire that gradually develops in between the pericarp and the husks or glumes. In addition, record the percent germination from each of the Petri dishes by determining the percentage of kernels with evidence of rootlet growth. Determine the percent germination using the following equation = (number of germinated kernels/number of total kernels) × 100.

10. After germination, collect samples for kilning. Dehydrate samples in a convection oven set at 60°C. Construct a dehydration curve by taking samples from the sampling barley malt sheet. Determine residual moisture using the procedure in Section 2.2.1.1. The recommended sampling frequency from the convection oven is 5, 10, 20, 40, 60, 90, 120, 150, 180, 240, and 360 minutes. The optimum kilning is required to lower the moisture content to approximately 5%–8%.

11. Allow samples to cool down at ambient temperature for at least 30 minutes and record the exact weight. Then, determine residual moisture, test weight, and 1,000 kernel weight.

12. Calculate the percent dry matter loss in the two unsampled lots of malt using the following equation: dry matter loss = [[(barley weight) × (100 − % barley moisture) − (malt weight) (100 − malt moisture)]/(barley weight) (100 − % barley moisture)] × 100.

13. Grind the resulting malts using a roller mill and determine particle size distribution (refer to procedure in Section 5.3.1.1) using a Rotap fitted with U.S. nos. 20, 35, 60, 80, and 100, and a collection pan. In addition, determine diastatic activity (refer to procedure in Section 14.2.1.3). Reserve the rest of the sample for nondiastatic malt, beer, or distilled spirit production.

14.2.1.2 Production of Nondiastatic and Dark Malts

Nondiastatic and dark malts are heat-treated or roasted at high temperatures to produce Maillard and caramelization reactions that greatly affect aroma, flavor, and color. During the heat treatment, caramelized sugar, dry, burnt, acid, and astringent flavors are produced, and malts lose all or most of their diastatic activity. These malts are used for the production of dark ale and lager beers, dark syrups, and flavorings for breakfast cereals and other foods.

A. *Samples, Materials, and Reagents*
- Different types of barleys
- Formaldehyde
- Sodium hypochlorite

B. *Materials and Equipments*
- Digital scale
- Winchester bushel meter
- Dockage tester with sieves to clean barley
- Air pump (aquarium)
- Germinator
- Stainless steel sheets
- Colander
- Beaker (2 L and 5 L)
- Roller or hammer mills
- Air-convection drier
- Aluminum dishes
- Desiccator
- Plastic bottle with sprayer
- Spatula
- Petri dishes

C. *Procedure*
Munich type of malt

1. Follow steps 1 to 8 described for production of diastatic malt (procedure in Section 14.2.1.1).

2. Kiln the malt first at low temperature (38°C) and when the moisture drops to 15%–25% increase the temperature to 75°C and then to 105°C.

3. Upon cooling or equilibration at room temperature, grind the Munich type of malt using a roller mill and determine particle size distribution (refer to procedure in Section 5.3.1.1) and diastatic activity (refer to procedure in Section 14.2.1.3). Reserve the sample for production of dark, aromatic, and full-bodied lager beer.

Chocolate or black nondiastatic malt

1. Follow steps 1 to 10 described for production of diastatic malt.

2. Kiln the lightly kilned malt at approximately 75°C for 30 minutes and then increase the temperature to 160°C–175°C for 15 minutes and then to 215°C for 10 minutes. The malt will acquire a dark blackish coloration (Figure 14.1).

3. Upon cooling or equilibration at room temperature grind the chocolate or black malt using a roller mill and determine particle size distribution (refer to procedure in Section 5.3.1.1) and diastatic activity (refer to procedure in Section 14.2.1.3).

Reserve the sample for production of nondiastatic malt typically used in grist formulations of Stouts to impart dark colors and special flavors.

14.2.1.3 Determination of Diastatic Activity of Malt (AACC 2000, Method 22-16)

A. *Samples, Ingredients, and Reagents*
- Different types of diastatic malts
- Distilled water
- Soluble starch
- Acetic acid
- Sodium acetate ($CH_3COONa \cdot 3H_2O$)
- Sodium hydroxide
- Potassium ferricyanide ($K_3[Fe(CN)_6]$)
- Sodium carbonate (Na_2CO_3)
- Sodium thiosulfate ($Na_2S_2O_3$)
- Potassium chloride (KCl)
- Sodium borate ($Na_2B_4O_7 \cdot 10H_2O$)
- Zinc sulfate ($ZnSO_4 \cdot 7H_2O$)
- Potassium iodide

B. *Materials and Equipments*
- Digital scale
- Graduated cylinders (25 mL, 100 mL, and 500 mL)
- Hot stirring plate
- Magnetic stirrer
- Shaking water bath
- Volumetric flasks (100 mL and 1 L)
- Pipettes (1 mL, 5 mL, and 10 mL)
- Dark bottle
- Refrigerator
- Funnel
- Whatman No. 1 filter paper
- Erlenmeyer flasks (100 mL, and 150 mL, and 1 L)
- Burette
- Chronometer
- Thermometer

C. **Procedure**
1. Prepare the following reagents:
   a. Starch buffer solution. Weigh exactly 2 g of soluble starch (dry weight) and blend it with a small amount of water (no more than 5% of total volume). Stir to form a smooth paste. Then, while stirring add the starch paste to 70 mL distilled water. Keep heating the water for two more minutes and then add approximately 10 mL of regular distilled water. Transfer contents to a 100-mL volumetric flask and then wash the empty starch container with 5 mL water. Add the wash water to the volumetric flask. Stir contents of the volumetric flask and allow it to cool down to 30°C. Then, with distilled water bring to the 100 mL mark. Then, add 2 mL of the sodium acetate buffer solution and stir contents.
   b. Buffer acetate solution. In a 1-L volumetric flask, dissolve 68 g trihydrated sodium acetate ($CH_3COONa \cdot 3H_2O$) in 500 mL acetic

acid. Then bring to the 1-L mark with distilled water. Stir contents before use.
   c. Sodium hydroxide (0.5 N). In a 1-L volumetric flask dissolve 20 g of sodium hydroxide with distilled water. Then bring to volume with more distilled water.
   d. Alkaline ferricyanide solution. In a 1-L volumetric flask, dissolve 16.5 g of potassium ferricyanide and 22 g anhydrous sodium carbonate in water. Then bring to exact volume with more distilled water. Stir contents and then store in a dark bottle.
   e. Sodium thiosulfate (0.05 N) titrating solution. In a 1-L volumetric flask, dissolve 12.41 g of sodium thiosulfate and 3.8 g sodium borate (borax) in distilled water. Then bring to exact volume with more distilled water.
   f. Acetic acid salt solution. In a 1-L volumetric flask, dissolve 70 g of potassium chloride (KCl) and 20 g zinc sulfate ($ZnSO_4 \cdot 7H_2O$) in 750 mL distilled water. Then gradually add 200 mL glacial acetic acid. Then bring to volume with more distilled water.
   g. Concentrated sodium hydroxide solution. Dissolve 50 g sodium hydroxide in 50 mL distilled water. Allow hot solution to cool down before use.
   h. Potassium iodide solution. In a 100-mL volumetric flask, dissolve 50 g potassium iodide with distilled water. Add one or two droplets of concentrated sodium hydroxide.
2. Prepare the malt extract as follows:
   a. Weigh 25 g of ground malt and place it in a 1-L Erlenmeyer. Determine the moisture content of the malt sample.
   b. Add 500 mL of a 0.5% salt solution. Stir contents, place solution in an incubator and allow the mix to rest for 2.5 hours at 30°C. Stir contents every 20 minutes.
   c. Filtrate the solution through Whatman No. 1 filter paper folded in a 15-cm diameter funnel.
   d. Collect and then return the first 50 mL of the filtrate for one second filtration.
   e. Collect the filtrate after 30 minutes.
   f. Minimize water evaporation during the filtration process by placing a watch glass on top of the funnel.
   g. Place filtrate in a closed container and immediately place it in a refrigerator (5°C).
3. Place 200 mL of the starch buffer solution (1a) in a 250 mL Erlenmeyer. Then, add 8 mL distilled water and 2 mL of the malt extract of step 2.
4. Shake contents and place volumetric flask on a shaking water bath set at 30°C for exactly 30 minutes.

5. After hydrolysis, immediately add 20 mL 0.5 N NaOH and shake or stir to stop enzyme activity.

6. Pipette 5 mL of the hydrolyzate into a test tube.

7. Add 10 mL of the alkaline potassium ferricyanide (1 d), shake contents and the place tube in a boiling water bath for 20 minutes. Make sure that the boiling water level is slightly above the sample contained in the test tube.

8. Remove test tube from the boiling water bath and then immediately cool down with running tap water. Transfer the contents to a 125-mL Erlenmeyer flask.

9. Add 25 mL of the acetic acid salt solution (1f) and 1 mL of the potassium iodide solution (1 hour). Shake contents. The solution will turn blue.

10. Titrate with 0.05 N sodium thiosulfate (1e) until the blue color first disappears.

11. Register the mL of sodium thiosulfate used.

12. Prepare a blank following step 3 with the immediate addition of 20 mL of 0.5 N NaOH before adding the malt extract and steps 4, 6, 7, 8, 9, and 10.

13. Register the mL of sodium thiosulfate used for the blank.

14. Calculate the diastatic activity using the following equation:

Diastatic power (malt diastatic unit/g malt) = 40 (mL blank − mL of sample) × F/V × [100/(100 − malt moisture content)

where F is the factor according to sodium thiosulfate normality = 1.0 and V is the mL of malt extract used for hydrolysis.

15. Convert the diastatic power result to degrees Litner (°L) by multiplying the above value for 18 if 2 mL of the malt extract was used or 36 if 1 mL was used.

16. Convert diastatic power to maltose equivalents by multiplying °L times 4, or multiply the ferricyanide equivalents (mL blank − mL of sample) for 72 or 144 when used 2 or 1 mL of the malt extract, respectively.

14.2.2 PRODUCTION OF HOPPED BEERS

Beer is produced after four sequential major operations: malting, mashing, hop addition, and fermentation. The malting process starts by cleaning the selected kernels to remove dockage, shriveled, and broken kernels, and other contaminating grains. The cleaned barley kernels are steeped in cold water (15°C) for an average of 24 hours to start activating the grain. The key step is germination of the hydrated kernels until achieving the maximum diastatic activity that usually takes from 3 to 5 days followed by kilning to stop activity and develop important flavorful and colorful compounds. The aim of the process is to achieve the maximum percentage of germination

and diastatic activity and conclude the process with the lowest possible dry matter loss (MacGregor and Batty 1993; Palmer 1989; Briggs 1998; Hardwick 1995; Hough et al. 1993). The resulting malt is coarsely ground immediately before mashing because the husks protect it against insects and its enzymes are more stable when not exposed to the air. It is important that the glumes remain as intact as possible because they will act more efficiently as a filtrating bed. Generally, the malt is ground in roller mills into endosperm particles with different granulations. The ground malt contains large and small grits (0.6–0.15 mm), semolina, and flour with particle size of approximately 0.15 mm. Generally, the ratio among large, intermediate, and fine particles is 27:35:38. Mashing has the main objective of hydrolyzing the starch and protein associated to the brewing adjuncts into fermentable carbohydrates, dextrins, and soluble nitrogen. The fermentable carbohydrates and soluble nitrogen are important yeast substrates whereas dextrins impart the typical body or texture associated to regular beers. Mashing consists of mixing the malt, water, and brewing adjuncts that are gradually heated to enhance starch and protein conversion. The temperature program usually starts at 35°C and after 30 minutes holds increases to 50°C, 65°C, and 75°C. Next, the mash is transferred to the lauter tun to separate the sweet wort from spent grains.

Most lager beers are produced by the double-mashing procedure because the brewers grist formulations usually contain a high amount of starchy adjuncts. These starchy materials require cooking to achieve complete starch gelatinization. The mashing consists of two distinctive stages. In the first, commonly known as adjunct mash, the brewing adjuncts are mixed with water and heated to 35°C. After a 30- to 60-minute stand, the contents are heated first to 70°C for about 30 minutes and followed by 100°C for 30–45 minutes. The aim is to first hydrate the adjuncts and malt and then promote starch gelatinization and conversion since most cereal starches gelatinize at temperatures higher than 65°C. Boiling is required to denature proteins and inactivate all microbes and enzymes. Once the adjunct mashing program is underway, the second mash is prepared by mixing and heating to 35°C, most of the malt and water. Then, the contents of the two vessels are mixed. The aim of the second mashing step is to convert starch and proteins into simpler carbohydrates and soluble proteins. This is optimally achieved by programming a gradual temperature increase that starts at 35°C for approximately 30 minutes. The temperature is usually ramped to 10°C–15°C until achieving 70°C. The sequential temperature increase favors the proteolytic enzymes, followed by β-amylase (optimum temperature of 60°C) and α-amylase (optimum temperature of 70°C). The high temperature of the last mashing stage stops most enzymatic activity, reduces viscosity, and improves the fluidity and filtering capacity of the resulting mash. During this operation, the contents are agitated to achieve a better malt solubilization and better exposure of adjuncts to enzymatic hydrolysis. Then, the mash is transferred to a lauter tun or filtrating vessel where the sweet wort is separated from spent grains. The filtering is usually performed at temperatures of 65°C–70°C and sparged with hot water (75°C–80°C). The higher temperature of the water used for sparging is efficient to remove the remaining extract from the mash. In most operations, lautering is considered the bottleneck of the process. Thus, the more rapidly the wort can be recovered the more brews can be daily performed (MacGregor and Batthy 1993; Palmer 1989; Briggs 1998; Hardwick 1995; Hough et al. 1993).

Hops are added to the sweet wort to impart the characteristic European beer flavor. The process simply consists of adding the hops to the wort to promote the extraction of solubles by boiling and lixiviation for 1.5–2.5 hours. Generally, half to two thirds of the hops are added at the beginning of the program and the rest at the end of the process with the objective of keeping key volatiles that enhances beer flavor and aroma. During boiling, the enzymes are inactivated, the wort becomes darker due to intrinsic wort compounds and caramelization reactions and the hopped wort becomes sterile. During this treatment, some soluble proteins will bind to tannins and precipitate decreasing turbidity. The hopped wort is cooled to about 6°C for traditional lagers and as high as 15°C–20°C for ales. The wort is also aerated with sterile air to increase its oxygen content, which is critically important for yeast growth and budding especially during the early phase of fermentation. During cooling more proteins becomes insoluble and removed by centrifugation (MacGregor and Batthy 1993; Palmer 1989; Briggs 1998; Hardwick 1995; Hough et al. 1993).

The wort is fermented into beer in special tanks or reactors equipped with cooling coils or cooling jackets. The most common equipment consists of a 3-m to 5-m-high stainless steel conical and hermetically sealed tank with 150- to 500-hL capacity. The wort is pitched with 1.5–2.5 g dry yeast/L. During the first stage of fermentation, the yeast reproduces asexually by budding, increasing the biomass from 4 to 5 times, and utilizes the available oxygen. Thus, the conditions gradually switch from aerobic to anaerobic. It is considered that after 12–24 hours fermentation the reactor conditions are anaerobic. During the anaerobic phase, the yeast metabolizes fermentable carbohydrates and free amino nitrogen producing ethanol and fusel alcohols (isopropanol, amylic, isoamylic, and butanol), respectively. During this stage, carbon dioxide is also produced and intermediate organic products that help to impart the characteristic beer flavor. For production of lagers, the fermentation process is carried out at 7°C–15°C during 8 to 10 days and for Pilsners at approximately 20°C for 3 to 5 days. Lagers are almost always fermented with bottom yeast whereas Pilsners with top yeast. Most beers are kept in closed tanks at a temperature of 0°C for 4 to 6 additional weeks to further reduce oxygen to a level of less than 0.2 ppm and enhance bouquet and aroma due to chemical changes such as the generation of diacetyl, dimethylsulfide, and hydrogen sulfide. During fermentation, yeast cells transform maltose and maltotriose into glucose, which is further metabolized into carbon dioxide, energy, ethanol, and other organic metabolites such as organic acids and volatile compounds. Approximately one third of the fermentable sugars are transformed into carbon dioxide. The progress of fermentation is usually followed using a refractometer that measures beer density. The initial wort density is about 1.040 and the finished product between 1.008 and 1.010 g/cm³. The organic acid production decreases pH to a level of 4.2. The change in the acidity coagulates some proteins and decreases even more the solubility of some acidic hop resins. Also during fermentation important quantities of FAN or soluble nitrogen are metabolized into fusel alcohols that affect the organoleptic properties of beer (MacGregor and Batthy 1993; Palmer 1989; Briggs 1998; Hardwick 1995; Hough et al. 1993).

14.2.2.1 Production of Regular Lager Beer

A. Samples, Ingredients, and Reagents

- Diastatic malt
- Distilled water
- Brewing adjuncts (refined grits or starches)
- Yeast for lager fermentation
- Hops (*Humulus lupulus*)
- Hydrochloric acid (HCl)
- Sodium bicarbonate (NaHCO₃)
- Active carbon
- Silica

B. Materials and Equipments

- Digital scale
- Roller mill
- Hot plate
- Shaking water bath with temperature control
- Lauter tun or filtering device
- Beakers (2 L)
- Fermentation reactor (5 L)
- Thermometer (0°C–100°C)
- pH meter
- Refractometer (0°C–30°Brix)
- Pycnometer (0%–10% alcohol)
- Centrifuge
- Exhauster (belt-steamer)
- Beer bottles with caps or lids
- Air pump (aquarium)

C. Procedure

1. Obtain a commercial barley malt or produce the desired malt following procedures in Section 14.2.1.1 or 14.2.1.2.

2. Mashing procedure

    a. In a 2-L beaker, mix 1 L distilled water with 433 g of brewing adjuncts (maize grits or starch, roller milled barley, rice grits) and 43 g diastatic malt.

    b. Place beaker with contents for 30 minutes in a shaking water bath set at 35°C. Increase the la temperature to 50°C and maintain it for 30 additional minutes. Remove beaker form the water bath and place it on a hot plate to raise the temperature to 95°C–100°C for 30 minutes. At the end of this cooking step add 270 mL water tempered to 40°C. Mix contents and allow the mix to drop the temperature to approximately 50°C.

c. In another 2 L beaker, mix 1.2 L water with 340 g ground malt. Place the beaker in a shaking water bath adjusted to 45°C for 30 minutes.

d. In a 5-L container, mix contents of steps b and c and place them in a water bath adjusted to 65°C for 30 minutes. Make sure that the temperature gradually increases during the 30 minutes. Change the temperature of the water bath to 75°C and allow contents to hydrolyze for 30 additional minutes.

e. Increase the temperature of the mash to 95°C–100°C on a hot plate. A sample of the mash can be obtained to determine °Plato, fermentable sugars, color, FAN, and % extract.

3. Lautering:

a. In a lauter tun or other filtering device, filter the resulting mash contents when the temperature drops to 65°C–70°C. The acrylic filtering device has a bottom place with 1 mm diameter holes that is furnished with a 1-cm-thick sponge and a system to apply vacuum (Figure 14.2). Drop the mash contents into the filtering device, allow insolubles to settle on the sponge, and then apply vacuum during the first 5 minutes lautering. Recycle the first 500 mL of filtered wort.

b. After lautering, sparge spent grains with 250 mL hot water (75°C–80°C).

c. Register the total lautering and sparge times required to obtain the sweet wort.

d. Recover the wet spent grains and put them in a convection oven set at 100°C. Measure the volume of the sweet wort.

e. Adjust to 13°Plato and 6.2 the soluble sugar content and pH of the sweet wort. The soluble sugar is adjusted by adding distilled water and pH by adding 0.1 N HCl or sodium bicarbonate.

f. Determine the total volume, °Plato, pH, FAN, % extract, and color of the sweet wort.

4. Addition of hops:

a. Weigh the required amount of hops considering the addition of 0.8 to 1 g/L sweet wort. Divide the hops into two lots, one containing

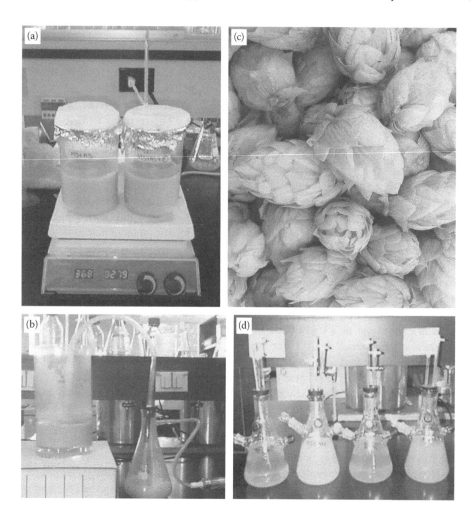

FIGURE 14.2 Sequential steps for the production of hopped beers. (a) Mashing of barley malt and brewing adjuncts; (b) lautering or filtration of mash to obtain spent grains and sweet wort; (c) illustration of hops; and (d) fermentation of beers.

70% of the weight, and the other the remaining 30%. Add the 70% of the hops to the sweet wort and heat contents to near boiling (95°C–100°C) for 90 minutes. Place a lid on top of the cooking container to minimize water losses. After discontinuing heat immediately add the rest of the hops and allow them to solubilize for 30 minutes.

b. Filter contents to remove spent hops. Recover the wort and adjust its volume to 13°Plato.

c. Place wort in a refrigerator for cooling (5°C). Then first filter and then centrifuge (5,000 rpm for 10 minutes at 5°C–10°C) the wort to remove insolubilized protein and reduce turbidity (Figure 14.2).

d. Aerate for 5 minutes the hopped wort preferably with sterile air using an air pump.

e. Determine the total volume, °Plato, pH, FAN, bittering units, polyphenols, and color of the resulting hopped wort.

f. To minimize microbial contamination, place the hopped wort in a sterile closed container in a refrigerator.

5. Yeast pitching and fermentation:

a. Take out from the refrigerator the hopped wort and allow contents to increase their temperature to 15°C.

b. Place hopped wort in a fermentation reactor that has been previously sterilized (Figure 14.2). Register the exact volume of the hopped wort added to the fermentation vessel.

c. Pitch dry or fresh compressed yeast at rates of 1.5 and 4.5 g/L hopped wort, respectively.

d. Ferment contents first at 15° for 1 day and then drop 1°C every day during 7–10 days. The first stage of fermentation (the first two days) is carried at aerobic conditions whereas the second under anaerobic conditions. After fermentation, drop the temperature of the green beer to 1°C and mature the beer for at least 1 week. During fermentation and maturation, sample the beer to calculate ethanol and amyl alcohol contents, residual fermentable sugars, available oxygen, yeast population, viscosity, pH, color, turbidity, FAN, foaming and beer metabolites such as diacetyl, dimethyl sulfide, ethyl acetate, and butyl acetate.

e. Filter the resulting beer to remove and recover yeast biomass. Then, centrifuge the beer at 5,000 rpm for 10 minutes at 5°C–10°C. Weigh the yeast biomass and determine its moisture content. Express biomass yield as fresh and dried. Alternatively, beer could be further clarified by filtration through active carbon or silica beds.

f. Measure the total beer volume and fill cleaned bottles with the resulting beer, leaving the typical head space. Place caps and pasteurize filled bottles in a exhauster for 20 minutes (internal temperature of 68°C). Cool down the pasteurized bottles with cold water and immediately store under refrigeration.

14.2.2.2 Production of Dark Beer

Dark beers are produced with a combination of diastatic and dark or toasted malts and higher amounts of hops to produce darker and stronger flavored beers. Some dark beers are supplemented with syrups rich in soluble sugars that upon heating produce Maillard and caramelization reactions.

A. *Samples, Ingredients, and Reagents*
- Diastatic and nondiastatic malts
- Distilled water
- Brewing adjuncts (refined grits or starches)
- Yeast for lager fermentation
- Hops (*Humulus lupulus*)
- Hydrochloric acid (HCl)
- Sodium bicarbonate ($NaHCO_3$)
- Active carbon
- Silica

B. *Materials and Equipments*
- Digital scale
- Roller mill
- Hot plate
- Shaking water bath with temperature control
- Lauter tun or filtering device
- Beakers (2 L)
- Fermentation reactor (5 L)
- Thermometer (0°C–100°C)
- pH meter
- Refractometer (0°C–30°Brix)
- Pycnometer (0%–10% alcohol)
- Centrifuge
- Exhauster (belt-steamer)
- Beer bottles with caps or lids
- Air pump (aquarium)

C. *Procedure*
1. Obtain a commercial barley malt or produce the desired malt following the procedures in Sections 14.2.1.1 and 14.2.1.2.

2. Mashing Procedure:

a. In a 2-L beaker, mix 1 L distilled water with 350 g of brewing adjuncts (maize grits, roller milled barley, malt, or glucose syrups) and 43 g diastatic malt and 33 g of dark or toasted malt.

b. Place beaker with contents for 30 minutes in a shaking water bath set at 35°C. Increase the la temperature to 50°C and maintain it for 30 additional minutes. Remove beaker form the water bath and place it on a hot plate to raise the temperature to 95°C–100°C for

30 minutes. At the end of this cooking step add 270 mL water tempered to 40°C. Mix contents and allow the mix to drop the temperature to approximately 50°C.

c. In another 2-L beaker, mix 1.2 L water with 250 g of malt and 140 g of dark or toasted malt. Place the beaker in a shaking water bath adjusted to 45°C for 30 minutes.

d. In a 5-L container, mix contents of steps b and c and place them in a water bath adjusted to 65°C for 30 minutes. Make sure that the temperature gradually increases during the 30 minutes. Change the temperature of the water bath to 75°C and allow contents to hydrolyze for 30 additional minutes.

e. Increase the temperature of the mash to 95°C–100°C on a hot plate.

3. Lautering:

a. Refer to process described for regular lager beer (refer to procedure in Section 14.2.2.1).

4. Addition of hops:

a. Refer to procedure in Section 14.2.2.1 described for regular lager beer but instead of using 0.8 use 1.5 g hops/L wort.

5. Yeast pitching and fermentation:

a. Follow the same procedure described for regular lager beer (refer to procedure in Section 14.2.2.1).

14.2.2.3 Production of Light Beer

Light beers that are low in dextrins and calories and are usually light colored are low in flavor and less viscous or with less body. Dextrins are usually converted during mashing into fermentable carbohydrates with amyloglucosidase. These beers usually contain one third less calories and cause less filling compared to regular beers.

A. *Samples, Ingredients, and Reagents*
- Diastatic malt
- Distilled water
- Brewing adjuncts (refined grits or starches)
- Amyloglucosidase
- Yeast for lager fermentation
- Hops (*Humulus lupulus*)
- Hydrochloric acid (HCl)
- Sodium bicarbonate (NaHCO$_3$)
- Active carbon
- Silica

B. *Materials and Equipments*
- Digital scale
- Roller mill
- Hot plate
- Shaking water bath with temperature control
- Lauter tun or filtering device
- Beakers (2 L)
- Fermentation reactor (5 L)

- Thermometer (0°C–100°C)
- pH meter
- Refractometer (0–30°Brix)
- Pycnometer (0%–10% alcohol)
- Centrifuge
- Exhauster (belt-steamer)
- Beer bottles with caps or lids
- Air pump (aquarium)

C. *Procedure*

1. Obtain a commercial barley malt or produce the desired malt following the procedures in Section 14.2.1.1 or 14.2.1.2.

2. Mashing Procedure:

a. In a 2-L beaker, mix 1 L distilled water with 433 g of brewing adjuncts (maize grits or starch, roller milled barley, rice grits) and 43 g light colored diastatic malt and 0.5 g of amyloglucosidase.

b. Place beaker with contents for 30 minutes in a shaking water bath set at 35°C. Increase the la temperature to 50°C and maintain it for 30 additional minutes. Remove beaker form the water bath and place it on a hot plate to raise the temperature to 95°C–100°C for 30 minutes. At the end of this cooking step add 270 mL water tempered to 40°C. Mix contents and allow the mix to drop the temperature to approximately 50°C.

c. In another 2-L beaker, blend 1.2 L water with 340 g light colored malt. Place the beaker in a shaking water bath adjusted to 45°C for 30 minutes.

d. In a 5-L container, mix contents of steps b and c and place them in a water bath adjusted to 65°C for 30 minutes. Make sure that the temperature gradually increases during the 30 minutes. Change the temperature of the water bath to 75°C and allow contents to hydrolyze for 30 additional minutes.

e. Increase the temperature of the mash to 95°C–100°C on a hot plate.

3. Lautering:

a. Refer to procedure in Section 14.2.2.1 described for regular lager beer.

4. Addition of hops:

a. Refer to procedure in Section 14.2.2.1 described for regular lager beer.

5. Yeast pitching and fermentation

a. Adjust °Plato of hopped wort to 12 and follow the same procedure described for regular lager beer. If beer exceeds 5° of alcohol, then add distilled water to drop the alcoholic content to 4.5° to 5°. Make sure to measure viscosity because this beer is less viscous compared to regular or dark beers.

14.2.2.4 Production of Ale Beers

Ale beers are produced from malted barley, hops, and top fermenting yeast using a warm fermentation (18°C–20°C). Compared to lager fermentations, the ale yeast will ferment the beer quickly giving it a sweet, full bodied, and fruity taste. These beers are especially popular in Europe. The most popular classes of ale beers are pale, bitter, Flanders brown, Altbier, Rauchbier, and brown.

A. Samples, Ingredients, and Reagents
- Diastatic malt
- Distilled water
- Brewing adjuncts (refined grits or starches)
- Yeast for ale fermentation
- Hops (*Humulus lupulus*)
- Hydrochloric acid (HCl)
- Sodium bicarbonate (NaHCO₃)
- Active carbon
- Silica

B. Materials and Equipments
- Digital scale
- Roller mill
- Hot plate
- Shaking water bath with temperature control
- Lauter tun or filtering device
- Beakers (2 L)
- Fermentation reactor (5 L)
- Thermometer (0°C–100°C)
- pH meter
- Refractometer (0–30°Brix)
- Pycnometer (0%–10% alcohol)
- Centrifuge
- Exhauster (belt-steamer)
- Beer bottles with caps or lids
- Air pump (aquarium)

C. Procedure
1. Obtain a commercial barley malt or produce the desired malt following the procedures in Section 14.2.1.1 or 14.2.1.2.
2. Mashing procedure:
   a. Refer to procedure in Section 14.2.2.1 for regular lager beer.
3. Lautering:
   a. Refer to procedure in Section 14.2.2.1 described for regular lager beer.
4. Addition of hops:
   a. Refer to procedure in Section 14.2.2.1 described for regular lager beer.
5. Yeast pitching and fermentation:
   a. Take out from the refrigerator the hopped wort and allow contents to increase their temperature to 18°C–20°C.
   b. Place hopped wort in a fermentation reactor that has been previously sterilized. Register the exact volume of the hopped wort added to the fermentation vessel.

c. Pitch top fermenting dry or fresh compressed ale yeast at rates of 1.5 g/L and 4.5 g/L hopped wort, respectively.
d. Ferment contents at 18°C–20°C for 3 days. During fermentation and maturation, sample the ale beer to calculate ethanol and amyl alcohol contents, residual fermentable sugars, available oxygen, yeast population, viscosity, pH, color, turbidity, FAN, foaming and beer metabolites such as diacetyl, dimethyl sulfide, ethyl acetate, and butyl acetate.
e. Filter the resulting beer to remove and recover yeast biomass. Then, centrifuge the beer at 5000 rpm for 10 minutes. Weigh the yeast biomass and determine its moisture content. Express biomass yield as fresh and dried. Alternatively, beer could be further clarified by filtration through active carbon or silica beds.
f. Measure the total beer volume and fill cleaned bottles with the resulting beer leaving the typical head space. Place caps and pasteurize filled bottles in a exhauster for 20 minutes (internal temperature of 68°C). Cool down the pasteurized bottles with cold water and immediately store under refrigeration.

14.2.3 Production of Rice Wine or Sake

Sake is classified as a noncarbonated alcoholic beverage widely consumed in Japan. The alcoholic spirit that contains from 14% to 16% ethanol is produced from refined rice. For sake production, four basic raw materials are used: refined polished white rice, water, an *Aspergillus oryzae* culture, commonly known as *koji-kin*, and yeast.

The traditional sake-making procedure consists of first the production of a highly refined white rice. Sake rice is extensively milled to remove from 30% to 50% of the weight of the brown kernel. Then, polished kernels are washed and steeped in pure water. About 25 kL of water are used for every ton of rice. The soaked rice is steam-cooked for approximately 45–50 minutes, allowed to cool down, and inoculated with the koji culture. Koji is industrially produced from a pure culture of *A. oryzae* that is inoculated in previously soaked and cooked rice and fermented at 35°C for 5 to 6 days. The mold culture produces various types of enzymes being the most relevant amylases and proteases that hydrolyze gelatinized starch and proteins, respectively. When the koji is ready, the next step is to create the starter mash, known as shubo or colloquially moto. Mashing consists of mixing cooked rice with lactic acid bacteria or simply with water containing lactic acid (0.7 L/1000 L water). The lactic acid impedes the growth of undesirable microorganisms. The ratio of steam cooked rice and koji rice is 75:25. During mashing, the starch is hydrolyzed into fermentable carbohydrates at temperatures close to 10°C. More steamed rice, water, and koji are added once a day for three days, doubling the volume of the mash each time. The mixture is now known as the main mash or *moromi*. Next, the mash is fermented with special strains of osmotolerant yeast that resist high alcohol concentrations. Fermentation is usually carried out at 20°C with intermittent agitation for 10 to 15 days. After two to six weeks fermentation, the fermenting sake is deliberately slowed down by lowering the temperature to less than 10°C. At the end of fermentation, sake is pressed to separate the liquid from the solids. With some sake, a small amount of distilled alcohol, called brewer's alcohol is added before pressing to extract flavors and aromas that would otherwise stay in the solids. The press-filtered alcoholic beverage with about 20% ethanol is in most instances pasteurized to inactivate yeast and denature enzymes. The unpasteurized sake, known as *namazake*, retains more flavorful compounds but it should be kept under refrigeration. The most common pasteurized sake is usually stored for periods of up to eight months to two years. Water is subsequently added to reduce the alcohol percentage from 20% back down around 15%–16% and finally the sake is pasteurized for the second time and bottled. Sake contains between 12% and 16% alcohol, 0.7%–0.8% acids, and 3.5% reducing sugars (Yoskizawa and Kishi 1985).

14.2.3.1 Production of Sake

A. *Samples, Ingredients, and Reagents*
- White polished rice
- Distilled water
- *Aspergillus oryzeae* culture
- Yeast (sake osmotolerant)
- Lactic acid
- Active carbon
- Filter paper

B. *Materials and Equipments*
- Digital scale
- Fermentation cabinet
- Hot plate
- Shaking water bath with temperature control
- Steamer or steam cooker (koshiki)
- Beakers (2 L and 5 L)
- Containers (2 L and 5 L)
- Fermentation reactor or vat (5 L and 10 L)
- Thermometer (0°C–100°C)
- pH meter
- Refractometer (0–30°Brix)
- Pycnometer (0%–30% alcohol)
- Kitasato flask
- Buchner filter
- Centrifuge
- Exhauster (belt-steamer)
- Bottles with caps or lids

C. *Procedure (Yoskizawa and Kishi 1985)*
1. Produce or obtain a highly refined white polished rice (refer to procedure in Section 5.2.3.1). The best sake rice is milled to remove from 30% to 50% of the weight of the brown rice.

2. Washed and steep the polished white rice in pure water. About 2.5 L of water is used for each kg of polished white rice.

3. Steam-cooked the tempered rice for approximately 45–50 minutes. Then, allow the cooked or gelatinized rice to equilibrate at room temperature.

4. Inoculate part of the cooked rice (25% of the total) with koji culture (*A. oryzae*). The pure culture of *A. oryzae* is sprinkled on previously soaked and cooked rice and fermented in a fermentation cabinet set at 35°C for 5 to 6 days. The mold culture produces various types of enzymes being the most relevant amylases and proteases that hydrolyze gelatinized starch and proteins, respectively.

5. Mix the rest of the cooked rice (75%) with a lactic acid bacteria culture or simply add lactic acid (0.7 mL/L water). The lactic acid impedes the growth of undesirable microorganisms. Determine the pH and acidity of the mash (refer to procedures in Section 2.10). Mash the koji and cooked rice at a temperature of approximately 10°C. Every day, add more steamed rice, water, and koji so to double the mash volume. This mixture is known as *moromi*.

6. Add more water and pitch the mash with a special strain of osmotolerant sake yeast (*Saccharomyces* sp.) and ferment at 20°C with intermittent agitation for 10 to 32 days.

7. Lower the temperature to less than 10°C to stop the fermentation.

8. Filter the fermenting mash through a filter cloth and discard the solids. Refilter the sake through a finer cloth to remove fine particles. Allow the sake to sit for a day and remove the solids that settle out.

9. Pass the sake through a Buchner filter containing filter paper and a 2-cm thick active carbon. Determine the alcohol content of the alcoholic beverage.

10. Place the resulting alcoholic beverage with approximately 20% ethanol in close containers in preparation for pasteurization aimed to inactivate yeast and bacteria and denature enzymes. Place the unpasteurized sake in an exhauster for 5 minutes or immerse the containers in a water bath adjusted to 80°C for 10 minutes.

11. After pasteurization, immediately cool down the container with running water and age the sake for several months.

12. Add distilled water to the sake to reduce or adjust the alcohol content to 15%–16%.

13. Pasteurize the sake again as in step 10.

14. Determine the pH, acidity, A_w, and ethanol and fusel alcohol contents (refer to Chapter 2).

14.2.4 RESEARCH SUGGESTIONS

1. Produce ale and lager beers using the same amounts and types of brewing adjuncts and hops. Compare the properties of the beers fermented with special strains of yeast for each type of wort and beer in terms of reducing sugars, FAN, ethanol and fusel alcohol contents, pH, color, flavor, haze, foaming capacity, and sensory properties.

2. Produce lager beers using the same formulation with the only difference of using regular maize starch or waxy maize starch as the main source of brewing adjuncts. Compare the properties of worts and beers in terms of fermentable sugar content, FAN, lautering time, ethanol and fusel alcohol contents, pH, color, flavor, haze, foaming capacity, and sensory properties.

3. Produce lager beers using the regular barley malt formulation and the substitution of the barley malt with a combination of microbial enzymes α-amylase, β-amylase, amyloglucosidase, and proteases. Compare the properties of worts and beers in terms of extraction, fermentable sugar content, FAN, lautering time, ethanol and fusel alcohol contents, pH, color, flavor, haze, foaming capacity, and sensory properties.

4. Produce lager beers using the same formulation with the only difference of using pelleted hops or the equivalent of a hop extract. Compare the properties of beers in terms of color, ethanol and fusel alcohol contents, pH, haze, foaming capacity, and sensory properties.

5. Produce ale beers using the same formulation with the only difference of using β-glucanases during the mashing process. Compare the properties of worts and beers in terms of fermentable sugar content, lautering time, ethanol and fusel alcohol contents, pH, color, flavor, haze, foaming capacity, and sensory properties.

6. Produce a 100% sorghum lager beer using malted sorghum, decorticated sorghum grits as brewing adjuncts and hops. Compare the properties of the sorghum wort and beer with counterparts obtained from barley malt in terms of reducing sugars, lautering, or filtration time, ethanol and fusel alcohol contents, pH, color, flavor, haze, foaming capacity, and sensory properties.

7. Produce and compared three 100% sorghum lager beers using malted sorghum, decorticated sorghum grits as brewing adjuncts and hops with the same formulation except for the addition of β-amylase or amyloglucosidase during the mashing process. Compare the properties of the three different types of worts and beers in terms of reducing sugars, viscosity, FAN, lautering time, ethanol and fusel alcohol contents, pH, color, flavor, haze, foaming capacity, and sensory properties.

8. Compare properties of sake produced with a regular (long) and waxy (short) polished rice in terms of water absorption during steaming, ease of hydrolysis with *Aspergillus oryzeae* and ethanol and fusel alcohol contents, pH, and sensory properties of the two different types of sake.

9. Compare properties of sake produced with a regular yeast and an osmotolerant sake yeast especially in terms of ethanol and fusel alcohol contents, pH, and sensory properties.

10. Produce sochu by distilling sake and determine the ethanol and fusel alcohol contents of the sake wine and distilled sochu.

14.2.5 RESEARCH QUESTIONS

1. Define the following terms:
   a. Gibberellic acid
   b. Malting
   c. Brewing adjunct
   d. Kilning
   e. Lautering
   f. Extraction rate
   g. Humulone
   h. Lupulone
   i. Sweet wort
   j. Free amino nitrogen
   k. Pitching
   l. Green beer
   m. Gushing
   n. Sun-struck beer
   o. Koji

2. Why is barley the preferred cereal for malting? What is the difference between a malt for beer and a malt for Scotch whiskey?

3. Describe at least five physicochemical changes that suffer during barley germination.

4. What is the principle of the tetrazolium assay used to test barley grain viability?

5. What is diastatic activity? What are the practical and analytical criteria generally used to determine the maximum diastatic activity?

6. Describe the general industrial operations used to produce barley malt. How is kilning modified to produce pale, chocolate, and caramel malts?

7. What are the main differences between the malting processes of sorghum and barley?

8. What are the most demanded brewing adjuncts by the brewing industry? What are the main chemical characteristics of these brewing adjuncts?

9. What is mashing? What are major differences, advantages, and disadvantages of infusion, temperature-programmed, and decoction mashing procedures?

10. What are differences and similarities between °Brix and °Plato?

11. What is the main rationale of programming a gradual temperature profile during mashing?

12. Why is lautering after mashing one of the most critical unit operations in the brewing process? What are the main factors affecting rate of wort filtration?

13. What are the main functionalities of hops in lager beer production? Describe at least three different types of chemical compounds associated to hops and their functionality.

14. What are the different stages during fermentation of lager beers? In which stage yeast reproduces and in which most of the ethanol is produced?

15. How yeast is harvested after beer or whiskey fermentation?

16. What are differences in terms of processing and caloric value among regular, dark, light, and alcohol free lager beers?

17. What is the relationship between wort or beer density and alcohol content?

18. What is sake? Explain and detail the typical process to transform white polished rice into sake.

19. What are the main biochemical changes that occur to temperature-abused beers? What are the main chemical compounds related to flavor and aroma of well-preserved and bad preserved beer?

20. What are the most common methods used to pasteurize beer? What is cold pasteurization?

14.3 PRODUCTION OF CEREAL-BASED ALCOHOLIC SPIRITS AND BIOETHANOL

For the manufacture of cereal-based alcoholic spirits, the following operations are practiced: starch gelatinization in preparation for hydrolysis with diastatic malt or enzymes, fermentation, distillation, and aging. There is a wide assortment of alcoholic spirits manufactured from cereals (Bathgate 1989; Lyons 1995; Ralph 1995; Yoneya 2007).

14.3.1 Distilled Spirits

Scotch malt whisky is made exclusively from an all-barley malt grist, whereas grain whiskies use a high proportion of cereal adjuncts. For instance, bourbon, rye, and Scotch grain whiskies contain at least 51% maize, rye, or wheat/maize, respectively.

Scotch whiskey is made from light-kilned and high-diastatic malt that is peated or smoked to various extents to yield spirits with characteristic flavors. Many distillers procure the raw material already cooked and mashed. However, some distilleries mill and process from scratch. Malting is a critical operation because it affects the process downstream and the organoleptic attributes of the beverage. As brewing malt, the barley is steeped in cold water (12°C–15°C) to increase the moisture to around 44% or 48%. The soaking operations usually last 48–60 hours in vessels that have aeration capabilities. During steeping air is applied in cycles. The air volumes applied vary from 0.5 to 17 m³/minutes/ton depending on the type of steep tank. The objective of the air is to provide oxygen, which promotes the physiological

activation of the grain. After steeping, the steeped barley is placed on germination beads for 4 to 5 days at 15°C. The temperature differential across the bed is minimized by forcing humidified air and turning the malt. The malt is kilned after achieving the desired diastatic activity. Scotch whisky malts are kilned using peat smoke. The tradition of using peat started a long time ago when it was the only available fuel for drying malt. Peat forms in bogs, from the decomposed roots, and foliage of moorland plants, principally heather. On very old moors, these layers may be several meters deep. After draining off as much water as possible, the top layer of actively growing heather is stripped and the underlying black peat is manually or machine-cut into blocks. The soggy wet peat blocks are allowed to dry to around 60% moisture. Generally, malt for whiskey production is dried with high air flows at relatively low temperature. Kilning cycles of 24–36 hours are common with initial air temperatures of 60°C–65°C and then rising to 70°C–75°C at the end of the cycle (Bathgate 1989). Peat smoke is introduced to the kiln from burners. The resulting malt with 4 to 5% moisture is allowed to rest for several weeks before mashing. The malt is ground with roller mills that are adjusted to obtain 15% husks, 75% grits, and 10% flour. The ground malt is mashed alone or with adjuncts depending on the type of alcoholic beverage. If adjuncts are used these are generally provided as grits. A uniform particle size distribution is desired to have a homogenous hydration, an adequate enzymatic conversion and spent grains that are not too difficult to filter. Generally, when adjuncts are used, the starch is gelatinized or cooked at atmospheric pressure or using pressure cookers. Pressure cooking generally improves alcohol yields. Different flavors that end up in the finished distilled beverage are produced during cooking. The temperature profile and duration of the thermal treatment affects the generation of flavorful compounds.

The gelatinized starch from the adjuncts and/or enzymatically damaged starch from the malt is converted into fermentable carbohydrates with the malt diastatic enzymes. The malt α-amylase and β-amylase yield worts rich in fermentable carbohydrates maltose and maltotriose and nonfermentable dextrins. The grist may be mashed three times at successive higher temperatures (63°C, 75°C, and 85°C) to maximize fermentable sugars in the extract.

Generally, the first and second worts are mixed and fermented and the third is used to mash the next batch of grits. During mashing, the starch of the ground malt and adjuncts is converted to fermentable carbohydrates and dextrins and the protein broken down into simpler and soluble molecules. The fermentable carbohydrates and FAN are important substrates form the subsequent step of yeast fermentation. The mashing protocol is aimed first toward the hydration of the malt and then applying a gradual temperature increase to enhance enzyme activity and conversion of the different substrates. When malt is used alone the most critical temperatures are 60°C, 70°C, and 80°C, and when adjuncts are utilized the mash is kept at lower initial temperatures to enhance their starch and protein conversion. After mashing, the contents are filtered to separate the wort from the spent grains. The most critical step for production of alcoholic spirits is fermentation. After cooling the wort to 20°C to 30°C, a pure strain or a mixture strains of yeast is pitched to convert fermentable carbohydrates into ethanol, soluble protein into fusel alcohols, and a wide array of metabolites that affect the flavor, aroma, and overall acceptability of the finished distilled product. Most fermentation processes are carried at temperatures lower than 32°C for 48 to 72 hours. During the first stage of fermentation, the yeast activates, consumes the available oxygen, and reproduces. Then, fermentable sugars and soluble nitrogen are gradually converted into ethanol and fusel alcohols, respectively. The fermentation ceases due to the osmotic pressure caused by the generated alcohol and when the substrate is fully utilized. Full attenuation is complete in 36 to 48 hours when the final gravity falls 2 to 3 degrees under that of water, giving an alcohol yield of around 8%. It is known that alcohol concentrations greater than 10%–12% inhibit the fermenting yeast. However, there are new yeast strains that are osmoresistant and are able to ferment high-specific-density worts. The rule of thumb applied in distilleries is that the raw material is transformed into one third carbon dioxide, one third alcohol, and one third spent grains. One of the major differences between distillery operations and brewing is the omission of a wort boiling stage after wort runoff. Consequently, amylases continue to be active during fermentation so higher amounts of dextrins are first hydrolyzed into simpler compounds and later on into ethanol.

All alcoholic spirits are obtained after distillation of the fermented beer. During this operation, the ethanol and other volatile compounds are separated from the beer in copper pot stills or modern continuous distillation towers. The alcohol concentration depends on the temperature and the type of distiller. The distillate from the pot still has an alcohol content of over 20% and is commonly known as low wines. The low wines are distilled in a second pot still and during this operation low fractions are obtained. The foreshots contain volatile organic compounds, which are deleterious to the flavor of the finished product. The degree to which vapors are rectified before condensation regulates the composition and flavor of the spirit. The second fraction contains about 68% ethanol, and this is considered the green whiskey. The final step in alcoholic beverage production is aging. The alcoholic beverage is usually adjusted to the desired alcoholic content or °Proof and placed in wood barrels or casks. The type of wood and the use of secondhand casks affect flavor development and *bouquet*. The amounts of acids, aldehydes, esters, and ketones increase during aging. Generally, the factors to control during aging are: beverage alcohol content, temperature of the cellar or aging room, and aging time. Aging varies according to the distilled beverage and desired quality. Aging times varies from 1 year up to 12 years or more. Scotch whiskies are produced from peat-smoked barley malt to impart the characteristic flavor and should be made exclusively from barley. On the other hand, other whiskeys such as bourbon are produced using maize grits as adjuncts (Bathgate 1989; Lyons 1995; Ralph 1995; Yoneya 2007).

14.3.1.1 Production of Distilled Spirits

A. *Samples, Ingredients, and Reagents*
- Grits from various types of cereals (i.e., maize, rice)
- Barley malt (peat smoked)
- Thermostable α-amylase (Termamyl®)
- Amyloglucosidase
- Yeast
- Cacium hydroxide

B. *Materials and Equipments*
- Digital scale
- Roller or hammer mil
- Hot plate or shaking water bath
- Beakers (2 L and 5 L)
- Filter cloth
- Lauter tun
- Thermometer
- pH meter
- Refractometer (0 to 30 to 40°Brix or Plato)
- Spatula
- Fermentation cabinet
- Pycnometer or densimeter for alcohol
- Fermentastion reactor
- Rotavapor or glass distilling unit
- Charred oakwood barrels or casks

C. *Procedure*
1. Mill the dehydrated barley malt using preferably a roller mill. Recover all fractions and mix them.
2. If an analog of Scotch whiskey is produced the malt has to be peat smoked. For Scotch whiskey, mill barley using the same procedure described above. For bourbon whiskey, mill maize grits into a fine flour using a roller or hammer mill.
3. In a 2-L beaker, mix 1 L distilled water with 433 g adjuncts and 43 g diastatic malt. For Scotch and bourbon whiskies, the adjuncts are ground barley and maize meal, respectively.
4. Place beaker in a shaking water bath set at 35°C and maintain the maintain the temperature for 30 minutes. Increase the temperature to 50°C for 30 additional minutes. During these programmed temperature steps the contents should be frequently agitated. Finally, transfer beaker to a hot plate and raise the temperature to 100°C for 30 minutes. After the cooking step add 270 mL water to drop the temperature to 50°C–55°C.
5. In other 2-L container, mix 1.2 L distilled water with 340 g malt and place beaker for 30 minutes in a shaking water bath adjusted to 45°C.
6. In a 5-L beaker, mix contents of steps 4 and 5 and heat the resulting mash to 65°C for 30 minutes in a shaking water bath. Make sure to gradually increase the temperature so to optimize enzyme hydrolysis. Finally, increase the temperature to 75°C for 30 minutes.

7. Determine pH, °Plato, and the amounts of glucose (refer to the glucose oxidase method in Section 2.8.6), reducing sugars (refer to procedure in Section 2.8.5) and FAN (refer to procedure in Section 2.5.2.1).

8. Before yeast pitching, sterilize the mash by boiling (100°C) for 5 minutes. Place mash in a sterile fermentation reactor and allow contents to cool down to 30°C.

9. Pitch the yeast at a rate of 1.5 g/L to 2.5 g/L of fresh compressed or 0.5 g/L to 0.8 g/L of dry yeast.

10. Set the temperature of the fermentation reactor to 30°C and allow contents to ferment for 5 days. During fermentation, sample the fermenting beer to calculate ethanol and amyl alcohol contents, residual fermentable sugars, available oxygen, yeast population, pH, and FAN (refer to Chapter 2).

11. Filter the resulting beer to remove spent grains and yeast biomass. The operation can be performed with a filter cloth or by centrifugation.

12. Place the fermenting beer in the distillation unit or rotavapor. Make sure all fittings of the distillation unit or rotavapor are sealed and the condenser has the proper water or refrigerant temperature. Heat the beer to first evaporate the alcohol and then recondensate. The optimum temperature for the rotavapor operating at 1.05 kg/cm^2 or 15 psi of vacuum is between 35°C and 40°C.

13. Recover the distilled alcoholic solution and determine ethanol content with an alcohol pycnometer.

14. Adjust alcoholic content to 31% to 35% or 68°Proof with distilled water.

15. Place the adjusted distilled spirit in a wood barrel for maturing at 14°C–18°C for at least 1 year. The optimum cask should be made from charred oak wood.

14.3.2 Production of Fuel Ethanol from Cereals

The continuous depletion of the fossil reserves and consequent escalation in their prices has stimulated an extensive evaluation of alternative technologies and substrates to meet the global energy demand. As a result, alternative sources of energy like methane, hydrogen, and ethanol are increasingly being considered as potential substitutes for fossil fuels. During the past decade, there has been special interest in the production of fuel ethanol from starchy grains especially in the United States. In this country, approximately 122 million tons of maize were transformed into 49 billion L of fuel ethanol in 2010 (Renewable Fuels Association, http://ethanolrfa.org). About 30% of the gasoline in the United States currently is blended with ethanol, and the percentage is still growing. This makes the fuel ethanol industry the fastest growing energy industry in the world.

The huge production is mainly due to the high price of petroleum, the environmental concerns related to the use of MTBE and that the renewable ethanol is friendlier to the environment in terms of CO_2, suspended air particles, and sulfur and nitrogen emissions.

The technologies to produce alcoholic beverages and fuel ethanol are similar and consist of first converting starch into fermentable carbohydrates in preparation for yeast fermentation and distillation. The main differences between potable and fuel alcohol are that distilled spirits contain significant amounts of water and other organic compounds that are aged under controlled conditions, whereas fuel ethanol consists of denatured anhydrous alcohol. Starchy grains such as maize, wheat, and sorghum are viable renewable resources for ethanol production. Maize is an excellent source of starch for a glucose platform. The starch is hydrolyzed in two sequential steps: liquefaction and saccharification. In the liquefaction step, starch granules are slurried in water, gelatinized with heat, and hydrolyzed to soluble dextrins with thermostable α-amylase. In the saccharification step, these oligosaccharides are further hydrolyzed to glucose. The saccharification and fermentation steps are often integrated to reduce the effect of glucose inhibition in the two process steps (BBI International 2003; Coble et al. 1981; Katzen et al. 1995; Madson and Monceaux 1995; Maisch 1987).

A. Samples, Ingredients, and Reagents
- Yellow maize or refined starch
- Thermostable α-amylase (Liquozyme®)
- Amyloglucosidase (Dextrozyme®)
- Yeast (active dry yeast)
- Yeast extract
- Zeolite

B. Materials and Equipments
- Digital scale
- Hammer mil
- Jet cooker or hot plate or shaking water bath
- Beakers (2 L and 5 L)
- Filter cloth
- Thermometer
- pH meter
- Refractometer (0 to 30°Brix or °Plato)
- Spatula
- Fermentation cabinet
- Pycnometer or densimeter for alcohol
- Fermentation reactor
- Rotavapor or glass distilling unit
- Column for zeolite

C. Procedure
1. Grind yellow maize with a hammer mill equipped with a 2.0-mm sieve.
2. Weigh 500 g of the ground maize or 500 g of maize starch and mix with 785 mL water at 35°C to obtain a slurry with approximately 35% solids. Adjust the pH of the suspension to 5.5 with HCl 0.1 N.
3. Place the beaker containing the slurry in a shaking water bath adjusted to 60°C. Add 0.7 mL

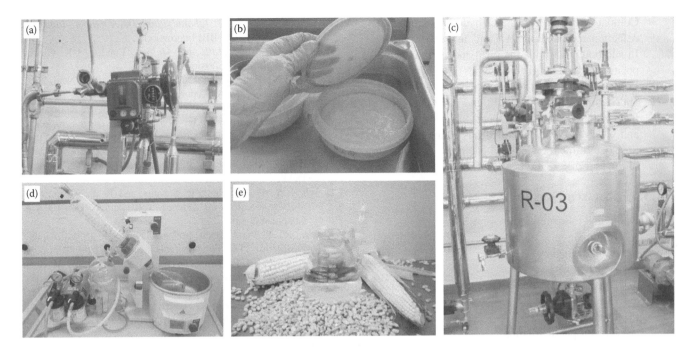

FIGURE 14.3 Sequential steps for the production of bioethanol from cereal grains. (a) Jet cooker used for the continuous gelatinization of ground grains; (b) liquefaction of gelatinized mashes with thermostable α-amylase; (c) simultaneous saccharification and fermentation of mashes; (d) first distillation step with a rotavapor; and (e) anhydrous ethanol obtained from maize.

of thermoresistant α-amylase and incubate the slurry for 20 minutes at 60°C. Then, increase the temperature of the slurry to 85°C for 195 minutes with continuous agitation. During hydrolysis determine the amount of reducing sugars (Figure 14.3).

4. After liquefaction, allow hydrolyzates to cool down to 35°C and adjust to 13°Plato, 150 mg/L FAN and pH 5.5. The °Plato is adjusted with distilled water, FAN by adding yeast extract and the pH with 0.1 N HCl. Place the diluted and adjusted mash in the reactor and add 0.25 g of amyloglucosidase and 0.35 g dry yeast (*Saccharomyces cerevisiae*).

5. Ferment for 48 to 72 hours at 35°C. Sample the fermenting beer throughout fermentation to determine oxygen, residual glucose, pH, FAN, ethanol, fusel alcohols, and yeast biomass.

6. Filter the beer using a filter cloth. Recover the distilled wet grains/yeast and place them in an oven set at 100°C for drying. Weigh the dried distilled grains/yeast.

7. Distill the beer using a glass distillation unit or a rotavapor system operating under vacuum at 35°C (Figure 14.3). Then, dehydrate the resulting ethanol solution by passing through a molecular sieve. Use microporous particles such as zeolite or aluminum silicates that selectively adsorb water. The zeolite should have a porous diameter of 3Å that traps water molecules.

8. Weigh and measure the volume of the total anhydrous ethanol produced and determine

yield. Ethanol yield (volume based) = (mL anhydrous ethanol/dry sample weight) or % ethanol yield (weight based) = (g anhydrous ethanol/g dry sample weight) × 100.

9. Regenerate the used zeolite column by forcing overheated anhydrous ethanol vapors through the packed bed.

14.3.3 RESEARCH SUGGESTIONS

1. Produce and compare fuel ethanol yields of regular ground yellow maize, fractionated maize (free of germ and pericarp), and maize starch. Compare the properties of enzyme hydrolyzates and beers in terms of glucose, FAN, and ethanol concentration. In addition, determine the yield and chemical composition of DDG.

2. Produce and compare fuel ethanol yields of regular ground yellow maize and regular ground sorghum. Compare the properties of enzyme hydrolyzates and beers in terms of glucose, FAN, and ethanol concentration. In addition, determine the yield and chemical composition of DDG.

3. Produce and compare fuel ethanol yields of sound, insect-damaged, and mold-damaged ground yellow maize. Compare the properties of enzyme hydrolyzates and beers in terms of glucose, FAN and ethanol concentration. In addition, determine the yield, and chemical composition of DDG.

4. Produce and compare fuel ethanol yields of whole, decorticated grain sorghum with and without supplementation of proteases during starch liquefaction.

Compare the kinetics of starch hydrolysis during liquefaction and yields of FAN and anhydrous ethanol. In addition, determine the yield and chemical composition of the four different types of DDG.

5. Produce and compare fuel ethanol yields of whole and steamed flaked sorghum and maize. Compare the kinetics of starch hydrolysis during liquefaction and yields of FAN and anhydrous ethanol. In addition, determine the yield and chemical composition of the four different types of DDG.

14.3.4 RESEARCH QUESTIONS

1. Define the following terms:
   a. Peat malt
   b. Scotch whiskey
   c. Bourbon whiskey
   d. Dry distilled grains (DDG)
   e. Fuel E15
   f. Zeolite
   g. Azeotropic distillation
   h. Fusel alcohols

2. In a flowchart summarize the process to produce Scotch Whiskey. How does this process vary in relation to production of bourbon whiskey?

3. In a flowchart summarize the process to produce fuel ethanol form maize. What is the regular yield of fuel ethanol from 1 ton of yellow maize?

4. What are advantages or disadvantages of the fractionated maize fuel ethanol process? What is the regular yield of fuel ethanol from this feedstock?

5. What are the main biochemical changes that occur during aging of distilled alcoholic spirits? What are the main chemical compounds related to flavor and aroma of distilled spirits?

6. What sorts of compounds are responsible for the *bouquet* of aged whiskeys? How can you determine amounts of these compounds?

REFERENCES

American Association of Cereal Chemists. 2000. *AACC Approved Methods of Analysis.* 10th ed. St. Paul, MN: AACC.

American Society of Brewing Chemists. 2009. *Methods of Analysis.* 10th ed. Chicago, IL: American Society of Brewing Chemists.

Bathgate, G. N. 1989. "Cereals in Scotch Whiskey Production." In *Cereal Science and Technology*, edited by G.H. Palmer, Chapter 4. Aberdeen, UK: Aberdeen University Press.

BBI International. 2003. *Ethanol Plant Development Handbook.* Grand Forks, ND: BBI International.

Briggs, D. E. 1998. *Malts and Malting.* London, UK: Blackie Academic and Professional.

Coble, C. G., E. A. Hiler, J. M. Sweeten, H. P. O'Neal, V. G. Reidenback, W. A. Lepori, W. H. Aldred, G. T. Schelling, and R. D. Kay. 1981. "Small Scale Ethanol Production from Cereals Feedstocks." In *Cereals a Renewable Resource. Theory and Practice*, edited by Y. Pomeranz and L. Munck, Chapter 30. St. Paul, MN: AACC.

Hardwick, W. 1995. *Handbook of Brewing.* New York, NY: Marcel Dekker.

Hough, J. S., D. E. Briggs, R. Stevens, and T. W. Young. 1993. *Malting and Brewing Science.* Vol. I and II. London, UK: Chapman & Hall.

Katzen, R., P. W. Madson, and G. D. Moon. 1995. "Alcohol Distillation. The Fundamentals." In *The Alcohol Textbook*, edited by T. P. Lyons, D. R. Kelsall, and J. E. Murtagh, Chapter 10. Nottingham, UK: Nottingham University Press.

Lyons, T. P. 1995. "The Production of Scotch and Irish Whiskies." In *The Alcohol Textbook*, edited by T. P. Lyons, D. R. Kelsall, and J. E. Murtagh, Chapter 11. Nottingham, UK: Nottingham University Press.

MacGregor, A. W., and R. S. Bhatty. 1993. *Barley: Chemistry and Technology.* St. Paul, MN: AACC.

Madson, P. W., and D. A. Monceaux. 1995. "Fuel Ethanol Production." In *The Alcohol Textbook*, edited by T. P. Lyons, D. R. Kelsall, and J. E. Murtagh, Chapter 16. Nottingham, UK: Nottingham University Press.

Maisch, W. F. 1987. "Fermentation Processes and Products." In *Corn Chemistry and Technology*, Chapter 19. St. Paul, MN: AACC.

Munroe, J. H. 2006. "Fermentation." In *Handbook of Brewing*, edited by F. G. Priest and G. G. Stewart, Chapter 12. Boca Raton, FL: CRC Taylor & Francis.

Palmer, G. H. 1989. "Cereal in Malting and Brewing." In *Cereal Science and Technology*, edited by G. H. Palmer, Chapter 3. Aberdeen, UK: Aberdeen University Press.

Ralph, R. 1995. "The Production of American Whiskies (Bourbon, Corn, Rye, Wheat and Tennessee)." In *The Alcohol Textbook*, edited by T. P. Lyons, D. R. Kelsall, and J. E. Murtagh, Chapter 12. Nottingham, UK: Nottingham University Press.

Steward, G. C. 2006. "Beer Stability." In *Handbook of Brewing*, edited by F. G. Priest and G. G. Stewart, Chapter 19. Boca Raton, FL: CRC Taylor & Francis.

Yoneya, T. 2007. "Manufacture of Whisky." In *Handbook of Food Products Manufacturing. Principles, Bakery, Beverages, Cereals, Cheese, Confectionary, Fats, Fruits, and Functional Foods*, edited by Y. H. Hui, Chapter 21. Hoboken, NJ: Wiley Interscience.

Yoshizawa, K., and S. Kishi. 1985. "Rice in Brewing." In: *Rice: Chemistry and Technology*, edited by B.O. Juliano, Chapter 17. St. Paul, MN: AACC.

Index